Ion Channel Localization

METHODS IN PHARMACOLOGY AND TOXICOLOGY

Mannfred A. Hollinger, PhD, *Series Editor*

Ion Channel Localization: Methods and Protocols
edited by **Anatoli N. Lopatin** and **Colin G. Nichols,** 2001

METHODS IN PHARMACOLOGY AND TOXICOLOGY

Ion Channel Localization

Methods and Protocols

EDITED BY

Anatoli N. Lopatin

University of Michigan, Ann Arbor, MI

AND

Colin G. Nichols

Washington University Medical School, St. Louis, MO

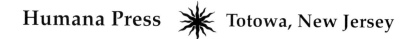

Humana Press ✳ Totowa, New Jersey

© 2001 Humana Press Inc.
999 Riverview Drive, Suite 208
Totowa, New Jersey 07512

For additional copies, pricing for bulk purchases, and/or information about other Humana titles, contact Humana at the above address or at any of the following numbers: Tel.: 973-256-1699; Fax: 973-256-8341; E-mail: humana@humanapr.com or visit our Website: http://humanapress.com

This publication is printed on acid-free paper. ◯
ANSI Z39.48-1984 (American Standards Institute) Permanence of Paper for Printed Library Materials.

Cover illustration: Autoradiograms showing the widespread distribution of [^{3}H]Ro 15-1788 binding sites in mouse brain. *See* Fig. 3 on page 49.

Cover design by Patricia F. Cleary.

Production Editor: Mark J. Breaugh.

Printed in the United States of America. 10 9 8 7 6 5 4 3 2 1

Library of Congress Cataloging-in-Publication Data

Ion channel localization: methods and protocols/edited by Anatoli N. Lopatin and Colin G. Nichols.
    p. cm.
  Includes bibliographical references and index.
  ISBN 0-89603-833-5 (alk. paper)
  1. Ion channels—Research—Methodology.   I. Lopatin, Anatoli N. II. Nichols, Colin G.
QH603.I54 I54 2001
  571.6'4—dc21   00-053983

Preface

Since the pioneering discoveries of Hodgkin, Huxley, and Katz, it has been clear that specific ion conductance pathways underlie electrical activity. Over the ensuing 50 years, there has been ever increasing, and occasionally explosive, changes in the scope of efforts to understand ion channel behavior. The introduction of patch clamp technology by Erwin Neher and Bert Sakmann about 20 years ago led to the realization of the great variety of novel ion channel species, and the subsequent revolution in cloning has revealed an even greater diversity of the underlying molecular entities.

Today, advances in the study of ion channel structure and function continue at a high pace, from angstrom resolution imaging of crystallized channels to their genetic manipulations in animals. In this regard, the field is a balanced one that inquires not only *what* ion channel entities are there, or how they operate, but also *where* are these molecular electronic switches? However, this balance is not particularly well presented to the general scientific audience or to specialists in the field. There are plenty of wonderful and useful books and monographs, as well as conferences and meetings on virtually every aspect of ion channel structure and function. However, we are unaware that the channel localization theme has been considered in a unified forum. In *Ion Channel Localization: Methods and Protocols*, therefore, we have invited leading specialists to contribute to a comprehensive review of methods in ion channel localization, to bring together in a single collection different aspects of the versatile potentials of today's technologies.

Pharmacological tools for ion channel localization are the core topics of the book. They have offered, and will continue to offer, probably the most specific way of localizing channels and receptors beyond and in addition to what can be accomplished by immunochemical and other technologies. Part I of the book deals with both fluorescent and radioligand applications of pharmacological tools. In Part II readers will find a detailed description of methods employing green fluorescent protein (GFP), a novel tool that is now facilitating an explosion of research in many areas, including the mapping of ion channels and receptors. We hope readers will find here the "exciting" part of the technology as well as warnings of pitfalls and data misinterpretation. In Part III of the book we have attempted to pull together assays in ion channel localization that utilize their functional properties, i.e., ion conduction, as a marker of their localization. Though channel function can only be found where there is underlying channel protein, the reciprocal is not necessarily true. The search for where active channels are to be found is the true goal of many localization studies, and this ultimately requires a function-based assay. Atomic force microscopy is a potentially revolutionary tool for understanding localization and organization in virtually every field of biological research, including ion channels. Detailed description of this technology and its application to ion channel localization, as well as discussion of some pioneering studies and perspectives, are considered in Part IV.

The potential scope of *Ion Channel Localization: Methods and Protocols* is enormous, and various aspects relevant to the issue of channel localization are not considered in detail. Standard techniques of molecular biology and protein biochemistry, including descriptions of immunochemical technology of antibody labeling, epitope tagging, biotinylation, in both fluorescent and radiolabeled versions, and electron microscopy are discussed elsewhere in detail (*see Immunochemical Protocols*, J. Pound, ed. and *Electron Microscopy Methods and Protocols*, M. A. N. Hajibagheri, ed. *Methods in Molecular Biology* series).

We would like to give our sincere thanks to all of the specialists who have contributed chapters to the book. It has been a pleasure and a privilege to work with them. We hope that the outcome will be useful to researchers interested in the localization of ion channels in cells, tissues, and organisms.

Anatoli N. Lopatin
Colin G. Nichols

Contents

Contributors

CRISTÓVÃO ALBUQUERQUE • *Department of Physiology and Cellular Biophysics, Columbia University, New York, NY*

JOHN ATACK • *Department of Biochemistry, Neuroscience Research Centre, Merck Sharp and Dohme Research Laboratories, Essex, UK*

GEORGE J. AUGUSTINE • *Department of Neurobiology, Duke University Medical Center, Durham, NC*

BALTAZAR BECERRIL • *Instituto de Biotecnología-UNAM, Avenida Universidad, Cuernavaca, Mexico*

GEULA M. BERNSTEIN • *Playfair Neuroscience Unit, Toronto Hospital Research Institute, Toronto, Ontario, Canada*

XUENONG BO • *Autonomic Neuroscience Institute, Royal Free and University College Hospital Medical School, London, UK*

MARC BORSOTTO • *Institut de Pharmacologie Moléculaire et Cellulaire, Valbonne, France*

THOMAS BUDDE • *Institute of Physiology, Otto-von-Guericke University, Magdeburg, Germany*

GEOFFREY BURNSTOCK • *Autonomic Neuroscience Institute, Royal Free and University College Hospital Medical School, London, UK*

GUNNAR BUYSE, *Laboratory of Physiology, Catholic University of Leuven, Leuven, Belgium*

DANIEL M. CZAJKOWSKY • *Department of Molecular Physiology and Biological Physics and Biophysics Program, University of Virginia School of Medicine, Charlottesville, VA*

ZHENGSHAN DAI • *Department of Cell Biology and Anatomy, University of North Carolina at Chapel Hill, Chapel Hill, NC*

MURIEL DELEPIERRE • *Laboratoire de Résonance Magnétique Nucléaire, Pasteur Institute, Paris, France*

GUY DROOGMANS • *Laboratory of Physiology, Catholic University of Leuven, Leuven, Belgium*

JAN EGGERMONT • *Laboratory of Physiology, Catholic University of Leuven, Leuven, Belgium*

HOLLY S. ENGELMAN • *Department of Physiology and Cellular Biophysics, Columbia University, New York, NY*

PHILIP G. HAYDON • *Department of Zoology and Genetics, Iowa State University, Ames, IA*

FRITJOF HELMCHEN • *Biological Computation Research Department, Bell Laboratories, Lucent Technologies, Murray Hill, NJ*

ROBERT M. HENDERSON • *Department of Pharmacology, University of Cambridge, Cambridge, UK*

UTA C. HOPPE • *Department of Medicine III, University of Cologne, Cologne, Germany*

SCOTT A. JOHN • *UCLA Cardiovascular Research Laboratory, UCLA School of Medicine, Los Angeles, CA*

DAVID C. JOHNS, *Department of Neurosurgery, The Johns Hopkins University, Baltimore, MD*

OWEN T. JONES • *Playfair Neuroscience Unit, Toronto Hospital Research Institute, Toronto, Ontario, Canada*

HOEON KIM • *Neuroscience Research Institute, University of California, Santa Barbara, CA*

JOSEPH C. KOSTER • *Department of Cell Biology and Physiology, Washington University Medical School, St. Louis, MO*

RATNESHWAR LAL • *Neuroscience Research Institute, University of California, Santa Barbara, CA*

C. JUSTIN LEE • *Department of Physiology and Cellular Biophysics, Columbia University, New York, NY*

HAI LIN • *Neuroscience Research Institute, Department of Molecular, Cellular and Developmental Biology, University of California, Santa Barbara, CA*

DIOMEDES E. LOGOTHETIS • *Department of Physiology and Biophysics, Mount Sinai School of Medicine, New York, NY*

ANATOLI N. LOPATIN • *Department of Physiology, University of Michigan, Ann Arbor, MI*

AMY B. MACDERMOTT • *Department of Physiology and Cellular Biophysics, Columbia University, New York, NY*

ELENA N. MAKHINA • *Department of Cell Biology and Physiology, Washington University Medical School, St. Louis, MO*

EDUARDO MARBÁN • *Institute of Molecular Cardiobiology, The Johns Hopkins University, Baltimore, MD*

DANIEL W. MCPHERSON • *Nuclear Medicine Group, Life Sciences Division, Oak Ridge National Laboratory, Oak Ridge, TN*

TOORAJ MIRSHAHI • *Department of Physiology and Biophysics, Mount Sinai School of Medicine, New York, NY*

BRYAN D. MOYER • *Department of Cell Biology, The Scripps Research Institute, San Diego, CA*

COLIN G. NICHOLS • *Department of Cell Biology and Physiology, Washington University Medical School, St. Louis, MO*

BERND NILIUS • *Laboratory of Physiology, Catholic University of Leuven, Leuven, Belgium*

HANS OBERLEITHNER • *Department of Physiology, University of Muenster, Muenster, Germany*

BRIAN O'ROURKE, *Division of Cardiology, The Johns Hopkins University, Baltimore, MD*

H. BENJAMIN PENG • *Department of Cell Biology and Anatomy, University of North Carolina at Chapel Hill, Chapel Hill, NC*

DIANA L. PETTIT • *NIEHS-NIH, Research Triangle Park, NC*

MARC PORTER • *Department of Zoology and Genetics, Iowa State University, Ames, IA*

LOURIVAL D. POSSANI • *Instituto de Biotechnología-UNAM, Avenida Universidad, Cuernavaca, Mexico*

FREDERICK SACHS • *Department of Physiology and Biophysics, SUNY Buffalo, Buffalo, New York*

MASSIMO SASSAROLI • *Department of Physiology and Biophysics, Mount Sinai School of Medicine, New York, NY*

HERMANN SCHILLERS • *Department of Physiology, University of Muenster, Muenster, Germany*

STEFAN W. SCHNEIDER • *Department of Physiology, University of Muenster, Muenster, Germany*

ZHIFENG SHAO • *Department of Molecular Physiology and Biological Physics and Biophysics Program, University of Virginia School of Medicine, Charlottesville, VA*

KENNETH SNYDER • *School of Medicine and Biomedical Sciences, SUNY Buffalo, Buffalo, New York*

BRUCE A. STANTON • *Department of Physiology, Dartmouth Medical School, Hanover, NH*

CYRILLE SUR • *Department of Biochemistry, Neuroscience Research Centre, Merck Sharp and Dohme Research Laboratories, Essex, UK*

HAJIME TAKANO • *Department of Zoology and Genetics, Iowa State University, Ames, IA*

DOMINIQUE TROUET • *Laboratory of Physiology, Catholic University of Leuven, Leuven, Belgium*

JAN TYTGAT • *Laboratory of Toxicology, University of Leuven, Leuven, Belgium*

RUDI VENNEKENS • *Laboratory of Physiology, Catholic University of Leuven, Leuven, Belgium*

JAMES N. WEISS • *UCLA Cardiovascular Research Laboratory, UCLA School of Medicine, Los Angeles, CA*

PING C. ZHANG • *Department of Biophysical Sciences, SUNY Buffalo, Buffalo, New York*

COLOR PLATES

Color plates 1–6 appear as an insert following p. 238.

PLATE 1   Fig. 2. Pseudocolor images of autoradiograph of [^{3}H]α,β-methyleneATP binding sites in rat brain. (*See* full caption on p. 62, Chapter 4.)

Fig. 4. Immunostaining of recombinant P2X$_4$ receptors in 1321N1 cells with a mouse monoclonal antibody. (*See* full caption on p. 62, Chapter 4.)

Fig. 7. Whole mount *in situ* hybridization of chick embryos (Day 4) with digoxigenin-labeled cP2X$_8$ RNA probe. (*See* full caption on p. 62, Chapter 4.)

PLATE 2   Fig. 3. Crystal growth is determined by the flow of Tl+ ions through K+ channels. (*See* full caption on p. 318, Chapter 17.)

PLATE 3   Fig. 2. Theoretical improvement in axial resolution with double-caged glutamate. (*See* full caption on p. 353, Chapter 19.)

PLATE 4   Fig. 2. Fluorescence of GFP-tagged K$_{ATP}$ channels in isolated islets from transgenic mice. (*See* full caption on p. 255, Chapter 13.)

PLATE 5   Fig. 4. Plasma membrane of *Xenopus laevis* oocyte spread on glass and studied by AFM in air. (*See* full caption on p. 418, Chapter 22.)

PLATE 6   Fig. 8. Plasma membrane patch of *Xenopus laevis* oocyte imaged by AFM in air (size: 0.09 μm^2). (*See* full caption on p. 422, Chapter 22.)

Part I

PHARMACOLOGICAL LABELING OF ION CHANNELS AND
RECEPTORS

Fluorescent Calcium Antagonists

Tools for Imaging of L-Type Calcium Channels in Living Cells

Thomas Budde

1. INTRODUCTION

Different types of voltage-dependent calcium (Ca^{2+}) channels (VCCs) in the plasma-membrane control depolarization-induced Ca^{2+} entry into cells, thereby serving important physiological functions, including excitation-contraction coupling, neurotransmitter and hormone release, and neuronal plasticity (for review, *see* refs. *1–4*). Their function is fine-tuned by a variety of modulators, such as enzymes and G-proteins *(5)*. In addition the spatial distribution of VCCs over the plasma membrane seems to be of fundamental importance for their contribution to cellular function *(6)*. On the molecular level, VCCs are complexes of a pore-forming α1 subunit, an extracellular α2 subunit attached to the membrane by linkage to the transmembrane δ subunit, and a γ subunit, which is a transmembrane glycoprotein (for review, *see* ref. *4*). At the time of this writing 10 genes encoding α1 subunits are known: α1A–α1I, and α1S *(7–9)*. Four of these (α1C, α1D, α1F, and α1S) encode L-type calcium channels (LTCCs), which are defined by distinct physiological and pharmacological properties, including activation at strong depolarized voltages, slow inactivation, large single channel conductance, and block by Ca^{2+} antagonists *(10,11)*. A number of chemically unrelated drugs, such as nifedipine (a dihydropyridine, DHP; Fig. 1A), verapamil (a phenylalkylamine, PAA; Fig. 1B), and diltiazem (a benzothiazepine, BTZ) belong to the group of Ca^{2+} antagonists, which are widely used in the therapy of cardiovascular disorders (for review, *see* ref. *12*). LTCCs are expressed in most neuronal cell types, are the primary type

From: *Ion Channel Localization Methods and Protocols*
Edited by: A. Lopatin and C. G. Nichols © Humana Press Inc., Totowa, NJ

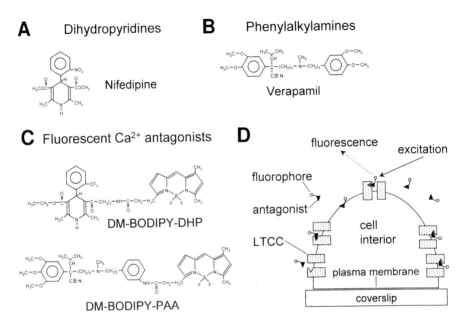

Fig. 1. Representative structures of Ca^{2+} antagonists and experimental strategy. Prototypic examples of dihydropyridines (**A**), phenylalklyamines (**B**), and fluorescent Ca^{2+} antagonists (**C**) are shown. (**D**) During incubation of living cells, fluorescent Ca^{2+} antagonists bind to LTCCs. After removal of unbound ligands only specific label remains (for possible complications *see* Section 2.).

in skeletal muscle cells, and are responsible for the inward movement of calcium ions that initiates contraction of cardiac and smooth muscle cells. The functional role of LTCCs in neurons is still under investigation. Several lines of evidence indicate that LTCCs have a crucial role in regulation of gene transcription by activation of the Ca^{2+}- and cAMP-dependent transcription factor CREB *(13)*.

The diversity of VCCs might suggest that different cell types would express a single or very limited number of VCC subtypes. However, the general theme revealed by immunocytochemical and molecular studies on neurons is that several VCCs are expressed by most neuronal cell types *(14–16)*. Therefore it has been suggested that different VCC subtypes are localized in different regions of the cell to serve specific functions. In order to examine the location of Ca^{2+} channels several different techniques have been used, including electrophysiological techniques, Ca^{2+} imaging, and immunocytochemical staining *(14,17–21)*. Although calcium imaging gives only indirect evidence for the location of VCCs, antibody staining reveals the

Table 1
Fluorescent Probes for LTCCs

Ca^{2+} antagonist	Absorption maximum (nm)	Emission maximum (nm)
DM-BODIPY-DHP[a]	504	511
ST-BODIPY-DHP[a]	565	570
DM-BODIPY-PAA[a]	504	511
DM-BODIPY-BAZ[b]	511	515

[a]Excitation and emission spectra were obtained in methanol (cf. Molecular Probes catalog).

[b]Excitation and emission spectra were obtained in buffer (cf. Molecular Probes catalog).

location of VCCs precisely, but is only used in fixed tissue. Electrophysiological techniques, like single channel recordings from somata and dendrites of neurons, need a great number of recordings to get the complete pattern of the VCC distribution. In addition, such techniques are not feasible for a number of neuronal cell types possessing very fine dendrites.

To overcome these disadvantages, fluorescence techniques have been developed for the direct detection of LTCCs in living cells, based on the development of fluorescent Ca^{2+} channel blockers (Fig. 1C), which are conjugates of Ca^{2+} antagonists with fluorophores. During incubation of living cells with fluorescent Ca^{2+} antagonists, the channel probe binds to LTCCs (Fig. 1D). After excitation with light of the appropriate wavelength (Table 1) the channel-bound fluorescence can be detected by means of an imaging system disclosing the localization of LTCC in a living cell (Fig. 1D).

2. MATERIALS AND METHODS

The strategy of labeling LTCCs in living cells involved the synthesis of fluorescent Ca^{2+} antagonists *(22,23)*. Ca^{2+} antagonists were coupled to the fluorophore BODIPY® (4,4-difluoro-4-bora-3a,4a-diaza-s-indacene; Molecular Probes). Primary amine precursors of PAA and DHP were synthesized and carbon spacer arms were inserted between the Ca^{2+} antagonists and the fluorescent moiety, a procedure based on the synthesis of fluorescent strychnine derivatives *(24)*. Recently a fluorescent BTZ was synthesized (DM-BODIPY-BAZ; 25). Solutions of alkyl-substituted derivatives of BODIPY have similar excitation and emission spectra for fluorescein but have significantly improved photostability, higher quantum yield, and low pH sensitivity *(24)*. BODIPY fluorophores with different fluorescence spectra could be synthesized by changing substitutes on the parent molecule, completing a family of fluorescent Ca^{2+} antagonists (*see* Table 1). The spectral properties of fluorescent Ca^{2+} antagonists allow the use of visible light in combination with standard filter sets for fluorescein or rhodamine. BODIPY dyes are available as fluorescent conjugates of proteins, nucleotides, enzyme substrates, receptor ligands, and channel blocker suitable for a large scale of biological applications.

BODIPY dyes are typically not water-soluble and dimethylsulfoxide (DMSO) should be used as solvent for stock solutions. Thereafter aliquots are added to the extracellular medium and dissociated cells, cell cultures, or slices are incubated for an appropriate amount of time in order to achieve sufficient cell staining. Thereafter unbound fluorescence should be removed by changing the extracellular medium or even using charcoal for adsorption (cf. *23*). During registration of channel-bound fluorescence there is only little loss of label in the range of 0.1%/min (*23*).

Because fluorescent Ca^{2+} antagonists may give rise to unspecific fluorescence owing to non-negligible lipid solubility, a ratio method was developed to overcome this problem (*26*). This method takes advantage of the homogenous staining of the plasma membrane by the voltage-sensitive dye RH414. Using a confocal laser-scanning microscope connected to an argon ion laser, the excitation was set to 488 nm. The fluorescence emitted from olfactory bulb neurons stained with DM-BODIPY-DHP and RH414 was split into two wavelengths by use of a dichroic mirror with a corner wavelength of 580 nm. The green fluorescence of DM-BODIPY-DHP was measured at $\lambda < 580$ nm, whereas the fluorescence of RH414 was measured at $\lambda > 580$ nm. By use of adequate software, ratio images were obtained by subtracting a constant background value from each image and dividing pixelwise the DM-BODIPY-DHP image by the corresponding RH414 image. Using this procedure, ratio images were normalized for the membrane surface area, and the distribution of fluorescence corresponds to the membrane surface density of LTCCs. Later this technique was adapted for the use with conventional fluorescence microscopy (*27*). For DM-BODIPY-DHP and RH414, the excitation wavelength was set to 496 nm and 531 nm, respectively. The fluorescence emitted from stained thalamic neurons was collected consecutively by switching the beam splitter/emission filter combination from dichroic mirror 510 nm/bandpass 510–560 nm for DM-BODIPY-DHP to dichroic mirror 580 nm/long pass 590 nm for RH414. With this filter configuration, a good separation of DM-BODIPY-DHP and RH414 fluorescence could be achieved because fluorescence of RH414 at $\lambda < 560$ nm and fluorescence of DM-BODIPY-DHP at $\lambda > 590$ nm, respectively, is negligible. In general, confocal microscopy is preferable when subcellular locations of LTCCs are imaged, because these methods allows optical sectioning of the specimen and reconstruction of three-dimensional images. When the ratio method is used, excitation wavelengths of DM-BODIPY-DHP and RH414 are different and thus excite the specimen at different focal planes. Again confocal microscopy is advantageous because modern laser scanning microscopes allow the adjustment of parfocality for the two images. Nevertheless reliable results can be obtained with standard fluorescence microscopy *(27)*.

The membrane solubility of Ca^{2+} antagonists may lead to an intracellular accumulation of fluorophores, causing falsified results, or may even make measurements impossible. To prevent these complications, incubation times (on the order of a few minutes) and antagonist concentrations (submicromolar or low micromolar) should be kept at a minimal level. It may even be advantageous to incubate only a single cell by means of a fast application system usually used for drug application during electrophysiological recording. By empirically finding the optimal loading conditions for a given preparation, it is possible to restrict DM-BODIPY-DHP fluorescence to the membrane *(27)*.

3. FLUORESCENT LABELING OF LTCC IN LIVING CELLS

3.1. Specificity of Fluorescent Antagonists

Several lines of evidence indicate that BODIPY conjugates of Ca^{2+} antagonists keep their ability to bind to LTCCs with high affinity and block ion permeation through the channels.

1. The interactions of fluorescent Ca^{2+} antagonists with membrane bound and partially purified LTCCs from skeletal muscle and cerebral cortex were assessed by determining their ability to inhibit binding of radiolabeled (+)-[^{3}H]PN200-110, which is a newer generation DHP *(22)*. DM- and ST-BODIPY-DHP recognized neuronal LTCCs with higher affinity than those of skeletal muscle. For neuronal LTCCs, (+)-DM- and (+)-ST-BODIPY-DHP exhibited K_d values of 2.8 nM and 26.3 nM, respectively, whereas the (−) optical antipodes each have a K_d of 0.9 nM. These binding constants are in the same range as those of the first-generation DHPs, like nifedipine ($K_d = 4.9$ nM for skeletal muscle LTCCs; *28*). For DM-BODIPY-PAA, K_d values were obtained by means of ligand saturation studies. Fixed concentrations of the fluorescent Ca^{2+} antagonist were saturated with increasing concentrations of LTCCs and channel-bound fluorescence was quantified directly. The K_d value derived from this type of analysis (5.6 nM) was even lower than for other PAAs. In addition it could be demonstrated, that only about 50% of DM-

BODIPY-PAA bound to LTCCs with high affinity. Until now, the optical enantiomers have not been separated and it is not known if (R)- or (S)-DM-BODIPY-PAA is the "bindable" enantiomer, although (S)-enantiomers are usually the more potent LTCC blocker *(29)*.

2. Labeling of LTCC with fluorescent Ca^{2+} antagonist is blocked by nonfluorescent agonist or antagonists, which compete for the same binding site. In GH_3 cells, LTCCs were visualized using the enantiomers of ST-BODIPY-DHP, which have identical physicochemical properties but were well-discriminated by LTCCs with an eudismic ratio of about 39 for the biological activity *(22)*. The eutomer, (–)-ST-BODIPY-DHP, stained GH_3 cells with much brighter fluorescence than the distomer, (+)-ST-BODIPY-DHP. In addition, using the optical antipodes of PN200–110, with (+)-PN200–110 being the more active enantiomer, a stereoselective inhibition of ST-BODIPY-DHP enantiomers could be demonstrated. These results are a proof for LTCC interaction with the fluorescent DHPs. Similar results were obtained in ectoderm cells from early gastrula stage *(30)* and thalamic slices *(27)*. In these studies labeling of the multicellular tissue by ST-BODIPY-DHP could be blocked by preincubation with BAYK 8644, a Ca^{2+} agonist of the DHP type *(31)*. Moreover, labeling observed with DM-BODIPY-PAA in perisynaptic Schwann cells of the frog neuromuscular junction was abolished when the preparations were incubated with verapamil *(32)*. Interestingly, similar results were obtained in sunflower protoplasts where verapamil inhibits DM-BODIPY-PAA fluorescence in a dose-dependent manner *(33)*.

3. The proof that DM-BODIPY-DHP binds to functional LTCCs comes from electrophysiological studies *(27)*. When high voltage-activated Ca^{2+} currents were elicited in thalamic relay cells by using depolarizing steps to 0 mV from a holding potential of –50 mV, repeated stimulation gave rise to Ca^{2+} currents of constant peak amplitude (Fig. 2). To assess the participation of LTCCs in the total current, the effects of DHP derivatives were tested. Application of the DM-BODIPY-DHP (0.5 μM) resulted in ~30% reduction of Ca^{2+} current amplitudes, an effect that was only partially reversible (Fig. 2). Although similar in structure to Ca^{2+} antagonists of the DHP type, BAYK promotes calcium entry through L-type channels *(34)*. Application of 5 μM BAYK enhanced high voltage-activated currents by about 50% (Fig. 2). These results demonstrated that fluorescent derivatives of Ca^{2+} antagonists are able to block ion flux through LTCCs, indicating the block of functional channels.

3.2. Ratio Measurements

There is a general problem related to fluorescence measurements in living cells because of their three-dimensional cell geometry. The plasma membrane at the edge of a cell is inclined and, near the ground of the recording chamber, almost vertically oriented (Fig. 1D). This means that there is a stacking of membrane at the edge of a cell, and after excitation of fluorophores, an objective is collecting more fluorescence light from the edge region than from the center of a cell. To overcome this dependency of

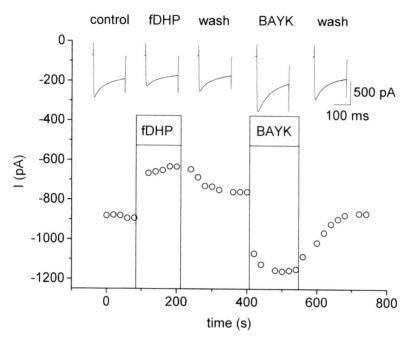

Fig. 2. Effect of Ca^{2+} channel agonists and antagonist on high voltage-activated Ca^{2+} current. Recording was obtained from a thalamocortical cell after acute isolation. Voltage commands (200 ms duration) to 0 mV from a holding potential of –50 mV were delivered every 20 s. A plot of the maximal inward current amplitude against time is shown. Representative current traces for each recording condition are plotted above the main panel. Application of DM-BODIPY-DHP (fDHP) results in a decrease of Ca^{2+} currents, while wash-in of BAYK leads to an increase of HVA current amplitude. Boxes indicate the duration of substance application.

the collected light on the orientation of the plasma membrane, a ratio technique was developed *(26)*. In this technique the fluorescence of DM-BODIPY-DHP (Fig. 3A) is normalized by the fluorescence of a dye that homogeneously stains the plasma membrane, e.g., RH414 (Fig. 3C). Normalization can be achieved by dividing pixelwise an DM-BODIPY-DHP image by an RH414 image, resulting in a ratio image that is corrected for the geometry of the plasma membrane and proportional to the density of LTCCs (Fig. 3B). DM-BODIPY-DHP images and corresponding ratio images are usually not identical, indicating the effectiveness of the ratio method (Fig. 3A,B). Using this method, it was shown that LTCC density in olfactory-bulb neurons is highest on somata, in particular at the base of dendrites, and decreased with distance from this maximum *(26)*. That this expression pat-

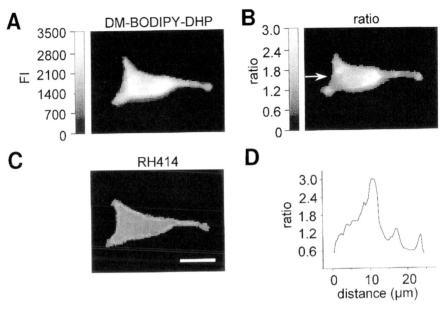

Fig. 3. Acutely isolated TC cell stained with DM-BODIPY-DHP and RH414. Scale bar = 10 μm. Gray-scale bar in **(A)** represents fluorescence intensity (FL) and applies for **(A)** and **(C)**. In **(B)**, ratio values are coded with 4096 shades of gray from black to white. **(A)** Conventional image of a neuron taken during excitation of DM-BODIPY-DHP and measuring the emitted fluorescence for 520 nm < λ < 560 nm. In this wavelength band the fluorescence originates predominantly from DM-BODIPY-DHP. **(B)** The ratio image was determined by dividing pixelwise A by C. **(C)** Image of the same neuron as in **(A)** taken during excitation of RH414. Fluorescence for λ > 590 nm was measured. In this range of wavelength the fluorescence originates mainly from RH414. **(D)** Ratio values on a line (position indicated by the arrow [B]) across the soma and the dendrite were plotted against the distance from the left edge of the cell. Note that the density of LTCCs is maximal at the somato-dendritic junction.

tern may apply more generally to central neurons was demonstrated by ratio measurements in thalamic neurons *(27)*. At least one main type of thalamic neurons, namely the thalamocortical relay cells, exhibit a similar distribution of LTCCs as olfactory neurons (Fig. 3B,D). These data indicate that the interpretation of channel-bound fluorescence in terms of exact channel location and density is improved by applying the ratio technique.

3.3. Localization of LTCCs Revealed by Fluorescent Ca^{2+} Antagonists

Several studies performed on very different tissues used fluorescent Ca^{2+} antagonists to reveal the subcellular location of LTCCs. The first study using fluorescent DHPs more generally described the presence of LTCCs in cultured GH_3 cells *(22)*. Later studies were performed with higher spatial resolution, indicating that LTCCs are localized in distinct cellular regions. Laser scanning confocal microscopy revealed an inhomogeneous fluorescent staining pattern of the basolateral membrane of cochlear outer hair cells, suggesting a heterologous distribution of LTCCs in the plasma membrane. Using the same technique it could also be demonstrated that LTCCs are arranged in clusters on olfactory-bulb *(26)* and thalamic neurons *(27)*. Neurons that make ribbon synapses are among a distinct group of nerve cells whose presynaptic vesicle release is linked to LTCCs. By use of DM-BODIPY-DHP, it has recently been shown that LTCCs are localized in the outer plexiform layer of the retinal section and in presynaptic terminals of rod ribbon synapses *(35)*. In addition to neurons and receptor cells, LTCCs are expressed by glial cells *(36)*. A study investigating the localization of LTCCs in the frog neuromuscular junction by the use of DM-BODIPY-PAA indicated that these channels are clustered at the finger-like processes of perisynaptic Schwan cells *(32)*. This location is appropriate to sense depolarization induced by neurotransmitters resulting in an opening of LTCCs and subsequent reduction of the Ca^{2+} concentration in the synaptic cleft. Because of the steep sensitivity of transmitter release on the extracellular Ca^{2+} concentration, this would result in a reduction in the amount of transmitter released.

Expression of LTCCs was also followed in the temporal dimension, indicating that neuronal developmental processes depend on the timed appearance of Ca^{2+} channels. Already very early in amphibian development, ectoderm cells of gastrula stages acquire neuronal competence (i.e., the ability to differentiate toward neuronal tissue) in relation to the appearance of LTCCs *(30)*. The highest density of LTCCs is reached when competence is optimal. Decrease of LTCCs occurs simultaneously with the loss of competence. In addition to this early developmental role, LTCCs may be involved in the differentiation of neurons. Treatment of fetal hippocampal neurons with basic fibroblast growth factor (bFGF), a single-chain polypeptide composed of 146 amino acids, results in an increase of high voltage-activated Ca^{2+} currents *(37)*. Visualization using ST-BODIPY-DHP revealed that bFGF-treated neurons expressed increased amounts of LTCCs on the cell body. In addition, bFGF-treated neurons acquired distinct morphology characterized by increased neuritic branching. Branching points were associated with clusters of LTCCs.

Besides investigations of neuronal structures, fluorescent Ca^{2+} antagonists were used for studying LTCC influence on renal blood flow *(38)*. Bifurcations of resistance arteries are important sites of hemodynamic regulation. These structures contain pacemaker cells sensitive to Ca^{2+} antagonists and appear to initiate vasoconstriction. Staining of renal resistance arteries with DM-BODIPY-DHP showed enhanced binding at branching points, indicating enhanced expression of LTCCs at the sites of bifurcation. LTCCs are not only expressed in the wall of blood vessels but also in cells transported with the blood stream. With the help of DM-BODIPY-DHP, it could be demonstrated that peripheral blood-derived dendritic immune cells express LTCCs *(39)*.

3.4. Other Applications Using Fluorescent Ca²⁺ Antagonists

Besides determination of LTCC location, fluorescent Ca^{2+} antagonists have successfully been used as tools for studying drug interactions with the channel and the interdependence of Ca^{2+} and drug binding. Addition of (+)-PN200-110 to purified LTCCs lowers their affinity to DM-BODIPY-PAA and accelerates its dissociation, indicating a tight coupling of the PAA and DHP binding domain in the folded structure of the $\alpha 1$ subunit *(23)*. Later a fluorescent diltiazem analog (DM-BODIPY-BAZ) was used to develop a novel binding assay based on fluorescent resonance energy transfer (FRET, *25*; *see* also Chapter 14). In this assay DM-BODIPY-BAZ was not excited directly at 488 nm but instead by radiationless energy transfer from trypophan residues of the LTCC molecules excited at 285 nm. This energy transfer between the BODIPY fluorophore (acceptor) and the tryptophan residues (donor) only occurs within close distance and requires tight binding to the protein. Therefore the fluorescent signal is mainly restricted to the bound ligand. Changes in the concentration of bound DM-BODIPY-BAZ can be monitored in real time without removing the unbound ligand. As a consequence, binding equilibrium remains unchanged. Using this technique, it was shown that DHPs decrease association and dissociation kinetics of DM-BODIPY-BAZ, indicating a direct interaction between DHP and BTZ compounds *(40)*. Detailed binding studies of DM-BODIPY-DHP to LTCCs also used the FRET signal *(41)*. Although the quantum yield of DM-BODIPY-DHP was high in solvent, it was low in buffer but increased upon specific binding to LTCCs. This indicates the existence of binding-induced changes of intramolecular quenching of the BODIPY fluorophore by the DHP moiety. Furthermore, measurements of the FRET signal at high time resolution revealed complex association and dissociation kinetics of DM-BODIPY-DHP indicating one or more intermediate conformational states for the formation of the DHP-LTCC complex. In addition to these drug-LTCC interactions the relationship between Ca^{2+} antagonists and Ca^{2+} binding was investigated using DM-BODIPY-PAA *(23)*. It was demonstrated that LTCCs lose their ability to bind PAAs or DHPs with high affinity when the channels were converted to a Ca^{2+} depleted state by addition of chelators. It has been shown that permeation of Ca^{2+} through VCCs requires selective high-affinity binding of the divalent cation to the selectivity filter of the channel *(42–44)*. These findings indicate that the selectivity filter of LTCCs also represents the Ca^{2+} binding site responsible for stabilization of drug binding. Altogether these findings lead to a concept of close reciprocal interactions between all types of Ca^{2+} antagonists, which probably bind to the same region of LTCCs, and Ca^{2+} ions *(12)*.

An alternative way for labeling of LTCCs is the use of Ca^{2+} antagonists displaying inherent fluorescence. Felodipine is unique among the DHPs in that it is fluorescent *(45)*. Fluorescence can be excited either directly at 380 nm or indirectly via energy transfer from the membrane protein at 290 nm *(46)*. Fluorescence of felodipine is enhanced by high affinity binding to LTCCs from skeletal muscle sarcoplasmic reticulum preparations, as was concluded from competition experiments with the DHP analog isradipine *(47)*. These studies demonstrate that felodipine is also a useful tool for probing LTCCs.

4. CONCLUSION

Fluorescent Ca^{2+} antagonists allow targeting LTCCs with a broad range of spectral and ligand properties and to characterizing LTCCs by measuring channel bound fluorescent label. Using confocal fluorimetric imaging systems, the location of LTCCs can be determined with high resolution in living cells. With the aid of a spectrofluorometer, association and dissociation kinetics, equilibrium saturation experiments, and drug interaction studies can be performed. In particular the latter features of fluorescent Ca^{2+} antagonists may lead to the replacement of "hot" radioligand studies by fluorimetric techniques. Following recent discoveries of LTCC structure, interactions with anchoring proteins, mechanisms of drug binding, permeation, and gating, fluorescent Ca^{2+} antagonists will be involved in a new area of studying these channels. These studies will explore the exact pattern of LTCC distribution, their co-localization with anchoring and regulating proteins, and the temporal sequence of channel expression.

ACKNOWLEDGMENTS

I thank Dr. T. Munsch for helpful discussions and his comments on an earlier version of this manuscript. This work was supported by the DFG (BU 1019/4–1) and the Kultusministerium des Landes Sachsen-Anhalt.

REFERENCES

1. Miller, R. J. (1988) Calcium signaling in neurons. *TINS* **11,** 415–419.
2. Kennedy, M. B. (1989) Regulation of neuronal function by calcium. *TINS* **12,** 417–420.
3. Bliss, T. V. P. and Collingridge, G. L. (1993) A synaptic model of memory: long-term potentiation in the hippocampus. *Nature* **361,** 31–39.
4. Catterall, W. A. (1998) Structure and function of neuronal Ca^{2+} channels and their role in neurotransmitter release. *Cell Calcium* **24,** 307–323.
5. Dolphin, A. C. (1998) Mechanisms of modulation of voltage-dependent calcium channels by G proteins. *J. Physiol. (Lond.)* **506,** 3–11.
6. Destexhe, A., Contreras, D., Steriade, M., Sejnowski, T. J., and Huguenard, J. R. (1996) In vivo, in vitro, and computational analysis of dendritic calcium currents in thalamic reticular neurons. *J. Neurosci.1* **16,** 169–185.
7. Birnbauer, L. (1994) The naming of voltage-gated calcium channels. *Neuron* **13,** 505–506.
8. Perez-Reyes, E., Cribbs, L. L., Daud, A., Lacerda, A. E., Barclay, J., Williamson, M. P., et al. (1998) Molecular characterization of a neuronal low-voltage-activated T-type calcium channel. *Nature* **391,** 896–900.
9. Lee, J. H., Daud, A. N., Cribbs, L. L., Lacerda, A. E., Pereverzev, A., Klockner, U., et al. (1999) Cloning and expression of a novel member of the low voltage-activated T- type calcium channel family. *J. Neurosci.* **19,** 1912–1921.
10. Reuter, H. (1983) Calcium channel modulation by neurotransmitters, enzymes and drugs. *Nature* **301,** 569–574.
11. Nowycky, M. C., Fox, A. P., and Tsien, R. W. (1985) Three types of neuronal calcium channel with different calcium agonist sensitivity. *Nature* **316,** 440–443.
12. Mitterdorfer, J., Grabner, M., Kraus, R. L., Hering, S., Prinz, H., Glossmann, H., and Striessnig, J. (1998) Molecular basis of drug interaction with L-type Ca^{2+} channels. *J Bioenerg. Biomembr.* **30,** 319–334.
13. Bading, H., Ginty, D. D., and Greenberg, M. E. (1993) Regulation of gene expression in hippocampal neurons by distinct calcium signaling pathways. *Science* **260,** 181–186.
14. Hell, J. W., Westenbroek, R. E., Elliott, E. M., and Catterall, W. A. (1994) Differential phosphorylation, localization, and function of distinct alpha 1 subunits of neuronal calcium channels. Two size forms for class B, C, and D alpha 1 subunits with different COOH-termini. *Ann. N. Y. Acad. Sci.* **747,** 282–293.
15. Yan, Z. and Surmeier, D. J. (1996) Muscarinic (m2/m4) receptors reduce N- and P-type Ca^{2+} currents in rat neostriatal cholinergic interneurons through a fast, membrane- delimited, G-protein pathway. *J. Neurosci.* **16,** 2592–2604.

16. Plant, T. D., Schirra, C., Katz, E., Uchitel, O. D., and Konnerth, A. (1998) Single-cell RT-PCR and functional characterization of Ca^{2+} channels in motoneurons of the rat facial nucleus. *J. Neurosci.* **18,** 9573–9584.

17. Westenbroek, R. E., Sakurai, T., Elliott, E. M., Hell, J. W., Starr, T. V., Snutch, T. P., and Catterall, W. A. (1995) Immunochemical identification and subcellular distribution of the alpha 1A subunits of brain calcium channels. *J. Neurosci.* **15,** 6403–6418.

18. Christie, B. R., Eliot, L. S., Ito, K. I., Miyakawa, H., and Johnston, D. (1995) Different Ca^{2+} channels in Soma and dendrites of hippocampal pyramidal neurons mediate spike-induced Ca2+ influx. *J. Neurophysiol.* **73,** 2553–2557.

19. Magee, J. C. and Johnston, D. (1995) Characterization of single voltage-gated Na^+ and Ca^{2+} channels in apical dendrites of rat CA1 pyramidal cells. *J. Physiol. (Lond.)* **487.1,** 67–90.

20. Markram, H., Helm, P. J., and Sakmann, B. (1995) Dendritic calcium transients evoked by single back-propagating action potentials in rat neocortical pyramidal neurons. *J. Physiol. (Lond.)* **485.1,** 1–20.

21. Munsch, T., Budde, T., and Pape, H.-C. (1997) Voltage-activated intracellular calcium transients in thalamic relay cells and interneurons. *Neuroreport* **8,** 2411–2418.

22. Knaus, H. G., Moshammer, T., Friederich, K., Kang, H. C., Haugland, R. P., and Glossmann, H. (1992) In vivo labeling of L-type channels by flourescent dihydropyridines: evidence for a functional, extracellular heparin-binding site. *PNAS* **89,** 3586–3590.

23. Knaus, H. G., Moshammer, T., Kang, H. C., Haugland, R. P., and Glossmann, H. (1992) A unique fluorescent phenylalkylamine probe for L-type Ca^{2+} channels. Coupling of phenylalkylamine receptors to Ca^{2+} and dihydropyridine binding sites. *J. Biol. Chem.* **267,** 2179–2189.

24. Srinivasan, Y., Guzikowski, A. P., Haugland, R. P., and Angelides, K. J. (1990) Distribution and lateral mobility of glycine receptors on cultured spinal cord neurons. *J. Neurosci.* **10,** 985–995.

25. Brauns, T., Cai, Z. W., Kimball, S. D., Kang, K. C., Haugland, R. P., Berger, W., et al. (1995) Benzothiazepine binding domain of purified L-type calcium channels: direct labeling using a novel fluorescent diltiazem analogue. *Biochemistry* **34,** 3461–3469.

26. Schild, H., Geiling, H., and Bischofberger, J. (1995) Imaging of L-type channels in olfactory blub neurons using flourescent dihydropyridine and a styryl dye. *J. Neurosci. Methods* **59,** 183–190.

27. Budde, T., Munsch, T., and Pape, H.-C. (1998) Distribution of L-type calcium channels in rat thalamic neurons. *Eur. J. Neurosci.* **10,** 586–597.

28. Ferry, D. R., Goll, A., and Glossmann, H. (1983) Differential labelling of putative skeletal muscle calcium channels by [^{3}H]-nifedipine, [^{3}H]-nitrendipine, [^{3}H]-nimodipine and [^{3}H]-PN 200 110. *Naunyn Schmiedebergs Arch. Pharmacol.* **323,** 276–277.

29. Rios, E. and Pizarro, G. (1991) Voltage sensor of excitation-contraction coupling in skeletal muscle. *Physiol. Rev.* **71,** 849–908.

30. Leclerc, C., Duprat, A. M., and Moreau, M. (1995) In vivo labelling of L-type Ca^{2+} channels by flourescent dihydropyridine: correlation between ontogen-

esis of the channels and the acquisition of neural competence in ectoderm cells from Pleurodeles waltl embryos. *Cell Calcium* **17**, 216–224.

31. Bechem, M., Hebisch, S., and Schramm, M. (1988) Ca^{2+} agonists: new, sensitive probes for Ca2+ channels. *TIBS* **9**, 257–261.

32. Robitaille, R., Bourque, M. J., and Vandaele, S. (1996) Localization of L-type Ca^{2+} channels at perisynaptic glia cells of the frog neuromuscular junction. *J. Neurosci.* **16**, 148–158.

33. Vallee, N., Briere, C., Petitprez, M., Barthou, H., Souvre, A., and Alibert, G. (1997) Studies on ion channel antagonist-binding sites in sunflower protoplasts. *FEBS Lett.* **411**, 115–118.

34. Nowycky, M. C., Fox, A. P., and Tsien, R. W. (1985) Long-opening mode of gating of neuronal calcium channels and its promotion by the dihydropyridine calcium agonist Bay K 8644. *PNAS* **82**, 2178–2182.

35. Nachman-Clewner, M., St Jules, R., and Townes-Anderson, E. (1999) L-type calcium channels in the photoreceptor ribbon synapse: localization and role in plasticity. *J. Comp. Neurol.* **415**, 1–16.

36. Puro, D. G., Hwang, J. J., Kwon, O. J., and Chin, H. (1996) Characterization of an L-type calcium channel expressed by human retinal Muller (glial) cells. *Mol. Brain. Res.* **37**, 41–48.

37. Shitaka, Y., Matsuki, N., Saito, H., and Katsuki, H. (1996) Basic fibroblast growth factor increases functional L-type Ca^{2+} channels in fetal rat hippocampal neurons: implications for neurite morphogenesis in vitro. *J. Neurosci.* **16**, 6476–6489.

38. Goligorsky, M. S., Colflesh, D., Gordienko, D., and Moore, L. C. (1995) Branching points of renal resistance arteries are enriched in L-type calcium channels and initiate vasoconstriction. *Am. J. Physiol.* **268**, F251–257.

39. Poggi, A., Rubartelli, A., and Zocchi, M. R. (1998) Involvement of dihydropyridine-sensitive calcium channels in human dendritic cell function. Competition by HIV–1 Tat. *J. Biol. Chem.* **273**, 7205–7209.

40. Brauns, T., Prinz, H., Kimball, S. D., Haugland, R. P., Striessnig, J., and Glossmann, H. (1997) L-type calcium channels: binding domains for dihydropyridines and benzothiazepines are located in close proximity to each other. *Biochemistry* **36**, 3625–3631.

41. Berger, W., Prinz, H., Striessnig, J., Kang, H. C., Haugland, R., and Glossmann, H. (1994) Complex molecular mechanism for dihydropyridine binding to L-type Ca(2+)-channels as revealed by fluorescence resonance energy transfer. *Biochemistry* **33**, 11,875–11,883.

42. Tsien, R. W., Hess, P., McCleskey, E. W., and Rosenberg, R. L. (1987) Calcium channels: mechanisms of selectivity, permeation, and block. *Annu. Rev. Biophys. Biophys. Chem.* **16**, 265–290.

43. Tang, S., Mikala, G., Bahinski, A., Yatani, A., Varadi, G., and Schwartz, A. (1993) Molecular localization of ion selectivity sites within the pore of a human L-type cardiac calcium channel. *J. Biol. Chem.* **268**, 13,026–13,029.

44. Yang, J., Ellinor, P. T., Sather, W. A., Zang, J. F., and Tsien, R. W. (1993) Molecular determinants of Ca^{2+} selectivity and ion permeation in L-type Ca^{2+} channels. *Nature* **366**, 158–161.

45. Johnson, J. D. (1983) Allosteric interactions among drug binding sites on calmodulin. *Biochem. Biophys. Res. Commun.* **112,** 787–793.
46. Dunn, S. M. and Bladen, C. (1992) Low-affinity binding sites for 1,4-dihydropyridines in skeletal muscle transverse tubule membranes revealed by changes in the fluorescence of felodipine. *Biochemistry* **31,** 4039–4045.
47. Minarovic, I. and Meszaros, L. G. (1998) Fluorescent probing with felodipine of the dihydropyridine receptor and its interaction with the ryanodine receptor calcium release channel. *Biochem. Biophys. Res. Commun.* **244,** 519–524.

2

Targeting Cerebral Muscarinic Acetylcholine Receptors with Radioligands for Diagnostic Nuclear Medicine Studies

Daniel W. McPherson

1. INTRODUCTION

Nerve cells communicate via the release of chemical messengers (neurotransmitters) which bind to a site (receptor) on another or the same cell causing an effect. The various neuroreceptor classes are responsible for important functions such as movement, memory, and learning. Naturally occurring neurotransmitters are agonists, molecules that trigger an effect in the target cell after binding to the receptor site. In most cases, the binding period of an agonist to the receptor is short and after release from the receptor, the agonist is rapidly taken up by the same nerve cell (reuptake) or metabolized by various bioenzymes. Antagonists are artificial "false" neurotransmitters that bind to a receptor, often with similar or higher affinity compared to an agonist, but do not cause an effect in the target receptor other than preventing the binding of the agonist. Typically, antagonists are designed to increase the binding affinity to the receptor site, to delay release from the receptor pocket, and inhibit the metabolism by bioenzymes.

The investigation of a receptor complex utilizing a false neurotransmitter labeled with an appropriate radio isotope has allowed nuclear medicine the opportunity to image noninvasively various receptor complexes in vivo. There currently exist two imaging modalities routinely utilized in nuclear medicine studies; single photon emission computed tomography (SPECT) and positron emission tomography (PET). Radionuclides utilized in SPECT decay via the emission of relatively low energy gamma ray (~160 KeV) and

From: *Ion Channel Localization Methods and Protocols*
Edited by: A. Lopatin and C. G. Nichols © Humana Press Inc., Totowa, NJ

the distribution of radioactivity is monitored utilizing an external detector. SPECT suffers from the relatively long time required to obtain sufficient counts for image processing in addition to contributions from regions that are not of interest owing to the planar-imaging aspect inherent in the technique. In contrast, PET radionuclides decay with the emission of a low-energy, positively charged beta particle (positron) that subsequently collides with an electron, resulting in annihilation of the electron with a release of two 511 KeV gamma rays emitted at 180° with respect to each other. An external ring of detectors detects this dual emission and allows the instantaneous processing of the event, affording a higher quality image with greater resolution in a shorter acquisition time. This attractive property allows for the modeling of kinetic binding parameters of the ligand-receptor interaction for a better understanding of receptor viability in healthy and diseased tissues. Advances in SPECT hardware and software technology has resulted in the development of two-head, three-head, and ring systems with increased sensitivity and resolution, affording imaging time, quality, and resolution similar to that obtained with PET instrumentation.

This chapter will discuss radiolabeled antagonists that demonstrate selective binding to the muscarinic acetylcholinergic receptor (mAChR) in preclinical and clinical trials for the noninvasive in vivo imaging of cerebral mAChR. In addition, the development of subtype-selective antagonists for the individual evaluation of the various mAChR subtypes will be addressed.

2. MUSCARINIC RECEPTOR COMPLEX

Many properties of mAChR have been known since ancient times and the physiological neurotransmitter signal molecule, acetylcholine—first observed as a contaminant in various biological preparations—was identified in 1914. This was followed by the discovery of an enzyme, cholinesterase, which degrades acetylcholine in vivo (*1*). The mAChR protein consists of seven putative membrane-spanning regions that are characteristic of the super family of G-protein-coupled receptors. They are incorporated into the sarcolemma, protruding into both the extra and intracellular spaces with the amino terminus of the peptide located outside the cell and the carboxyl terminus localized inside the cell.

An important advancement in the study of mAChR was the development of subtype-selective ligands in the late 1970s that allowed for the identification of four subtypes, designated M_1–M_4, by classical pharmacological methods (*2*). Recently, five isoforms (m1–m5) were identified utilizing molecular cloning technique (*3*). Subsequent studies have shown the correlation between the pharmacologically and genetically defined subtypes: M_1 = m1, m4, m5; M_2 = m2; M_3 = m3. (In this chapter, the pharmacological receptor subtypes will be designated as M_1 and the cloned subtypes designated as m1.) The m1, m3, and m5 subtypes preferentially activate phospholipase C via a pertussis toxin insensitive G-protein ($G_{q/11}$ family of proteins) catalyzing phosphoinositide breakdown and the m2 and m4 subtypes inhibit adenyl cyclase activity via a different pertussis toxin-sensitive G-protein ($G_{i/o}$ family of proteins) *(4)*. Receptor desensitization via phosphorylation is a reversible process, can occur within seconds, and involves phosphorylation of the receptor and its associated G protein.

Cerebral M_1 binding sites are localized postsynaptically and M_2 sites are predominately located presynaptically. The mAChR subtypes are located in various concentrations in cortical and subcortical brain regions *(5)*. The m1 subtype is most abundant in the cortex (40%), striatum (31%), and hippocampus (35–60%). Lower levels of the m1 subtype are reported in the nucleus basalis (15–20%). The m2 subtype is enriched in the occipital cortex (36%), nucleus basalis (41%), thalamus (50%), cerebellum (88%), and pons/medulla (81%). The m4 subtype is enriched in the putamen (50%), with lower amounts in cortical regions, hippocampus, and nucleus basalis (13–23%). The m3 and m5 subtype proteins have been detected at significantly lower levels in these cerebral regions.

Change in density or function of cerebral mAChR have been implicated in aging, sudden infant death syndrome (SIDS), memory, sleep disorders, alcoholism, Parkinson's disease (PD), and various dementias such as Alzheimer's disease (AD) or *(6–11)*. This has spurred interest in the development of radiolabeled false neurotransmitters for imaging cerebral mAChR to aid in a greater understanding of the role of mAChR in normal and disease processes.

3. LABELING CHEMISTRY

Fluorine-18 (F-18, $t_{1/2}$ = 110 min) and carbon-11 (C-11, $t_{1/2}$ = 20 min) are two widely utilized radio isotopes for labeling PET neurotransmitters, owing to their favorable decay properties, and are cyclotron produced in high specific activity (to stable isotopes). However, their short half-lives often preclude distribution to other sites and necessitates the need to produce these isotopes onsite increasing the cost for their use.

The development of SPECT ligands is important owing to the large number of medical centers routinely using SPECT systems, allowing this technology to benefit a larger patient population at a lower cost. Iodine-123

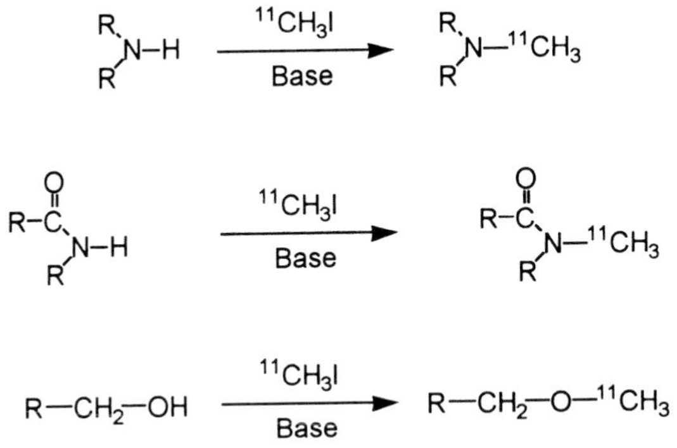

Scheme 1. Incorporation of C-11 into an amide or ether position.

(I-123) is well suited for SPECT owing to its half-life (13.2 h) and imagable gamma ray (158.9 KeV). The longer half-life is advantageous because radiopharmaceuticals can be prepared in a regional pharmacy and shipped to various nuclear medicine centers in a large area, thereby lowering the cost and increasing the availability. In addition, there are two iodine radio isotopes, I-125 and I-131, which are commercially available at low cost with suitable specific activity for the initial development of new radioiodinated ligands.

3.1. Carbon-11

The incorporation of C-11 is routinely investigated because many neurotransmitters contain a functional group that C-11 can be readily incorporated into under mild conditions. Owing to the short half-life, many facile methods have been optimized for rapid C-11 incorporation (Scheme 1). A widely utilized method is the addition of a labeled methyl group via C-11 labeled methyl iodide or methyl triflate to a secondary nitrogen or hydroxyl moiety to afford a tertiary amine, amide, or ether, respectively *(12)*. The introduction of the radiolabeled group at the final stage of synthesis affords a purified radiopharmaceutical with high specific activity. Another routinely utilized method is the introduction of the C-11 into a carbonyl moiety via C-11 labeled carbon dioxide (Scheme 2) *(13)*. However, in many cases, the C-11 label is introduced earlier in the synthesis, resulting in a longer synthesis time and affording a lower radiochemical yield and specific activity owing to the decay of the C-11.

3.2. Fluorine-18

The introduction of F-18 is not as straightforward because naturally occurring neurotransmitters do not contain a fluorine atom. However the

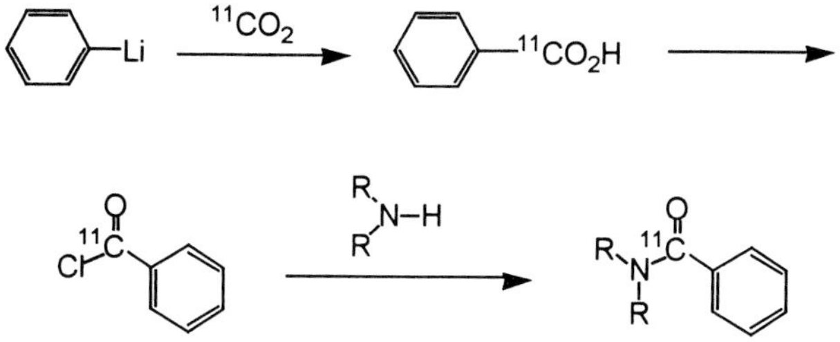

Scheme 2. Incorporation of C-11 into a carbonyl moiety.

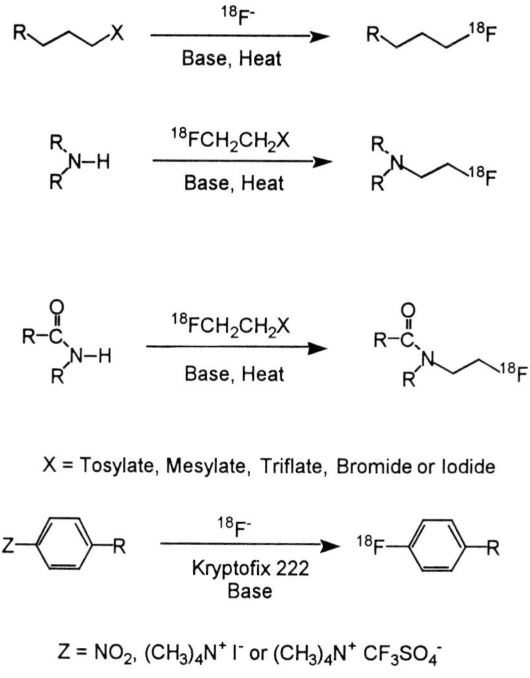

X = Tosylate, Mesylate, Triflate, Bromide or Iodide

Z = NO_2, $(CH_3)_4N^+ I^-$ or $(CH_3)_4N^+ CF_3SO_4^-$

Scheme 3. Incorporation of F-18 into an alkyl, amine, amide, or aromatic position.

longer half-life allows for F-18 incorporation at an earlier stage in the synthesis and more elegant chemistry can be utilized. F-18 is usually introduced as a fluoroalkyl group or placed in a biologically inactive position on a phenyl ring via a nucleophilic displacement of a suitable leaving group (Scheme 3) *(14,15)*.

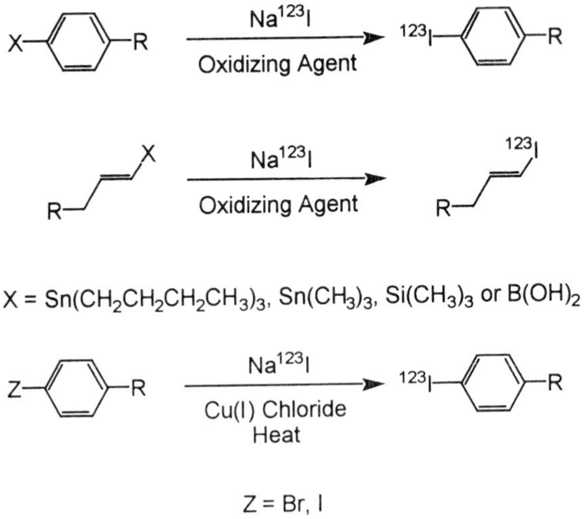

Scheme 4. Incorporation of radioiodine into an alkenyl or aromatic moiety.

3.3. Iodine-123

Analogous to F-18, naturally occurring neurotransmitters do not contain an iodine atom. The introduction of an iodine moiety can cause a dramatic increase in the lipophilicity hindering the ability of the ligand to effectively cross the blood-brain barrier (BBB) and thus lowering the level of tracer available for binding. In addition, the relatively large size of iodine has the potential to interfere in the receptor-binding pocket interactions. Iodine is typically placed in a metabolically stable position on an aromatic ring or an alkenyl group via electrophilic iododemetallation of an alkyl stannyl, silyl, or boronic intermediate with sodium iodine (Scheme 4) *(16)*. An alternative method for iodine incorporation is via a halogen exchange reaction *(17)*. However, a decrease in specific activity of the radiopharmaceutical is realized when iodine for iodine exchange is utilized and may hinder its use as a suitable tracer owing to competition of the unlabeled ligand for the receptor site.

4. SPECT IMAGING STUDIES

4.1. R,S-IQNB

R-1-Azabicyclo[2.2.2]oct-3-yl α-hydroxy-α,α-phenylacetate (QNB) has been shown to be a potent mAChR antagonist, and a proposed "three points of attachment" model for binding of QNB to the receptor did not explain the role of the second phenyl ring *(18,19)*. The addition of an iodine atom to one

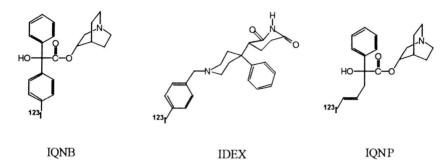

IQNB   IDEX   IQNP

Fig. 1. Radioiodinated ligands developed for SPECT studies of mAChR.

of the phenyl rings was observed to afford an analog, 3-quinuclidinyl 4-iodobenzilate, (IQNB, Fig. 1), which retained a high mAChR binding affinity in vitro *(20)*. This modification inferred chirality (i.e., absolute asymmetry in space) to the benzilic center and in addition to the chirality of the quinuclidinyl ring, racemic IQNB contains four stereoisomers. Upon separation (resolution) of the stereoisomers, R,S-IQNB was observed to be slightly m1 selective (12-fold) in vitro but did not demonstrate subtype selectivity in vivo *(21)*. (Throughout this chapter, the first stereochemical designation refers to the heterocycle ring and the second stereochemical designation refers to the benzilic moiety.) In initial animal studies, a positive correlation between the mAChR concentration and R,S-IQNB binding was demonstrated in various cerebral structures *(22)*.

R,S-IQNB was subsequently labeled with I-123 and the first in vivo imaging of cerebral mAChR in a healthy volunteer was reported and demonstrated the potential utility of nuclear medicine technology for the imaging of mAChR *(23)*. Subsequent studies followed in healthy individuals and patients with dementias *(24–29)*. These studies demonstrated a measured difference in the distribution of activity between IQNB binding and blood flow as measured by technetium-99m (Tc-99m) HMPAO, an established blood flow tracer. Another study compared regional glucose metabolism utilizing F-18-2-deoxyglucose (FDG) to IQNB binding and larger defects were observed in IQNB binding as compared to FDG utilization in patients diagnosed with dementia, although a better understanding of receptor quantification was required to determine various ligand-binding parameters.

Although in vitro binding assays indicate R,S-IQNB not to be subtype selective, owing to the delayed time between radiotracer administration and imaging required to allow sufficient localization of radiotracer and clearance of nonspecific uptake (approx 24 h), R,S-IQNB accumulated in cerebral regions containing a high concentration of the M_1 (m1, m4) subtype and does not allow for the imaging of the M_2 (m2) mAChR subtype.

4.2. Iododexetimide

The successful in vivo imaging of mAChR utilizing R,S-IQNB spurred the development of new radiopharmaceuticals to improve imaging properties, such as an increased ability to pass the BBB and a rapid clearance of nonspecific binding. Dexetimide, another established potent muscarinic antagonist, was reported to accumulate in cerebral regions containing a high concentration of mAChR in a stereospecific and saturable manner *(30)*. When labeled with I-123, dexetimide (IDEX, Fig. 1) retained a high specificity for cerebral mAChR in vitro and in vivo although not demonstrating mAChR subtype selectivity *(31)*.

In studies involving healthy individuals, IDEX showed favorable dosimetry, high specific binding, and a clear binding profile not related to blood flow, affording high quality images reflecting the known distribution of mAChR at 6 h postinjection *(32,33)*. As observed for R,S-IQNB, the activity accumulated in the cortex and striatum with minimal uptake in cerebellum and thalamus, indicating an apparent in vivo selectivity for M_1 rich cerebral regions.

IDEX has been utilized in studies of patients with temporal lobe epilepsy *(34–36)* and although these studies show IDEX binding to be decreased in the hippocampal region, no difference in IDEX binding was detected when a partial volume correction was applied to the image analysis. In a study involving patients diagnosed with mild AD, IDEX binding was observed to be reduced in patients with mild probable AD in the temporal and temporoparietal cortex as compared to controls *(37)*.

4.3. IQNP

Recently, we evaluated a novel QNB analog, 1-azabicyclo[2.2.2]oct-3-yl α-hydroxy-α-(1-iodo-1-propen-3-yl)-phenylacetate (IQNP, Fig. 1), in which the modification of one of the phenyl rings of QNB to an iodopropenyl moiety afforded a ligand with decreased lipophilicity and the potential for facile passage across the BBB *(38)*. Owing to the presence of two asymmetric centers and the *cis-trans* isomerization of the double bond, racemic IQNP contains eight stereoisomers. Upon resolution of the stereoisomers, E-R,R-IQNP was observed to have an 80-fold higher binding affinity for the M_1 (m1, m4) subtype over the M_2 (m2) subtype and Z-R,R-IQNP demonstrated a high nonsubtype selective binding affinity in vitro *(39)*.

Subsequent in vivo rat biodistribution studies utilizing E- and Z-R,R-IQNP supported this significant difference in binding to the various mAChR subtypes *(40,41)*. In vivo autoradiographic studies in rats showed that although both the E- and Z-R,R-isomers label the thalamic nuclei to the same degree, the E isomer labeled the pons, colliculis, and cerebellum to a lesser degree. An ex vivo autoradiographic study utilizing healthy human brain slices obtained at autopsy showed pretreatment with biperiden (M_1 selective antagonist) inhibited the binding of E-R,R-IQNP *(42)*. Subsequent nonhuman primate imaging studies have also confirmed a significant difference in E- and Z-R,R-IQNP binding to the M_1 and M_2 subtypes *(42–44)*.

A unique feature of iodine in the development of new radiopharmaceuticals is the availability of three radio isotopes with sufficient specific activity that can be employed in a single in vivo biological study. By individually analyzing the decay energy and half-life of each isotope, a direct in vivo comparison of different ligands or stereoisomers is possible, allowing each animal as its own control. In this manner the effects of age, injection technique, circadian rhythm, and diet; for example, do not distort the data and absolute differences in receptor binding can be evaluated. In a dual-label study, I-125-Z-R,R-IQNP and I-131-E-R,R-IQNP were administered to the same animal and, in agreement with previous individual studies, E-R,R-IQNP bound selectively to cerebral regions containing a high concentration of the M_1 (m1, m4) subtype and Z-R,R-IQNP demonstrated nonselective binding in vivo at 6 h postinjection *(41)*. A triple-label study was also performed utilizing I-123-Z-R,R-IQNP, I-131-IDEX, and I-125-R,S-IQNB and Z-R,R-IQNP was observed to accumulate to a higher degree in all mAChR regions. More importantly, Z-R,R-IQNP is the first example of an iodinated ligand demonstrating a significant and prolonged binding in cerebral regions containing a high concentration of the M_2 subtype. Initial SPECT studies in progress with I-123-E- and Z-R,R-IQNP in healthy volunteers have also confirmed the difference in subtype mAChR binding of these isomers (Fig. 2) *(45)*.

5. PET IMAGING STUDIES

5.1. Scopolamine

Because C-11 can be conveniently incorporated directly without a compromise in the biological behavior of the ligand, scopolamine (SCOP, Fig. 3), an established mAChR antagonist, was first investigated for imaging mAChR via PET *(46)*. Preliminary in vivo studies in rats suggested the cerebral distribution of radioactivity paralleled mAChR populations and a subsequent PET study performed in six healthy individuals demonstrated the potential for imaging mAChR via PET *(47)*. However, it was concluded the

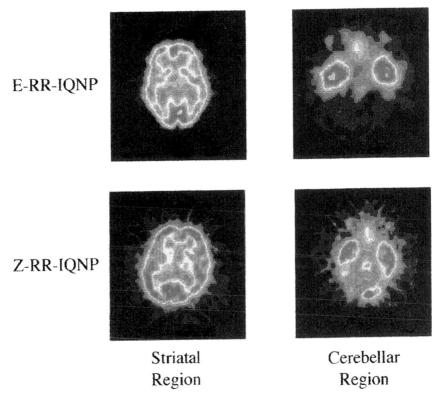

E-RR-IQNP

Z-RR-IQNP

Striatal   Cerebellar
Region   Region

Fig. 2. Initial human volunteer SPECT imaging study utilizing I-123-E- and Z-RR-IQNP (100 MBq) at 30 h postinjection. (Used with permission of Nobuhara, Halldin et al., Karolinska Institute, Stockholm, Sweden.)

use of SCOP was not an ideal tracer owing an unfavorable binding profile and lack of an appropriate compartmental kinetic binding model arising from the short half-life of C-11.

5.2. QNB, Dexetimide, Benzotropine

The promising results of SCOP lead to the subsequent C-11 labeling of QNB, dexetimide (DEX), and benztropine (BENZ) (Fig. 3) *(48–50)*. Of these ligands only C-11 BENZ has been utilized for the evaluation of mAChR in the human brain and the localization of radioactivity was shown to be specific for M_1 mAChR rich cerebral areas at 60 min postinjection *(50)*. In a study evaluating age-related changes in mAChR binding, a decrease in BENZ binding was observed in regions of high density as com-

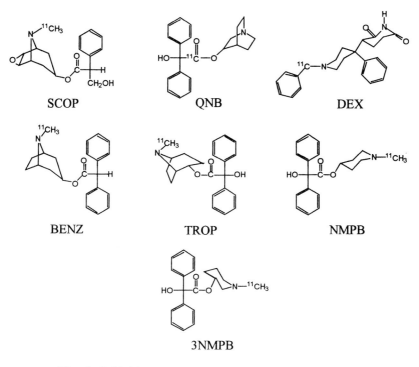

Fig. 3. C-11-labeled ligands developed for PET studies.

pared to regions containing a relatively low density *(51)*. However, as reported for SCOP, owing to the short half-life of C-11, the prolonged time required for clearance of nonspecific binding to allow a better delineation of receptor binding in receptor-rich areas was not achieved. As techniques for processing PET data have improved overcoming the limited study time of C-11 and the resultant poor receptor binding kinetics, a study involving six healthy volunteers reported the anatomical standardization of cerebral mAChR images obtained utilizing BENZ have the potential to delineate physiological or pathological alterations *(52)*.

5.3. Tropinyl Benzilate

To overcome long equilibration times as compared to transport rates that make it difficult to evaluate mAChR viability accurately, C-11 tropanyl benzilate (TROP, Fig. 3), was investigated *(53)*. Imaging studies conducted in female pigtail monkeys demonstrated at 50–80 min postinjection regional localization of activity was consistent with mAChR distribution. Subsequent imaging and kinetic analysis in six young, healthy volunteers demonstrated reliable receptor density information and an appropriate compartmental kinetic model could be obtained *(54)*. A subsequent study to quantify mAChR in normal aging was performed and, as opposed to other studies and clinical evidence, cerebral cortical cholinergic dysfunction in elderly subjects was not attributable to a major loss of total muscarinic cholinoceptive capacity *(55)*.

5.4. 4-N-Methylpiperidinyl Benzilate

A decrease in the ligand binding affinity may afford improved ligand-receptor binding profile required for the development of kinetic compartmental model for the determination of receptor function and viability. 4-*N*-Methylpiperidinyl benzilate (NMPB, Fig. 3), the simplest of a series of N-substituted benzilic esters, displays a lower binding affinity as compared to QNB *(56)*. An initial PET study utilizing C-11-NMPB allowed the development of an appropriate compartmental model for the quantification of mAChR and an accurate distinction of receptor binding parameter (K_3) to estimate tracer delivery with acceptable precision in both intra- and intersubject comparison *(57)*.

In an aging study, a 45% age-related decrease in K_3 was observed over the age range of 18–75 yr *(58)*. In another study, patients were evaluated for mAChR occupancy after administration of trihexyphenidyl (anticholinergic drug), L-dopa (antiparkinson drug), or triazolam (insomnia drug) to evaluate the effect of drug therapy in the treatment of various dementias *(59,60)*. It was observed the administration of a therapeutic dose of trihexyphenidyl caused a mean 28% inhibition of K_3 and after administration of L-dopa no significant change in K_3 was observed. Administration of triazolam, reported to decrease cortical acetylcholine release, also caused a decrease in the binding of NMPB in the temporal cortex and thalamus. This study demonstrates the potential of nuclear medicine for the measurement of drug-induced changes in mAChR occupancy for more effective management of drug therapies.

In patients diagnosed with PD, K_3 values were observed to be 20% higher in the frontal cortex as compared to age-matched controls *(61)*. However, alterations in cerebral blood flow (CBF) has the potential to impart a significant influence on the results and must be taken into account when interpreting the data, for example, an increase in CBF is expected to cause an increase in ligand delivery and a higher cerebral accumulation of activity. Because a decreased or unchanged CBF has been reported in patients diagnosed with PD, the increase in NMPB binding is owing to deviations in mAChR. It was postulated the increase in NMPB binding was a response to a loss of ascending cholinergic input to the frontal cortex and relates to frontal lobe dysfunction.

In another study addressing the important role of CBF on the interpretation of radiopharmaceutical-receptor binding studies, cerebral glucose metabolism (via F-18-FDG), CBF (via Tc-99m-HMPAO), and mAChR binding (via C-11 NMPB) were measured in 18 patients diagnosed with "probable AD" *(62)*. A significant decrease in NMPB binding, a greater decrease in glucose metabolism and a slight decrease in the CBF were observed in patients diagnosed with mild or moderate AD as compared to controls. This study suggests that although there was decrease in mAChR binding, FDG was a more sensitive tool for the detection of degenerative cerebral regions in AD.

In a study evaluating of the role of mAChR in human narcolepsy, NMPB uptake in the pons, thalamus, striatum, and cerebral cortex was measured in 11 patients and 21 normal controls *(63)*. In addition, 7 of the 11 patients underwent additional PET scans after alleviation of the symptoms by drug therapy. No difference in NMPB binding between the patients and controls before or after drug therapy was observed and does not support a major role for drug therapy targeted at mAChR for the clinical improvement of human cataplexy.

5.5. (+)-N-Methyl-3-Piperidinyl Benzilate

(+)-*N*-Methyl-3-piperidinyl benzilate (3NMPB, Fig. 3), an analog of NMPB, displays a decreased in vitro binding affinity as compared NMPB and may afford improved binding kinetic parameters for quantification of mAChR function *(64)*. Utilizing in vitro autoradiographic analysis in rats, 3NMPB exhibited high accumulation in the corpus striatum, hippocampus, colliculis, and cerebral cortex, but the issue of receptor binding equilibrium has not yet been addressed.

5.6. Fluorine-18-Labeled Ligands

F-18, with its longer half-life, has the potential for a longer imaging protocol to allow nonspecific binding to clear and to achieve ligand-binding equilibrium for a higher target to nontarget tissue ratio. Surprisingly, only the initial evaluation of fluorodexetimide (FDEX) *(65)*, 1-azabi–cyclo[2.2.2]oct-3-yl α-(1-fluoropentan-5-yl)-α-hydroxy-α-phenylacetate (FQNPe) *(66)* and *N*-fluoroethyl-4-piperidinyl benzilate (FNEPB) have been reported (Fig. 4) *(67)*.

6. DEVELOPMENT OF mAChR SUBTYPE-SPECIFIC LIGANDS

The radiopharmaceuticals discussed earlier demonstrate the potential for the noninvasive in vivo evaluation of mAChR function and viability utiliz-

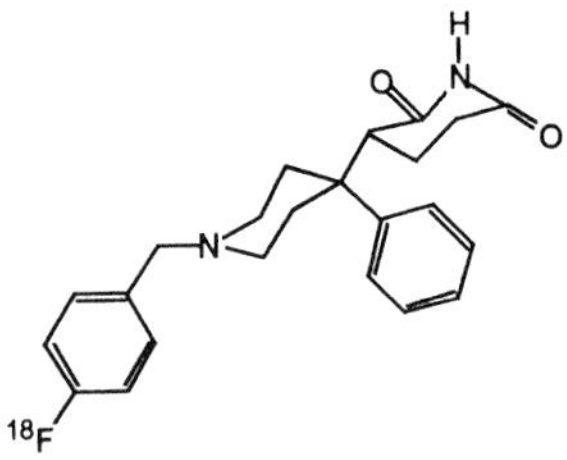

FDEX

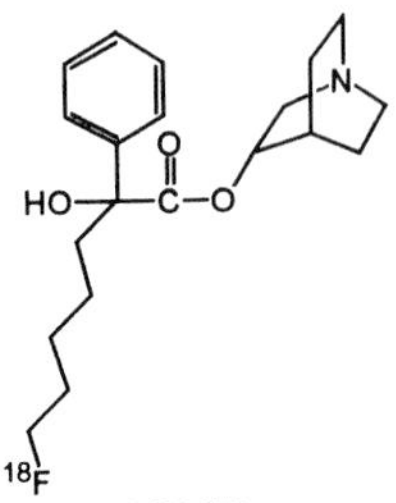

FQNPe

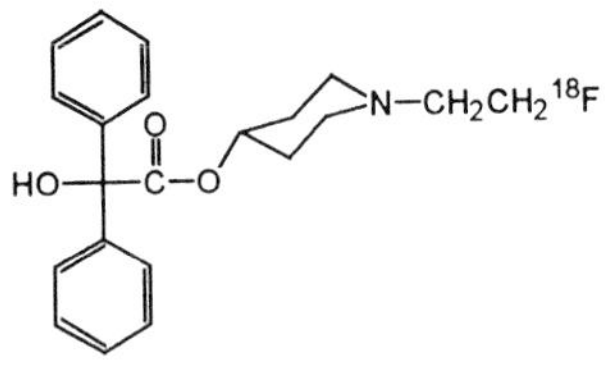

FNEPB

Fig. 4. F-18-labeled ligands developed for PET studies.

ing nuclear medicine protocols. However, a major disadvantage is the lack of demonstrated mAChR subtype selectivity of these radiopharmaceuticals. The ability to image the various mAChR subtypes independently is of importance owing to the role the mAChR subtypes are postulated to play in various biological processes and diseases. For example, the m2 subtype is postulated to decrease in the early stages and, as a response, the m1 subtype is postulated to be upregulated in later stages of AD. The ability to image selectively the m2 mAChR subtype is therefore of importance for an early diagnosis and a better understanding of the progression of AD. Another expected benefit for the selective subtype imaging of mAChR is the monitoring of various drug regiments to afford more effective treatments. Therefore, there is a need for the design and evaluation of new radiopharmaceuticals targeted to the individual mAChR subtypes.

6.1. PET Ligands

5,11-Dihyro-8-chloro-11-[4-[3-[(2,2-dimethyl-1-oxopentyl)ethylamino]-propyl]-1-piperidinyl]-acetyl]–6H-pyrido[2,3-b][1,4]benzodiazepin-6-one (BIBN 99, Fig. 5) is a lipophilic M_2 antagonist with central nervous system (CNS) activity, able to cross the BBB, and demonstrates a m2/m1 selectivity of 33 to 1 in vitro *(68)*. C-11-BIBN 99 has recently been reported although the in vivo biological evaluation was not discussed *(69)*.

A fluorinated QNB analog, R-1-azabicyclo[2.2.2]oct-3-yl S-α-hydroxy-α-(4-fluoromethyl)phenyl-α-phenylacetate (FMeQNB, Fig. 5), was shown to have a m2/m1 selectivity of 7 to 1 in vitro *(70)*. In rats studies, F-18-FMeQNB uptake was nearly uniform in all brain regions, reflecting the reported m2 subtype concentration, and was reduced by 36–54% in all cerebral regions following co-injection of unlabeled FMeQNB. In subsequent monkey PET imaging studies, FMeQNB demonstrated cerebral uptake with slow clearance that was displaced by QNB to a greater extent in the thalamus (high m2 concentration) as compared to the cortex (low m2 concentration). These results support the assumption that FMeQNB displays selective m2 binding in vivo but until the development of a proven m2 subtype selective ligand able to cross the BBB, the subtype selectivity of FMeQNB cannot be firmly established. As observed for other QNB analogs, FMeQNB demonstrates a slow receptor binding off-rate that prohibits the determination of various kinetic parameters required for the evaluation of mAChR viability.

6.2. SPECT Ligands

The modest ability of E-R,R-IQNP to differentiate between the M_1 and M_2 mAChR subtypes in vitro and in vivo is encouraging in the development of radioiodinated subtype ligands. Changes in the benzilic or the heterocycle moieties of QNB have been shown to influence mAChR binding affinity and subtype selectivity of new analogs. An IQNP analog, 1-methylpiperidin-4-yl α-hydroxy-α-(1-iodo-1-propen-3-yl)-α-phenylacetate (IPIP, Fig. 5) has been prepared in which the quinuclidinyl ring was modified to a 1-methylpiperidin-4-yl ring and resulted in a decrease in the lipophilicity allowing a more effective passage across the BBB *(71)*. The individual I-125 IPIP isomers were evaluated in vivo in rats and demonstrated a rapid and high accumulation in regions of the brain containing mAChR. Although not demonstrating an increased cerebral uptake, E-R-IPIP selectively accumulated in M_1 rich cerebral regions by 4 h postinjection. Z-S- and Z-R-IPIP initially demonstrated a significant and uniform uptake in cerebral regions containing mAChR indicating nonsubtype selectivity with Z-S-IPIP demonstrating similar kinetic binding as observed for Z-R,R-IQNP. Z-R-IPIP, however, demonstrated a faster release from the M_2 site and may have potential in the evaluation of changes in receptor function in M_2 rich cerebral regions.

IPIP is a member of a unique class of radiopharmaceuticals that can be radiolabeled either with I-123 on the allyl position for SPECT studies or by C-11 in the N-methyl position for PET studies. Ex vivo metabolic studies with Z-S-IPIP demonstrated the N-methyl group to be stable in vivo and the desmethyl compound does not cross the BBB. In addition, if IPIP is metabo-

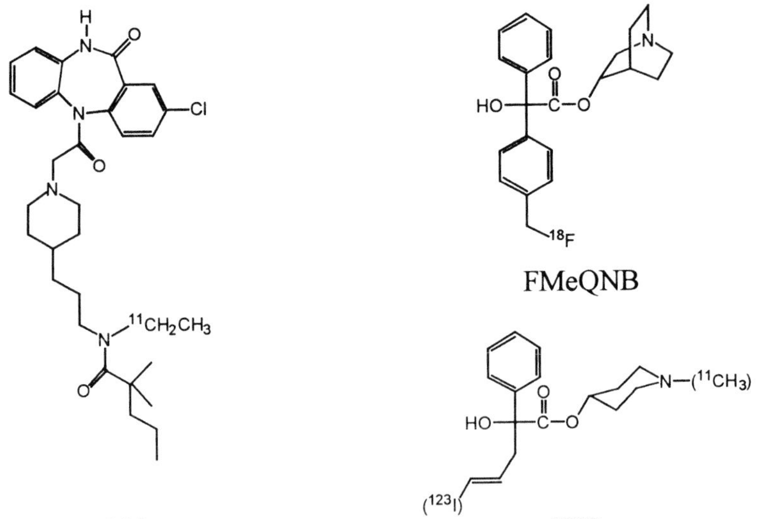

Fig. 5. Ligands investigated for evaluation of mAChR subtypes.

lized after release from the receptor pocket, potential metabolites were not observed to compete with IPIP binding at the receptor site making this position attractive for C-11 labeling. Initial studies have shown E-R-IPIP is readily radiolabeled with C-11 under mild conditions *(72)*.

7. CONCLUSIONS

The development of radiopharmaceuticals targeted to mAChR have demonstrated the potential for the detailed study of mAChR density and viability by nuclear medicine imaging techniques for a variety of biological processes and disease states. The evolution of appropriate kinetic binding models for interpretation of imaging studies have allowed a better understanding of the radiopharmaceutical-receptor binding kinetics in vivo. Although a variety of "false" neurotransmitters labeled with either C-11, F-18, or I-123 have been developed, these radiopharmaceuticals do not possess ideal receptor binding properties to allow a complete understanding of kinetic binding parameters of the ligand-receptor interaction. Future developments in radiopharmaceutical selectively design include the ability to bind the radiopharmaceutical to individual mAChR subtypes for a better understanding of the role of the mAChR subtypes in aging, memory, movement, and disease processes. Improved imaging protocols to optimize ligand-receptor kinetic models will afford a more detailed modeling and understanding of the receptor binding parameters. In addition, this new generation of mAChR subtype selective radiopharmaceuticals will allow for an increased role of nuclear medicine studies as an accepted tool in the early diagnosis and treatment of various dementias and diseases. Nuclear medicine protocols will also serve as an important tool in the monitoring of various drug regiments affording improved drug therapy and an efficient, cost-effective modality of treatment leading to an improvement in the quality of life.

ACKNOWLEDGMENT

Work supported at Oak Ridge National Laboratory by the Office of Science, United State Department of Energy, under contract DE-AC05-96OR22464 with Lockheed Martin Energy Research Corporation.

REFERENCES

1. Burgen, A. S. V. (1995) The background of the muscarinic system. *Life Sci.* 11/12: 801–806.
2. Mutschler, E., Moser, U., Wess, J., and Lambrecht, G. (1989) Muscarinic receptor subtypes: agonists and antagonists, in *Progress in Pharmacology and Clinical Pharmacology*, vol. 7/1, (Zwieten, P. A. and vanand Schonbaum, E., eds.), Gustav Fischer Verlag, Stuttgart, pp. 13–31.
3. Buckley, N. J., Bonner, T. I., Buckley, C. M., and Brann, M. R. (1989) Antagonist binding properties of five cloned muscarinic receptors expresses in CHO-K$_1$ cells. *Mol. Pharmacol.* **35,** 469–476.
4. Gainetdinov, P. R. and Caron, M. G. (1999) Delineating muscarinic receptor functions. *Proc. Natl. Acad. Sci. USA* **96,** 12,222–12,223.
5. Levey, A. I. (1993) Immunological localization of m1-m5 muscarinic acetylcholine receptors in peripheral tissues and brain. *Life Sci.* **52,** 441–448.
6. Levey, A. I. (1996) Muscarinic acetylcholine receptor expression in memory circuits: implications for treatment of Alzheimer disease. *Proc. Natl. Acad. Sci. USA* **93,** 13,541–13,546.
7. Brown, J. H. and Taylor, P. (1996) Muscarinic receptor agonists and antagonists, in *The Pharmacological Basis of Therapeutics* (Hardman, J. G. and Limbird, L. E., eds.), McGraw-Hill, NY, pp 141–160.
8. Baghdoyan, H. A. and Lydic, R. (1999) M$_2$ muscarinic receptor subtype in the feline medial pontine reticular formation modulates the amount of rapid eye movement sleep. *Sleep* **22,** 835–847.
9. Nordberg, A., Alaguzoff, I., and Winblad, B. (1992) Nicotinic and muscarinic subtypes in the human brain: changes with aging and dementia. *J. Neurosci. Res.* **31,** 103–111.

10. Freund, G. and Ballinger, W. E. (1991) Loss of synaptic receptors can precede morphologic changes induced by alcoholism. *Alcohol Alcoholism* (**Suppl. 1**), 385–391.

11. Kinney, H. C., Filiano, J. J., Sleeper, L. A., Mandel, L. F., Valdes-Dapena, M., and White, W. F. (1995) Decreased muscarinic receptor binding in the arcuate nucleus in sudden infant death syndrome. *Science* **269**, 1446–1450.

12. Nagren, K., Halldin, C., Muller, L., Swahn, C. G., and Lehikoinen, P. (1995) Comparison of [^{11}C]methyl triflate and [^{11}C]methyl iodide in the synthesis of PET radioligands such as [^{11}C]beta-CIT and [^{11}C]beta-CFT. *Nucl. Med. Biol.* **22**, 965–979.

13. Prenant, C., Barre, L., and Crouzel, C. (1989) Synthesis of [^{11}C]–3-quinuclidinyl benzilate (QNB). *J. Labelled Comp. Rad.* **27**, 1257–1265.

14. Halldin, C., Farde, L., Hogberg, T., Hall, H., Strom, P., Ohlberger, A., and Solin, O. (1991) A comparative PET-study of five carbon-11 or fluorine-18 labelled salicylamindes. Preparation and in vitro dopamine D-2 receptor binding. *Nucl. Med. Biol.* **18**, 871–881.

15. Lang, L., Jagoda, E., Schmall, B., Vuong, B. K., Adams, R., Nelson, D. L., Carson, R. E., and Eckelman, W. C. (1999) Development of fluorine-18-labeled 5HT$_{1A}$ antagonists. *J. Med. Chem.* **42**, 1576–1586.

16. Seevers, R. H. and Counsell, R. E. (1982) Radioiodination techniques for small organic molecules. *Chem. Rev.* **82**, 575–590.

17. Kampfer, I., Heinicke, J., Sorger, D., Schulze, K., Schliebs, R., and Knapp, W. H. (1996) Novel preparation of (R,R)bromo-3-quinuclidinyl benzilate (Br-QNB), a precursor for the synthesis of (R,R)[^{123}I]iodo-QNB. *J. Labelled Comp. Rad.* **38**, 1047–1052.

18. Sternbach, L. H. and Kaiser, S. (1952) Antispasmodics. I. Bicyclic basic alcohols. *J. Am. Chem. Soc.* **74**, 2215–2218.

19. Beckett, A. H., Lan, N. T., and Khokhar, A. Q. (1971) Anti-acetylcholinesterase activity of some stereoisomeric aminoboranes. *J. Pharm. Pharmacol.* **23**, 528–533.

20. Rzeszotarski, W. J., Eckelman, W. C., Francis, B. E., Simms, D. A., Gibson, R. E., Jagoda, E. M., et al. (1984) Synthesis and evaluation of radioiodinated derivatives of 1-azabicyclo[2.2.2]oct-3-yl α-hydroxy-α-(4-iodophenyl)-α-phenylacetate as potential radiopharmaceuticals. *J. Med. Chem.* **27**, 156–159.

21. Kiesewetter, D. O., Silverton, J. V., and Eckelman, W. C. (1995) Synthesis and biological properties of chiral fluoroalkyl quinuclidinyl benzilates. *J. Med. Chem.* **38**, 1711–1719.

22. Gibson, R. E. (1990) Muscarinic acetylcholine receptors, in *Quantitative Imaging. Neuroreceptors, Neurotransmitters, and Enzymes* (Frost, J. J., Wagner, H. N., Jr., eds.), Raven Press, Boston, MA, pp. 129–152.

23. Eckelman, W. C., Reba, R. C., Rzeszotarski, W. J., Gibson, R. E., Hill, T., Holman, B. L., et al. (1984) External imaging of cerebral muscarinic acetylcholine receptors. *Science* **223**, 291–294.

24. Holman, B. L., Gibson, R. E., Hill, T. C., Eckelman, W. C., Albert, M., and Reba, R. C. (1985) Muscarinic acetylcholine receptors in Alzheimer's disease,

in vivo imaging with iodine 123-labeled 3-quinuclidinyl 4-iodobenzilate and emission tomography. *JAMA* **254,** 3063–3066.

25. Weinburger, D. R., Gibson, R., Coppola, R., Jones, D. W., Molchan, S., Sunderland, T., et al. (1991) The distribution of cerebral muscarinic acetylcholine receptors *in vivo* in patients with dementia. A controlled study with [123]IQNB and single photon emission computed tomography. *Arch. Neurol.* **48,** 169–176.

26. Owens, J., Murray, T., McCulloch, J., and Wyper, W. (1992) Synthesis of (R,R)-[^{123}I]-QNB, a SPECT imaging agent for cerebral muscarinic acetylcholine receptors *in vivo. J. Labelled Comp. Rad.* **31,** 45–60.

27. Weinburger, D. R., Jones, D., Reba, R. C., Mann, U., Coppola, R., Gibson, R., et al. (1992) A comparison of FDG PET and IQNB SPECT in normal subjects and in patients with dementias. *J. Neuropsychiatry Clin. Neursci.* **4,** 239–248.

28. Wyper, J., Brown, D., Patterson, J., Owens, J., Hunter, R., Teasdale, E., and McCulloch, J. (1993) Deficits in iodine-labelled 3-quinuclidinyl benzilate binding in relation to cerebral blood flow in patients with Alzheimer's disease. *Eur. J. Nucl. Med.* **20,** 379–386.

29. Sunderland, T., Esposito, G., Molchan, S. E., Coppola, R., Jones, D. W., Gorey, J., et al. (1995) Differential cholinergic regulation in Alzheimer's patients compared to controls following chronic blockade with scopolamine: a SPECT study. *Psychopharmacology* **121,** 231–241.

30. Laduron, P. M. and Janssen, P. F. M. (1979) Characterization and subcellular localization of brain muscarinic receptors labelled *in vivo* by [^{3}H]dexetimide. *J. Neurochem.* **33,** 1223–1231.

31. Wilson, A. A., Dannals, R. F., Ravert, H. T., Frost, J. J., and Wagner, H. N., Jr. (1989) Synthesis and biological evaluation of [^{125}I]- and [^{123}I]-4-iododexetimde, a potent muscarinic cholinergic receptor antagonist. *J. Med. Chem.* **32,** 1057–1062.

32. Boundy, K. L., Barnden, L. R., Rowe, C. C., Reid, M., Kassiou, M., Katsifis, A. G., and Lambrecht, R. M. (1995) Human dosimetry and biodistribution of iodine-123-iododexetimide: a SPECT imaging agent for cholinergic muscarinic neuroreceptors. *J. Nucl. Med.* **36,** 1332–1338.

33. Muller-Gartner, H. W., Wilson, A. A., Dannals, R. F., Wagner, H. N., Jr., and Frost, J. J. (1992) Imaging muscarinic cholinergic receptors in human brain in vivo with SPECT, [I-123]-4-iododexetimide and [I-123]–4-iodolevetimide. *J. Cereb. Blood Flow Metab.* **12,** 562–570.

34. Muller-Gartner, H. W., Mayberg, H. S., Fisher, R. S., Lesser, R. P., Wilson, A. A., Ravert, H. T., et al. (1993) Decreased hippocampal muscarinic cholinergic receptor-binding measured by I-123 iododexetimide and single photon emission computed tomography in epilepsy. *Ann. Neurol.* **34,** 235–238.

35. Boundy, K. L., Rowe, C. C., Black, A. B., Kitchener, M. I., Barnden, L. R., Sebben, R., et al. (1996) Localization of temporal lobe epileptic foci with iodine-123 iododexetimide cholinergic neuroreceptor single-photon emission computed tomography. *Neurology* **47,** 1015–1020.

36. Weckesser, M., Hufnagel, A., Ziemons, K., Griessmeier, M., Sonnenberg, F., Hacklander, T., et al. (1997) Effect of partial volume correction on muscarinic

cholinergic receptor imaging with single-photon emission tomography in patients with temporal lobe epilepsy. *Eur. J. Nucl. Med.* **24,** 1156–1161.

37. Claus, J. J., Dubois, E. A., Booij, J., Habraken, J., de Munck, J. C., van Herk, M., et al. (1997) Demonstration of a reduction in muscarinic receptor binding in early Alzheimer's disease using iodine-123 dexetimide single-photon emission tomography. *Eur. J. Nucl. Med.* **24,** 602–608.

38. McPherson, D. W., DeHaven-Hudkins, D. L., Callahan, A. P., and Knapp, F. F., Jr. (1993) Synthesis and biodistribution of iodine-125-labeled 1-azabicyclo[2.2.2]oct-3-yl α-hydroxy-α-(1-iodo-1-propen-3-yl)-α-phenylacetate. A new ligand for the potential imaging of muscarinic receptors by SPECT. *J. Med. Chem.* **36,** 848–854.

39. McPherson, D. W., Lambert, C. R., Jahn, K., Sood, V., McRee, R. C., Zeeberg, B., et al. (1995) Resolution, in vitro and in vivo evaluation of isomers of iodine-125-labeled 1-azabicyclo[2.2.2]oct-3-yl α-hydroxy-α-(1-iodo-1-propen-3-yl)-α-phenylacetate (IQNP). A high affinity ligand for the muscarinic receptor. *J. Med. Chem.* **38,** 3908–3917.

40. Rayeq, M. R., Boulay, S. F., Sood, V. K., McPherson, D. W., Knapp, F. F., Jr., Zeeberg, B. R., and Reba, R. C. (1996) *In vivo* autoradiographic evaluation of isomers of I-125-labeled 1-azabicyclo[2.2.2.]oct-3-yl α-hydroxy-α-(1-iodo-1-propen-3-yl)-α-phenylacetate (IQNP). Direct evidence for enhanced *in vivo* M_2 muscarinic subtype selectivity for Z-(-) (-)-[^{125}I]-IQNP. *Receptors Signal Transduction* **6,** 13–34.

41. McPherson, D. W., Greenbaum, M., Luo, H., Beets, A. L., and Knapp, F. F., Jr. (2000) Evaluation of Z-(R,R)-IQNP for the potential imaging of the m2 mAChR rich regions of the brain and heart. *Life Sci.* **66,** 885–896.

42. Bergstrom, K. A., Halldin, C., Hiltunen, J., Swahn, C. G., Ito, H., Ginovert, N., et al. (1998) I-125 and I-123-labeled E-(-,-)-IQNP: potential radioligand for visualization of M_1 acetylcholinergic receptors in brain. Determination of metabolites using HPLC. *Nucl. Med. Biol.* **25,** 209–214.

43. Bergstrom, K., Halldin, C., Savonen, A., Okubo, Y., Hiltunen, J., Nobuhara, K., et al. (1999) Iodine-123 labelled Z-(R,R)-IQNP: A potential radioligand for visualization of M_1 and M_2 muscarinic acetylcholine receptors in Alzheimer's disease. *Eur. J. Nucl. Med.* **26,** 1482–1485.

44. Nobuhara, K., Halldin, C., Hall, H., Karlsson, P., Farde, L., Hiltunen, J., et al. (2000) Z-IQNP: A potential radioligand for SPECT imaging of muscarinic acetylcholine receptors in Alzheimer's disease. *Pyschopharmacology (Berl.)* **149(1),** 45–55.

45. Nobuhara, K., Farde, L., Halldin, C., Karlsson, P., Swahn, C. G., Olsson, H., et al. (2000) SPECT imaging of central muscarinic acetylcholine receptors with iodine-123 labelled E-IQNP and Z-IQNP. *Eur. J. Nucl. Med,* in press.

46. Vora, M. M., Finn, R. D., Boothe, T. E., Liskwosky, D. R., and Potter, L. T. (1983) [N-Methyl-^{11}C]scopolamine: synthesis and distribution in rat brain. *J. Labelled Comp. Rad.* **20,** 1229–1236.

47. Frey, K. A., Koeppe, R. A., Mulholland, G. K., Jewett, D., Hichwa, R., Ehrenkaufer, R. L. E., et al. (1992) *In vivo* muscarinic cholinergic receptor imaging in human brain with [^{11}C]scopolamine and positron emission tomography. *J. Cereb. Blood Flow Metab.* **12,** 147–154.

48. Varastet, M., Brouillet, E., Chavoix, C., Prenant, C., Crouzel, C., Stulzaft, O., et al. (1992) In vivo visualization of cerebral muscarinic receptors using [^{11}C]quinuclidinyl benzilate and positron emission tomography in baboons. *Eur. J. Pharmacol.* **213**, 275–284.
49. Dannals, R. F., Langstrom, B., Ravert, H. T., Wilson, A. A., and Wagner, H. N., Jr. (1988) Synthesis of radiotracers for studying muscarinic cholinergic receptors in the living human brain using positron emission tomography: [^{11}C]dexetimide and [^{11}C]levetimide. *Appl. Radiat. Isot.* **39**, 291–295.
50. Dewey, S. L., MacGregor, R. R., Brodie, J. D., Bendriem, B., King, P. T., Volkow, N. D., et al. (1990) Mapping muscarinic receptors in human and baboon brain using [N-^{11}C-methyl]-benztropine. *Synapse* **5**, 213–223.
51. Dewey, S. L., Volkow, N. D., Logan, J., MacGregor, R. R., Fowler, J. S., Schlyer, D. J., and Bendriem, B. (1990) Age-related decreases in muscarinic cholinergic receptor binding in the human brain measured with positron emission tomography (PET). *J. Neurosci. Res.* **27**, 569–579.
52. Ono, S., Kawashima, R., Ito, H., Koyama, M., Goto, R., Inoue, K., et al. (1996) Regional distribution of the muscarinic cholinergic receptor in the human brain studies with ^{11}C-benztropine and PET using an anatomical standardization technique. *Kaku Igaku* **33**, 721–727.
53. Mulholland, G. K., Otto, C. A., Jewett, D. M., Kilbourn, M. R., Koeppe, R. A., Sherman, P. S., et al. (1992) Synthesis, rodent biodistribution, dosimetry, metabolism, and monkey images of carbon-11-labeled (+)-2αtropanyl benzilate: A central muscarinic receptor imaging agent. *J. Nucl. Med.* **33**, 423–430.
54. Koeppe, R. A., Frey, K. A., Mulholland, G. K., Kilbourn, M. R., Buck, A., Lee, K. S., and Kuhl, D. E. (1994) [^{11}C]Tropanyl benzilate-binding to muscarinic cholinergic receptors: methodology and kinetic modeling alternatives. *J. Cereb. Blood Flow Metab.* **14**, 85–99.
55. Lee, K. S., Frey, K. A., Koeppe, R. A., Buck, A., Mulholland, G. K., and Kuhl, D. E. (1996) In vivo quantification of cerebral muscarinic receptors in normal human aging using positron emission tomography and [^{11}C]tropanyl benzilate. *J. Cereb. Blood Flow Metab.* **16**, 303–310.
56. Mulholland, G. K., Kilbourn, M. R., Sherman, P., Carey, J. E., Frey, K. A., Koeppe, R. A., and Kuhl, D. E. (1995) Synthesis, in vivo biodistribution and dosimetry of [^{11}C]N-methylpiperidinyl benzilate ([^{11}C]NMPB), a muscarinic acetylcholine receptor antagonist. *Nucl. Med. Biol.* **22**, 13–17.
57. Zubieta, J. K., Koeppe, R. A., Mulholland, G. K., Kuhl, D. E., and Frey, K. A. (1998) Quantification of muscarinic cholinergic receptors with [^{11}C]NMPB and positron emission tomography: method development and differentiation of tracer delivery from receptor binding. *J. Cereb. Blood Flow Metab.* **18**, 619–631.
58. Suhara, T., Inoue, O., Kobayashi, K., Suzuki, K., and Tateno, Y. (1993) Age-related changes in human muscarinic acetylcholine receptors measured by positron emission tomography. *Neurosci. Lett.* **149**, 225–228.
59. Suhara, T., Inoue, O., Kobayashi, K., Satoh, T., and Tateno, Y. (1994) An acute effect of triazolam on muscarinic cholinergic receptor binding in the human brain measured by positron emission tomography. *Psychopharmacology (Berl.)* **113**, 311–317.

60. Shinotoh, H., Asahina, M., Inoue, O., Suhara, T., Hirayama, K., and Tateno, Y. (1994) Effects of trihexyphenidyl and L-dopa on brain muscarinic cholinergic receptor binding measured by positron emission tomography. *J. Neural. Transm. [P-D Sect]* **7,** 35–46.

61. Asahina, M. and Shinotoh, H. (1997) Muscarinic cholinergic receptor imaging of parkinsonian brains using ^{11}C-NMPB and PET. *Nippon Rinsho.* **55,** 233–237.

62. Yoshida, T., Kuwabara, Y., Ichiya, Y., Sasaki, M., Fukumura, T., Ichimiya, A., et al. (1998) Cerebral muscarinic acetylcholinergic receptor measurement in Alzheimer's disease patients on ^{11}C-N-methyl-4-piperidinyl benzilate. Comparison with cerebral blood flow and cerebral glucose metabolism. *Ann. Nucl. Med.* **12,** 35–42.

63. Sudo, Y., Suhara, T., Honda, Y., Nakajima, T., Okubo, Y., Suzuki, K., et al. (1998) Muscarinic cholinergic receptors in human narcolepsy: a PET study. *Neurology* **51,** 1297–1302.

64. Takahashi, K., Murakami, S., Miura, S., Iida, H., Kanno, I., and Uemura, K. (1999) Synthesis and autoradiographic localization of muscarinic cholinergic antagonist (+)-N-methyl-3-piperidinyl benzilate as a potent radioligand for positron emission tomography. *Appl. Rad. Isot.* **50,** 521–525.

65. Wilson, A. A., Scheffel, U. A., Dannals, R. F., Stathis, M., Ravert, H. T., and Wagner, H. W., Jr. (1991) *In vivo* biodistribution of two [^{18}F]-labelled muscarinic cholinergic receptor ligands: 2-[^{18}F]- and 4-[^{18}F]fluorodexetimide. *Life Sci.* **48,** 1385–1394.

66. Luo, H., Beets, A. L., McAllister, M. J., Greenbaum, M., McPherson, D. W., and Knapp, F. F., Jr. (1998) Resolution, in vitro and in vivo evaluation of fluorine-18-labeled isomers of 1-azabicyclo[2.2.2]oct-3-yl α-fluoroalkyl-α-hydroxy-α-phenylacetate (FQNPe) as new PET candidates for the imaging of muscarinic-cholinergic receptor. *J. Labelled Comp. Rad.* **41,** 681–704.

67. Takahashi, K., Miura, S., Hatazawa, J., Shimosegawa, E., Kinoshita, T., Ito, H., et al. (1999) Synthesis of [^{18}F]fluoroethyl-4-piperidinyl benzilate, a muscarinic receptor antagonist, for use in receptor activation studies with PET. *J. Labelled Comp. Rad.* **42,** S497–S499.

68. Doods, H., Entzeroth, M., Ziegler, H., Schiavi G., Engel, W., Mihm, G., et al. (1993) Characterization of BIBN 99: a lipophilic and selective muscarinic M_2 receptor antagonist. *Eur. J. Pharmacol.* **242,** 23–30.

69. Aubert, C., Perrio-Huard, C., and Lasne, M. C. (1997) Synthesis of [^{11}C]BIBN 99, a new selective radioligand for the in vivo studies of M_2 muscarinic receptors by PET. *J. Labelled Comp. Rad.* **40,** 752–754.

70. Kiesewetter, D. O., Carson, R. E., Jagoda, E., Endres, C. J., Der, M. G., Herscovitch, P., and Eckelman, W. C. (1997) In vivo muscarinic binding selectivity of (R,S)- and (R,R)-[^{18}F]-fluoromethylQNB. *Bioorgan. Med. Chem.* **5,** 1555–1567.

71. McPherson, D. W., Breeden, W., Luo, H., Beets, A., and Knapp, F. F., Jr. (1998) Resolution, radiolabeling and in vivo evaluation of the isomers of IPIP. An attractive ligand for imaging mAChR. *J. Nucl. Med.* **39,** 49.

72. McPherson, D., Halldin, C., Hall, H., Nobuhara, K., Sandell, J., Knapp, F. F., Jr., and Farde, L. (1999) Evaluation of carbon-11 labeled E-(R)-IPIP for the potential PET imaging of muscarinic receptors. *J. Labelled Comp. Rad.* **42,** S378–S380.

3

GABA$_A$ Receptors

Autoradiographic Localization of Different
Ligand Sites and Identification of Subtypes
of the Benzodiazepine Binding Site

Cyrille Sur and John Atack

1. INTRODUCTION

GABA is generally accepted as the major inhibitory neurotransmitter within the vertebrate brain. Pharmacologically, the responses to GABA were initially characterized in terms of their sensitivity to a variety of agonists and antagonists. Thus, fast, ion channel-mediated effects that can be blocked by bicuculline, SR 95531 (both of which act at the GABA binding site), and picrotoxin and stimulated by GABA, muscimol, and isoguvacine, are mediated by GABA$_A$ receptors. On the other hand, bicuculline-insensitive effects which are stimulated by GABA and baclofen and inhibited by phaclofen, are mediated by G-protein linked, metabotropic GABA$_B$ receptors. In addition, a third type of GABA receptor, the so-called GABA$_C$ receptor, has been identified on the basis of its bicuculline and baclofen insensitivity *(1)*. In the present chapter, we will concentrate on the autoradiographic identification of bicuculline-sensitive GABA$_A$ receptors.

The bicuculline-sensitive GABA$_A$ receptor possesses a rich pharmacology. Thus, there are two agonist (GABA) binding sites defined in terms of their low and high agonist affinity, which can be labeled using either [^{3}H]GABA, [^{3}H]muscimol, [^{3}H]bicuculline, or [^{3}H]SR 95531. In addition, the GABA$_A$ receptor contains a convulsant (picrotoxinin) binding site that lies within the ion channel itself and can be labeled with [^{35}S]*t*-butylbicyclophosphorothionate ([^{35}S]TBPS), [^{3}H]*t*-butylbicycloorthobenzoate ([^{3}H]TBOB), or [^{3}H]4'-ethynyl-4-*n*-propylbicycloorthobenzoate ([^{3}H]EBOB).

From: *Ion Channel Localization Methods and Protocols*
Edited by: A. Lopatin and C. G. Nichols © Humana Press Inc., Totowa, NJ

In addition to GABA and convulsant binding sites, the $GABA_A$ receptor also contains binding sites for a number of different classes of compounds, which can act either by direct activation of the receptor (e.g., barbiturates) or by modulation of the actions of GABA *(2)*. This latter class includes compounds that act at the steroid, loreclezole, anaesthetic, ethanol, and benzodiazepine binding sites, all of which exert their actions via allosteric modulation of the activation by GABA or opening of the channel. Because binding to the benzodiazepine site of the $GABA_A$ receptor mediates the anxiolytic, anticonvulsant and muscle-relaxant effects of clinically used benzodiazepines (such as diazepam), this binding site has been the most intensively studied binding site on the $GABA_A$ receptor and has resulted in a classification of $GABA_A$ receptor subtypes based on their affinity for different benzodiazepine site ligands *(2)*. A more detailed understanding of this heterogeneous benzodiazepine binding pharmacology in vertebrate brain tissue has emerged from a characterization of the pharmacological properties of recombinant $GABA_A$ receptors.

$GABA_A$ receptors are pentamers made up of subunits assembled from the 16 members ($\alpha1$–6, $\beta1$–3, $\gamma1$–3, δ, ε, π, and θ) of this gene family *(1,3)*. The majority of $GABA_A$ receptors in the brain contain α, β, and γ subunits in the stoichiometry of 2 α, 2 β, and 1 γ proteins *(4,5)*. The benzodiazepine binding site of the $GABA_A$ receptor occurs at the interface of the α and γ subunits and thus these subunits define the pharmacology of this binding site with the type of β subunit having little effect *(1,2)*. Because the predominant γ subunit in the brain is $\gamma2$, the major contributor to heterogeneity of benzodiazepine site pharmacology of native $GABA_A$ receptors must therefore be variations in the subunit composition. For example, [^{3}H]Ro 15-4513 labels the benzodiazepine site of $GABA_A$ receptors containing $\alpha1$, $\alpha2$, $\alpha3$, $\alpha4$, $\alpha5$, and $\alpha6$ receptors but diazepam (and other classical benzodiazepine agonists as well as the antagonist Ro 15-1788) only displaces binding from receptors containing the $\alpha1$, $\alpha2$, $\alpha3$, or $\alpha5$ subunit, with the $\alpha4$ and $\alpha6$ subunits conferring diazepam insensitivity *(6)*. Thus, classical benzodiazepines only bind to $GABA_A$ receptors containing $\alpha1$, $\alpha2$, $\alpha3$, or $\alpha5$ subunits.

To summarize, although heterogeneity of binding at the agonist (GABA) and convulsant binding sites of $GABA_A$ receptor subtypes have been reported *(7,8–10)*, no subtype-selective compounds for these binding sites are available. Similarly, although loreclezole is known to preferentially interact with $GABA_A$ receptors containing $\beta2$ and $\beta3$ but not $\beta1$ *(11)*, no radioligand is available to exploit this selectivity. In contrast, the pharmacology of the benzodiazepine binding site has been extensively studied and has yielded a variety of ligands that can be employed to distinguish between the benzodiazepine site of GABA receptors containing different α subunits. The use of various ligands available to anatomically localize either the total population of GABA_A receptors or more specific subtypes based on benzodiazepine pharmacology is described later.

2. GABA_A RECEPTOR BINDING SITES: METHODS AND APPLICATIONS

2.1. GABA Binding Site

2.1.1. Methods

Adult mice were killed by decapitation and the brains were carefully removed and frozen in iso-pentane cooled to –60°C with dry ice following which brains were stored at –70°C. Twelve μm thick sections of brain mounted in Lipshaw M-1 embedding matrix were cut at –15°C using a Leica Cryocut 1800 cryostat. Sections were thaw-mounted onto microscope slides and allowed to dry at room temperature. Air-dried sections were then stored at –70°C until required for autoradiography.

For autoradiography, sections were thawed at room temperature and washed in three changes of ice-cold 10 m*M* Tris/1 m*M* EDTA, pH 7.4, for 30 min. and then allowed to dry. Air-drying after this preincubation is not essential but is often more convenient, especially if a large number of sections are to be processed. Thus, sections can be washed in batches rather than on a timed schedule as would be required if the incubation started immediately following the preincubation. Sections were then incubated for 45 min at 4°C in Tris/EDTA buffer containing 5 n*M* [³H]muscimol (NEN, specific activity: 20.0 Ci/mmol). Nonspecific binding was defined using 100 μ*M* GABA and specific binding is generally >95% of total binding. Sections were washed twice for 1 min in ice-cold Tris/EDTA buffer. The use of a relatively long (2 min) wash time results in dissociation of [³H]muscimol from low affinity sites such that only the high-affinity GABA binding sites are labeled *(8)*. After washing, sections are dipped in distilled water and dried in a stream of cold air. It is important that drying is performed as quickly as possible to prevent diffusion of ligand away from the site of the receptor. Once dry, sections were apposed to [³H]Hyperfilm (Amersham) for 8 wk. Films are then developed using Kodak D19 developer.

2.1.2. Distribution

The distribution of rat brain [³H]muscimol binding sites is shown in Fig. 1A. Thus, [³H]muscimol binding has a relatively widespread distribution in cortical and subcortical regions. Nevertheless, this distribution is more

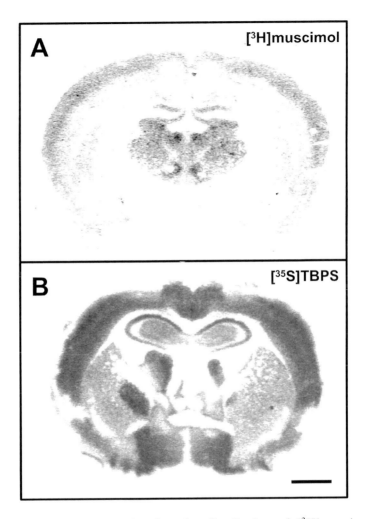

Fig. 1. Autoradiograms showing the distribution of [³H]muscimol (**A**) and [³⁵S]TBPS (**B**) binding sites in coronal sections of mouse brain. Calibration bar, 1.5 mm.

restricted than that of either [³⁵S]TBPS (Fig. 1B) or [³H]Ro 15-1788 (Fig. 3A). For example, muscimol preferentially labels the more superficial (layers I–IV) compared to deeper layers of the cortex, whereas [³H]benzodiazepines and [³⁵S]TBPS have high levels of binding in all regions of the cortex *(8)*. Discrepancies are also seen in the hippocampus, globus pallidus, and hypothalamus, where [³H]muscimol binding is relatively low (Fig. 1A *[8]*), yet there is appreciable [³H]Ro 15-1788 and

[^{35}S]TBPS binding. In addition to the divergence of the distribution of [^{3}H]muscimol-labeled GABA binding sites and the convulsant and benzo-diazepine binding sites, there is also a discrepancy between the distribution of GABA binding sites labeled with either [^{3}H]muscimol and [^{3}H]bicuculline *(8)*.

This latter anomaly is probably related to the different affinity and ago-nist-preferring states of the GABA binding sites labeled with [^{3}H]muscimol and [^{3}H]bicuculline. Hence, the agonist binding site of the GABA$_A$ receptor can be labeled by either at the high-affinity GABA site using the agonists [^{3}H]GABA (in the presence of baclofen to block binding to GABA$_B$ recep-tors) and [^{3}H]muscimol or by using antagonists at the low-affinity GABA binding site, [^{3}H]bicuculline or [^{3}H]SR 95531. It is important to note that since, by definition, all GABA$_A$ receptors contain a GABA binding site, then these ligands should bind to GABA$_A$ receptors irrespective of whether or not they contain a benzodiazepine binding site. However, the abundance of GABA$_A$ receptors in the brain that do not contain a benzodiazepine bind-ing site, either because they do not contain a γ subunit or because they con-tain a γ1 (which confers relative insensitivity to benzodiazepines *(1,2)* is relatively small *(4)*. Accordingly, the biggest discrepancies between the binding of [^{3}H]benzodiazepines and GABA biding site ligands occurs in regions, such as the cerebellum *(8)*, where there is a relatively large propor-tion of GABA$_A$ receptors that do not possess a γ2 subunit.

Although there is a modest degree of agreement between the distribution of the binding of different GABA binding site ligands, for example [^{3}H]GABA and [^{3}H]SR 95531 *(12)* or between [^{3}H]GABA *(13)* and [^{3}H]muscimol *(14)*, discrepancies do occur and are probably related to a heterogeneity of GABA$_A$ receptor subtypes *(8)*. These differences appear to be most striking in the cer-ebellum, where there is a marked difference in the distribution of high- and low-affinity GABA binding sites, labeled with [^{3}H]muscimol *(14)* and [^{3}H]bicuculline *(15)*, respectively. Furthermore, although the distribution of binding sites labeled with [^{3}H]GABA and [^{3}H]SR 95531 are generally similar *(12)* in certain regions of the brain, there is a discrepancy because [^{3}H]SR 95531 also binds to monamine oxidase-A *(16)*.

2.2. Convulsant Binding Site

2.2.1. Methods

Mouse brain sections were prepared as described earlier (Section 2.1.1.). Frozen sections were thawed and washed at 4°C for 30 min in 3 changes of buffer 50 m*M* Tris-HCl/1 m*M* ethylenediaminetetracetic acid (EDTA), pH 7.4) and then air-dried. Sections were then incubated for 90 min at 25°C in buffer (50 mM Tris-HCl/120 mM NaCl, pH 7.4) containing 10 nM [^{35}S]TBPS (NEN, specific activity 68.7 Ci/mmol) and nonspecific binding was established using 10 µM picrotoxin. Under these conditions, specific binding is >98% of total binding. Following incubation, slices are given two 5 min washes in incubation buffer followed by rapid dipping in de-ionized water and drying under a stream of cool air. When dry, sections are apposed to Kodak X-OMat film for 2 d.

2.2.2. Distribution

The convulsant (picrotoxinin) binding site lies with the ion channel of the GABA$_A$ receptor and can be labeled with [^{35}S]TBPS *(17)* and Fig. 1B shows the distribution of these binding sites in mouse brain. There are high levels of binding in the cortex, globus pallidus, amygdala, and stratum oriens of the hippocampus and lower levels are found in the caudate/putamen and hypothalamus (Fig. 1B *[17]*). The distribution of [^{35}S]TBPS binding sites differs from the distribution of [^{3}H]muscimol binding sites in so far as the globus pallidus, which has high levels of [^{35}S]TBPS binding has low levels of [^{3}H]muscimol and in the cerebellum the molecular layer is enriched in [^{35}S]TBPS binding sites, whereas [^{3}H]muscimol binding sites are highly expressed in the granular layer *(18)*. Discrepancies between [^{3}H]muscimol and [^{35}S]TBPS binding may in part be related to heterogeneity of [^{35}S]TBPS binding, because α and γ subunit composition can affect the [^{35}S]TBPS binding properties of the GABA$_A$ receptor *(7)*.

The convulsant (picrotoxinin) binding site can also be labeled with either [^{3}H]t-butylbicycloorthobenzoate ([^{3}H]TBOB *[10]*) or [^{3}H]4'-ethynyl-4-*n*-propylbicycloorthobenzoate ([^{3}H]EBOB *[19]*). Although the distribution of [^{35}S]TPBS, [^{3}H]TBOB, and [^{3}H]EBOB binding sites are at a gross level generally in agreement (i.e., a widespread distribution throughout cortical and subcortical regions), discrepancies do occur *(8,19)*. On the other hand, the distributions of [^{3}H]TBOB and [^{3}H]EBOB are in very good agreement with each other *(10,19)*, suggesting that these two ligands bind to common determinants of the convulsant binding site but that these features are only partially shared with [^{35}S]TPBS.

[^{3}H]TBOB binding also correlates poorly with the distribution of [^{3}H]muscimol binding sites but correlates well with the distribution of the benzodiazepine sites ligands [^{3}H]zolpidem and [^{3}H]oxoquazepam, which preferentially label the benzodiazepine binding site of GABA$_A$ receptors containing an α1 subunit *(8,10,20)*.

An addition factor to be considered in the choice of radioligand for identifying the convulsant binding site of the GABA$_A$ receptor is the fact that being a higher energy β-emitter, the exposure times for [^{35}S]TBPS (2–3 d) are appreciably shorter than for [^{3}H]TBOB or [^{3}H]EBOB (2–3 wk). On the other hand, the anatomical resolution obtained using [^{3}H]TBOB or [^{3}H]EBOB is much higher than that for [^{35}S]TBPS.

3. BENZODIAZEPINE BINDING SITE SUBTYPES: METHODS AND APPLICATIONS

The relationship between a specific benzodiazepine pharmacological profile and the presence of a given α subunit in the GABA$_A$ receptors provides a unique opportunity to use selective [^{3}H]benzodiazepine site ligands to visualize specific GABA$_A$ receptor subtypes in the central nervous system (CNS). To this end, several radiolabeled benzodiazepine site ligands have proven invaluable tools. For example, the combined population of GABA$_A$ receptors with a benzodiazepine binding site containing either and α1, α2, α3, α4, α5, or α6 subunit can be labeled with [^{3}H]Ro 15-4513. Inclusion of diazepam with [^{3}H]Ro 15-4513 restricts the labeling to α4 and α6 containing GABA$_A$ receptors. The difference between [^{3}H]Ro 15-4513 in the presence and absence of diazepam therefore represents GABA$_A$ receptors containing α1, α2, α3, and α5 subunits and this receptor population can be identified directly using [^{3}H]benzodiazepines, such as diazepam, flunitrazepam, or Ro 15-1788. More specific analysis of individual subtypes of GABA$_A$ receptor can be achieved using [^{3}H]zolpidem to label α1 subunit containing receptors, whereas more recently, [^{3}H]L-655,708 has been reported as a compound with selectivity for GABA$_A$ receptors containing an α5 subunit *(21,22)*. In the following section, the methods used for mapping subtypes of GABA$_A$ receptor in the mammalian CNS based on their benzodiazepine pharmacology (i.e., their α subunit composition) will be described.

3.1. Labeling of α1, α2, α3, α4, α5, α6 Receptors with [^{3}H]Ro 15-4513

3.1.1. Methods

Slide-mounted tissue sections kept at –70°C are thawed at room temperature and washed in three changes of ice-cold buffer (50 mM Tris-HCl/1 mM EDTA, pH 7.4) for 30 min. Slides are then air-dried for 15 min and incubated for 60 min at 4°C in Tris/EDTA buffer containing 8 nM [^{3}H]Ro 15-4513 (NEN, specific activity: 21.7 Ci/mmol). Nonspecific binding is determined by incubating sections in 8 nM [^{3}H]Ro 15-4513 plus 40 μM bretazenil, a benzodiazepine site ligand that interacts with all subtypes. Under these conditions specific binding represents >98% of total binding.

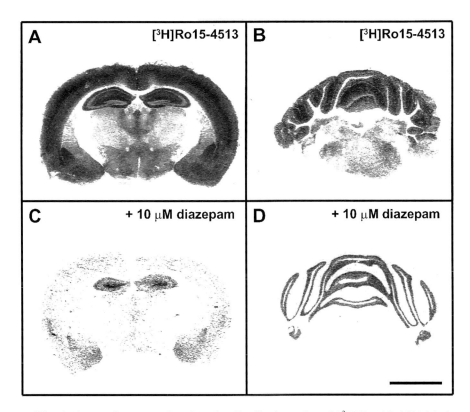

Fig. 2. Autoradiograms showing the distribution of total [³H]Ro 15-4513 binding sites in mouse forebrain (**A**) and cerebellum (**B**) as well as of diazepam-insensitive [³H]Ro 15-4513 binding sites (**C,D**). Calibration bar, 3 mm.

Labeled tissue sections are rinsed twice for 1 min each in cold Tris/EDTA buffer, dipped in distilled water and dried in a stream of cold air. They are then exposed in the dark to [³H]Hyperfilm (Amersham) for 3 wk.

3.1.2. Distribution

As previously reported *(23)* [³H]Ro 15-4513 binding sites have a widespread distribution in rat brain with high levels of expression in the cortex, cerebellum and hippocampal formation. As shown in Fig. 2A, a similar pattern is observed in mouse brain with, for instance, very intense [³H]Ro 15-4513 labeling in cortical layers III-IV, dentate gyrus, stratum oriens of CA1-CA3 fields of the hippocampus, lateral amygdaloid nucleus, olfactory bulb (not shown), and cerebellum granule cell layer (Fig. 2B). A moderate to intense [³H]Ro 15-4513 labeling is encountered in others brain regions.

The overall distribution of [^{3}H]Ro 15-4513 binding sites is in agreement with the localization of different GABA$_A$ receptor subunits determined by *in situ* hybridization *(24,25)* and immunocytochemistry *(26)*. It also closely matches the distribution of benzodiazepine sites visualized by [^{3}H]Ro 15-1788 autoradiography with the exception of cerebellar granule cells that are more labeled by [^{3}H]Ro 15-4513 because of the high expression (~30% of all GABA$_A$ receptors) of $\alpha6\beta\gamma2$ receptors in this brain area *(27)*. Similarly, one might expect that compared to [^{3}H]Ro 15-1788 binding there would be higher levels of [^{3}H]Ro 15-4513 binding in area expressing $\alpha4\beta\gamma2$ receptors such as thalamus and hippocampus (*see* Section 3.2.2.). However, the relatively low proportion of this subtype (~6–10% *[28,29]*) means that in these regions, the levels of [^{3}H]Ro 15-1788 and [^{3}H]Ro 15-4513 are comparable. In conclusion, [^{3}H]Ro 15-4513 is a versatile and easy to use radioligand for autoradiographic localization of all benzodiazepine binding sites. However, in routine experiments that do not specifically look at the cerebellum [^{3}H]Ro 15-1788 is usually preferred because of its similar pattern of labeling, its higher binding affinity, and specific radioactivity.

3.2. Labeling of $\alpha4$ and $\alpha6$ Receptors with [^{3}H]Ro 15-4513 in the Presence of 10 µM Diazepam

3.2.1. Methods

They are identical to those used for [^{3}H]Ro 15-4513 autoradiography except that 10 µ*M* of diazepam is included in the incubation solution and slides are exposed to [^{3}H]Hyperfilm for 6–8 wk. Bretazenil (40 µ*M*) is used to determine nonspecific binding.

3.2.2. Distribution

As shown in Fig. 2C, Diazepam-Insensitive (DIS) [^{3}H]Ro 15-4513 binding sites have a restricted and low-level expression in rodent telencephalon. A moderate to intense signal is observed in the CA1-CA3 fields of the hippocampus, amygdala nuclei, and the dentate gyrus, respectively. In cortical regions and thalamus, the expression of DIS [^{3}H]Ro 15-4513 binding sites is very low. Analysis of rodent-brain sagittal sections revealed also the presence of low levels of DIS [^{3}H]Ro 15-4513 binding sites in the olfactory bulb, striatum, hypothalamus, and brainstem *(23,28)*. In the CNS, with the exception of the cerebellum, DIS [^{3}H]Ro 15-4513 have been shown to correspond to the expression of $\alpha4\beta\gamma2$ receptors *(28,29)*. Although the expression pattern of DIS [^{3}H]Ro 15-4513 sites is relatively consistent with the distribution of $\alpha4$ mRNA *(24)* and protein *(28,30)*, the virtual absence of DIS [^{3}H]Ro 15-4513 sites in the thalamus despite the presence of $\alpha4$ mRNA suggests the existence of $\alpha4$ subunit-containing GABA$_A$ receptors that do not possess a [³H]Ro 15-4513-sensitive binding site. Indeed, in the thalamus as well as in the hippocampus the existence of $\alpha4\beta\delta$ receptors that lack a benzodiazepine site has been reported (29). Thus, although the combination of [³H]Ro 15-4513 plus diazepam easily allows the visualization of $\alpha4\beta\gamma2$ receptors it does not permit the study of all $\alpha4$ subunit-containing $GABA_A$ receptors.

In the cerebellum (Fig. 2D), an intense DIS [³H]Ro 15-4513 labeling is observed in the granule cell layer, where they account for around 35–50% of total [³H]Ro 15-4513 benzodiazepine binding sites (23). The localization of DIS [³H]Ro 15-4513 sites in cerebellum agrees well with the expression of $\alpha6$ mRNA and protein in the granule cell layer (25) and the proportion of $\alpha6\beta\gamma2$ receptors (27). However, as already stressed for $\alpha4$ receptors, this autoradiographic approach is not suitable to investigate the 30% of $\alpha6$ receptors co-assemble with a δ subunit (27).

3.3. Labeling of α1, α2, α3, and α5 Receptors with [³H]Ro 15-1788

3.3.1. Methods

The methods are very similar to those described earlier for [³H]Ro 15-4513. Following a 30-min preincubation and air-drying, sections are incubated 60 min at 4°C in Tris/EDTA buffer containing 2 nM [³H]Ro 15-1788 (NEN, specific activity: 87 Ci/mmol), washed twice for 2 min in cold Tris/EDTA buffer, dipped in distilled water, and dried. After 3 wk exposure, [³H]Hyperfilm was developed and autoradiograms analyzed. The nonspecific signal is defined by incubating sections in solution containing 2 nM [³H]Ro 15-1788 plus 10 μM Flunitrazepam.

3.3.2. Distribution

The benzodiazepine [³H]Ro 15-1788 has been widely used to study the distribution of benzodiazepine binding sites in human, rat, and mouse brain (17,22,31). [³H]Ro 15-1788 binding sites have a widespread distribution in rodent CNS (Fig. 3A,B) with high levels of expression in regions such as cortex, hippocampus, amygdala, globus pallidus, and cerebellum. This pattern of distribution is similar to that seen with the classical benzodiazepine agonists [³H]flunitrazepam and [³H]diazepam (20,32) as well as the atypical anxiolytic [³H]alprazolam (32) and is in agreement with the known distribution of the various α subunit mRNAs and polypeptides (24–26). For instance, [³H]Ro 15-1788 signal in the hippocampus arises from the high expression of $\alpha2$, $\alpha3$, and $\alpha5$ subunits, whereas in other brain regions it roughly follows the distribution of $\alpha1\beta\gamma2$ receptors, the predominant neuronal $GABA_A$ receptor subtype (4). In conclusion [³H]Ro 15-1788 is a very

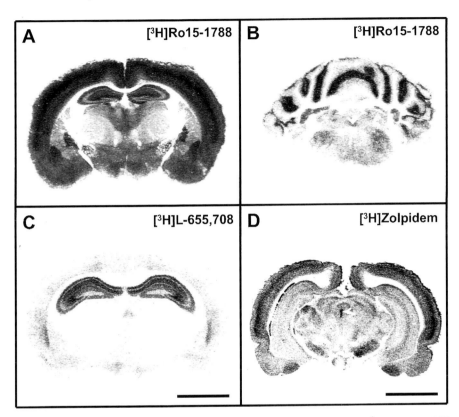

Fig. 3. Autoradiograms showing the widespread distribution of [³H]Ro 15-1788 binding sites **(A,B)** in mouse brain. As shown in **(C)**, α5 receptor expression visualized by [³H]L-655,708 is mostly restricted to the mouse hippocampal formation. As illustrated in **(D)**, [³H]zolpidem binding sites have a widespread expression in rat brain. Calibration bar: 3 mm (A–C) and 4 mm (D).

convenient and useful radioligand to study benzodiazepine sensitive GABA_A receptors given its high specific activity and the virtual lack of nonspecific labeling after 3 wk exposure.

3.4. Labeling of α1 Receptors with [³H]Zolpidem

3.4.1. Methods

Frozen sections were thawed at room temperature for 15 min and preincubated in 50 mM Tris-HCl, pH 7.9, for 30 min. Then they were incubated for 30 min at 4°C with 10 nM [³H]zolpidem. Nonspecific binding was determined on adjacent sections with 10 mM of zolpidem. Labeled sections were washed in cold Tris-HCl buffer for two times 30 s, dipped in distilled water and dried in a stream of cold air. Sections were exposed for 5 wk to [^{3}H]Hyperfilm.

3.4.2. Distribution

As illustrated in Fig. 3D, [^{3}H]zolpidem binding sites have a heterogeneous distribution in rat brain with, for example, intense autoradiographic signal being found in substantia nigra, layer IV of the cortex and amygdala areas. Extensive autoradiographic analysis have mapped the brain localization of [^{3}H]zolpidem binding sites and shown the correspondence between their distribution and the presence of α1 subunit containing GABA$_A$ receptors *(20)*. Furthermore, in an elegant study, Niddam and co-workers have determined the proportion of [^{3}H]zolpidem binding sites in various central nervous system areas by quantitatively comparing [^{3}H]zolpidem and [^{3}H]flunitrazepam autoradiographic signals *(20)*. They demonstrated that [^{3}H]zolpidem binding sites account for more than two third of total benzodiazepine binding sites in regions such as olfactory bulb, cortex, septal nucleus, globus pallidus, substantia nigra, colliculus, and molecular layer of the cerebellum.

[^{3}H]oxo-quazepam has also been used as a ligand to selectively identify α1 subunit containing GABA$_A$ receptors *(33)*. However, this radioligand has relatively high levels of nonspecific binding (in the region of 50% of total binding) and from that point of view [^{3}H]zolpidem is a better radioligand for autoradiographic studies.

In conclusion, the availability of the α1 subunit containing GABA$_A$ receptor selective ligand [^{3}H]zolpidem has been very useful in both mapping the brain distribution of this receptor isoform and quantitatively determining its contribution to the total benzodiazepine receptor population throughout the brain. Moreover, the distribution of α1 containing GABA$_A$ receptors forms the neuroanatomical basis for the understanding of the unique behavioral properties of drugs such as zolpidem *(34)*.

3.5. Labeling of α5 Receptors with [^{3}H]L-655,708

3.5.1. Methods

Following 30 min preincubation, incubation is carried out at 4°C for 2 h in Tris/EDTA containing 2 n*M* [^{3}H]L-655,708 plus 10 m*M* zolpidem to exclude low affinity binding to other a (i.e., α1, α2, and α3) subunit containing GABA$_A$ receptors. Slides are then washed twice for 1 min each in cold buffer, dipped in cold distilled water, dried, and exposed to [^{3}H]Hyperfilm for 8 wk. Nonspecific labeling is determined using 10 µ*M* flunitrazepam. Under these conditions, specific binding represents >95% of total binding.

3.5.2. Distribution

The distribution of [^{3}H]L-655,708 binding sites in rodent brain is highly regionalized. As illustrated in Fig. 3C, intense [^{3}H]L-655,708 labeling is observed in the hippocampus and the endopiriform nucleus, whereas a moderate to low labeling is present in the different cortical areas. [^{3}H]L-655,708 binding sites are virtually absent from the thalamus, with the exception of the paraventricular nucleus, which exhibits a moderate labeling. Extensive mapping study in rat brain with [^{3}H]L-655,708 revealed also the presence of moderate labeling in the olfactory bulb, amygdalo-hippocampal area, and some hypothalamic nuclei *(22)*. This pattern of [^{3}H]L-655,708 binding sites expression is in agreement with the distribution of both α5 subunit mRNA *(24,25)* and α5 polypeptide *(26,30)*. Comparative quantitative analysis of [^{3}H]L-655,708 and [^{3}H]Ro 15-1788 binding sites expression revealed that α5 subunit containing GABA$_A$ receptors account for around 25% of total benzodiazepine sites in CA1-CA3 fields of rat hippocampus, 13% in endopiriform nucleus, and less than 10% in brain regions such as cortex, amygdala, basal ganglia, and thalamus *(22)*.

In addition to [^{3}H]L-655,708, [^{3}H]RY-80 has also been used to specifically label α5 subunit containing GABA$_A$ receptors *(35)*. This compound has an α5 selectivity similar to that of [^{3}H]L-655,708 and a comparison of the autoradiographic distribution of binding sites identified by these two radioligands has demonstrated an essentially identical anatomical localization *(36)*. In summary, [^{3}H]L-655,708 is a useful α5 subunit selective radioligand that allows a precise qualitative and quantitative analysis of α5 subunit containing GABA$_A$ receptors in the CNS. Not only should this radioligand prove useful in understanding the role of this GABA$_A$ receptor subtype in physiological and pathophysiological situations, but it should aid the interpretation of the behavioral properties of α5 subtype selective drugs in the same way that [^{3}H]zolpidem has aided in the elucidation of the mechanism of action of the novel pharmacological properties of zolpidem.

4. APPLICATIONS OF GABA AND BENZODIAZEPINE SITE AUTORADIOGRAPHY

Besides the mapping and the quantification of specific receptor subtypes described above, GABA and benzodiazepine sites autoradiography can be used to analyze GABA$_A$ receptors in various physiological and pathological conditions. In this chapter, we do not intend to give an exhaustive list of all the applications of GABA$_A$ receptor autoradiography, but rather we shall present selected examples that should raise the awareness of the reader about the multiple applications of this technique. More detailed examples of the application of autoradiography to the study of the physiology and pathophysiology of benzodiazepine binding sites is available elsewhere *(37)*.

In addition to GABA and benzodiazepine sites, $GABA_A$ receptors possess binding sites for steroids such as alphaxalone, 3α-OH-5α-pregnan-20-one or pregnenolone sulfate *(2)* that enhance GABA-induced chloride flux. Autoradiographic analysis of [^{35}S]TBPS binding modulation is a method of choice to study functional interactions between neurosteroids and $GABA_A$ receptors in a brain region selective manner *(38)*.

$GABA_A$ receptor autoradiography has been shown to be a technique of choice to investigate the regulation of this inhibitory ligand-gated channel in human pathological brain samples. In Alzheimer's patient hippocampus, no change was observed in the number of $GABA_A$ receptors labeled with [^{3}H]muscimol *(39)*. Similarly, autoradiographic studies with [^{3}H]flunitrazepam failed to demonstrate any reduction of benzodiazepine binding sites in Alzheimer's disease hippocampus, whereas there was a 40% decrease in entorhinal cortex *(39,40)*. More recently, [^{3}H]L-655,708 has been used to demonstrate a relative preservation of α5 subunit containing $GABA_A$ receptors in the hippocampal formation of Alzheimer's patients *(41)*. Similar autoradiographic approaches has been used to study $GABA_A$ receptors in the brain of schizophrenic *(42)* or epileptic *(43)* patients. The autoradiographic analysis of $GABA_A$ receptor system has also been widely employed in animal models of epilepsy *(44)*, paroxysmal dystonia *(45)*, and Parkinson's disease *(10,46)*.

Finally, $GABA_A$ receptor autoradiography has proved to be an invaluable tool in confirming the loss or modification of specific $GABA_A$ receptor subunits in transgenic mice as well as the regional specificity of such changes along with establishing compensatory up- or downregulation of other receptor subunits *(47–49)*.

5. CONCLUSIONS

Autoradiography is a versatile and powerful method to explore not only the distribution but also the quantity, regulation, and modulation of $GABA_A$ receptors in the CNS. As discussed, the molecular resolution of this approach relies heavily on the availability of high-affinity radioligands with selectivity for any given receptor subtype. At present, $GABA_A$ receptor subtypes have been defined in terms of their benzodiazepine pharmacology. Although there is no doubt that this has greatly enhanced our understanding of the function of GABA$_A$ receptor subtypes, there is a continuing need to further define the roles of these different subtypes (for example, there is currently no compounds available to differentiate between α2 vs α3 subunit-containing GABA$_A$ receptors). Moreover, there is undoubtedly heterogeneity in the agonist and convulsant binding sites of GABA$_A$ receptors that remain unexplored and additional insights may come from transgenic mice. For instance, if [^{3}H]TBOB and [^{3}H]EBOB appear to be associated with α1 subunit containing GABA$_A$ receptors, are these binding sites lost in α1 subunit knockout mice?

Subtype selective ligands have proved extremely useful in untangling the complex pharmacology of benzodiazepine receptor isoforms. Future goals should be the development of selective ligands, whether binding at the agonist, convulsant, or benzodiazepine binding site, that will allow an even more precise dissection of the roles of the multiplicity of GABA$_A$ receptor subtypes, including those containing recently discovered subunits such as θ or ε *(3,50)*.

REFERENCES

1. Barnard, E. A., Skolnick, P., Olsen, R. W., Mohler, H., Sieghart, W., Biggio, G., et al. (1992) International Union of Pharmacology. XV. Subtypes of γ-aminobutyric acid$_A$ receptors: classification on the basis of subunit structure and receptor function. *Pharmacol. Rev.* **50,** 291–313.
2. Sieghart, W. (1995) Structure and pharmacology of γ-aminobutyric acid$_A$ receptor subtypes. *Pharmacol. Rev.* **47,** 181–234.
3. Bonnert, T. P., McKernan, R. M., Farrar, S., Le Bourdelles, B., Heavens, R. P., Smith, D. W., et al. (1999) θ, a novel γ-aminobutyric acid type A receptor subunit. *Proc. Natl. Acad. Sci. USA* **96,** 9891–9896.
4. McKernan, R. M. and Whiting, P. J. (1996) Which GABA$_A$-receptor subtypes really occur in the brain? *Trends Neurosci.* **19,** 139–143.
5. Tretter, V., Ehya, N., Fuchs, K., and Sieghart, W. (1997) Stoichiometry and assembly of a recombinant GABA$_A$ receptor subtype. *J. Neurosci.* **17,** 2728–2737.
6. Luddens, H., Pritchett, D. B., Kohler, M., Killisch, K., Monyer, H., Sprengel, R., and Seeburg, P. H. (1990) Cerebellar GABA$_A$ receptor selective for a behavioural alcohol antagonist. *Nature (Lond.)* **346,** 648–651.
7. Korpi, E. R. and Luddens, H. (1993) Regional γ-aminobutyric acid sensitivity of t-butylbicyclophosphoro[^{35}S]thionate binding depends on γ-aminobutyric acid$_A$ receptor subunit. *Mol. Pharmacol.* **44,** 87–92.
8. Olsen, R. W., McCabe, R. T., and Wamsley, J. K. (1990) GABAA receptor subtypes: autoradiographic comparison of GABA, benzodiazepine, and convulsant binding sites in the rat central nervous system. *J. Chem. Neuroanat.* **3,** 59–76.

9. Ebert, B., Wafford, K. A., Whiting, P. J., Krogsgaard-Larsen, P., and Kemp, J. A. (1994) Molecular pharmacology of γ-aminobutyric acid type A receptor agonists and partial agonists in oocytes injected with different α, β and γ receptor subunit combinations. *Mol. Pharmacol.* **46,** 957–963.

10. Sakurai, S. Y., Kume, A., Burdette, D. E., and Albin, R. L. (1994) Quantitative autoradiography of [^{3}H]t-butylbicycloorthobenzoate binding to the γ-aminobutyric acid receptor$_A$ complex. *J. Pharmacol. Exp. Ther.* **270,** 362–370.

11. Wingrove, P. B., Wafford, K. A., Bain, C., and Whiting, P. J. (1994) The modulatory action of loreclezole at the γ-aminobutyric acid type A receptor is determined by a single amino acid in the β2- and β3-subunit. *Proc. Natl. Acad. Sci. USA* **91,** 4569–4573.

12. Bristow, D. R. and Martin, I. L. (1988) Light microscopic autoradiographic localisation in rat brain of the binding sites for the GABAA receptor antagonist [^{3}H]SR 95531: comparison with the [^{3}H]GABAA receptor distribution. *Eur. J. Pharmacol.* **148,** 283–288.

13. Bowery, N. G., Hudson, A. L., and Price, G. W. (1987) GABA$_A$ and GABA$_B$ receptor site distribution in the rat central nervous system. *Neuroscience* **20,** 365–383.

14. Palacios, J. M., Wamsley, J. K., and Kuhar, M. J. (1981) High affinity GABA receptors: autoradiographic localization. *Brain Res.* **222,** 285–307.

15. Olsen, R. W., Snowhill, E. W., and Wamsley, J. K. (1984) Autoradiographic localization of low affinity GABA receptors with [^{3}H]bicuculline methochloride. *Eur. J. Pharmacol.* **99,** 247,248.

16. Luque, J. M., Erat, R., Kettler, R., Cesura, A., Da Prada, M., and Richards, J. G. (1994) Radioautographic evidence that the GABAA receptor antagonist SR 95531 is a substrate inhibitor of MAO-A in the rat and human locus coeruleus. *Eur. J. Neurosci.* **6,** 1038–1049.

17. Wamsley, J. K., Gehlert, D. R., and Olsen, R. W. (1986) The benzodiazepine/barbiturate-sensitive convulsant/GABA receptor/chloride ionophore complex: autoradiographic localization of individual components, in *Benzodiazepine/GABA Receptors and Chloride Channels: Structural and Functional Properties* (Olsen, R. W. and Venter, J. C., eds.), Liss, New York, pp. 299–313.

18. Palacios, J. M., Young, W. S., and Kuhar, M. J. (1980) Autoradiographic localization of γ-aminobutyric acid (GABA) receptors in the rat cerebellum. *Proc. Natl. Acad. Sci. USA* **77,** 670–674.

19. Kume, A. and Albin, R. L. (1994) Quantitative autoradiography of 4'-ethynyl-4-n-[2,3-^{3}H$_2$]propylbicycloorthobenzoate binding to the GABA$_A$ receptor complex. *Eur. J. Pharmacol.* **263,** 163–173.

20. Niddam, R., Dubois, A., Scatton, B., Arbilla, S., and Langer, S. Z. (1987) Autoradiographic localization of [^{3}H]zolpidem binding sites in the rat CNS: comparison with the distribution of [^{3}H]flunitrazepam binding sites. *J. Neurochem.* **49,** 890–899.

21. Quirk, K., Blurton, S., Fletcher, S., Leeson, P., Tang, F., Mellilo, D., et al. (1996) [^{3}H]L-655,708, a novel ligand selective for the benzodiazepine site of GABA$_A$ receptors which contain the α5 subunit. *Neuropharmacology* **35,** 1331–1335.

22. Sur, C., Fresu, L., Howell, O., McKernan, R. M., and Atack, J. R. (1999) autoradiographic localization of α5 subunit-containing GABA_A receptors in rat brain. *Brain Res.* **822**, 265–270.

23. Turner, D. M., Sapp, D. W., and Olsen, R. W. (1991) The benzodiazepine/ alcohol antagonist Ro 15-4513: binding to a GABA receptor subtype that is insensitive to diazepam. *J. Pharmacol. Exp. Ther.* **257**, 1236–1242.

24. Wisden, W., Laurie, D. J., Monyer, H., and Seeburg, P. H. (1992) The distribution of 13 GABA_A receptor subunit mRNAs in the rat brain. I. Telencephalon, diencephalon, mesencephalon. *J. Neurosci.* **12**, 1040–1062.

25. Laurie, D. J., Seeburg, P. H., and Wisden, W. (1992) The distribution of 13 GABA_A receptor subunit mRNAs in the rat brain. II. Olfactory bulb and cerebellum. *J. Neurosci.* **12**, 1063–1076.

26. Fritschy, J. M. and Mohler, H. (1995) GABA_A-receptor heterogeneity in the adult rat brain: differential regional and cellular distribution of seven major subunits. *J Comp Neurol* **359**, 154–194.

27. Jechlinger, M., Pelz, R., Tretter, V., Klausberger, T., and Sieghart, W. (1998) Subunit composition and quantitative importance of hetero-oligomeric receptors: GABA_A receptors containing α6 subunits. *J. Neurosci.* **18**, 2449–2457.

28. Benke, D., Michel, C., and Mohler, H. (1997) GABA_A receptors containing the α4-subunit: prevalence, distribution, pharmacology, and subunit architecture in situ. *J. Neurochem.* **69**, 806–814.

29. Sur, C., Farrar, S., Kerby, J., Whiting, P. J., Atack, J. R., and McKernan, R. M. (1999a) Preferential coassembly of α4 and δ subunits of the γ-aminobutyric acid_A receptor in rat thalamus. *Mol. Pharmacol.* **56**, 110–115.

30. Sperk, G., Schwarzer, C., Tsunashima, K., Fuchs, K., and Sieghart, W. (1997) GABA_A receptor subunits in the rat hippocampus: I. Immuncytochemical distribution of 13 subunits. *Neuroscience* **80**, 987–1000.

31. Houser, C. R., Olsen, R. W., Richards, J. G., and Mohler, H. (1988) Immunohistochemical localization of benzodiazepine/GABA_A receptors in the human hippocampal formation. *J. Neurosci.* **8**, 1370–1383.

32. Wamsley, J. K., Longlet, L., Hunt, M. E. Mahan, D. R., and Alburges, M. E. (1993) Characterization of the binding and comparison of the distribution of benzodiazepine receptors labeled with [^{3}H]diazepam and [^{3}H]alprazolam. *Neuropsychopharmacology* **8**, 305–314.

33. Yezuita, J. P., McCabe, R. T., Barnett, A., Iorio, L. C., and Wamsley, J. K. (1988) Use of the selective benzodiazepine-1 (BZ-1) ligand [^{3}H]oxo-quazepam (SCH 15-725) to localize BZ-1 receptors in the rat brain. *Neurosci. Lett.,* **88**, 86–92.

34. Sanger, D. J. and Depoortere, H. (1998) The pharmacology and mechanism of action of zolpidem. *CNS Drug Rev.* **4**, 323–340.

35. Skolnick, P., Hu, R. J., Cook, C. M., Hurt, S. D., Trometer, J. D., Liu, R., et al. (1997) [^{3}H]RY 80: A high-affinity, selective ligand for γ-aminobutyric acid_A receptors containing *alpha*-5 subunits. *J. Pharmacol. Exp. Ther.* **283**, 488–493.

36. Li, M., Szabo, A., and Rosenberg, H. C. (1999) Evaluation of alpha-5 subunit-containing GABAA receptors using selective ligands. *Soc. Neurosci. Abstr.* **25**, 1482.

37. Fernández-López, M. A., Chinchetru, M. A., and Fernández, P. C. (1997) The autoradiographic perspective of central benzodiazepine receptors: a short review. *Gen. Pharmacol.* **29**, 173–180.

38. Nguyen, Q., Sapp, D. W., Van Ness, P. C., and Olsen, R. W. (1995) Modulation of GABA$_A$ receptor binding in human brain by neuroactive steroids: species and brain regional differences. *Synapse* **19,** 77–87.

39. Greenamyre, J. T., Penney, J. B., D'Amato, C. J., and Young, A. B. (1987) Dementia of the Alzheimer's type: changes in hippocampal L-[^{3}H]glutamate binding. *J. Neurochem.* **48,** 543–551.

40. Jansen, K. L. R., Faull, R. L. M., Dragunow, M., and Synek, B. L. (1990) Alzheimer's disease: changes in hippocampal N-methyl-D-aspartate, quisqualate, neurotensin, adenosine, benzodiazepine, serotonin and opiod receptors: an autoradiographic study. *Neuroscience* **39,** 613–627.

41. Howell, O., Atack, J., McKernan, R., and Sur, C. (1999) Mapping of the α5 subunit containing GABA$_A$ receptor in the human hippocampus and its preservation in Alzheimer's disease. *Br. J. Pharmacol.* **128,** 292.

42. Benes, F. M., Khan, Y., Vincent, S. L., and Wickramasinghe, R. (1996) Differences in the subregional and cellular distribution of GABA$_A$ receptor binding in the hippocampal formation of schizophrenic brain. *Synapse* **22,** 338–349.

43. Hand, K. S. P., Baird, V. H., Van Paesschen, W., Koepp, M. J., Revesz, T., Thom, M., et al. (1997) Central benzodiazepine receptor autoradiography in hippocampal sclerosis. *Br. J. Pharmacol.* **122,** 358–364.

44. Clark, M., Massenburg, G. S., Weiss, S. R. B., and Post, R. M. (1994) Analysis of the hippocampal GABA$_A$ receptor system in kindled rats by autoradiographic and in situ hybridization techniques: contingent tolerance to carbamazepine. *Mol. Brain Res.* **26,** 309–319.

45. Nobrega, J. N., Richter, A., McIntyre Burnham, W., and Loscher, W. (1995) alterations in the brain GABA$_A$/benzodiazepine receptor-chloride ionophore complex in a genetic model of paroxysmal dystonia: a quantitative autoradiographic analysis. *Neuroscience* **64,** 229–239.

46. Pan, H. S., Penney, J. B., and Young, A. B. (1985) γ-aminobutyric acid and benzodiazepine receptor changes induced by unilateral 6-hydroxydopamine lesions of the medial forebrain bundle. *J. Neurochem.* **45,** 1396–1404.

47. Gunther, U., Benson, J., Benke, D., Fritschy, J. M., Reyes, G., Knoflach, F., et al. (1995) Benzodiazepine-insensitive mice generated by targeted disruption of the γ2 subunit gene of γ-aminobutyric acid type A receptor. *Proc. Natl. Acad. Sci. USA* **92,** 7749–7753.

48. Makela, R., Uusi-Oukari, M., Homanics, G. E., Quinlan, J. J., Firestone, L. L., Wisden, W., and Korpi, E. R. (1997) Cerebellar g-aminobutyric acid type A receptors: pharmacological subtypes revealed by mutant mouse lines. *Mol. Pharmacol.* **52,** 380–388.

49. Crestani, F., Lorez, M., Baer, K., Essrich, C., Benke, D., Laurent, J. P., et al. (1999) Decreased GABA$_A$-receptor clustering results in enhanced anxiety and a bias for threat cues. *Nature Neurosci.* **2,** 833–839.

50. Whiting, P. J., McAllister, G., Vasilatis, D., Bonnert, T. P., Heavens, R. P., Smith, D. W., et al. (1997) Neuronally restricted RNA splicing regulates the expression of a novel GABAA receptor subunit conferring atypical functional properties. *J. Neurosci.* **17,** 5027–5037.

4

Localization of ATP P2X Receptors

Xuenong Bo and Geoffrey Burnstock

1. INTRODUCTION

The biological effects of extracellular purine compounds were first observed 70 years ago *(1)*. The first evidence that ATP might be a neurotransmitter came from the studies of sensory innervation in the 1950s *(2)*. It was found that antidromic stimulation of sensory nerves led to vasodilatation of rabbit ear artery, which was accompanied by ATP release. In the early 1960s, a nonadrenergic, noncholinergic (NANC) neurotransmission was recognized in the autonomic nervous system. Early evidence indicated that the principal active substance released from at least some of these nerves was ATP *(3)*. The concept of purinergic neurotransmission was proposed by Burnstock in 1972 *(4)*. It is now recognized that ATP acts as a neurotransmitter, cotransmitter, or neuromodulator in many systems *(5)*.

In 1978, Burnstock proposed the basis for subclassifying the receptors mediating the actions of extracellular purines into P_1- (adenosine as the endogenous ligand) and P_2-purinoceptors (ATP and ADP as the endogenous ligands) *(6)*. This was based on agonist potency order, specific antagonism, and cross-membrane signal transduction mechanism. P_1-purinoceptors were further divided into A_1 and A_2 adenosine receptors according to their effects on adenylate cyclase *(7)*. An A_3 subtype was proposed in 1986 *(8)*.

Diverse effects of ATP and its analogs on peripheral tissues have also been observed. In 1985, subclassification of P_2-purinoceptors into P_{2X}- and P_{2Y}-subtypes was proposed by Burnstock and Kennedy *(9)*. After that a number of other P2 subtypes were proposed including P_{2T} on platelets, P_{2Z} on mast cells *(10)*, and P_{2U} for a receptor responsive to both ATP and UTP *(11)*. In 1993 two P2Y purinoceptors were cloned and recognized to belong

From: *Ion Channel Localization Methods and Protocols*
Edited by: A. Lopatin and C. G. Nichols © Humana Press Inc., Totowa, NJ

to the G protein-coupled receptor family *(12,13)*. In the following year, two P2X receptors were cloned and recognized as ATP-gated cation channels *(14,15)*. It then became clear that, like many other neurotransmitters, ATP also acts through two subfamilies of receptors, one is via the G protein-coupled receptors, and the other is via ion channel receptors. Therefore, the P2 purinoceptors were reclassified into two subfamilies, i.e., the P2X (ion channel) and P2Y (G protein-coupled) receptors *(16)*. The P2Y receptor subfamily encloses the former P_{2Y} and P_{2U} receptors, whereas the P2X subfamily encloses the former P_{2X} and P_{2Z} receptors. So far, 10 P2Y and seven P2X receptor subtypes have been cloned. Recently, we have cloned another novel P2X receptor subtype from embryonic chick skeletal muscle *(17)*. Molecular cloning and characterization of P2 receptor subtypes have expanded our knowledge about this receptor family *(18,19)*.

Great progress has been made in the study of P2 receptors, including their classification, distribution, biological functions, selective agonists and antagonists, signal transduction mechanisms, biochemical characteristics, and molecular properties *(19)*. The development of potential therapeutic agents targeting P2 receptors is undergoing rapid expansion. Conditions being explored include cystic fibrosis, asthma, inflammation, hypertension, incontinence, cancer, and pain. In order to reduce side-effects of potential drugs, tissue distribution of targeted receptors is an important factor to be considered in addition to the selectivity of the drugs. In this chapter, we provide protocols of the commonly used experimental techniques for localization of ATP P2X receptors in our laboratory. Similar techniques with modification by individual researchers have been used in many other laboratories.

2. METHODS

2.1. Autoradiography

2.1.1. Development of Radioligand

Before the cloning of P2X receptor subtypes, the existence of P2X receptors was supported by evidence from pharmacological and electrophysiological studies *(20)*. No information was available about the tissue distribution of P2X receptors. Because α,β-methyleneATP (α,β-MeATP) was considered the most potent P2X receptor agonist in pharmacological studies due to its resistance to ATPases, we had this compound tritiated by Amersham International plc. Radioligand binding studies showed that [^{3}H]α,β-MeATP bound specifically to P2X receptors in smooth muscle of urinary bladder with a K_d value of 10 n*M* *(21,22)*. Autoradiogaphy with this radioligand showed specific binding sites were localized in smooth muscle of urinary bladder, vas deferens, and blood vessels *(21,23,24)*. For the first time, P2X receptors could be quantitated and the distribution visualized. After molecular cloning of P2X receptor subtypes, it was recognized that only $P2X_1$, $P2X_3$, and chick $P2X_8$ *(17)* receptors are responsive to α,β-MeATP, so the radioligand binding sites we reported were mainly for $P2X_1$ receptors. Although eight P2X receptor subtypes have been cloned so far, few selective agonists and antagonists for the subtypes are currently available. $[^3H]$α,β-MeATP still remains the main radioligand available to study P2X receptors responsive to α,β-MeATP. $[^{35}S]$Adenosine 5'-O-(3-thiotriphosphate) (ATPγS) has been used to study P2X receptors in the absence of Ca^{2+} in radioligand binding assay *(25)*, but not for autoradiographic localization of P2X receptors.

$[^3H]$α,β-MeATP is now commercially available from both Amersham Pharmacia Biotech AB (Uppsala, Sweden) and NEN Life Science Products Inc. (Boston, MA).

2.1.2. Tissue Preparation

Fresh tissues were dissected, embedded in OCT compound (Sakura Finetech, The Netherlands), and frozen in isopentane precooled in liquid nitrogen. Cryostat sections (14 μm in thickness) were cut and thaw-mounted onto gelatin-coated slides. Sections can be stored at –80°C for 2 mo without significant loss of binding sites.

2.1.3. Radioligand Binding

Slide-mounted sections were preincubated in 50 mM Tris-HCl buffer with protease inhibitors (1 mM ethylene glycol-bis N,N,N',N'-tetraacetic acid (EGTA), 1 mM benzamidine hydrochloride, 0.1 mM phenylmethylsulfonyl fluoride (PMSF), 0.01% bacitracin, and 0.002% soybean trypsin inhibitors, Buffer A, pH 7.4) at 30°C for 10 min to remove endogenous ligands and the embedding matrix. They were then transferred to Buffer A containing 1–10 nM $[^3H]$α,β-MeATP and incubated at 30°C for 15 min. Nonspecific binding was determined in the presence of 100 μM β,γ-methyleneATP. At the end of the incubation the sections were washed in ice-cold 50 mM Tris-HCl buffer and rinsed in ice-cold distilled water. The sections were dried rapidly under a stream of cold air.

2.1.4. Generation of Autoradiograms

2.1.4.1. EMULSION-COATED COVERSLIPS

Autoradiograms were produced by the method of Young and Kuhar *(26)*. Nuclear emulsion (Ilford K5, diluted 1:1 with distilled water) was melted in a hot water bath. Coverslips were coated with the emulsion and dried overnight at room temperature. The emulsion-coated coverslips were attached to one end of each slide with cyanoacrylate adhesive. The assemblies were packed tightly and exposed for 2 wk at 4°C in a desiccator. The emulsion was developed in Kodak D-19 (20°C, 3 min) and fixed in Ilford Hypam for 5 min. After being washed in running water for 30 min, the slides were soaked in double-distilled water for 5 min, and then the sections were stained with 0.5% Toluidine blue. Sections were dehydrated in graded ethanol (from 70–100%) and cleared in Histo-Clear (National Diagnostics, Manville). The coverslips and the slides were bound together tightly with D.P.X. Mountant (BDH). The autoradiograms were examined under a microscope. Both bright- and dark-field images of the same field of view were photographed for comparison.

2.1.4.2. HYPERFILM-^{3}H

After the sections were incubated with the radioligand, washed, and dried, Hyperfilm-^{3}H (Amersham Pharmacia) was applied over the sections and exposed for 2 mo at room temperature. The films were developed and fixed those for emulsion-coated coverslips.

2.1.5. Semi-Quantitation of Autoradiograms

Autoradiographic slides were viewed under a photomicroscope with an oil immersion objective lens. The images were captured by a video camera attached to the microscope. Video signals were processed by a Seescan I3000 image processing system using the software Solitaire Plus (Seescan Ltd., Cambridge, UK). Autoradiographic grains over the sections and the background were counted. Grain densities in different tissues were compared.

For autoradiograms generated with Hyperfilm-^{3}H, the images were captured with a video camera and processed with the same Seescan image analysis and the optical densities of the labeling in different tissues or structures were measured and compared.

2.1.6. Examples of P2X Receptor Localization by Autoradiography

P2X receptors were found to be highly expressed in smooth muscle of rat, guinea pig, and rabbit urinary bladder and vas deferens in radioligand binding assays *(21–23)*, therefore, the exposure time was much shorter than for the autoradiography of many other neurotransmitter receptors. In 2 wk high density silver grains were generated over the smooth muscle of rat urinary bladder, vas deferens and blood vessels (Fig. 1). The specific binding was displaced by an excessive amount of unlabeled β,γ-methyleneATP. In the brain and spinal cord, the density of [^{3}H]α,β-MeATP binding sites was much lower than that of in urinary bladder smooth muscle, therefore, exposure time of 2 mo was required to generate the autoradiograms with Hyperfilm-

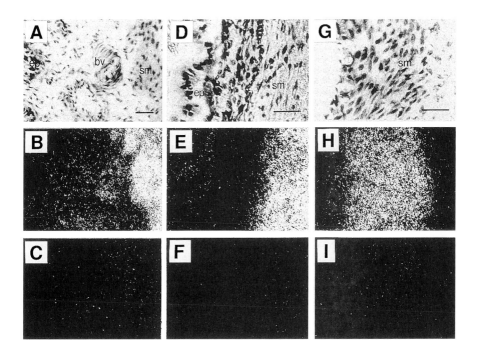

Fig. 1. Autoradiograph of $[^3H]\alpha,\beta$-methyleneATP binding sites in rat tissues. Bright field views of sections of urinary bladder **(A)**, vas deferens **(D)**, and ear artery **(G)**, stained with 0.5% Toluidine blue; **(B)**, **(E)**, and **(H)** are dark-field views of the same fields of **(A)**, **(D)**, and **(G)**, respectively, showing the total binding of $[^3H]\alpha,\beta$-methyleneATP to the sections; **(C)**, **(F)**, and **(I)** are dark-field views of the sections adjacent to **(A)**, **(D)**, and **(G)**, respectively, showing the nonspecific binding to the sections after displacement with β,γ-methyleneATP. (bv, blood vessel; ep, epithelium; sm, smooth muscle) Scale bar, 50 µm. (Reprinted with permission from ref. *21*).

^3H *(27)*. Pseudocolor images in Fig. 2 show the binding site densities in different regions of rat brain. The specific binding was also displaced by unlabeled β,γ-methyleneATP (Fig. 2C) and the antagonist pyridoxalphosphate-6-azophenyl-2',4'-disulfonic acid (PPADS) (Fig. 2B).

2.2. Immunocytochemistry

2.2.1. Light Microscopy

2.2.1.1. TISSUE PREPARATION

Animals were killed by asphyxiation with CO_2 and perfused immediately with 4% paraformaldehyde. The tissues of interest were dissected and postfixed in the same fixative overnight. They were then saturated with 20%

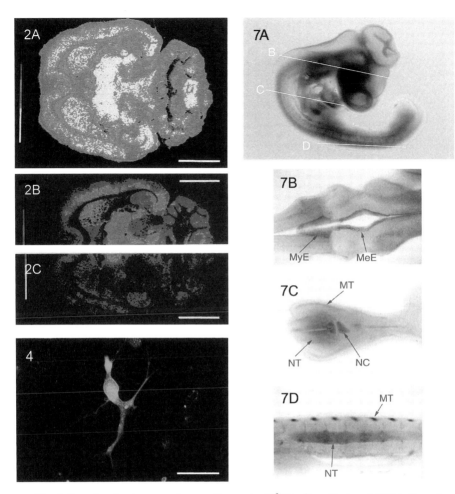

Fig. 2. Pseudocolor images of autoradiograph of $[^3H]\alpha,\beta$-methyleneATP binding sites in rat brain. Yellow represents the area with the highest density, followed by orange, red, pink, and blue. Indigo shows the background. **(A)** The image of a horizontal section showing the total binding of $[^3H]\alpha,\beta$-methyleneATP; **(B)** The image of an adjacent section of **(A)** showing binding after the displacement by 100 mM PPADS; **(C)** The image of an adjacent section of **(A)** showing the binding after the displacement by 100 µM β,γ-methyleneATP. Scale bars, 5 mm. (Reprinted with permission from ref. 27).

Fig. 4. Immunostaining of recombinant $P2X_4$ receptors in 1321N1 cells with a mouse monoclonal antibody. 1321N1 cells were transfected with pcDNA3.1/Zeo-$P2X_4$ and left for two days before immunostaining with FITC-conjugated secondary antibody. Scale bar = 100 µm.

Fig. 7. Whole mount *in situ* hybridization of chick embryos (Day 4) with digoxigenin-labeled $cP2X_8$ RNA probe. **(A)** Lateral view of the whole embryo. **(B)** Section over the brain showing the expression of $cP2X_8$ RNA in mesencephalon (MeE) and myelencephalon (MyE). **(C)** Section over the middle part of the embryo showing the expression of $cP2X_8$ RNA in myotome (MT), neurotube (NT) and notochord (NC). **(D)** Longitudinal section along lower spine showing the expression of $cP2X_8$ RNA in myotome and neurotube. (Reprinted with permission from ref. 27.)

sucrose in phosphate-buffered saline (PBS). Thereafter, the tissues were rapidly frozen, cut into sections of 10-μm in thickness, and thaw-mounted on *poly*-L-lysine-coated slides.

2.2.1.2. SOURCES OF ANTIBODIES

Anti-P2X receptor polyclonal antibodies (PAbs) used in our laboratory were provided by Roche Bioscience Institute (Palo Alto, CA). They were raised in New Zealand rabbits by multiple injections of synthetic peptides corresponding to 15 amino acids of the carboxyl termini of the cloned rat P2X receptors *(28)*. Several other laboratories have used PAbs against P2X receptors from other sources *(29–32)*. Some antibodies were generated using the extracellular loops of P2X receptor protein as antigens *(32)*.

PAbs against rat and human $P2X_1$, rat $P2X_2$, rat $P2X_4$, and rat $P2X_7$ receptors are available commercially from Alomone Labs Ltd. (Jerusalem, Israel) and Chemicon International, Inc. (Temecula).

We have produced an anti-$P2X_4$ receptor monoclonal antibody (MAb) using a polypeptide corresponding to the extracellular loop. A species of Ig*M* antibody was found to bind specifically to $P2X_4$ receptors. However, the affinity of the antibody was low, therefore a high concentration of antibody was required to generate detectable signal, which also created high background staining. We have used it successfully on cell lines transfected with $P2X_4$ receptor cDNA. However, its usage on tissue sections is limited.

2.2.1.3. IMMUNOSTAINING WITH THE EXTRAVIDIN PEROXIDASE-CONJUGATED COMPLEX PROCEDURE

Standard procedures were followed with some modifications according the operator's personal experience (*see* refs. *33* and *34* for reference). 3,3'-Diaminobenzidine (DAB) was used to generate a color product. Because of the low level of expression of some P2X receptors in certain tissues, several intensification methods were used that are described in Sections 2.2.1.4.–2.2.1.6.

2.2.1.4. NICKEL INTENSIFICATION METHOD

To enhance the DAB-generated immunostaining signals with nickel, sections bound with Extravidin peroxidase were incubated in a solution containing 0.05% DAB, 0.04% nickel ammonium sulfate, 0.2% β-D-glucose, 0.004% ammonium nitrate, and 1.2 U/mL glucose oxidase in PBS to generate immuno-signals.

2.2.1.5. SILVER-GOLD INTENSIFICATION METHOD

The DAB color product in the sections can be enhanced by the silver-gold intensification method *(35)*. After color development, the sections were washed in PBS for 3 × 5 min and in 2% sodium acetate for 2 × 15 min. They were then treated with 10% thioglycolic acid for 6–12 h at room temperature, followed by 2% sodium acetate washes for 2 × 15 min. A developer was prepared by mixing Solution A (5% sodium carbonate) and Solution B (0.2% ammonium nitrate, 0.2% silver nitrate, 1% tungstosilicic acid, and 5 mL formaldehyde) in a ratio of 1:1. The sections were developed for 6–10 min. Close monitoring under the microscope is essential to prevent over-reaction. The development was stopped with 1% acetic acid for 5 min, followed by a wash in 2% sodium acetate for 5 min. The sections were treated in 0.05% tetracholoauric acid for 5 min, followed by another wash in 2% sodium acetate for 5 min. The sections were then washed in 3% sodium thiosulfate for 2 × 10 min and finally in 2% sodium acetate for 5 min and PBS for 10 min.

Alternatively, following the PBS and sodium acetate wash after the color reaction, the sections were treated in 0.1 mM cupric sulfate for 10 min. After being washed in 2% acetic acid for 2 × 5 min, the sections were treated with 1% hydrogen peroxide in 2% sodium acetate for 30 min. The other steps were the same as described earlier.

2.2.1.6. TYRAMIDE SIGNAL AMPLIFICATION METHOD

The principle of this technique is to use horseradish peroxidase to catalyze the deposition of biotin-labeled tyramide onto tissue sections close to the enzyme, which will significantly enhance the signal. A kit called TSA-Indirect can be purchased from NEN Life Science Products. The manufacturer's protocol was followed closely in our experiment.

2.2.1.7. IMMUNOSTAINING OF TRANSFECTED CELLS FOR FLUORESCENT MICROSCOPY

Cells of the human astrocytoma cell line, 1321N1, were first grown to 80% confluence in vented flasks and then seeded in chambered coverglass (Nalge Nunc International, Rochester, NY). After 2 d, the cells were transfected with a mixture of 1 μg pcDNA3.1/Zeo-P2X$_4$ and 5 μL SuperFect Transfection Reagent (Qiagen GmbH, Hilden, Germany). One to two days after the transfection, the cells were fixed in 4% paraformaldehyde and 0.2% picric acid and processed for standard fluorescent immunostaining *(33,34)*. Anti-P2X$_4$ receptor monoclonal antibody was partially purified from the culture medium of the hybridoma. It was diluted at a ratio of 1:30 with the blocking solution consisting of 5% normal goat serum, 0.1% bovine serum albumin (BSA), and 0.1 M glycine in PBS. Fluorescein-5-isothiocyanate (FITC)-conjugated goat anti-mouse immunoglobulin (DAKO, Glostrup, Denmark) was diluted 1:300 in PBS with 0.1% BSA. After the final wash, the chambers were removed carefully and coverslips were mounted with Citifluor (Ted Pella Inc., Redding).

2.2.2. Electron Microscopy

The protocols for electron microscopic immunocytochemistry of P2X receptors are standard peroxidase-antiperoxidase complex and Extravidin-perioxidase conjugated complex methods (*see* refs. *36* and *37*).

2.2.3. Examples of Immunolabeling of P2X Receptors

Using the nickel-intensified Extravidin-perioxidase conjugated complex method, a population of neurons in rat dorsal root ganglion, mainly the small-sized, were heavily stained with anti-$P2X_3$ receptor antibody, whereas another population showed a moderate level of staining (Fig. 3A). Many large neurons were immunonegative. In the trigeminal ganglion, similar pattern was observed and the nerve fibers were shown with higher magnification (Fig. 3B).

Using the tyramide signal amplification method, large nerve bundles in the connective tissues in the circumvallate papillae and a dense network of nerve fibers at the base of taste buds were stained strongly with the anti-$P2X_3$ receptor antibody (Fig. 3C) *(38)*. The nerve fibers penetrated the basal lamina of the taste buds and many varicose fibers reached the tips of the buds. Some nerve fibers also appeared in the epithelium where no taste buds were seen. With the silver-gold intensification method, the $P2X_3$ receptor immuno-signal in the taste buds was even more stronger than the tyramide amplification method (Fig. 3D), therefore, the silver-gold amplification method is quite useful when the level of protein expression or the affinity of the primary antibody is low.

Owing to the higher level of expression of recombinant P2X receptors in transfected cells, amplification of immuno-signals may not be needed. Immunostaining with fluorescent secondary antibody is an easy and fast method to detect the expression of the recombinant receptors expressed in cell lines. Figure 4 shows the staining of a single 1321N1 cell transfected with $P2X_4$ cDNA with an anti-$P2X_4$ receptor monoclonal antibody. Dense labeling on the membrane is visible.

Electron microscopic immunostaining revealed immunoreactivity to $P2X_1$ in rat cerebellum (Fig. 5) *(36)*. The most prominent immunoreactivity was observed in the molecular layer of the cerebellar cortex, where it labeled a small subpopulation of spines/thorns of Purkinje cell dendrites. The immuno-positive dendritic spines of Purkinje cells synapsed with immuno-negative axon varicosities of granule cells. In some labeled dendritic spines, the pronounced $P2X_1$ immunoreactivity was concentrated at the postsynap-

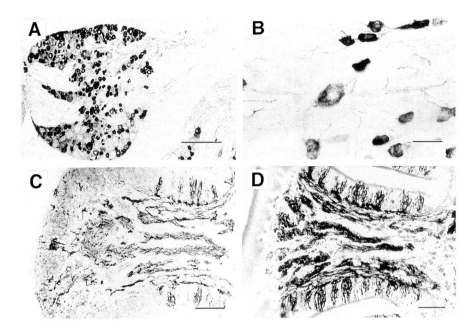

Fig. 3. Immunostaining of P2X$_3$ receptors with rabbit polyclonal antibodies in rat tissues. The standard procedure used was the Extravidin-perioxidase-conjugated complex method. **(A)** Immunopositive neurons in the dorsal root ganglion with nickel intensification. **(B)** Immunopositive neurons and nerve fibers in trigeminal ganglion with nickel intensification. **(C)** Immunopositive nerve fibers in circumvallate papillae in rat tongue with tyramide amplification. (Reprinted with permission from ref. *38*) **(D)** Immunopositive nerve fibers in circumvallate papillae in the tongue with silver-gold intensification. Scale bars, (A), 500 μm; (B), 50 μm; (C, D), 100 μm.

tic density of the junction, leaving the other region of the dendrite less well labeled (Fig. 5B).

2.3. In Situ *Hybridization*

Many books describing the protocols for *in situ* hybridization are available *(39,40)*. Although the basic procedures are the same, individual protocols vary significantly, based on the operator's personal experience. The following describes the experimental protocol used in our laboratory.

2.3.1. *Synthesis of Digoxigenin-Labeled Probes*

Segments of cDNAs (450–1100 bp) from the coding regions of P2X receptors were subcloned into vectors such as pBluescript SKII (Stratagene,

La Jolla, CA) or pcDNA II (Invitrogen, Carlsbad). Digoxigenin-UTP-labeled cRNA probes were synthesized as run-off transcripts on linearized plasmid DNA using a DIG-RNA labeling kit (Roche Diagnostics). The yields and the sizes of the DIG-probes were checked with agarose electrophoresis. The probes were kept at $-80°C$ and can be used within 1 yr.

2.3.2. In Situ *Hybridization on Cryostat Sections*

Cryostat sections (10–20 μm in thickness) were cut, thaw-mounted onto silanized microscope glass slides, and fixed immediately in freshly prepared 4% paraformaldehyde for at least 30 min. The slides were washed in PBS for 3×10 min and then soaked in 70% ethanol (slides can be stored in this solution for several days at 4°C). The slides were rinsed in ultra-pure water for 2×10 min and in 0.1 M HCl for 10 min. After a further wash in PBS for 2×10 min, the slides were placed in a mixture of 0.1 M triethanolamine, pH 8.0 (adjust pH with HCl) and 0.25% acetic acid anhydride (mixed just before use) for 20 min. Sections were then washed with PBS for 2×5 min, dehydrated in an ascending ethanol series (70, 80, and 95% ethanol) for 5 min respectively and air-dried. Sections were incubated in prehybridization buffer containing 50% formamide, 50 mM Tris-HCl, 20 mM NaCl, 25 mM ethylenediaminetetraacetic acid (EDTA), 2.5x Denhardt's solution, and 0.25 mg/mL tRNA in a humidified chamber for at least 3 h at 37°C. Hybridization was performed in a buffer containing 50% formamide, 20 mM Tris-HCl, 1 mM EDTA, 1x Denhardt's solution, 0.5 mg/mL tRNA, 0.1 mg/mL polyA$^+$ RNA, and 0.1 M dithiothreitol (DTT) with various concentrations of antisense probe at 55–70°C overnight. After hybridization the sections were washed in 0.2x SSC solution at 55°C for 30 min, in 0.1x SSC/50% formamide solution at 55°C for 3×60 min, and finally rinsed in 0.2x SSC for 10 min at room temperature.

The hybridization signal was detected with an anti-digoxigenin antibody conjugated to alkaline phosphatase (anti-DIG-AP antibody) (Roche Diagnostics) using 4-nitroblue tetrazolium chloride (NBT) and 5-bromo-4-cloro-3-indolylphosphate (BCIP) (Roche Diagnostics) as substrates. The sections were equilibrated in Buffer 1 (100 mM Tris-HCl, 150 mM NaCl, pH 7.5) for 10 min, and then blocked for 30 min in Buffer 2 consisting of 1% Blocking reagent (Roche Diagnostics) and 0.5% BSA dissolved in Buffer 1. Slides were placed in the humidified chamber and anti-DIG-AP antibody (1:1000–2000 diluted in Buffer 2) was applied and incubated at 4°C overnight. After incubation, the sections were washed in Buffer 1 for 2×15 min, equilibrated for 3 min in Buffer 3 (100 mM Tris-HCl, 100 mM NaCl, 50 mM MgCl$_2$, pH 9.5), and then developed in the dark with Buffer 3 consisting of 0.35 mg/mL NBT, 0.175 mg/mL BCIP, and 0.25 mg/mL levamisole. When an appropriate level of color reaction appeared (from 30 min to overnight), the development was stopped by washing the slides in TE buffer (10 mM Tris-HCl, 1 mM EDTA, pH 8.0). For permanent storage the slides were washed in water, air-dried overnight, rinsed briefly in Histo-Clear, and then mounted in DPX mountant. It should be noted that mounting medium containing any kind of alcohol can lead to fading of hybridization signal. Background control experiments included substitution of the specific antisense probe with the corresponding sense probe, or omission of the specific riboprobe.

2.3.3. Whole Mount In Situ Hybridization

Chick embryos (up to 6 d old) were dissected and fixed in freshly prepared 4% paraformaldehyde in PBS at 4°C for 2 h to overnight (embryos can be stored in the fixative at 4°C for several weeks without significant loss of signal). Collected embryos were washed in PBT buffer (PBS with 0.1% Tween-20) for 2 × 10 min. They were dehydrated in 25, 50, and 75% methanol in PBT (10 min in each solution) and in 100% methanol for 2 × 10 min (embryos can also be stored at this stage at –20°C for several months). Embryos were rehydrated in the reverse order in methanol solutions, bleached with 6% hydrogen peroxide in PBT for 1 h, and washed in PBT three times. For better penetration of probes, embryos were treated with protease K (10 μg/mL in PBT) for 20 min (digestion time can be adjusted according to the age of the embryos) and washed twice in PBT. They were postfixed in 0.2% gluteraldehyde/4% paraformaldehyde in PBT for 20 min, followed by three washes in PBT.

Prehybridization was carried out in a buffer containing 50% formamide, 5× SSC, 50 μg/mL yeast RNA, 1% sodium dodecyl sulfate (SDS), and 50 μg heparin at 55°C for 2 h, followed by overnight hybridization with 1 μg/mL DIG-RNA probe at 55°C (longer hybridization time is required for older embryos). After hybridization, the embryos were first washed with Solution 1 (50% formamide, 5× SSC, and 1% SDS) at 55°C for 30 min, in Solution 2 (50% formamide and 2× SSC) at 55°C for 2 × 60 min, and finally in TBST (0.8% NaCl, 0.02% KCl, 1% Tween-20, 25 mM Tris-HCl, pH 7.5, with levamisole added to 2 mM on the day of use) for three times.

To detect the hybridization signals, the embryos were first preblocked with 10% normal goat serum in TBST for 60–90 min and then incubated with 1:2000 diluted anti-DIG-AP antibody in 10% normal goat serum in TBST and rocked lightly overnight at 4°C. The antibody can be preabsorbed with chick embryo powder to reduce background staining. However, this step may not be needed. After antibody binding, the embryos were washed in TBST for 3 × 15 min, and then, the buffer was changed hourly throughout the day. The wash was continued overnight with light shaking. On the following day, the embryos were washed 3×15 min with freshly prepared NTMT buffer (100 mM NaCl, 100 mM Tris-HCl, pH 9.5, 50 mM MgCl$_2$, 0.1% Tween-20, 2 mM levamisole). Color reaction was carried out in the dark with NTMT containing 0.35 mg/mL NBT and 0.175/mL BCIP until desired color intensity was achieved. To stop the reaction, the embryos were washed in PBT with 20 mM EDTA. Finally, the embryos were fixed in 4% paraformaldehyde before storing.

The embryos can be photographed with a dissection microscope fitted with a camera. To help the orientation, the embryos were placed into a trough made in 1% agarose gel in a petri dish. Whole embryos were photographed and then embedded in gelatin-albumin gel. Sections of the embryos (100-μm thick) were obtained with a vibratome.

2.3.4. Examples of In Situ Hybridization

Individual cells can be clearly labeled with digoxigenin-labeled probes as the color reaction only occurs close to the fixed mRNAs inside the cells. In Fig. 6A, Purkinje cells in rat cerebellum were labeled by a P2X$_4$ receptor DIG-RNA probe *(41)*. Neurons in rat mesenteric ganglion were also labeled with the same probe (Fig. 6B). In rat nodose ganglion (Fig. 6C) and trigeminal ganglion (Fig. 6D), neurons were labeled with a P2X$_3$ receptor DIG-RNA probe. Some neurons were stained more heavily than others, reflecting the different level of expression of P2X$_3$ mRNA transcript in different neurons. Similar pattern were also observed in immunocytochemical studies *(42,43)*.

Whole mount *in situ* hybridization of the newly cloned chick P2X$_8$ receptors showed discrete pattern of expression of cP2X$_8$ RNA transcript in Day 4 embryo (Fig. 7). The hybridization signals were observed in myotome, brain, the ventral part of the neural tube, and notochord.

3. CONCLUSION

So far, only the conventional methods have been used for localization of P2X receptors. Autoradiography with [^{3}H]α,β-MeATP has provided a lot of information about the distribution of P2X receptors before data from the molecular cloning of P2X receptor subtypes became available. This radioligand labels all α,β-MeATP responsive P2X receptors without the problem of species specificity. However, autoradiography with the tritium-labeled ligand is a time-consuming process. Moreover, the inability to distinguish the P2X receptor subtypes also limits its use. The development of subtype-specific agonists and antagonists will solve the latter problem.

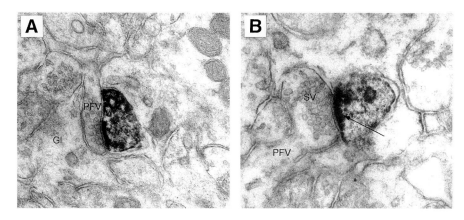

Fig. 5. Electron microscopic immunostaining of $P2X_1$ receptor with rabbit polyclonal antibodies in rat cerebellum. Molecular layer of rat cerebellum processed for perioxidase anti-perioxidase conjugated complex (A) and Extravidin-perioxidase-conjugated complex immunocytochemistry (B) showing $P2X_1$-positive dendritic spines of Purkinje cells involved in the formation of asymmetric axo-dendritic synapses. (A) Note the $P2X_1$-negative varicosity of the parallel fiber (PFV) of the ascending granule cell axon upon the $P2X_1$-positive dendritic spine (Gl, neuroglia process). × 56,000. (B) A $P2X_1$-positive postsynaptic dendritic spine displaying labeling mostly at the postsynaptic density (arrow) (SV, spherical synaptic vesicles). × 97,000. (Reprinted with permission from ref. *36*.)

The development of anti-P2X receptor polyclonal antibodies in several laboratories has significantly expanded the tools available to study the distribution of P2X receptors. Simple immunocytochemistry procedures allow researchers to process a large amount of tissue in a short time. The availability of many signal enhancement techniques has provided the opportunity to reveal the existence of P2X receptors in very fine structures such as the sensory nerve fibers in the skin. They are also the only tools used to study the subcellular distribution of the receptors. The immunostaining of $P2X_1$ receptor found on the postsynaptic membrane has provided further evidence that ATP acts as a neurotransmitter. The main drawback is the possible nonspecific binding of the antibodies to other proteins, and therefore, caution should be exercised in carrying out the experiments and interpreting the results.

In situ hybridization is usually the first method to be used to study the cellular expression of newly cloned receptors. With high stringency hybridization and proper controls, the results should be quite reliable. However, this technique is more complicated than immunocytochemistry and requires RNase-free operation. It can identify the cells which express the RNA transcripts, but is unable to locate the target organ.

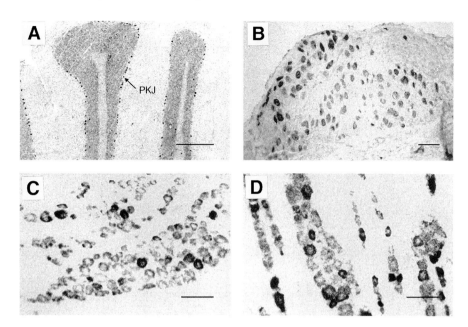

Fig. 6. *In situ* hybridization of rat tissues with digoxigenin-labeled RNA probes. Purkinje cells in the cerebellum (**A**) and neurons in mesenteric ganglion (**B**) were labeled with a $P2X_4$ receptor RNA probe. Neurons in nodose ganglion (**C**) and trigeminal ganglion (**D**) were labeled with a $P2X_3$ receptor RNA probe. Scale bars, (A), 500 μm, (B) = 50 μm, (C, D) = 100 μm.

REFERENCES

1. Drury, A. N. and Szent-Györgyi, A. (1929) The physiological activity of adenine compounds with special reference to their action upon the mammalian heart. *J. Physiol. (Lond.)* **68,** 213–237.
2. Holton, P. (1959) The liberation of adenosine triphosphate on antidromic stimulation of the sensory nerves. *J. Physiol. (Lond.)* **145,** 494–504.
3. Burnstock, G., Campbell, G., Satchell, D. G., and Smythe, A. (1970) Evidence that adenosine triphosphate or a related nucleotide is the transmitter substance released by non-adrenergic inhibitory nerves in the gut. *Br. J. Pharmacol.* **40,** 668–688.
4. Burnstock, G. (1972) Purinergic nerves. *Pharmacol. Rev.* **24,** 509–581.
5. Burnstock, G. (1997) The past, present and future of purine nucleotides as signalling molecules. *Neuropharmacology* **36,** 1127–1139.
6. Burnstock, G. (1978) A basis for distinguishing two types of purinergic receptor, in *Cell Membrane Receptors for Drugs and Hormones: A Multidisciplinary Approach* (Straub, R. W. and Bolis, L., eds.), Raven Press, New York, pp. 107–118.

7. van Calker, D., Müller, M., and Hamprecht, B. (1979) Adenosine regulates via two different types of receptors, the accumulation of cyclic AMP in cultured brain cells. *J. Neurochem.* **33,** 999–1005.

8. Ribeiro, J. A. and Sebastiao, A. M. (1986) Adenosine receptors and calcium: basis for proposing a third (A_3) adenosine receptor. *Prog. Neurobiol.* **26,** 179–209.

9. Burnstock, G. and Kennedy, C. (1985) Is there a basis for distinguishing two types of P_2-purinoceptor? *Gen. Pharmacol.* **5,** 433–440.

10. Gordon, J. L. (1986) Extracellular ATP: effects, sources and fate. *Biochem. J.* **233,** 309–319.

11. O'Connor, S. E., Dainty, I. A. and Leff, P. (1991) Further subclassification of ATP receptors based on agonist studies. *Trends Pharmacol. Sci.* **12,** 137–141.

12. Webb, T. E., Simon, J., Krishek, B. J., Bateson, A. N., Smart, T. G., King, B. F., et al. (1993) Cloning and functional expression of a brain G protein-coupled ATP receptor. *FEBS Lett.* **324,** 219–225.

13. Lustig, K. D., Shiau, A. K., Brake, A. J., and Julius, D. (1993) Expression cloning of an ATP receptor from mouse neuroblastoma cells. *Proc. Natl. Acad. Sci. USA* **90,** 5113–5117.

14. Valera, S., Hussy, N., Evans, R. J., Adami, N., North, R. A., Surprenant, A., and Buell, G. (1994) A new class of ligand-gated ion channel defined by P2X receptor for extracellular ATP. *Nature* **371,** 516–519.

15. Brake, A. J., Wagenbach, M. J., and Julius, D. (1994) New structural motif for ligand-gated ion channels defined by iontropic ATP receptor. *Nature* **371,** 519–523.

16. Abbracchio, M. P. and Burnstock, G. (1994) Purinoceptors: are there families of P2X and P2Y purinoceptors? *Pharmacol. Ther.* **64,** 445–475.

17. Bo, X., Schoepfer, R., and Burnstock, G. (2000) Molecular cloning and characterization of a novel ATP P2X receptor subtype ($cP2X_8$) from embryonic chick skeletal muscle. *J. Biol. Chem.* **275,** 14,401–14,407.

18. Buell, G., Collo, G., and Rassendren, F. (1996) P2X receptors: an emerging channel family. *Eur. J. Neurosci.* **8,** 2221–2228.

19. Ralevic, V. and Burnstock, G. (1988) Receptors for purines and pyrinidines. *Pharmacol. Rev.* **50,** 413–492.

20. Burnstock, G. (1993) Physiological and pathological roles of purines: an update. *Drug Dev. Res.* **28,** 195–206.

21. Bo, X. and Burnstock, G. (1989) [^{3}H]α,β-methylene ATP: a radioligand for P_2-purinoceptors. *J. Auton. Nerv. Syst.* **28,** 85–88.

22. Bo, X. and Burnstock, G. (1990) High- and low-affinity binding sites for [^{3}H]α,β-methylene ATP in rat urinary bladder membranes. *Br. J. Pharmacol.* **101,** 291–296.

23. Bo, X. and Burnstock, G. (1992) Species differences in characteristics and distribution of [^{3}H]α,β-methylene ATP binding sites in urinary bladder and urethra of rat, guinea-pig and rabbit. *Eur. J. Pharmacol.* **216,** 59–66.

24. Bo, X. and Burnstock, G. (1993) Heterogeneous distribution of [^{3}H]α,β-methylene ATP binding sites in blood vessels from rat, guinea-pig, and rabbit. *J. Vasc. Res.* **30,** 87–101.

25. Michel, A. D. and Humphrey, P. P. A. (1996) High affinity P2X-purinoceptor binding sites for [^{35}S]-adenosine 5'-O-[3-thiotriphosphate] in rat vas deferens membranes. *Br. J. Pharmacol.* **117,** 63–70.

26. Young, W. S. III and Kuhar, M. J. (1979) A new method for receptor autoradiography: [³H]opioid receptors in rat brain. *Brain Res.* **179,** 255–270.
27. Bo, X. and Burnstock, G. (1994) Distribution of [³H]α,β-methylene ATP binding sites in rat brain and spinal cord. *NeuroReport* **5,** 1601–1604.
28. Oglesby, I. B., Lachnit, W. G., Burnstock, G., and Ford, A. P. D. W. (1999) Subunit specificity of polyclonal antisera to the carboxy terminal regions of P2X receptors, P2X₁ through P2X₇. *Drug Dev. Res.* **47,** 189–195.
29. Kanjhan, R., Housley, G. D., Thorne, P. R., Christie, D. L., Palmer, D. J., Luo, L., and Ryan, A. F. (1996) Localization of ATP-gated ion channels in cerebellum using P2x₂R subunit-specific antisera. *NeuroReport* **7,** 2665–2669.
30. Vulchanova, L., Riedl, M. S., Shuster, S. J., Buell, G., Surprenant, A., North, R. A., and Elde, R. (1997) Immunohistochemical study of the P2X₂ and P2X₃ receptor subunits in rat and monkey sensory neurons and their central terminal. *Neuropharmacology* **36,** 1229–1242.
31. Lê, K. T., Villeneuve, P., Ramjaun, A. R., McPherson, P. S., Beaudet, A., and Seguela, P. (1998) Sensory presynaptic and widespread somatodendritic immunolocalization of central ionotropic P2X ATP receptors. *Neuroscience* **83,** 177–190.
32. Hansen, M. A., Bennett, M. R., and Barden, J. A. (1999) Distribution of purinergic P2X receptors in the rat heart. *J. Auton. Nerv. Syst.* **78,** 1–9.
33. Polak, J. M. and Van Noorden, S. (eds.) (1997) *Introduction to Immunocytochemistry.* BIOS Scientific, Oxford, UK.
34. Beesley, J. E. (ed.) (1993) *Immunocytochemistry: A Practical Approach.* IRL Press at Oxford University Press, Oxford, UK.
35. Liposits, Z., Setalo, G., and Flerko, B. (1984) Application of the silver-gold intensified 3,3'-diaminobenzidine chromogen to the light and electron microscopic detection of the luteinzing hormone releasing hormone system of the rat brain. *Neuroscience* **13,** 513–524.
36. Loesch, A. and Burnstock, G. (1998) Electron-immunocytochemical localization of P2X₁ receptors in the rat cerebellum. *Cell Tissue Res.* **294,** 253–260.
37. Llewellyn-Smith, I. J. and Burnstock, G. (1998) Ultrastractural localization of P2X₃ receptors in rat sensory neurons. *NeuroReport,* **9,** 2545–2550.
38. Bo, X., Alavi, A., Xiang, Z., Oglesby, I. B., Ford, A. P. D. W., and Burnstock, G. (1999) Distribution of ATP-gated P2X₂ and P2X₃ receptor immunoreactive nerves in rat taste buds. *NeuroReport* **10,** 1107–1111.
39. Polak, J. M. and McGee, J. O'D. (eds.) (1998) *In Situ Hybridization: Principles and Practice.* Oxford University Press, Oxford, UK.
40. Wilkinson, D. G. (ed.) (1998) *In Situ Hybridization: A Practical Approach.* Oxford University Press, Oxford, UK.
41. Bo, X., Zhang, Y., Nassar, M., Burnstock, G., and Schoepfer, R. (1995) A P2X purinoceptor cDNA with novel pharmacological profile. *FEBS Lett.* **375,** 129–133.
42. Xiang, Z., Bo, X., and Burnstock, G. (1998) Localization of ATP-gated P2X receptor immunoreactivity in rat sensory and sympathetic ganglia. *Neurosci. Lett.* **256,** 105–108.
43. Bradbury, E. J., Burnstock, G., and McMahon, S. B. (1998) The expression of P2X₃ purinoceptors in sensory neurons: effects of axotomy and glial-derived neurotrophic factor. *Mol. Cell. Neurosci.* **12,** 256–268.

5

Small Conductance Calcium-Activated Potassium Channels in Rat Brain

Autoradiographic Localization Using Two Specific Toxins, Apamin and Scyllatoxin

Marc Borsotto

1. INTRODUCTION

Calcium-dependent potassium channels (KCa channels) are involved in numerous physiological processes such as neurosecretion, action potential, and regulation of repetitive activity *(1,2)*. As regards to their biophysical and pharmacological properties, KCa channels can be divided into three groups called BKCa, IKCa, and SKCa channels.

BKCa channels have a large unitary conductance (150–200 pS) *(3,4)*, and are present in the plasma membrane of numerous excitable and nonexcitable cells. These channels are voltage-sensitive, and are blocked by TEA *(5)* and by scorpion toxins such as charybdotoxin *(6,7)* and iberiotoxin *(8)*. They are responsible for the fast component of the afterhyperpolarization phase (a phase that follows an action potential) and then they help to repolarize the cell membrane *(2,9,10)*.

IKCa channels exhibit a single channel conductance of 20–80 pS, and are present in blood cells *(11)* and in smooth muscle cells *(12,13)*. They are voltage-sensitive. IKCa channels are weakly sensitive to TEA and are blocked by charybdotoxin but not by iberiotoxin *(14)*. It was proposed that these channels could help set the cell resting potential and regulate electrogenic processes *(15)*.

SKCa channels have smaller single-channel conductances of 8–20 pS *(16,17)*. They are activated in a voltage independent manner by submicromolar calcium concentrations, and are TEA-insensitive *(4)*. They

From: *Ion Channel Localization Methods and Protocols*
Edited by: A. Lopatin and C. G. Nichols © Humana Press Inc., Totowa, NJ

are found in a wide variety of excitable and nonexcitable cells where they play fundamental roles. These channels are activated by the calcium increase, which occurs during an action potential, and their activation produces a membrane hyperpolarization, which results in an inhibition of the cell firing. The decrease of the intracellular calcium concentration is slow, indicating that SKCa channels opening generates a long-lasting hyperpolarization also called slow afterhyperpolarization (sAHP) *(16)*. Controlling sAHP is essential to control spike frequency of repetitive action potentials and necessary for a normal neurotransmission by protecting the cell from tetanic activity.

SKCa channels can be divided into two classes *(18)*, channels that are sensitive to the bee-venom toxin apamin and those that are apamin insensitive. Apamin-insensitive SKCa channels are rare; the most studied and the best characterized are those present in hippocampal pyramidal neurons *(2,19)*. Some cells, such as vagal neurons, express both apamin-sensitive and -insensitive SKCa channels *(18,20,21)*.

Apamin, a peptidic neurotoxin isolated from the honey bee *Apis mellifera* venom, was the first purified and characterized toxin acting on potassium channels. Apamin is a highly basic peptide of 18 amino acids (MW = 2000) tightly bridged by two disulfide bounds *(22)*. Apamin is one of the rare toxins able to pass through the blood–brain barrier (BBB). Structure-function studies demonstrated that the two arginine residues at positions 13 and 14 are essential for the apamin activity *(23,24)*. It was also shown that the integrity of the histidine residue 18 is not required for toxin activity. These observations allowed the preparation of a radioactive monoiododerivative of apamin *(23)*, which was widely used to characterize the biochemical properties of the apamin receptor. Using ^{125}I-apamin it was determined that the affinity of apamin for its receptors was very high, Kd = 10–60 pM, but that the number of apamin receptors was very low; the maximal number of sites (B$_{max}$) ranged from 1–60 fmol/mg of protein *(23,25–28)*. Only the pheochromocytoma cell line (PC12) possess apamin binding sites with different properties, high number of sites (B$_{max}$ = 600 fmol/mg of protein), and low affinity (Kd = 350 pM) *(29,30)*. Apamin-sensitive SKCa channels are also blocked by a neurotoxin purified from the venom of the scorpion *Leiurus quinquestriatus hebraeus* called scyllatoxin (or leiurotoxin). Scyllatoxin (ScyTx) is a 31 amino acid peptide (MW = 3400) bridged by three disulfide bounds, structurally and immunologically unrelated to apamin *(31,32)*. Structure-function studies using chemical modifications of ScyTx have shown that the arginine residues at positions 6 and 13 were essential for both the binding and functional effect of the toxin *(33)*. The integrity of the histidine residue 31 is necessary for a fully active toxin *(32,33)*, thus to obtain a iodinated peptide, the preparation of a synthetic derivative of ScyTx where the Phe residue at position 2 was replaced by a Tyr residue, Tyr2-ScyTx, was necessary *(32)*.

[125]I-Tyr2-ScyTx binding experiments indicate that the affinity of the toxin for its receptors is also very high, Kd = 80 to 150 pM, and that the number of the receptor sites is in the same range as that of apamin; B_{max} = 1–50 fmol/mg protein *(32)*. ScyTx acts as a competitive inhibitor for the ^{125}I-apamin and its receptor, and conversely apamin competitively inhibits ^{125}I-Tyr2-ScyTx binding *(32)*.

In the central nervous system (CNS), apamin-sensitive SKCa channels are involved in a number of important processes. Injection with sublethal doses of apamin produces: 1) an accelerated acquisition and a better retention of learned tasks in rats and mice *(34,35)*, associated with an increase in the amounts of c-fos and c-jun mRNAs in the hippocampus *(36)*; and 2) a modification of the sleep patterns and a disturbance of the circadian cycle *(37)*.

From mammalian brain, three cDNAs encoding SK channels have been cloned *(10)*. These channels, called SK1, SK2, and SK3, belong to the potassium channel family with one P domain (the pore-forming region) and six transmembrane domains *(10)*. Cloned SK channels display the same toxin-sensitivity difference, SK1 is apamin-insensitive (no effect for concentrations up to 100 nM), whereas SK2 and SK3 are both apamin sensitive. Nevertheless, their sensitivities are different; $K_{0.5}$ for apamin (concentration that inhibits 50% of the channel activity) are 60 pM and 1 nM for SK2 and SK3, respectively *(10,38)*. Molecular biology approaches have confirmed the heterogeneity of the SKCa channels seen with the biochemical and electrophysiological investigations.

Apamin receptors also exist in peripheral tissues. Apamin induces contractions of smooth muscles previously relaxed by epinephrin or neurotensin *(26)*. Normal adult skeletal muscle does not contain apamin receptors, however, on denervated skeletal muscles *(16,39)*, or on muscles from patients suffering of myotonic dystrophy (MD), apamin binding sites can be measured *(40)*. Apamin was shown to be able to abolish myotonia induced on arm muscles of patients with MD *(41)*; nevertheless, it appeared that MD is not owing to a defective gene of one of the cloned SKCa channels *(42)*.

Here we describe the use of apamin and scyllatoxin for localization of apamin sensitive SKCA channels in CNS by the *in situ* hybridization technique on rat brain sections.

2. MATERIALS AND METHODS

2.1. Animals

Adult male Sprague Dowley rats weighing 150–200 g were used. They were kept at constant room temperature under standardized light/dark condition (12 h/12 h). Food and water were given ad libitum.

2.2. Rat Brain Membrane Preparations

Synaptosome membranes were prepared from rat brains by the method described in Abita et al. *(43)*. Protein concentration was determined by the Hartree method *(44)*.

2.3. Radioactive Toxin Labeling

Iodinations at high specific radioactivity of toxins were obtained as described in *(23)* for apamin and in *(32)* for scyllatoxin.

2.4. Binding Experiments

Rat brain synaptosomes (0.3 mg/mL) were incubated with increasing concentrations of ^{125}I-apamin in a buffer containing 10 mM Tris-HCl at pH 8.0, 5.4 mM KCl and 0.1% bovine serum albumin (BSA). Samples were incubated for 30 min at 0°C and then 0.8 mL aliquots were filtered under reduced pressure through a GF/C filter (Whatman) presoaked for at least 1 h in 0.5% PolyEthylenImine (PEI) in water. Each filter was rapidly washed twice with 5 ml of cold 10 mM Tris-HCl, pH 8.0, and then counted in a gamma counter apparatus. Nonspecific binding was measured in parallel experiments in presence of an excess (1 μM) of unlabeled apamin.

2.5. Brain Section Preparation

Rats were halothane-anesthetized and sacrificed by decapitation; their brains were immediately removed and frozen in isopentan at –40°C. Brain sections 15-μm thick were cut on a cryostat microtome, and thaw-mounted onto polylysine- (or cold chromalun/gelatin-) coated glass slides. Slides were stored at –20°C until used.

Brain sections were preincubated 15 min at 4°C in a buffer containing 140 mM choline chloride, 5.4 mM KCl, 2.8 mM CaCl$_2$, 1.3 mM MgSO$_4$, 20 mM Tris-HCl, pH 7.4, and 0.1% BSA. Then sections were incubated 30 min at 4°C in the same buffer with 20 pM of ^{125}I-apamin dissolved in 100 mM Tris-HCl, pH 7.4/0.1%BSA. The nonspecific component was determined by using a large excess (1 μM) of unlabeled apamin added 15 min before adding 25 pM of ^{125}I-apamin. Scyllatoxin competition experiments were performed by adding to the binding buffer increasing concentrations, 10 pM to 10 µM, of synthetic unlabeled scyllatoxin instead of unlabeled apamin.

At the end of the incubation times, sections were washed 3 times for 20 s in 100 mM Tris-HCl pH 7.4/0.1% BSA and once in distilled water. Slides were dried with a cold stream of air and exposed on autoradiographic film for 12 d at room temperature.

2.6. *Autoradiogram Quantification*

Sets of ^{125}I standards were prepared as followed. Known amounts of inactivated ^{125}I-apamin were mixed with brain tissue aliquots previously crushed to an homogenous degazed paste; another alternative is to use commercial autoradiographic ^{125}I microscales (Amersham). Blocks were frozen in the same way as described for rat brains. 15-µm thick sections were cutted in a cryostat microtome and thaw-mounted onto glass slides. A set of ^{125}I standard slides was exposed on the same autoradiographic film as the labeled sections. Then standards were used to quantify the radioactivity by analyzing the film with a computer image analysis system (Pericolor 2000, Numelec).

Labeled slides were prepared by incubating sections with increasing concentrations, 6–400 pM, of ^{125}I-apamin in the same buffer as mentioned previously. Nonspecific binding was determined with 1 µM of unlabeled apamin. The nonspecific binding was homogenous over the whole brain. Specific binding component was calculated by subtracting the nonspecific component from the total binding. For each area a mean value was calculated from 6–8 measurements in three different animals. Biochemical parameters were calculated using the Scatchard plot analysis of the equilibrium binding data.

3. BRAIN DISTRIBUTION OF APAMIN RECEPTORS

The distribution of apamin-sensitive SKCa channels was approached using the quantitative autoradiographic analysis. Quantitative autoradiography is a particularly efficient technique to analyze mutual interaction in different parts of the brain (but also in a number of other tissues) of different types of toxins associated with one (or more) class of ionic channels. This type of technique is very dependent on the quality of the ligand used. The high affinity of apamin to its receptor was revealed as a very convenient characteristic to study the localization of apamin receptors on rat brain sections. Equilibrium binding studies on rat brain synaptosomes preparations indicated that the nonspecific binding of ^{125}I apamin is very low, less than 10% at a concentration corresponding approximately to the Kd value, 20 pM (Fig. 1A).

First kinetic of association of ^{125}I apamin to its receptor on rat brain sections was measured by using 20 pM of labeled toxin. The half-life of association determined was 11 min and the maximal binding was reached at 30 min. The nonspecific binding was homogeneously distributed and corresponded to less than 20% (Fig. 2B) at this concentration of iodinated apamin. A time of incubation of 30 min was chosen because it was long enough to reach equilibrium and short enough to preserve the integrity of the brain sections.

[125]I apamin binding to rat brain sections was found to be saturable and of high affinity. The Scatchard plot of these data indicated a Kd value of 25 pM and a Bmax value of 15.5 fmol/mg protein (Fig. 1B). These values are in good agrement with those measured on rat brain synaptosomes, Kd = 18 pM and Bmax = 12.5 fmol/mg protein (Fig. 1A).

Similar measurements can be performed with each brain area using the autoradiographic procedure; typical curves of equilibrium binding experiments are given in Fig. 1C,D. When brain sections were incubated with increasing concentrations of ^{125}I-apamin, the optical densities (ODs) of autoradiograms for the different brain structures increased. Computerization of these ODs by comparison with ODs of the radioactive standards allowed the calculation of the concentration of bound apamin on each area. Kd values measured with this protocol ranged from 15.0–26.1 pM; however, in the majority of the structures Kd values are in the 20 pM range. The Bmax value is dependent from the structure observed and varied from 2.0–61.6 fmol/mg of protein. The lower Bmax value is measured in the white matter tracts and the higher in the lateral septum area (for detailed results, *see* ref. *45*). The fact that Kd values are similar indicates that the observed variations in the autoradiographic labeling corresponds to a difference in the number of apamin binding sites between brain areas.

In the olfactory bulb, the higher site density was observed for the anterior nucleus (Fig. 2A) and the lower for the olfactory tubercle (Fig. 2B). As for the other white matter tracks, a very low-grain density was observed in the corpus callosum (Fig. 2B). Small differences of apamin binding sites were observed in different frontoparietal cortex regions (Fig. 2B,C). In the basal ganglia a moderate level of specific apamin binding was associated with the caudate putamens and with the accumbens nucleus and ventral pallidus (Fig. 2C,D). The globus pallidus presented a very low labeling (Fig. 2E). In the amygdala structure, only the basolateral and basomedial nuclei had a high

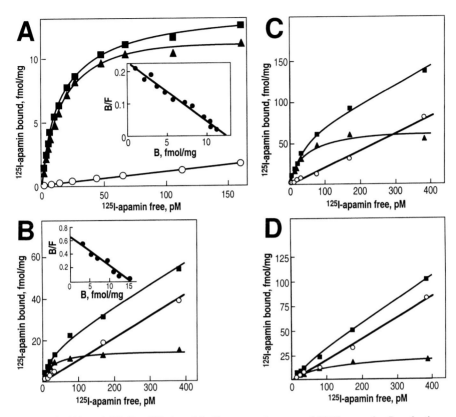

Fig. 1. (A) and **(B)** Equilibrium binding experiments of 125I-apamin. Incubations were performed as described in Section 2. **(A)** On rat brain synaptosomes. Each value is the mean of four determinations obtained from two separate experiments. Specific binding (▲) correspond to the difference between the total binding (■) and the non-specific binding (○). Inset, Scatchard plot of these data. **(B)** Specifically bound ^{125}I-apamin; F, free ^{125}I-apamin. Kd = 18 pM, Bmax = 12.5 fmol/mg of protein. **(B)** On coronal brain sections. For each concentration three section levels were used: 1) fore-brain with cerebral cortex and basal ganglia, 2) lower midbrain with hippocampus, and 3) hindbrain with cerebellum and medula oblongata. Each value is the mean of four determinations obtained with three separate experiments. (■) Total binding, (○) nonspecific binding, (▲) specific binding. Inset, Scatchard plot of these data, **(B)** specifically bound ^{125}I-apamin; F, free ^{125}I-apamin. Kd = 25 pM, Bmax = 15.5 fmol/mg of protein. **(C)** and **(D)** Autoradiogram determination of ^{125}I-apamin binding to coronal rat brain sections. Autoradiogram were obtained and quantified as described in Section 2. Each value represent the mean of 4–6 measurements for three studied animals. (■) Total binding, (○) nonspecific binding, (▲) specific binding. **(C)** Lateral septal nucleus. **(D)** Intermediate septal nucleus. Note the large difference in the specific binding between the two structures, Scatchard plots (not shown) indicate Kd values of 21.2 and 26.2 pM, and Bmax values of 29.4 and 8.0 fmol/mg of protein for lateral and intermediate septal nucleus, respectively.

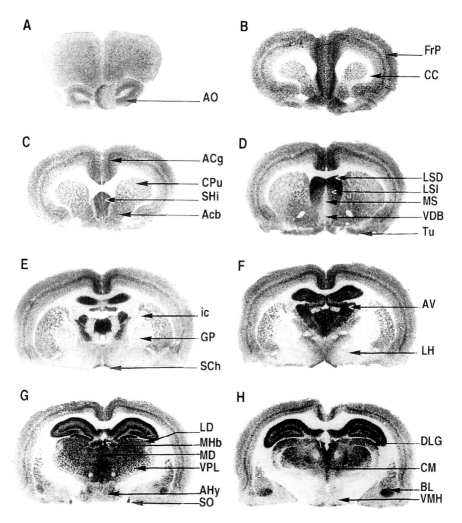

Fig. 2. Autoradiographic distribution of apamin receptors in rat brain. Coronal sections were incubated with 20 p*M* of ^{125}I-apamin in absence **(A–O)** or in presence **(nonspecific binding)** of 1 μ*M* of unlabeled apamin. Abbreviations: AO, anteror olfactory nucleus; FrP, frontoparital cortex; Acg, cingular cortex anterior area; Cpu, caudate putamen; Shi, septohippocampal nucleus; Acb, accumbes nucleus; LSD, dorsal lateral septum; LSI, intermediate lateral septum; MS, medial septum; VDB, diagonal band of the septum; Tu, olfactory tubercle; ic, internal capsule; GP, globus pallidus; SCh, suprachiasmatic nucleus; AV, anteroventral thalamic nucleus; LH, lateral hypothalamic area; LD, laterodorsal thalamic nucleus; MHb, medial habenula; MD, mediodorsal thalamic nucleus; VPL, ventroposterior thalamic nucleus; AHy, anterior hypothalamic area; SO, supraoptic hypothalamic nucleus;

(continued)

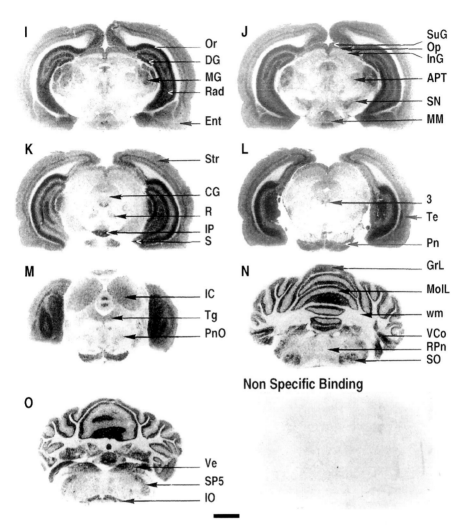

Non Specific Binding

DLG, dorsal lateral geniculate nucleus; CM, central medial thalamic nucleus; VMH, ventromedial hypothalamic nucleus; Or, stratum oriens; DG, dendate gyrus; MG, medial lateral geniculate nucleus; Rad, stratum radiatum; Ent, entorhinal cortex; SuG, superior colliculus; Op, optic nerve layer; InG, intermediate grey layer; APT, anterior pretectal area; SN, substancia nigra; MM, median mammilary nuclei; Str, striate cortex; CG, central grey; R, red nucleus; IP, interpeduncular nucleus; S, subiculum; 3, oculomotor nucleus; Te, temporal cortex auditory area; Pn, pontine nuclei; IC, inferior colliculus; Tg, tegmental dorsal nuclei; PnO, pontine reticular nucleus; GrL, cerebellar granular layer; Mol L, cerebellar molecular layer; wm, cerebellar fibers white matter tracts; Vco, ventral cochlear nucleus; RPn, raphe pontis nucleus; SOl, superior olive; Ve, vestibular nuclei; SP5, nucleus of the spinal tract of the trigeminal nerve; IO, inferior olive.

density of apamin receptor (Fig. 2G,H). Differences in the apamin binding site densities were seen in the septal region. The dorsal, ventral, and septohippocampal nuclei presented very high densities, whereas a moderate level of binding was observed over the intermediate lateral septal nucleus and a low level over the medial septal nucleus and the vertical limb of the diagonal band (Fig. 2D). Distribution of apamin binding sites was also heterogenous in the hippocampal formation. Stratum oriens and the subiculum possessed very high densities, whereas other hippocampal structures presented high to moderate levels of labeling (Fig. 2G–L). The majority of thalamus nuclei showed a moderate amount of apamin binding sites, whereas habenula showed a high density (Fig. 2G,H). A low level was found in the pretectal area (Fig. 2F–K) and in the hypothalamus (Fig. 2E–H). In the suprachiasmatic and supraoptic nuclei a very high labeling was observed (Fig. 2E–H). Moderate levels of apamin binding sites were seen in the inferior colliculus (Fig. 2M) and in the superficial gray layer of the superior colliculus; conversely, the deep layers presented only a low level (Fig. 2J–L). The cerebelar cortex presented a high apamin binding-site density in the granular layer and only a low density in the molecular layer (Fig. 2N,O).

Owing to a very fast dissociation kinetic ($t_{1/2}$ = 60 s) of ScyTx from its receptors, it was impossible to localize the ScyTx binding sites directly. However when ScyTx is used instead of apamin to inhibit the ^{125}I-apamin binding, three main groups of apamin binding sites can be distinguished by their ScyTx affinities (Fig. 3). The first group correspond to structures where ScyTx have high affinities for apamin receptors; $K_{0.5}$ comprised between 30–70 pM. The second group correspond to areas with intermediate affinities, $K_{0.5}$ of 100–500 pM, and the third group to areas with the lower affinities, $K_{0.5}$ of 800–1200 pM.

The first group contains regions like basolateral amygdaloid nucleus, striate cortex, central medial thalamic nucleus, medial septal nucleus, parietal cortex, central medial thalamic nucleus, ventral tegmental area, and temporal cortex, auditory area. Spinal tract of trigeminal nerve, lateral septum, and lateral peoptic area constitute the third group. All other brain structures containing apamin binding sites belong to the second group.

Apamin receptors identified in these experiments could in principle be present on several cell types existing on brain sections such as neuronal and neuroglial cells, and endothelial and smooth muscle cells of blood vessels. Apamin receptors have been found in smooth muscle *(25)* and the Kd values for the association of apamin are nearly the same as these found on nerve membranes *(23)*. However, for several reasons apamin receptors identified here are probably not related to the smooth muscle cells. First, the propor-

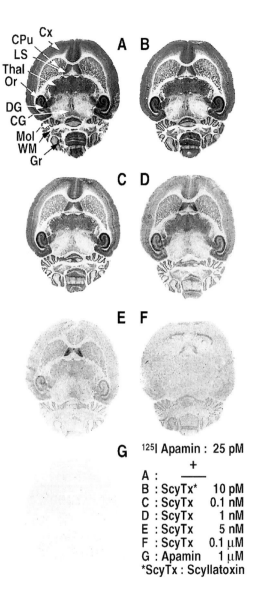

Fig. 3. Autoradiographic distribution of scyllatoxin binding sites in rat brain. Brain sections were incubated with 20 p*M* of ^{125}I-apaminin in the absence (**A**) or in the presence (**B–F**) of synthetic scyllatoxin or unlabeled apamin (**G**). Abbreviations: CG, central grey; Cpu, caudate putamen; Cx, neocortex; DG, dentate gyrus; Gr, cerebellar granular layer; LS, lateral septum; Mol, cerebellar molecular layer; Or, stratum oriens; Thal, thalamus; WM, white matter.

tion of muscular cells is negligible compared with the neuronal cells. Second, no correlation appeared between the number of apamin binding sites and the capillar density in different brain regions. Glial cell paticipation in ^{125}I-apamin binding cannot be evaluated unambiguously by the autoradiographic analysis used here. Nevertheless, the white matter of cerebellum, which contains oligodendrocytes and fibrous astrocytes in high densities, only presents a very low level of apamin binding. Moreover, the cerebellar cortex, which is rich in astrocytes, is poor in apamin binding sites, whereas the granular layer where the glial cell density is very low, is much richer in apamin binding sites. These observations suggest that the presence of apamin receptors on rat brain sections is associated with the neuronal cells.

Confirmation was brought by the cloning of cDNAs encoding SKCa channels where one of them, SK1, is apamin insensitive and two of them, SK2 and SK3, are apamin sensitive *(10)*. *In situ* hybridization performed with antisense RNA probes indicates an excellent correlation between radioactive toxin labeling and nucleic acid probe labeling *(10)*. SK1-mRNAs are mainly localized, as expected, in hippocampal formations, but also in the anterior olfactory nucleus, and to a lesser extent in olfactory tubercule, in cerebellum, and in cortex. SK2-mRNAs are the most widely expressed, particularly in the hippocampus formations, in anterior olfactory nucleus, and in granular layer of cerebellum. SK3-mRNA are also widely distributed, with a maximal labeling in the lateral septum and the supraoptic nucleus of the thalamus.

Autoradiographic studies performed on rat brain sections with ^{125}I-apamin demonstrated a very heterogenous distribution of the apamin receptors. In the whole brain, apamin binds to its receptors with the same affinity, whereas ScyTx affinities allows the discrimination between the three different groups of apamin receptors. Several hypotheses could explain the existence of these three types of structures: 1) three types of receptors, one for each group; 2) two types of receptors, one with a high affinity and another with a low affinity. (The group two [intermediate affinities] would be a mixture of the two types; the low number of binding sites would explain the reason why they are undifferentiated by the classical equilibrium binding experiment analysis); and 3) only one type of receptors would exist, the ScyTx binding affinities, then, would be modulated by different associated proteins.

Identification of endogenous equivalent of apamin in pig brain *(46)* and scyllatoxin in PC12 cells *(30)* argued in favor of the existence of several apamin-sensitive SKCa subtypes. Recent cloning of the three cDNAs encoding SKCa channels *(10)* clearly indicates that more than one receptor type exists because both SK2 and SK3 are able to bind apamin, although with different affinity. At the time of this writing, no other cloning of SKCa channels was published (the SK4 isolated from fetal human brain *[15]* corresponded to an IKCa channel); however, we cannot exclude the existence of other members of this channel family. Intermediate affinities could also be supported by the formation of heteromultimeric channels. It was shown that SK1 (apamin-insensitive) and SK2 (apamin-sensitive) could assemble and give rise to channels with intermediate sensitivities for apamin inhibition *(38)*. Heteromultimeric channel formation, together with the post-translation modifications such as phosphorylation by protein kinases *(47,48)*, could account for differences seen in sAHP in different brain regions *(49,50)*.

4. CONCLUSION

Quantitative autoradiography analysis allowed the identification of brain structures that contain apamin receptors. The use of two highly specific toxins, apamin and scyllatoxin, led to discrimination between three different groups as a function of their affinities for scyllatoxin, because apamin has equivalent affinities for receptors belonging to the three groups. These results indicated that apamin-sensitive potassium channels do not correspond to a unique channel protein but to a family of channel proteins. These observations revealed the increased complexity of the SKCa channels, because it was already established the existence of channels that were or were not sensitive to apamin. These hypotheses were recently confirmed by the cloning of three cDNAs encoding SKCa channels. One of them is apamin-insensitive and the two others are differently sensitive to apamin. The complexity was even further increased by the fact that these proteins could assemble to form heteromultimeric channels with intermediate biophysical and pharmacological properties.

Existence of both specific toxins and cDNAs offer real opportunities to understand the contribution of the different sAHP in physiological processes where SKCa (apamin-sensitive and -insensitive) participate. This is of particular interest because SKCa channels are described to be involved in functions as different as learning, memory, circadian-rhythm control, and sleep-wake cycle duration. SKCa channels could constitute an important target for therapeutic treatment of disorders concerning these different CNS functions, but also for some diseases affecting peripheral organs like smooth or skeletal muscles.

ACKNOWLEDGMENTS

We thank F. Aguila for his expert photographical assitance and V. Lopez for her skilled secretarial assistance. This work was supported by the Centre National de la Recherche Scientifique.

REFERENCES

1. Vergara, C., Latorre, R., Marrion, N. V., and Adelman, J. P. (1998) Calcium-activated potassium channels. *Curr. Opin. Neurobiol.* **8(3)**, 321–329.
2. Sah, P. (1996) Ca(2+)-activated K+ currents in neurones: types, physiological roles and modulation. *Trends Neurosci.* **19(4)**, 150–154.
3. Marty, A. (1989) The physiological role of calcium-dependent channels. *Trends Neurosci.* **12(11)**, 420–424.
4. Romey, G. and Lazdunski, M. (1984) The coexistence in rat muscle cells of two distinct classes of Ca^{2+}-dependent K^+ channels with different pharmacological properties and different physiological functions. *Biochem. Biophys. Res. Commun.* **118**, 669–674.
5. Latorre, R. (1986) Ion channel reconstitution, in *The Large Calcium-Activated Potassium Channel* (Miller, ed.), Plenum, New York, pp. 431–467.
6. Gimenez-Gallego, G., Navia, M. A., Reuben, J. P., Katz, G. M., Kaczorowski, G. J., and Garcia, M. L. (1988) Purification, sequence, and model structure of charybdotoxin, a potent selective inhibitor of calcium-activated potassium channels. *Proc. Natl. Acad. Sci. USA* **85 (10)**, 3329–3333.
7. McKinnon, R. and Miller, C. (1988) Mechanism of charybdotoxin block of the high-conductance, Ca^{2+}-activated K^+ channel. *J. Gen. Physiol.* **91**, 335–349.
8. Galvez, A., Gimenez-Gallego, G., Reuben, J. P., Roy-Contancin, L., Feigenbaum, P., Kaczorowski, G. J., and Garcia, M. L. (1990) Purification and characterization of a unique, potent, peptidyl probe for the high conductance calcium-activated potassium channel from venom of the scorpion Buthus tamulus. *J. Biol. Chem.* **265(19)**, 11,083–11,090.
9. Viana, F., Bayliss, D. A., and Berger, A. J. (1993) Multiple potassium conductances and their role in action potential repolarization and repetitive firing behavior of neonatal rat hypoglossal motoneurons. *J. Neurophysiol.* **69(6)**, 2150–2163.
10. Kohler, M., Hirschberg, B., Bond, C. T., Kinzie, J. M., Marrion, N. V., Maylie, J., and Adelman, J. P. (1996) Small-conductance, calcium-activated potassium channels from mammalian brain [see comments]. *Science* **273(5282)**, 1709–1714.
11. Grinstein, S., Dupre, A., and Rothstein, A. (1982) Volume regulation by human lymphocytes. Role of calcium. *J. Gen. Physiol.* **79(5)**, 849–868.
12. Ishii, T. M., Silvia, C., Hirschberg, B., Bond, C. T., Adelman, J. P., and Maylie, J. (1997) A human intermediate conductance calcium-activated potassium channel. *Proc. Natl. Acad. Sci. USA* **94(21)**, 11,651–11,656.
13. Morris, A. P., Gallacher, D. V., and Lee, J. A. (1986) A large conductance, voltage- and calcium-activated K+ channel in the basolateral membrane of rat enterocytes. *FEBS Lett.* **206(1)**, 87–92.
14. Castle, N. A. and Strong, P. N. (1986) Identification of two toxins from scorpion (Leiurus quinquestriatus) venom which block distinct classes of calcium-activated potassium channel. *FEBS Lett.* **209(1)**, 117–121.
15. Joiner, W. J., Wang, L. Y., Tang, M. D., and Kaczmarek, L. K. (1997) hSK4, a member of a novel subfamily of calcium-activated potassium channels. *Proc. Natl. Acad. Sci. USA* **94(20)**, 11,013–11,018.

16. Blatz, A. L. and Magleby, K. L. (1986) Single apamin-blocked Ca-activated K+ channels of small conductance in cultured rat skeletal muscle. *Nature* **323(6090)**, 718–720.

17. Maruyama, Y., Gallacher, D. V., and Petersen, O. H. (1983) Voltage and Ca2+-activated K+ channel in baso-lateral acinar cell membranes of mammalian salivary glands. *Nature* **302(5911)**, 827–829.

18. Sah, P. and McLachlan, E. M. (1991) Ca(2+)-activated K+ currents underlying the afterhyperpolarization in guinea pig vagal neurons: a role for Ca(2+)-activated Ca2+ release. *Neuron* **7(2)**, 257–264.

19. Lancaster, B. and Adams, P. R. (1986) Calcium-dependent current generating the afterhyperpolarization of hippocampal neurons. *J. Neurophysiol.* **55(6)**, 1268–1282.

20. Schwindt, P. C., Spain, W. J., and Crill, W. E. (1992) Effects of intracellular calcium chelation on voltage-dependent and calcium-dependent currents in cat neocortical neurons. *Neuroscience* **47(3)**, 571–578.

21. Lorenzon, N. M. and Foehring, R. C. (1992) Relationship between repetitive firing and afterhyperpolarizations in human neocortical neurons. *J. Neurophysiol.* **67(2)**, 350–363.

22. Vincent, J.-P., Schweitz, H., and Lazdunski, M. (1975) Structure-function relationships and site of action of apamin, a neurotoxic polypeptide of bee venom with an action on the central nervous system. *Biochemistry* **14**, 2081–2091.

23. Hugues, M., Duval, D., Kitabgi, P., Lazdunski, M., and Vincent, J.-P. (1982) Preparation of a pure monoiodo-derivative of the bee venom neurotoxin apamin and its binding properties to rat brain synaptosomes. *J. Biol. Chem.* **257**, 2762–2769.

24. Labbe-Jullie, C., Granier, C., Albericio, F., Defendini, M. L., Ceard, B., Rochat, H., and Van Rietschoten, J. (1991) Binding and toxicity of apamin. Characterization of the active site. *Eur. J. Biochem.* **196(3)**, 639–645.

25. Hugues, M., Duval, D., Schmid, H., Kitabgi, P., Lazdunski, M., and Vincent, J.-P. (1982) Specific binding and pharmacological interactions of apamin, the neurotoxin from bee venom, with guinea pig colon. *Life Sci.* **31**, 437–443.

26. Hugues, M., Schmid, H., Romey, G., Duval, D., Frelin, C., and Lazdunski, M. (1982) The Ca^{2+} dependent slow K^+ conductance in cultured rat muscle cells: characterization with apamin. *EMBO J.* **1**, 1039–1042.

27. Seagar, M. J., Deprez, P., Martin-Moutot, N., and Couraud, F. (1987) Detection and photoaffinity labelling of the Ca2+-activated K+ channel-associated apamin receptor in cultured astrocytes from rat brain. *Brain Res.* **411(2)**, 226–230.

28. Wu, K., Carlin, R., Sachs, L., and Siekevitz, P. (1985) Existence of a Ca2+-dependent K+ channel in synaptic membrane and postsynaptic density fractions isolated from canine cerebral cortex and cerebellum, as determined by apamin binding. *Brain Res.* **360(1–2)**, 183–194.

29. Schmid-Antomarchi, H., Hugues, M., and Lazdunski, M. (1986) Properties of the apamin-sensitive Ca^{2+}-activated K^+ channel in PC12 pheochromocytoma cells which hyper-produce the apamin receptor. *J. Biol. Chem.* **261**, 8633–8637.

30. Auguste, P., Hugues, M., Borsotto, M., Thibault, J., Romey, G., Coppola, T., and Lazdunski, M. (1992) Characterization and partial purification from

pheochromocytoma cells of an endogenous equivalent of Scyllatoxin, a scorpion toxin which blocks small conductance Ca^{2+}-activated K^+ channels. *Brain Res.* **599,** 230–236.

31. Castle, N. and Strong, P. (1986) Identification of two toxins from scorpion *(Leiurus quinquestriatus)* venom which block distinct classes of calcium-activated potassium channel. *FEBS Lett.* **209,** 117–121.

32. Auguste, P., Hugues, M., Grave, B., Gesquiere, J. C., Maes, P., Tartar, A., Romey, G., Schweitz, H., and Lazdunski, M. (1990) Leiurotoxin I (scyllatoxin), a peptide ligand for Ca2(+)-activated K+ channels. Chemical synthesis, radiolabelling, and receptor characterization. *J. Biol. Chem.* **265(8),** 4753–4759.

33. Auguste, P., Hugues, M., Mourre, C., Moinier, D., Tartar, A., and Lazdunski, M. (1992) Scyllatoxin, a blocker of Ca(2+)-activated K+ channels: structure-function relationships and brain localization of the binding sites. *Biochemistry* **31(3),** 648–654.

34. Deschaux, O., Bizot, J. C., and Goyffon, M. (1997) Apamin improves learning in an object recognition task in rats. *Neurosci. Lett.* **222(3),** 159–162.

35. Messier, C., Mourre, C., Bontempi, B., Sif, J., Lazdunski, M., and Destrade, C. (1991) Effect of apamin, a toxin that inhibits Ca(2+)-dependent K+ channels, on learning and memory processes. *Brain Res.* **551(1–2),** 322–326.

36. Heurteaux, C., Messier, C., Destrade, C., and Lazdunski, M. (1993) Memory processing and apamin induce immediate early gene expression in mouse brain. *Brain Res. Mol. Brain. Res.* **18(1–2),** 17–22.

37. Gandolfo, G., Schweitz, H., Lazdunski, M., and Gottesmann, C. (1996) Sleep cycle disturbances induced by Apamin, a selective blocker of Ca^{2+}-activated K^+ channels. *Brain Res.* **736,** 344–347.

38. Ishii, T. M., Maylie, J., and Adelman, J. P. (1997) Determinants of apamin and d-tubocurarine block in SK potassium channels. *J. Biol. Chem.* **272(37),** 23,195–23,200.

39. Schmid-Antomarchi, H., Renaud, J. F., Romey, G., Hugues, M., Schmid, A., and Lazdunski, M. (1985) The all-or-none role of innervation in expression of apamin receptor and of apamin-sensitive Ca2+-activated K+ channel in mammalian skeletal muscle. *Proc. Natl. Acad. Sci. USA* **82(7),** 2188–2191.

40. Renaud, J. F., Desnuelle, C., Schmid-Antomarchi, H., Hugues, M., Serratrice, G., and Lazdunski, M. (1986) Expression of apamin receptor in muscles of patients with myotonic muscular dystrophy. *Nature* **319(6055),** 678–680.

41. Behrens, M. I., Jalil, P., Serani, A., Vergara, F., and Alvarez, O. (1994) Possible role of apamin-sensitive K+ channels in myotonic dystrophy. *Muscle Nerve* **17(11),** 1264–1270.

42. Harley, H. G., Rundle, S. A., Reardon, W., Myring, J., Crow, S., Brook, J. D., et al. (1992) Unstable DNA sequence in myotonic dystrophy. *Lancet* **339 (8802),** 1125–1128.

43. Abita, J. P., Chicheportiche, R., Schweitz, H., and Lazdunski, M. (1977) Effects of neurotoxins (veratridine, sea anemone toxin, tetrodotoxin) on transmitter accumulation and release by nerve terminals in vitro. *Biochemistry* **16(9),** 1838–1844.

44. Hartree, E. F. (1972) Determination of protein: a modification of the Lowry method that gives a linear photometric response. *Anal. Biochem.* **48(2),** 422–427.
45. Mourre, C., Hugues, M., and Lazdunski, M. (1986) Quantitative autoradiographic mapping in rat brain of the receptor of apamin, a polypeptide toxin specific for one class of Ca^{2+}-dependent K^+ channels. *Brain Res.* **382,** 239–249.
46. Fosset, M., Schmid-Antomarchi, H., Hugues, M., Romey, G., and Lazdunski, M. (1984) The presence in pig brain of an endogenous equivalent of apamin, the bee venom peptide that specifically blocks Ca^{2+}-dependent K^+ channels. *Proc. Natl. Acad. Sci. USA* **81,** 7228–7232.
47. Lancaster, B., Nicoll, R. A., and Perkel, D. J. (1991) Calcium activates two types of potassium channels in rat hippocampal neurons in culture. *J. Neurosci.* **11(1),** 23–30.
48. Pedarzani, P. and Storm, J. F. (1996) Evidence that Ca/calmodulin-dependent protein kinase mediates the modulation of the Ca2+-dependent K+ current, IAHP, by acetylcholine, but not by glutamate, in hippocampal neurons. *Pflugers Arch.* **431(5),** 723–728.
49. Lancaster, B. and Zucker, R. S. (1994) Photolytic manipulation of Ca2+ and the time course of slow, Ca(2+)- activated K+ current in rat hippocampal neurones. *J. Physiol.* **475(2),** 229–239.
50. Sah, P. and McLachlan, E. M. (1992) Potassium currents contributing to action potential repolarization and the afterhyperpolarization in rat vagal motoneurons. *J. Neurophysiol.* **68(5),** 1834–1841.

6

Mapping N-Type Calcium Channel Distributions with ω-Conotoxins

Geula M. Bernstein and Owen T. Jones

1. INTRODUCTION

1.1. General Background

Natural toxins have revolutionized the study of ion channels (1). Owing to their specificity and potency, toxins form the basis of many of the most important ligands used by modern biologists to identify, discriminate, manipulate, or purify ion channels. An excellent example of the biological contribution of toxins is the use of analogs of ω-conotoxin GVIA (ω-CgTx) in visualizing the distribution of N-type voltage-dependent calcium channels (N-VDCCs) in neurons (Table 1). ω-conotoxin GVIA was first isolated from the venom of the Pacific cone snail *Conus geographus* by Olivera and colleagues (2). This toxin drew attention because of its unusual pharmacological properties, which electrophysiological (3,4) and biochemical studies (5,6) now indicate are owing to blockade of voltage-dependent Ca^{2+} influx into neurons by its exclusive interaction with N-VDCCs (*see* Section 1.2.2.). Surprisingly, native ω-CgTx proved to be a polypeptide of just 27 amino acids (Fig. 1A), much shorter than most previously identified polypeptide toxins (2). Preparation of a synthetic analog of ω-CgTx confirmed both its structure and activity (7).

1.2. Properties of ω-CgTx

1.2.1. Physical Properties

Owing to the commercial availability of pure ω-CgTx in radiolabeled and unlabeled forms and its small size, it is one of the most extensively charac-

From: *Ion Channel Localization Methods and Protocols*
Edited by: A. Lopatin and C. G. Nichols © Humana Press Inc., Totowa, NJ

Table 1
Examples of the Use of ω-CgTx-Based Labels in N-VDCC Mapping

Detection label	Preparation	Use	Refs.
Fl-ω-CgTx, Cy3-ω-CgTx	Rat hippocampal brain slices	Density and distribution of N-VDCCs in kindled model of temporal lobe epilepsy	(25,26)
Fl-ω-CgTx	Rat hippocampal brain slices	Spatio-temporal distribution of N-VDCCs in development	(6)
Fl-ω-CgTx	Rat hippocampal brain slices	Distribution of N-VDCCs — emphasis on dendritic spines	(20)
TmRhd-ω-CgTx	Mouse postnatal day 10 cerebellar brain slices	Temporal expression of granule cell N-VDCCs	(39)
TmRhd-ω-CgTx	Xenopus sartorius muscle	Spatial distribution of N-VDCCs along motor nerve terminal	(15)
TmRhd-ω-CgTx	Rat hippocampal CA1 cultured neurons	Spatial distribution and mobility (FRAP) of N-VDCCs	(13)
[^{125}I]-ω-CgTx	Rabbit brain slices	Distribution of centrally administered ω-CgTx in vivo	(36)
[^{125}I]-ω-CgTx	Rat brain slices	Spatio-temporal expression of N-VDCCs in development	(24)
[^{125}I]-ω-CgTx	Human hippocampal and cerebellar slices	Distribution of N-VDCCs	(27)
[^{125}I]-ω-CgTx	Rat brain slices	Distribution of N-VDCCs	(28)
[^{125}I]-ω-CgTx	Brain slices of cerebellar mutant mice (pcd and weaver)	Distribution of N-VDCCs	(29)
[^{125}I]-ω-CgTx	Rat brain slices	Distribution of N-VDCCs	(30)
[^{125}I]-ω-CgTx	Rat brain slices	Distribution of N-VDCCs	(31)
Biotinylated-ω-CgTx	Chick ciliary ganglion	Localization of N-VDCCs at presynaptic nerve terminal	(17)
Biotinylated-ω-CgTx	Membranes of electric organ of Torpedo marmorata	Colloidal gold labeling and freeze fracture of N-VDCCs at nerve terminals	(18)
Biotinylated-ω-CgTx	Frog neuromuscular junction	Distribution of N-VDCCs at synaptic terminal	(16)
Anti-ω-CgTx antibodies	Human sural nerve	Localization of N-VDCCs in C-fibers	(32)
Anti-ω-CgTx antibodies	Teleost neurons	Distribution of N-VDCCs in cerebellar and electrosensory neurons	(33)
Anti-ω-CgTx antibodies	Rat cerebellar brain slices	Distribution of N-VDCCs	(34)

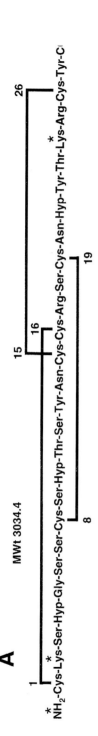

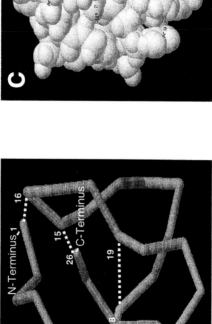

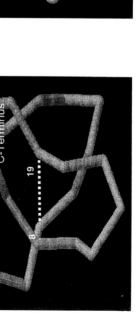

Fig. 1. Structure of ω-CgTx. (**A**) Primary amino acid sequence showing disulfide bonds (lines). (**B**) Conformation of ω-C polypeptide backbone showing positions of disulphide bonds. (**C**) Space filling model of ω-CgTx showing compact stru Note positions of nonpolar and basic residues. The structures in (B) and (C) were deduced from 2D NMR (8) and were gene from information in the Brookhaven database using the program RASMOL written by Roger Sayle.

terized toxins (2). The primary sequence of ω-CgTx is notable for its preponderance of hydrophilic residues, especially hydroxyproline. Also present are two lysine residues, which, together with two arginines and the amino terminus, give the toxin a basic character. Structural NMR (8) shows that, upon folding, the toxin adopts a compact structure stabilized by the formation of 3 disulfide bridges (Fig. 1).

1.2.2. Interaction with the N-Type Calcium Channel

The first evidence that ω-CgTx interacts with VDCCs came from its ability to block Ca^{2+} influx into synaptosomes. Such channels appeared distinct from those blocked by L-type VDCC ligands, notably dihydropyridines. Electrophysiology (3,4), biochemical purification (5), and direct pharmacological analysis of cloned VDCC subtypes expressed in transfected cells (9), indicates that the target for high-affinity ω-CgTx binding is the N-VDCC alone.

1.2.3. Structure-Activity Relationships

The binding of ω-CgTx seems to occur with a 1:1 stoichiometry at a binding pocket in the external face of N-VDCCs (4). In equilibrium binding studies, ω-CgTx interacts with N-VDCCs with extremely high affinity (K_d 40 pM) (6). Whether equilibrium is reached is equivocal, however. The association of ω-CgTx is rapid and largely complete within 10 min ($k_{on} = 3 \times 10^8 l \cdot mol^{-1} \cdot min^{-1}$), whereas any dissociation is extremely slow ($k_{off} = 5 \times 10^{-4}$ min^{-1}). The K_d's derived from the rates of binding are in the 0.1–5 pM range, much lower than the equilibrium values (6). This discrepancy may reflect binding to different channel conformations, consistent with biophysical data showing a preferential interaction with the inactivated state (10). For practical purposes, ω-CgTx binding is essentially irreversible. The high affinity probably reflects the ability of the toxin to make multipoint attachments with residues in the N-VDCC binding site.

1.3. Use of ω-CgTx-Based Labels in N-Channel Mapping Studies

1.3.1. General Background

The use of toxins in mapping ion channels has its origins in pioneering work on the nicotinic acetylcholine receptor (nAChR) and its selective, high affinity interaction with specific radio- or fluorescent-labeled analogs of snake-venom toxins (11,12). By labeling nAChRs with these toxin analogs, it became possible to visualize nAChR dynamics at the neuromuscular junction (NMJ) and, thus, define key aspects of synaptogenesis. Realizing the power of this strategy, several groups began to use toxin analogs to map neuronal voltage-dependent channels, a particularly difficult task owing to their much lower density than nAChRs at the NMJ. Even so, by 1989 developments in imaging permitted the mapping of N-VDCCs in central neurons *(13)*.

1.3.2. Mapping and the Distribution of N-type Calcium Channels

An immediate question is why one would want to map N-VDCCs? The answer lies in their key role in signal transduction *(14)*. Calcium channels, generally, represent the primary route by which voltage-changes are coupled to biochemical events. However, because Ca^{2+} diffusion is highly restricted in the nerve cytoplasm, the precise distribution of VDCCs is a major determinant of the local Ca^{2+} signaling and biochemical events defining nerve function. By targeting the appropriate VDCC subtypes to select regions, neurons can construct compartments with specific Ca^{2+} signaling properties. The highly polarized distribution of N-VDCCs is consistent with this notion.

N-VDCCs are concentrated at axon terminals but are absent from the axon shaft *(15–19)*. At the axon terminals, the voltage-dependent activation of presynaptic N-VDCCs provides, at least in part, the influx of Ca^{2+} that triggers neurotransmitter release at most central and some peripheral synapses *(18)*. A specific role for N-VDCCs in neurotransmission is supported by their alignment in bands at sites of transmitter release, at least in frog *(15,16)* and chick *(17)*. N-VDCCs are also found throughout most of the somata, dendrites, and discrete subsets of dendritic spines *(6,13,20–22)*. In dendrites, N-VDCCs seem to be involved in the back-propagation of action potentials and other plasticity-related phenomena *(23)*. Interestingly, in these locations N-VDCCs are often clustered *(6,13,20)*, indicating their possible recruitment into macromolecular signaling complexes. Significantly, N-VDCC distributions are highly dynamic and alter in synaptogenesis *(15)*, development *(6,24)*, and in models of seizure *(25,26)*. The distribution of N-VDCCs in tissues has also been determined for many species *(27–34)*.

1.3.3. Why Map N-Channels with ω-Conotoxins?

Diverse strategies have been employed for mapping N-VDCCs and other channels (Table 1), so why would one use ω-CgTx, i.e., visualization-based methods? In fact, there are numerous reasons. First, optical methods provide composite maps of N-VDCCs throughout the cell. In contrast, the major alternative — patch-clamp electrophysiology — involves "sampling" each region, an impossible feat for a single neuron. Second, ω-CgTx-based methods identify channels in regions of neurons that are too small to be accessed by recording electrodes and in any case are easily adapted for analysis at the electron microscopic level. Alternatives such as Ca^{2+} imaging are indirect, have poor resolution and sensitivity, and are restricted to regions with many active channels. Third, only ω-CgTx-based methods permit the live imaging needed to resolve the cellular dynamics of N-VDCCs and how they respond to factors such as electrical activity, cell contact, and disease. Antibodies cannot be used because live imaging demands labels that access external regions of the channels. This condition is satisfied by the polar membrane-impermeant ω-CgTx, but antibodies to external regions of N-VDCCs have proved difficult to make. Immunocytochemistry also suffers from a more subtle problem, especially relevant to mapping and trafficking studies, concerning its tendency to overestimate the disposition of channels at the cell surface. Specifically, the cell-permeabilization steps needed for immunocytochemistry allow antibodies access to channel populations that are both intracellular (for example on trafficking vesicles) and at the cell surface, that are hard to resolve by light microscopy. One powerful alternative is to use green fluorescent protein (GFP) technology to visualize GFP-tagged N-VDCCs in live cells *(35)*. However, the transfection of such large constructs and the resolution of their trafficking and distribution is presently almost impossible in primary neurons. Fourth, because ω-CgTxs bind selectively and with high affinity to N-VDCCs in diverse species, including humans, rats, mice, rabbits, bovines, and frogs *(2)*, they are applicable to diverse experimental models. In contrast, the utility of antibodies (especially those against N-VDCC peptides) across species requires careful consideration of the target sequence.

1.3.4. Mapping N-Channels with ω-CgTxs: The Types of Labels and Their Advantages and Disadvantages

Four classes of ω-CgTx-based methods have been used to map N-VDCCs: autoradiography, immunochemistry, avidin-biotin, and fluorescence. Examples of each are given in Tables 1 and 2. Autoradiography and immunochemistry have major limitations and are not dealt with in detail.

1.3.4.1. AUTORADIOGRAPHY

Several studies have used autoradiography to map N-VDCCs in brain *(24,27–31,36)*, but this method is limited by its poor subcellular resolution, especially with the more common [^{125}I]-ω-CgTx label.

1.3.4.2. IMMUNOCYTOCHEMISTRY

Antibodies to ω-CgTx are available commercially and have been used to map N-VDCCs by indirect immunocytochemistry *(32–34)*. However, in spite of its high resolution, this method is limited to fixed rather than live tissue.

Table 2
Comparison of Methods Used to Map N-VDCCs

Methods	Live cells	Resolution	Composite mapping	Sensitivity	Simplicity	Cost of equipment	Cost of reagents	Commercial availability
Non-ω-CgTx-based								
Patch clamp								
Electrophysiology	+	+++	–	+++++	+	V. high	Low	+++++
Calcium imaging	+	++++	+	+++	+++	High	Low	+++++
Immunocytochemistry	+/–	+++++	+	+++++	++++	Med–high	Med	++
GFP-tagged channels	+	++++(+)	+	++++	+(++++)	Med–high	Med	–
ω-CgTx-based								
Autoradiography	–	++	+	+++	+++	Med	Med	+++++
Immunocytochemistry	–	+++++	+	+++++	++++	Med–high	Med	+++++
Avidin-biotin	+	++++(+)	+	++++(+)	+++	Med–high	Med	+++++
Fluorescent	+	++++(+)	+	++++(+)	+++++	High	Med	+++++

1.3.4.3. Biotinylated ω-CgTx

Methods using biotinylated ω-CgTx (Bi-ω-CgTx) rely on the extraordinarily high affinity of biotin for avidin or related proteins (K_d $10^{-15}M$). Tissues labeled with Bi-ω-CgTx are treated with avidin conjugated to a suitable reporter and are then imaged appropriately *(16–18)*. There are many advantages to such methods. First, they are applicable to live or fixed samples. Second, a plethora of reporters is available. Useful reporters include fluorophores and gold particles, the latter being used for silver enhanced or electron microscopy. Third, such methods can provide considerable signal amplification because avidin-conjugates often bear multiple reporters *(37)*. Fourth, Bi-ω-CgTx is easy to make as the conjugation reaction is efficient and the conjugates easy to detect during purification by high-performance liquid chromatography (HPLC). Fifth, the binding properties of Bi-ω-CgTx are well-characterized *(38)*. The only real disadvantage of this method is the multiple steps needed for labeling and the tendency of avidin and streptavidin (but to a lesser extent neutravidin) to bind nonspecifically with some cell surface components *(37)*.

1.3.4.4. Fluorescent ω-CgTx Analogs

The identification of N-VDCCs labeled with fluorescent analogs of ω-CgTx is the simplest way to map N-VDCC distributions, especially in live cells and thus forms the focus of the rest of this chapter *(6,13,15,20,25,26,39)*. Their advantages over other ω-CgTx-based methods include the ease of labeling and detection, applicability to live imaging and the potential use of the fluorophore as an antigen in subsequent immunocytochemistry. Moreover, fluorescent-ω-CgTxs can be used for other specialized fluorescence applications such as fluorescence photobleach recovery (FPR) studies of N-VDCC mobility *(13)* and energy-transfer measurements. The major disadvantage is that fluorescent ω-CgTxs are not especially easy to prepare, although several are available commercially. The low number of fluorophores associated with each labeled channel is another potential disadvantage, but the severity of this problem largely depends on the sensitivity of the imaging microscope.

2. METHODS

For the sake of simplicity and their versatility, we will focus on the preparation, characterization and use of fluorescent ω-CgTxs. In addition, because fluorescent ω-CgTxs are somewhat more difficult to prepare than their biotinylated counterparts, they amply illustrate the bulk of pitfalls likely to be encountered. For a wider treatment of the design, construction, and use of fluorescent ligands, *see* ref. *40*.

2.1. Preparation of Fluorescent ω-Conotoxins

2.1.1. Some Basic Considerations

The ideal fluorescent ω-CgTx is a conjugate whose emission is well-resolved from any background fluorescence and whose high affinity limits the time-dependent decrease in specific fluorescence caused by dissociation and dilution into the surrounding medium. Both the fluorescence and the affinity depend on the choice of fluorophore. Ideal fluorophores are those that are bright, photostable, and have physicochemical properties that do not unduly influence the N-VDCC-ω-CgTx interaction or the solubility of the ω-CgTx. No particular fluorophore is ideal but some are considerably better than others, our preference is for those that are water-soluble and excited by the emission lines of our available microscopes. Fluorophores to avoid are those that emit <500 nm owing to cellular autofluorescence, ones that are very nonpolar such as most pyrene derivatives, and those that are extremely large such as phycocyanins (MW >700,000). Some fluorophores can give wholly unexpected problems. Thus, the Bodipy dyes are highly quenched when conjugated to ω-CgTx and are destroyed by many common HPLC solvents. Also important is whether the fluorophore is available in a suitable form for conjugation. Fortunately, most common fluorophores are available as reactive intermediates from suppliers such as Molecular Probes, Inc. (www.probes.com). Finally, fluorophores for which antibodies are available are useful as they can be used in immunocytochemistry. Moreover, because many anti-fluorophore antibodies quench the fluorescence of the fluorophore, and are cell-impermeant, they can be used to resolve cell surface (quenchable) and intracellular (nonquenchable) label. A list of excellent fluorophores and their structures is given in Table 3.

2.1.2. Labeling

The attachment of fluorophores to ω-CgTx relies upon the availability of chemically reactive amino acid functional groups in the polypeptide. Several potentially useful residues exist (notably the N-terminus, lysines, arginines, and tyrosine) but almost all ω-CgTx conjugation reactions target the primary amines of the N-terminus and the lysines (at positions 2 and 24) *(25,38)*. The reasons are twofold. First, the chemistry of amine conjugations is simple and well defined. Second, diverse fluorophores containing amine-reactive functional groups are available. The most useful functional groups are the *N*-hydroxysuccinimidyl (NHS) esters (or their more water-soluble Sulfo-NHS counterparts), because these are mild, efficient, and leave few

Table 3
Structures, Wavelengths of Maximum Excitation (λ_{ex}) and Emission (g_{em}), and Extinction Coefficients of Useful Fluorophores for Conjugation to ω-CgTx

Fluorophore	Structure	λ_{ex}	λ_{em}	ε (lit/mol/cm)
Cy3		550	570	150,000
5-Carboxyfluorescein (5-FAM)		494	517	78,000
Alexa Fluor 546		556	572	99,000
Texas Red		595	615	112,000
5-Carboxytetramethylrhodamine (5-TAMRA)		555	580	89,000

by-products. The basic conjugation reaction, shown in Fig. 2. involves aminolysis of the NHS-ester of the desired fluorophore. A reliable recipe that works every time is given in the accompanying flow chart for Fluorescein ω-CgTx (Fig. 3).

2.1.3. Resolution of the Labeling Reaction Mixture

Once terminated, the labeling reaction must be resolved to isolate the desired products. This is not always easy. Owing to the presence of three potentially reactive sites in ω-CgTx, there are as many as seven species of conjugate (3 singly-, 3 doubly-, and 1 triply-labeled) as well as unreacted ω-CgTx. There are also numerous dye products including the hydrolyzed

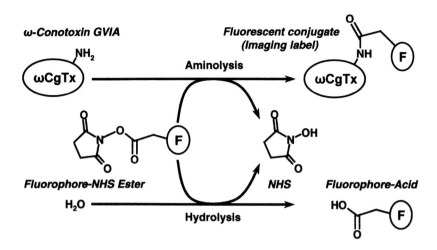

Fig. 2. Reaction for the conjugation of a fluorescent label to ω-CgTx. The desired labeling reaction involves aminolysis of the active N-hydroxysuccinimidyl (NHS) ester form of the fluorophore (F) with a lysine side chain or N-terminal amine in ω-CgTx. The competing reaction, involving hydrolysis of the NHS-label to the non-amine reactive fluorophore acid, is also shown.

fluorophore and its glycine adduct. To make matters worse, some labels are impure or isomeric mixtures.

The most important task is to remove any unreacted ω-CgTx, because this will compete with the fluorescent ω-CgTx for N-VDCC binding sites. Free dye products must also be removed to prevent nonspecific staining. The best way to achieve these objectives satisfactorily is through the use of HPLC (Fig. 3) *(6,13,20,25,38)*. The losses encountered with alternative chromatographic methods owing to nonspecific binding are enormous, even with columns equilibrated with eluents containing carrier proteins such as bovine serum albumin (BSA). The dye and unmodified toxin removal steps can be done in one step by reversed-phase HPLC (RP-HPLC) on a C_{18} column *(13)*. However, it is much easier to identify the products if the ω-CgTx-containing materials are first resolved from the dye components using an ion-exchange step *(6,40)*. The column we prefer is the sulfopropyl-based TSK SP5W. Once a useful elution profile has been established, it is usually possible to optimize the run time. One effective strategy for anionic labels is first to elute all the free dye products, then elute the protein-containing fractions in one step using a high salt solution. The protein-containing fraction,

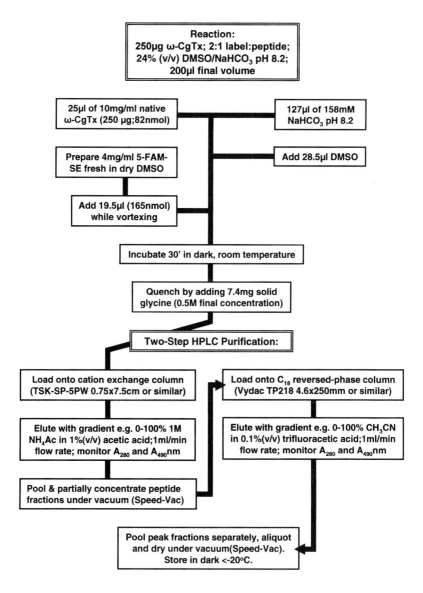

Fig. 3. Flow chart for the labeling and purification of fluoresceinated ω-CgTx (5-FAM-ω-CgTx). Note: The NHS (or sulfo-NHS) esters rapidly hydrolyze to the nonreactive fluorophore-carboxylate, especially at alkaline pHs. Thus, stock solutions of the NHS-labels should be made in dimethylsulphoxide (DMSO) and used fresh (preferable), or kept frozen until needed. The sulfo-NHS labels are best made in water and used immediately. Because NHS (or sulfo-NHS) esters react with unprotonated amines, the conjugation reaction is favoured by higher pHs but such

(continued)

now devoid of dye, can then be partially concentrated and resolved by the reversed-phase C_{18} column.

The simplest way to identify each species of product is to compare chromatograms corresponding to the conjugation reaction with those for parallel control reactions lacking either ω-CgTx or label *(40)* (Fig. 4). Because HPLC runs and solvents can vary slightly with time, it is best to run all chromatograms on the same day, the conjugation reaction being run after the controls. Peaks are best identified using an absorbance detector. Whereas pure ω-CgTx and most fluorophores can be detected <350 nm, the latter also possess characteristic absorbances at higher wavelengths where ω-CgTx cannot be detected. Consequently, multi-channel detectors are better than single-channel detectors because they can be set to wavelengths that discriminate between the fluorophore-containing components and native ω-CgTx, respectively. Peak identification can also be determined crudely. Fractions containing free and conjugated dye often have a different color to the naked eye. Moreover, once dried, unmodified and conjugated ω-CgTxs are white or colored powders, respectively, that are easily re-dissolved in water. In contrast, dry, free dye products usually form dark, water-insoluble patches or stains.

2.1.4. Storage and Handling of the Label

As peptides, ω-CgTx and its derivatives are prone to hydrolyze in aqueous solutions. Thus, they are best stored as lyophilized powders in sealed tubes. Concentrated stock solutions made in water and frozen and stored in aliquots at –20°C or lower are stable for several months. Repeated freeze-thaw cycles and storage at 4°C should be avoided rigorously. Solutions used in cell labeling can be frozen and re-used, but this is not wise owing to the risk of conjugate breakdown and increased nonspecific staining. Fluorescent analogs should be stored in foil or dark containers owing to their photosensitivity. Polypropylene plasticware or silanized glassware must always be used! This point cannot be emphasized too strongly. Through experience

---

pHs also enhance the undesirable hydrolysis reaction. At the optimum pH of around 8.0 the labeling reaction is extremely rapid and complete within a few minutes. Controlling the reaction stoichiometry is critical to prevent under- or overmodification and for simplifying purification. The stoichiometry we prefer is around 2 moles of label/mol of ω-CgTx. The reaction efficiency is sensitive to the concentration of both the label and ω-CgTx, thus dilute reactions (<0.1 m*M* toxin) should be avoided. Components containing amines other than ω-CgTx, such as buffers containing Tris or proteins like BSA, interfere and must be avoided. Too low or high a concentration of DMSO reduces the yield; we use 10–25% (v/v).

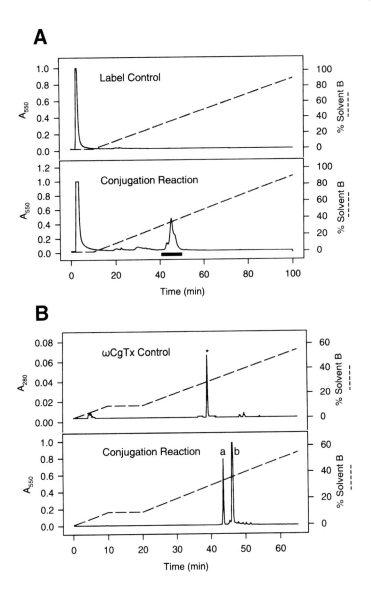

Fig. 4. Examples of HPLC Profiles obtained during purification of a Cy3-conjugated ω-CgTx. (**A**) Preliminary separation of free dye products from protein-containing fractions (underlined) by cation-exchange HPLC (TSK-SP–5PW). Flow rate 1 mL/min. Solvent B (95% ammonium acetate in water). (**B**) Resolution of peptidic fraction by HPLC on C$_{18}$ reversed phase column. Note appearance of two distinct mono-modified products (peaks I and II) and unmodified ω-CgTx (*).

we have found that ω-CgTx and its derivatives bind strongly to polystyrene, untreated glass, and even some metal syringe needles. Such nonspecific binding can often, but not always, be reduced using solutions containing proteins such as BSA (0.1–1%). The serum in cell culture media seems to have a similar effect.

2.2. Product Characterization

2.2.1. Quantitation and the Stoichiometry, Location, and Fidelity of Labeling

The amount of conjugate and the degree and sites of labeling are important parameters in determining the potency and predicting the biological activity of ω-CgTx analogs *(13,20,25,38)* (*see* below). The simplest way to determine the amount of conjugate and the degree of labeling, N_L (moles/ mole ω-CgTx) is through conventional spectrophotometry using the appropriate extinction coefficients for ω-CgTx and label. In principle, it is possible to determine N_L from the areas of the dye and dye + label product peak heights in HPLC runs. However, this can be risky as the dye extinction coefficients are often influenced by the composition of the HPLC solvent and can change markedly when eluting with a solvent gradient.

In some cases, the amount of product is too low to determine accurately by spectrophotometry and is, thus, best determined by amino acid analysis *(38)*. Determination of N_L and also the precise sites of labeling is done using one of two methods: amino acid analysis or mass spectrometry *(25)*. In both procedures, the labeled ω-CgTx is unfolded by reduction of its three disulfide bonds, alkylated to prevent re-oxidation, and then digested with a protease that cleaves at lysine residues (such as Lys C). To identify labeled sites by amino acid analysis, the digestion products are resolved by HPLC, and their amino acid compositions determined. Because conjugation of lysine residues blocks their sensitivity to cleavage by the protease, larger fragments of novel, but predictable, amino acid composition are generated. Although this approach has been applied to biotinylated ω-CgTx conjugates *(38)*, it is time-consuming and the data can be hard to interpret. A much more sophisticated approach relies on mass spectrometry to identify the sites of labeling from the molecular weights of the proteolytic fragments. Not only is this method unambiguous, but it is also highly sensitive and, with the widespread availability of mass spectrometry service facilities, convenient and cost-effective.

In some circumstances, the properties of the fluorophore may be altered undesirably (*see* Section 2.1.1.). Gross chemical changes introduced during labeling and purification can be resolved by mass spectrometry. Alterations in the optical properties of the fluorophore can also occur, in particular quenching of the fluorescence emission following conjugation. Such changes are best resolved through spectrofluorimetry, if possible using a well-characterized protein adduct of the fluorophore (e.g., a BSA or IgG conjugate) rather than the free dye, as a reference.

2.2.2. Biological Activity of the Product

The value of imaging labels depends on their biological activity and must be determined for each conjugate. Modification of ω-CgTx has two detrimental effects: elimination of bonding sites and interposition of the fluorophore between ω-CgTx and the N-VDCC binding pocket. The activity of the toxin is best assessed by membrane binding or electrophysiology assays *(13,20,25)*.

Membrane binding assays test the ability of the conjugated-ω-CgTx to displace $[^{125}I]$-ω-CgTx binding from synaptic membranes *(13,20,25,38)*. However, as successful labeling reflects the label's residence time on its target, it is more accurate to express the utility of the label in terms of its dissociation rate constant k_{off} rather than the more easily measured equilibrium affinity constant k_i *(38)*. Fortunately, the rate constants (k_{on}) for association of ω-CgTx labels with N-VDCCs are similar and, thus, differences in k_i's are an indirect, convenient, and largely valid reflection of k_{off}. To determine the relative potencies of competitors, it is best to compare dose-response curves for inhibition of binding with respect to those for unmodified ω-CgTx *(13,20,25)*. As a rule of thumb, modifications to ω-CgTx lower its affinity rather than its selectivity. Mono- and di-conjugated ω-CgTx derivatives typically bind 10- (Kd 0.4 nM) and 100- (Kd 4 nM) fold less well than native ω-CgTx (Kd 40 pM), respectively. Membrane-binding assays have numerous benefits: they are sensitive, reasonably cheap, do not require very expensive equipment to perform, and are ideal for screening large numbers of potential conjugates. The major criticism levelled at such assays is their limitation to measuring just one aspect of toxin function: binding.

Electrophysiology is the most widely used alternative to binding assays *(13,20)* and is often claimed to be a more appropriate way to monitor the biological activity of toxin conjugates because it tests the blockade of functional channels. This argument is specious, because no ω-CgTx conjugate has ever been made that is active in binding but not electrophysiological assays (or vice versa). More serious, electrophysiology is not straightforward, requires expensive equipment, is wasteful of conjugate, and is a poor estimate of ω-CgTx potency owing to difficulties in controlling the concentration owing to nonspecific binding, tissue permeation (brain slices), or mode of application.

2.3. Imaging with Fluorescent ω-Conotoxins

2.3.1. General Considerations

The density of N-VDCCs can be very low so the fluorescence emanating from neurons labeled with fluorescent ω-CgTxs is quite weak *(6,13,15,20,25,26,39)*. Thus, any step that improves the fluorescence signal-to-noise ratio is useful. How is this achieved? First, it is critical to use the right probes (*see* above). Second, even with an "ideal" conjugate, the appropriate hardware is essential. To attain the desired sensitivity, we collect images using laser-scanning confocal microscopes (LSCMs) *(6,20,25,26)*. Imaging systems fitted with high sensitivity cameras are also suitable *(13)*. Unfortunately, regular fluorescence microscopy rarely works and requires tissues such as the frog NMJ where N-VDCCs are highly concentrated *(15)*. Even then, long film-exposure times are necessary. Confocal imaging is ideal owing to its ability to remove contributions from out-of-focus light. In addition the ability of LSCM to obtain high-resolution images in optical sections <1 μm thick, to depths of up to 300 μm, is key to imaging labeled tissues, discriminating between fluorescence emanating from the cell surface rather than internally, and for reconstructing images in three dimensions.

2.3.2. Imaging Protocol

To map the distribution of N-VDCCs in tissues such as hippocampus, fresh brain slices are labeled with fluorescent ω-CgTx using conditions that aid survival but obviate internalization (Fig. 5) *(6,20,25,26)*. The tissue is then washed to remove free label. For live imaging, the slices are maintained using a specially adapted thermostatted and aerated microscope chamber. For more permanent, and often more crisp images, fluorescent ω-CgTx-labeled slices are fixed using 2–4% paraformaldehyde, cleared in methyl salicylate, and mounted prior to viewing. Fixation has no discernible effect on the fluorescence of any of the ω-CgTx conjugates we have tried. Images of labeled cells in culture are obtained identically *(13)*.

In general, the fluorescence emission is collected via epifluorescence optics, amplified, and displayed in real time. Image data is then stored on a computer for further processing and display. The analysis of the images is an entire discipline in itself, for which the reader is referred to excellent texts on digital image processing *(41)*. As a guideline, it is advisable to collect Z-series where possible. The image series provide a good impression of the disposition of the label and allow the creation of image stacks. Such stacks can be used to generate 3D images throughout the cell, thus, allowing one to follow fluorescent ω-CgTx labeling along processes such as dendrites as they thread above and below individual confocal planes *(20)*. The 3D images also aid in discriminating between cell surface and intracellular

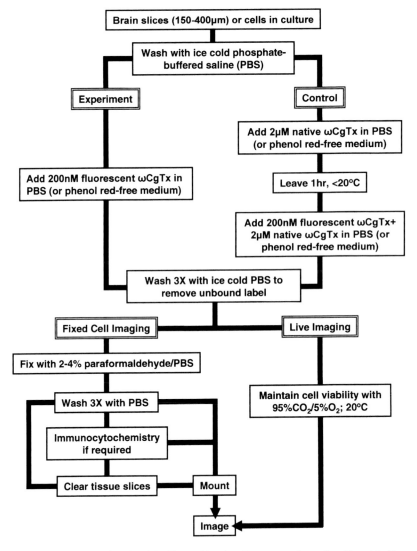

Fig. 5. Flow chart for the labeling of brain slices or cultured cells with fluorescent-ω-CgTx.

labeling. Image stacks also serve as important source data for many deconvolution algorithms used in image enhancement. Always note the type of objective, its numerical aperture, the refractive index of the immersion medium, e.g., oil, and the excitation wavelength. The precise image format is also important. We convert our BioRad PIC images into TIFF files and use these as source images for processing. Such files also serve as sources for generating 2D matrices of the pixel intensities at each X,Y coordinate. The resulting matrices allow one to develop user-defined image processing algorithms such as those used to show enhanced N-VDCC expression in epileptic brain tissue *(25,26)*. Processed images (as TIFF or JPEG files) are displayed in programs such as Powerpoint, CorelDraw, or Adobe Illustrator. Typical examples are shown in Fig. 6.

2.3.3. Issues for Successful Imaging

2.3.3.1. LABEL CONCENTRATION

The affinity of labeled ω-CgTx derivatives for N-VDCCs is lower than that of unmodified ω-CgTx and is further diminished by ions like Ca^{2+}, often present in label solutions. Thus, higher concentrations are often needed for labeling N-VDCCs than are used in ω-CgTx blocking experiments. Higher concentrations of label are also required for imaging brain slices (0.2–2 μM) vs dissociated cultures (50–500 nM) owing to poor tissue permeation.

2.3.3.2. SUITABLE CONTROLS

Specimens labeled with fluorescent-ω-CgTx must be processed in parallel with appropriate controls *(42)*, which include: (1) an unlabeled specimen and (2) a specimen preincubated with an excess of unmodified ω-CgTx prior to incubation with fluorescent ω-CgTx (*see* Fig. 5). The first control assesses the background fluorescence in the specimen, whereas the second control assesses the nonspecific binding of the fluorescent ω-CgTx. To preclude exchange between bound unmodified and fluorescent ω-CgTx excess unmodified ω-CgTx should be added before, during, and after the fluorescent ω-CgTx.

2.3.3.3. INTERNALIZATION

The lengthy incubation of live cells with fluorescent ω-CgTx facilitates nonspecific labeling via ligand internalization *(43)*. During labeling, most internalization occurs by fluid phase endocytosis. Once the free ligand has been washed off, internalization arises by endocytosis of labeled N-VDCCs. Because endocytosis is temperature and tonicity-dependent, incubating specimens at or below 20°C, or in hypertonic media, often curbs ligand internalization, although these conditions may affect the viability of the cells, especially in brain slices.

2.3.3.4. AUTOFLUORESCENCE

Intracellular or "auto" fluorescence is a persistent problem in neurons that arises from endogenous flavonoids and lipofuchsin *(20,42)*.

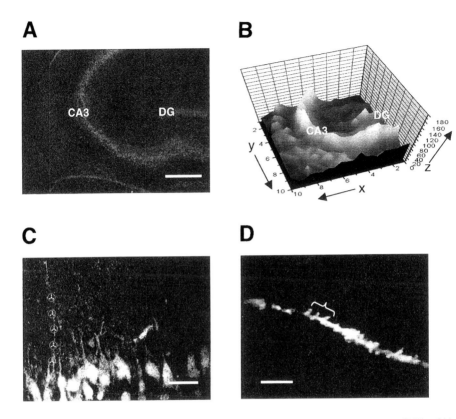

Fig. 6. Images of rat hippocampal neurons labeled with fluorescent-ω-CgTx. **(A)** Adult rat hippocampal brain slice showing subfields CA3 and dentate gyrus (DG) labeled with fluorescein-ω-CgTx at low magnification (6×). Scale bar, 300 μm. **(B)** Contour plot (128 level grayscale) showing the distribution of fluorescence in three dimensions for the slice shown in (A). **(C)** and **(D)** Images of dendrites (arrowheads) in CA1 hippocampal neurons labeled with fluorescein-ω-CgTx at intermediate ([C] Scale bar, 30 μm) and high ([D] Scale bar, 5 μm) resolution. A group of dendritic spines is indicated by the bracket. Images (C) and (D) were obtained in collaboration with Dr. L. Mills. For further images and details, *see* refs. *(6,20,25,26).*

Autofluorescence occurs over a wide spectral range and is worst in old or dying cells. Autofluorescence is best dealt with by recognizing its properties and distribution. For example, it usually decreases with increasing wavelength. Lipofuchsin fluorescence has a granular appearance.

2.3.3.5. PHOTOBLEACHING

Photobleaching refers to the decrease in fluorescence intensity seen upon sustained excitation and its extent reflects the fluorophore, the strength of, and period of exposure to, the excitation beam and buffer oxygenation *(42)*. Photobleaching is especially problematic with intense light sources such as the lasers used in LSCM. Most of those fluorophores shown in Table 3 do not photobleach excessively. Nevertheless, it is essential that sample exposure times are minimized and the light source attenuated as much as possible using the lowest apertures and the highest neutral-density filters giving acceptable images.

2.3.3.6. FIXATION AND MOUNTING

Background fluorescence can occur when fixing neurons *(42)*. Paraformaldehyde is better than glutaraldehyde and any background fluorescence is often removed by borohydride reduction and clearing agents like methylsalicylate *(20)*. Mounting should be done with a medium that contains anti-oxidants to reduce photobleaching.

2.3.3.7. IDENTIFICATION OF CELLS AND SUBCELLULAR COMPARTMENTS

Labeling with fluorescent ω-CgTxs is compatible with routine immunocytochemistry protocols. Standard markers that we use include GFAP and neurofilament L to resolve glia and neurons, respectively. Somatodendrites are reliably resolved using antibodies to MAP-2 *(13)*, whereas total neurites are visualized using anti-β-tubulin. In high magnification studies, the fluorescence of labeled N-VDCCs is related to processes using vital stains like DiI *(20)*. In disperse live cell cultures, the cell surface can be defined using fluorescent-tagged wheat-germ agglutinin.

2.3.3.8. OPTIMIZATION OF LABELING

Once a labeling method has been developed, it is highly reproducible and can be applied to tissues from different brain regions. Irreproducible labeling mainly arises via alterations in label concentration, incubation conditions, and tissue quality. Optimization is most useful when background fluorescences are high and usually only requires altering the labeling time, the concentration of label used, or the time taken to wash cells.

3. CONCLUSIONS AND FUTURE PROSPECTS

The use of ω-CgTx-based labels for mapping N-VDCCs makes possible experiments that simply cannot be addressed in other ways. Although the purification is involved, the ease and reliability of the conjugation reactions, and the labeling strategy offset any disadvantages. Moreover, the plethora of fluorophores that are currently available or being developed allows one to tailor and make probes for a variety of novel applications. Some future developments that we envisage include the coupling of ω-CgTx to pH or Ca^{2+}-sensitive indicators to follow N-VDCC trafficking. Other developments are likely to emphasize the live imaging of labeled N-VDCCs. The development of ever more sensitive ω-CgTx-based methods should ultimately lead to the mapping of individual N-VDCCs and our ability to define how their distributions are regulated. In summary, the future for labeled ω-CgTxs seems very bright.

ACKNOWLEDGMENTS

This work was supported by a research grant (OTJ) and Fellowship (GMB) from the Natural Sciences and Engineering Research Council of Canada.

REFERENCES

1. Adams, M. E. and Olivera, B. M. (1994) Neurotoxins: overview of an emerging research technology. *Trends Neurosci.* **17,** 151–155.
2. Olivera, B. M., Rivier, J., Scott, J. K., Hillyard, D. R., and Cruz, L. J. (1991) Conotoxins. *J. Biol. Chem.* **266,** 22,067–22,070.
3. Regan, L. J., Sah, D. W., and Bean B. P. (1991) Ca2+ channels in rat central and peripheral neurons: high-threshold current resistant to dihydropyridine blockers and omega-conotoxin. *Neuron* **6,** 269–280.
4. Ellinor, P. T., Zhang, J. F., Horne, W. A., and Tsien, R. W. (1994) Structural determinants of the blockade of N-type calcium channels by a peptide neurotoxin. *Nature* **372,** 272–275.
5. Witcher, D. R., De Waard, M., Sakamoto, J., Franzini-Armstrong, C., Pragnell, M., Kahl, S. D., and Campbell, K. P. (1993) Subunit identification and reconstitution of the N-type Ca^{2+} channel complex purified from brain. *Science* **261,** 486–489.
6. Jones, O. T., Bernstein, G. M., Jones, E. J., Jugloff, D. G., Law, M., Wong, W., and Mills, L. R. (1997) N-Type calcium channels in the developing rat hippocampus: subunit, complex, and regional expression. *J. Neurosci.* **17,** 6152–6164.
7. Rivier, J., Galyean, R., Gray, W. R., Azimi-Zonooz, A., McIntosh, J. M., Cruz, L. J., and Olivera, B. M. (1987) Neuronal calcium channel inhibitors. Synthesis of omega-conotoxin GVIA and effects on 45Ca uptake by synaptosomes. *J. Biol. Chem.* **262,** 1194–1198.
8. Davis, J. H., Bradley, E. K., Miljanich, G. P., Nadasdi, L., Ramachandran, J., and Basus, V. J. (1993) Solution structure of omega-conotoxin GVIA using 2-D NMR spectroscopy and relaxation matrix analysis. *Biochemistry* **32,** 7396–7405.
9. Williams, M. E., Brust, P. F., Feldman, D. H., Patthi, S., Simerson, S., Maroufi, A., et al. (1992) Structure and functional expression of an ω-conotoxin-sensitive human N-type calcium channel. *Science* **257,** 389–395.

10. Stocker, J. W., Nadasdi, L., Aldrich, R. W., and Tsien, R. W. (1997) Preferential interaction of ω-Conotoxins with inactivated N-type Ca^{2+} channels. *J. Neurosci.* **17,** 3002–3013.

11. Axelrod, D., Ravdin, P., Koppel, D. E., Schlessinger, J., Webb, W. W., Elson, E. L., and Podleski, T. R. (1976) Lateral motion of fluorescently labeled acetylcholine receptors in membranes of developing muscle fibers. *Proc. Natl. Acad. Sci. USA* **73,** 4594–4598.

12. Anderson, M. J., Cohen, M. W., and Zorychta, E. (1977) Effects of innervation on the distribution of acetylcholine receptors on cultured muscle cells. *J. Physiol. (Lond.)* **268,** 731–756.

13. Jones, O. T., Kunze, D. L., and Angelides, K. J. (1989) Localization and mobility of ω-conotoxin-sensitive Ca^{2+} channels in hippocampal CA1 neurons. *Science* **244,** 1189–1193.

14. Catterall, W. A. (1998) Structure and function of neuronal Ca^{2+} channels and their role in neurotransmitter release. *Cell Calcium.* **24,** 307–323.

15. Cohen, M. W., Jones, O. T., and Angelides, K. J. (1991) Distribution of Ca^{2+} channels on frog motor nerve terminals revealed by fluorescent ω-conotoxin. *J. Neurosci.* **11,** 1032–1039.

16. Robitaille, R., Adler, E. M., and Charlton, M. P. (1990) Strategic location of calcium channels at transmitter release sites of frog neuromuscular synapses. *Neuron* **5,** 773–779.

17. Haydon, P. G., Henderson, E., and Stanley, E. F. (1994) Localization of individual calcium channels at the release face of a presynaptic nerve terminal. *Neuron* **13,** 1275–1280.

18. Farinas, I., Egea, G., Blasi, J., Cases, C., and Marsal, J. (1993) Calcium channel antagonist omega-conotoxin binds to intramembrane particles of isolated nerve terminals. *Neuroscience* **54,** 745–752.

19. Dunlap, K., Luebke, J. I., and Turner, T. J. (1995) Exocytotic Ca^{2+} channels in mammalian central neurons. *Trends Neurosci.* **18,** 89–98.

20. Mills, L. R., Niesen, C. E., So, A. P., Carlen, P. L., Spigelman, I., and Jones O. T. (1994) N-type Ca^{2+} channels are located on somata, dendrites, and a subpopulation of dendritic spines on live hippocampal pyramidal neurons. *J. Neurosci.* **14,** 6815–6824.

21. Magee, J., Hoffman, D., Colbert, C., and Johnston, D. (1998) Electrical and calcium signaling in dendrites of hippocampal pyramidal neurons. *Ann. Rev. Physiol.* **60,** 327–346.

22. Westenbroek, R., Hell, J. W., Warner, C., Dubel, S. J., Snutch, T. P. and Catterall, W. A. (1992) Biochemical properties and subcellular distribution of an N-type calcium channel α1 subunit. *Neuron* **9,** 1099–1115.

23. Schiller, J., Schiller, Y., and Clapham, D. E. (1998) NMDA receptors amplify calcium influx into dendritic spines during associative pre- and postsynaptic activation. *Nature Neurosci.* **1,** 114–118.

24. Filloux, F., Schapper, A., Naisbitt, S. R., Olivera, B. M., McIntosh, J. M. (1994) Complex patterns of [^{125}I]omega-conotoxin GVIA binding site expression during postnatal rat brain development. *Brain Res. Dev. Brain Res.* **78,** 131–136.

25. Bernstein, G. M., Mendonca, A., Wadia, J., Burnham, W. M., and Jones, O. T. (1999) Kindling enhances N-type calcium channels in the rat hippocampus. *Neuroscience* **94,** 1083–1095.

26. Bernstein, G. M., Mendonca, A., Wadia, J., Burnham, W. M., and Jones, O. T. (1999) Kindling induces an asymmetric enhancement of N-type calcium channels in the dendritic fields of the rat hippocampus. *Neurosci. Lett.* **268,** 155–158.

27. Albensi, B. C., Ryujin, K. T., McIntosh, J. M., Naisbitt, S. R., Olivera, B. M., and Filloux, F. (1993) Localization of [^{125}I]omega-conotoxin GVIA binding in human hippocampus and cerebellum. *Neuroreport* **4,** 1331–1334.

28. Takemura, M., Kiyama, H., Fukui, H., Tohyama, M., and Wada, H. (1989) Distribution of the omega-conotoxin receptor in rat brain. An autoradiographic mapping. *Neuroscience* **32,** 405–416.

29. Maeda, N., Wada, K., Yuzaki, M., and Mikoshiba, K. (1989) Autoradiographic visualization of a calcium channel antagonist, [^{125}I]omega-conotoxin GVIA, binding site in the brains of normal and cerebellar mutant mice (pcd and weaver). *Brain Res.* **489,** 21–30.

30. Kerr, L. M., Filloux, F., Olivera, B. M., Jackson, H., and Wamsley, J. K. (1988) Autoradiographic localization of calcium channels with [^{125}I]omega-conotoxin in rat brain. *Eur. J. Pharmacol.* **146,** 181–183.

31. Takemura, M., Kiyama, H., Fukui, H., Tohyama, M., and Wada, H. (1988) Autoradiographic visualization in rat brain of receptors for omega-conotoxin GVIA, a newly discovered calcium antagonist. *Brain Res.* **451,** 386–389.

32. Quasthoff, S., Adelsberger, H., Grosskreutz, J., Arzberger, T., and Schroder, J. M. (1996) Immunohistochemical and electrophysiological evidence for omega-conotoxin-sensitive calcium channels in unmyelinated C-fibres of biopsied human sural nerve. *Brain Res.* **723,** 29–36.

33. Tharani, Y., Thurlow, G. A., and Turner, R. W. (1996) Distribution of omega-Conotoxin GVIA binding sites in teleost cerebellar and electrosensory neurons. *J. Comp. Neurol.* **364,** 456–472.

34. Fortier, L. P., Tremblay, J. P., Rafrafi, J., and Hawkes, R. (1991) A monoclonal antibody to conotoxin reveals the distribution of a subset of calcium channels in the rat cerebellar cortex. *Brain Res. Mol. Brain Res.* **9,** 209–215.

35. Grabner, M., Dirksen, R. T., and Beam, K. G. (1998) Tagging with green fluorescent protein reveals a distinct subcellular distribution of L-type and non-L-type Ca2+ channels expressed in dysgenic myotubes. *Proc. Natl. Acad. Sci. USA* **95,** 1903–1908.

36. Whorlow, S. L., Loiacono, R. E., Angus, J. A., and Wright, C. E. (1996) Distribution of N-type Ca^{2+} channel binding sites in rabbit brain following central administration of omega-conotoxin GVIA. *Eur. J. Pharmacol.* **315,** 11–18.

37. Wilchek, M. and Bayer, E. A. (eds.) (1990) *Methods in Enzymology,* vol. 184. Academic, San Diego.

38. Jones, O. T. and So, A. P. (1993) Preparation and characterization of biotinylated analogs of the calcium channel blocker omega-conotoxin. *Anal. Biochem.* **214,** 227–232.

39. Komuro, H. and Rakic, P. (1992) Selective role of N-type calcium channels in neuronal migration. *Science* **257,** 806–809.
40. Jones, O. T., Koncz, E. J., and So, A. P. (1994) Imaging ion channels in live central neurons using fluorescent ligands. I. Ligand construction, in *Three Dimensional Confocal Microscopy: Volume Investigation of Biological Specimens* (Stevens, J. K., Mills, L. R., and Trogadis, J. E., eds.), Academic, Orlando, FL, pp. 183–213.
41. Baxes, G. A., ed. (1994) *Digital Image Processing: Principles and Applications.* Wiley and Sons, New York.
42. Jones, O. T., Koncz, E. J., and So, A. P. (1994) Imaging ion channels in live central neurons using fluorescent ligands. II. Labelling of cells and tissues, in *Three Dimensional Confocal Microscopy: Volume Investigation of Biological Specimens* (Stevens, J. K., Mills, L. R., and Trogadis, J. E., eds.), Academic, Orlando, FL, pp. 215–232.
43. Mukherjee, S., Ghosh, R. N., and Maxfield, F. R. (1997) Endocytosis. *Physiol. Rev.* **77,** 759–803.

7

Fluorescent Imaging of Nicotinic Receptors During Neuromuscular Junction Development

Zhengshan Dai and H. Benjamin Peng

1. INTRODUCTION

Synaptic transmission at the vertebrate neuromuscular junction (NMJ) is accomplished by activity-dependent release of the neurotransmitter acetylcholine from the motor terminal and its detection by nicotinic acetylcholine receptors (AChRs) residing in the postsynaptic membrane of the skeletal muscle cell. The vesicular release at the nerve terminal is a highly efficient process that ensures the exocytosis of several hundred quanta upon each nerve impulse. The high fidelity of the ACh detection is based on the fact that AChRs are clustered to extremely high density at the postsynaptic membrane. Thus, the hallmark of NMJ development is the temporal and spatial registration of the vesicular release mechanism and the postsynaptic AChR clustering.

Fluorescently conjugated α-bungarotoxin (BTX) is the probe of choice for mapping the distribution of AChRs in skeletal muscle cells. The action of this toxin on skeletal muscle nicotinic receptors was first described by Lee and Chang over 30 years ago (1). As an alpha neurotoxin purified from the venom of the banded krait *Bungarus multicinctus*, this proteinaceous toxin binds with extremely high affinity in an essentially irreversible manner to the α-subunit of skeletal muscle AChRs. Because of its small size (M_r 8,000D) and high specificity for AChRs, it readily penetrates through tissue with minimal background labeling. Thus, it provides an ideal marker for AChRs in skeletal muscle. The application of fluorescent BTX in mapping AChRs constitutes the main topic of this chapter. Through the use of this

From: *Ion Channel Localization Methods and Protocols*
Edited by: A. Lopatin and C. G. Nichols © Humana Press Inc., Totowa, NJ

powerful reagent, great strides have been made in the exploration of AChR cluster formation that accompanies NMJ development. We are now beginning to unravel the cellular and molecular mechanisms involved in the assembly of this postsynaptic specialization. In this endeavor, the use of cultured skeletal muscle cells has stood out as one of the most fruitful approaches in deciphering the clustering process. In this chapter, the methodology and observations on producing AChR clusters in cultured muscle cells are used to illustrate AChR imaging with fluorescent BTX. In particular, experimental data from the use of cultured *Xenopus* myotomal muscle cells obtained in our laboratory are featured.

2. IMAGING ACHRS WITH FLUORESCENT BTX

Nicotinic AChRs in skeletal muscle are pentamers with a molecular mass of 250 kDa consisting of two α subunits and one each of β, δ, and γ subunit *(2)*. During vertebrate development, the γ subunit is replaced by ε subunit as the NMJ matures *(3,4)*. BTX binds with a 1:1 stoichiometry to the α subunit and thus each AChR can bind two BTX molecules. The site density of AChRs in skeletal muscle cells has been estimated by electron-microscopic autoradiography on specimens labeled with I^{125}-conjugated BTX to be on the order of 10,000 per μm^2 at the NMJ *(5)*. The density falls three orders of magnitude just a few micrometers away from the junction. At this high density, AChR clusters can be easily detected by light microscopy after labeling with fluorescently conjugated BTX. Because BTX's specificity for AChRs is extremely high, cell area away from the NMJ on the muscle cell generally shows very low background in adult muscle fibers. In noninnervated or denervated muscle fibers, a low background fluorescence is detected in nonjunctional region, reflecting the increased site density of diffusely distributed AChRs. Thus, the relative site density of AChRs can be readily quantified with the aid of fluorescent BTX.

The use of fluorescently conjugated BTX was pioneered by Anderson and Cohen *(6)* and by Ravdin and Axelrod *(7)*. The availability of lysine residues in this molecule allows it to be conveniently conjugated with conventional fluorophores such as fluorescein isothiocyanate or tetramethylrhodamine isothiocyanate. Fluorescent BTX is now available commercially in a number of fluorophores covering a wide spectral range (e.g., Molecular Probes, Eugene, OR).

The excellent tissue penetrability of BTX allows it to be used to label muscle cells in culture as well as in sectioned or whole-mount muscle specimen. This is in sharp contrast to antibody-based reagents, which generally penetrate poorly into tissues. Because BTX recognizes an extracellular epitope on AChR, cells can be conveniently labeled in the living state. However, this toxin remains highly specific for tissues fixed by aldehydes or by organic solvents such as ethanol or methanol. Thus, it is a versatile probe for AChRs.

3. EXPERIMENTAL STUDIES ON ACHR CLUSTERING

3.1. Spontaneously Formed AChR Hot Spots

In cultured muscle cells, AChRs spontaneously cluster in the absence of motor innervation *(8–10)*. These hot spots are functionally defined as nonsynaptic AChR clusters. Hot spots form more likely on the surface facing the substratum (ventral) as shown in Fig. 1A. Less frequently, they form on the top (dorsal) surface of the cells. Interestingly, the morphology of ventral vs dorsal hot spots is often different. The ventral hot spots tend to be more compact in appearance whereas the dorsal ones are more diffuse and often assume an elaborate spider web pattern (Fig. 1A inset). These hot spots bear a high degree of similarity in structure and in molecular composition to postsynaptic AChR clusters at the NMJ. The molecular complex consisting of transmembrane, cytoskeletal and extracellular-matrix proteins characteristic of the postsynaptic membrane are also present at the hot spot *(11)*. Membrane infoldings characteristic of mature NMJs, are also a prominent feature of the hot spots, in particular the ventral ones as observed with electron microscopy or fluorescence imaging (Fig. 1B) *(12,13)*.

Hot spots also develop in denervated muscle or in muscle that is prevented from innervation in vivo *(14–16)*. This indicates that they are not owing to artifactual condition of tissue culture. Recent studies have shed light on the signal involved in hot-spot formation. When the synaptic organizing molecule agrin (detailed in Section 3.3.) is expressed in the extrajunctional region of either innervated or denervated muscle, AChR clusters that are not associated with the motor terminal are also induced *(17,18)*. These agrin-induced clusters are structurally and molecularly similar to hot spots. This suggests that agrin may play a role in the formation of hot spots.

3.2. AChR Clusters Induced by Innervation

The formation of high-density AChR clusters in the postsynaptic membrane can be conveniently studied in tissue culture *(9,19–22)*. When muscle cells are cocultured with spinal motoneurons, AChR clusters are induced at nerve-muscle contacts (Fig. 2 and inset). This induction appears unique to

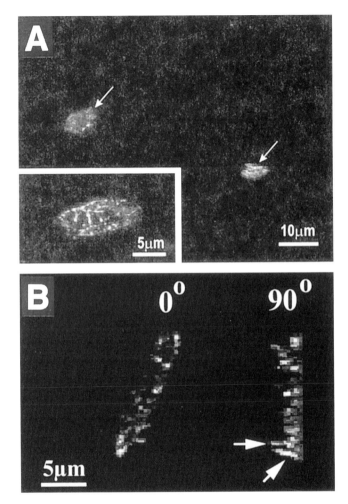

Fig. 1. AChR hot spots that form spontaneously in cultured *Xenopus* muscle cells after tetramethyl rhodamine-BTX (R-BTX) labeling. **(A)** Hot spots on the ventral surface. These clusters are more compact in shape. Inset, a hot spot on the dorsal surface. A more diffuse appearance is seen. **(B)** A hot spot seen in top (0°) and lateral (90°) view. The lateral view shows the localization of AChRs along membrane folds at the hot spot.

motoneurons as sensory or sympathetic neurons fail to induce cluster formation when cocultured with muscle cells *(19)*. Despite the presence of AChR hot spots as described earlier, neurons induce new clusters de novo and generally ignore those pre-existing receptor clusters *(8)*. In culture, the neurite generally grows along or underneath the muscle fiber and seldom

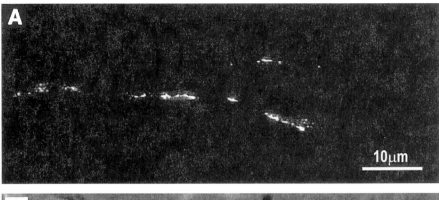

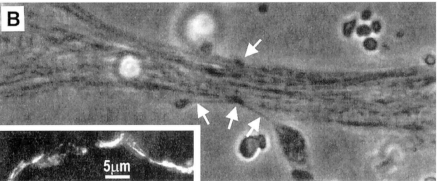

Fig. 2. AChR clustering induced by innervation in culture. **(A)** R-BTX image; **(B)** phase contrast (same for subsequent figures). Arrows point to sites of nerve-muscle contact along the edge of the muscle cell. Inset in (B) shows a cluster at a nerve-muscle contact beneath the muscle cell.

grows over it. By labeling muscle cells with fluorescent BTX either prior to or after spinal neuron coculture, the contribution of AChR pools either pre-existent at the cell surface or from the intracellular store to the cluster formation can be determined. From these studies, it has been shown the pre-existent surface AChRs are induced to aggregate under the neural signal *(8)*. In addition, there is evidence that local insertion of new receptors at the nerve-muscle contacts also contributes to the cluster formation in chick myotubes *(24)*.

3.3. AChR Clusters Induced by Agrin

First purified from the cholinergic synapse-rich electric organ of *Torpedo*, agrin is a heparan-sulfate proteoglycan that induces AChR cluster formation in vitro and in vivo *(25–28)*. Although it was first characterized as a

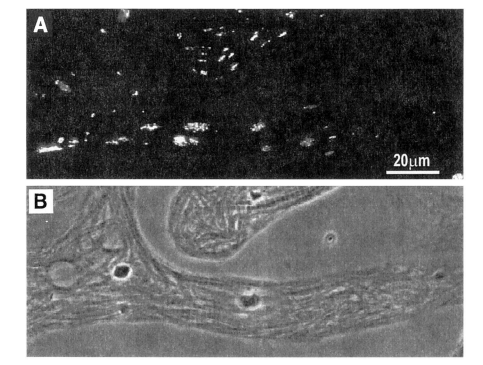

Fig. 3. AChR clusters induced by bath application of agrin. Clusters are induced along the entire muscle cells.

NMJ-organizing molecule, it has now been shown to be an ubiquitous component of the basement membrane of a number of tissues *(29–31)*. Through alternative splicing, several forms of agrin are produced. The form, which has an insert of 8, 11, or 19 amino acids at the Z position (also referred to as B position in chick), is especially potent in causing AChR clustering and is specifically expressed by neural tissue *(27,32,33)*. When agrin is bath-applied to cultured muscle cells, a large number of AChR clusters is induced (Fig. 3). These clusters tend to be smaller than hot spots in *Xenopus* muscle cells. The effective concentration of agrin necessary for inducing AChR clustering is in the nano- to picomolar range. Thus, it is a highly potent inducer of AChR clustering. Targeted deletion of the agrin gene in mice results in severe disruption of NMJs with a dramatic loss of AChR clusters at nerve-muscle contacts *(34,35)*. As described earlier, ectopic expression of agrin by plasmid injection into adult muscle also results in AChR cluster formation. These results have demonstrated the essentiality of agrin as a motoneuron-derived molecule for postsynaptic induction at the NMJ.

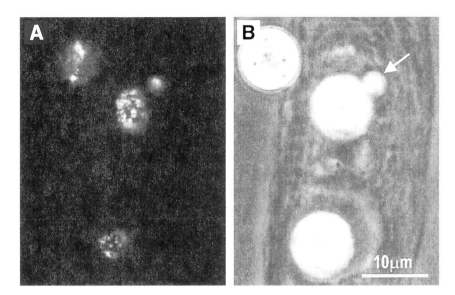

Fig. 4. AChR clusters induced by beads coated with HB-GAM. AChRs are aggregated discretely at the bead-muscle contact. The size of the cluster is proportional to the size of the bead. The arrow points to a small bead that is associated with a small cluster.

Unlike the spatially discrete process of nerve innervation, agrin's effect on AChR clustering is produced by a diffuse application to the bath in cultured muscle cells. Interestingly, although agrin application in the bath results in its binding to the entire muscle cell in culture, only a subset of these binding sites develop AChR clusters *(36,37)*. Thus, agrin may exert its stimulatory effect in conjunction with a muscle-derived cofactor, which has a nonuniform distribution at the cell surface and dictates the location of AChR clustering induced by agrin.

3.4. AChR Clusters Induced by Beads

Spatially discrete induction of AChR cluster formation can be produced by growth factor-coated microspheres in cultured *Xenopus* muscle cells (Fig. 4). A number of factors, including basic fibroblast growth factor (bFGF), heparin-binding growth-associated molecule (HB-GAM; also known as pleiotrophin), midkine, insulin, insulin-like growth factor-I (IGF-I) and polycations such as polylysine, were found to be strong inducers of AChR clustering when applied via beads *(38–43)*. AChRs are clustered discretely at the bead-muscle contacts in the same manner as nerve innervation. The size of the clusters is dictated by the size of the beads used (Fig. 4). Thus, clusters with diameter ranging from submicron range to more than 10 μm can be induced on muscle cells. The larger clusters generally consist of an ensemble of smaller aggregates (Fig. 4). The onset of AChR clustering follows immediately after bead-muscle contacts. In addition to AChR clustering, the beads also induce the formation of membrane invaginations resembling postsynaptic folds *(40)*. Thus, this offers a versatile system to study the molecular mechanisms underlying AChR cluster formation in muscle cells.

3.5. AChR Clusters Induced by Electric Fields

DC electric field is a potent stimulus to effect AChR clustering in cultured muscle cells. In response to experimentally imposed field on the order of 0.1– 0.5 mV/μm, AChRs become clustered along the cathodal edge of the muscle cell within several hours (Fig. 5) *(44,45)*. Recent studies suggest that the field is not the motive force for the migration of AChRs but appears to be a triggering mechanism that recruits AChRs to the cathodal side, because AChRs continue to cluster following the termination of the field exposure *(46)*.

In nonmuscle cells, DC electric field can also induce clustering of certain transmembrane proteins. For example, a recent study has shown that receptors for epidermal growth factor are concentrated on the cathodal face of keratinocytes in response to DC electric fields *(47)*. Although the mechanism involved in the field-induced clustering of transmembrane proteins is not clearly understood, recent studies have implicated the activation of tyrosine kinase receptors in the cases of AChRs and EGFRs *(46,47)*. As discussed later, tyrosine kinase activation appears to be the common denominator underlying all forms of AChR clustering processes.

3.6. AChR Clustering Induced by Rapsyn

Rapsyn is a peripheral membrane protein that specifically associates with AChRs in skeletal muscle and in *Torpedo* electric organ *(48–52)*. Biochemical and molecular studies have shown its association with the cytoplasmic domain of AChR subunits *(53–56)*. It exists in a 1:1 stoichiometry with the AChR *(57)*. Targeted deletion of rapsyn gene results in the abolishment of AChR clustering in skeletal muscle *(58)*. Thus, rapsyn is a key molecule involved in AChR cluster formation. Experimentally, when rapsyn is expressed in heterologous cell types, such as *Xenopus* oocytes and embryonic cells or fibroblasts together with AChR subunits, clustering of the receptors is observed *(59–61)*. Overexpression of rapsyn in cultured muscle cells also results in a large increase in AChR clusters which are generally smaller than spontaneously formed hot spots (Fig. 6). When rapsyn is expressed on its own without AChRs, it forms clusters by itself *(59–61)*.

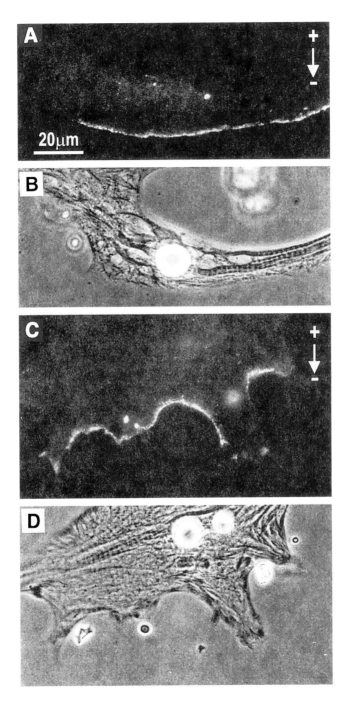

Fig. 5. AChR clusters induced by DC electric fields. A field of 0.5 mV/μm was applied to these muscle cells. The arrows indicate the field direction: +, anode; –, cathode. AChRs aggregate along the cathode-facing edge of these muscle cells. As shown in these examples, the entire cathodal edge is often populated by AChRs.

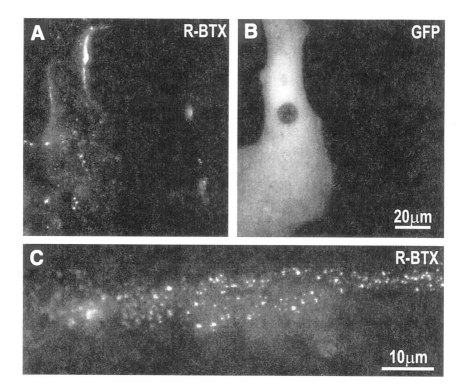

Fig. 6. Rapsyn-induced AChR clustering. Muscle cultures were prepared from *Xenopus* embryos injected with a mixture of rapsyn and GFP mRNAs at 1–2-cell stage. The GFP was used as a marker for rapsyn-expressing cells. **(A,B)** The left cell in this pair shows GFP fluorescence **(B)** and is thus overexpressing rapsyn. This cell shows a large number of microclusters, whereas the nonfluorescent cell on the right (without rapsyn overexpression) exhibits the normal hot-spot pattern. **(C)** Microclusters induced by rapsyn overexpression at a higher magnification.

Thus, rapsyn has the innate property of membrane association to form complexes *(62,63)*. Using antibodies against phosphorylated tyrosine, one can detect the concentration of phosphotyrosine-containing proteins at these rapsyn patches induced by its overexpression *(59,64)*. Thus, rapsyn is also capable of recruiting signaling molecules in addition to its interaction with AChRs. Its assembly in response to synaptogenic signal appears to be key to understanding the formation of AChR clusters in skeletal muscle cells.

3.7. AChR Microclusters Induced by Crosslinking

In addition to stimulus-induced clustering, AChRs can also be aggregated by crosslinking with multivalent ligands in cultured muscle cells. In one procedure, AChRs are first labeled with biotinylated BTX and then followed by fluorescently conjugated avidin, which presents four biotin-binding sites *(65,66)*. As shown in Fig. 7, microclusters of AChRs are observed following the crosslinking step. Other crosslinking method can also be used. For example, following BTX labeling, anti-BTX antibody is applied to be followed by a fluorescently conjugated secondary antibody. Crosslinking generally results in a decrease in the lateral mobility of AChRs and this causes an inhibition in the stimulus-induced clustering process *(67)*.

4. MECHANISM OF ACHR CLUSTER FORMATION

4.1. Lateral Mobility of AChRs and Diffusion-Mediated Trapping

In all procedures described earlier, the contribution of AChRs pre-existent on the cell surface to the experimentally induced clusters can be demonstrated by prelabeling AChRs with fluorescent BTX and following their accumulation after the stimulus is applied *(68)*. This indicates that AChRs on the cell surface undergo lateral migration and become concentrated at the clusters. Lateral diffusion of AChRs can be directly measured by FRAP (fluorescence recovery after photobleaching) method. Cultured muscle cells are first labeled with fluorescent BTX. A spot on the order of 1 μm on the cell surface is then photo-bleached by a laser beam delivered through the microscope objective. The recovery of fluorescence as a result of the exchange of bleached AChRs with the surrounding unbleached ones owing to the receptors" lateral diffusion in the plane of the membrane is monitored with a greatly attenuated excitation laser beam. From this measurement, the diffusion coefficient of diffusible AChRs on the cell surface is estimated to be on the order of 10^{-10} to 10^{-11} cm^2/s *(69–71)*. In comparison, AChRs within the cluster are essentially immobile, with a diffusion coefficient less than 10^{-12} cm^2/s. This sharp contrast in AChR mobility before and after clustering gives rise to the diffusion-mediated trap hypothesis, which depicts that AChRs at the surface of muscle cells are freely diffusible and their immobilization by traps induced by synaptogenic stimuli results in their clustering *(70,72)*. This hypothesis is generally supported by experimental data, although it has not yet been definitively tested. The observation that immobilization of AChRs by crosslinking agents abolishes AChR cluster formation lends support to this model.

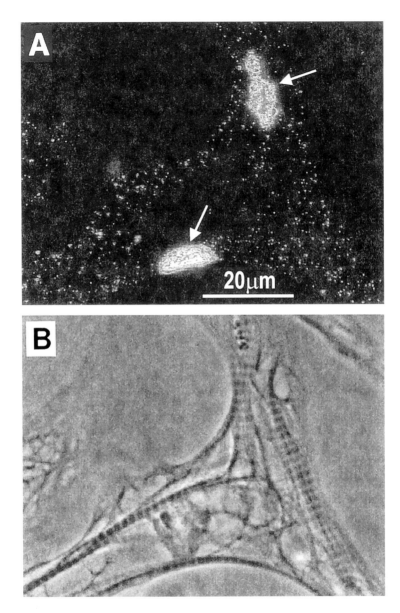

Fig. 7. Microclusters induced by AChR crosslinking. Muscle cells were first labeled with biotinylated BTX, then followed by fluorescently conjugated streptavidin. Diffuse AChRs form microclusters after this procedure. Arrows point to two hot spots.

4.2. The Role of Tyrosine Kinases in AChR Clustering

Recent studies have implicated the role of tyrosine kinase activation in the formation of AChR clusters. Using anti-phosphotyrosine antibodies, AChR clusters induced by nerve, agrin, growth factor-coated beads and DC electric fields are associated with phosphotyrosine labeling (Fig. 9B) *(46,66,73)*. Although several AChR subunits are substrates of tyrosine kinases, they cannot account for all the phosphotyrosine labeling at AChR clusters. This is shown by the fact that phosphotyrosine localization occurs prior to AChR accumulation at clusters induced by growth factor-coated beads in cultured muscle cells *(66)*. Recent studies from our lab have shown that when AChR clustering is inhibited by its crosslinking, phosphotyrosine is still clustered in response to bead or agrin stimulation *(67)*. In addition, inhibitors to tyrosine kinases block AChR clustering induced by several stimuli in cultured muscle cells *(46,66,74)*.

In nerve and agrin-induced AChR cluster formation, recent data have shown that muscle-specific kinase (MuSK) plays a key role in the signaling process *(75,76)*. MuSK is a receptor tyrosine kinase that is expressed in high level in skeletal muscle in a developmentally regulated fashion *(77–80)*. Its expression is high during embryonic development when synaptogenesis takes place but is downregulated after NMJs are formed. Denervation causes an upregulation in its expression in adult animals. Targeted deletion of MuSK results in severe disruption in NMJ formation with a total absence of AChR clustering *(75)*. In cultured myotubes, MuSK is activated as shown by its tyrosine phosphorylation by agrin. However, agrin by itself does not bind to the ectodomain of MuSK. This interaction is thought to be mediated by another yet unidentified component residing on the surface of the skeletal muscle *(76)*.

The tyrosine kinases responsible for AChR clustering induced by other stimuli are not known. Because several growth factors can induce AChR clustering when applied via beads as described earlier suggest that their cognate receptors are also capable of conveying the key signal for the assembly of AChRs. The fact that the electric field effect on AChR clustering is also blocked by tyrosine kinase inhibitors *(46)* suggests a novel kinase activation mechanism by ligand-independent process. Thus, despite the disparity in the nature of AChR cluster-inducing stimuli listed earlier, the involvement of tyrosine kinase is a common denominator for all of them. It will be of interest to decipher whether these stimuli elicit a common downstream signaling pathway after the tyrosine kinase activation.

4.3. The Role of the Cytoskeleton in AChR Clustering

As described earlier, rapsyn is a myristoylated peripheral membrane protein that is associated with the cytoplasmic domain of AChR subunits and is essential for the formation of AChR clusters. A recent study has shown distinct motifs within this molecule are involved in its membrane targeting and AChR clustering properties *(63)*. Although rapsyn is clearly associated with AChRs within the cluster, it is not yet clear whether diffusely distributed AChRs are also complexed with rapsyn. In addition to rapsyn, AChR clusters are associated with a large array of cytoskeletal proteins, most notably the dystrophin/utrophin complex. Whereas dystrophin is enriched along the postsynaptic folds at the NMJ, its close relative utrophin is localized at the AChR-rich domain of the postsynaptic membrane *(81)*. Despite their close relationship, AChR clusters still form when both dystrophin and utrophin are deleted in double-knockout mice *(82,83)*.

In addition to these specialized proteins, AChR clusters are also associated with ubiquitous cytoskeletal proteins such as F-actin and microtubules *(68,84–86)*. Because disruption of microtubule assembly does not affect the clustering process (our unpublished results), this cytoskeletal protein is unlikely involved directly in cluster assembly. F-actin concentration at AChR clusters has been shown by both light (Fig. 8) and electron microscopy. Our recent study has shown that local actin polymerization is elicited by signals that elicit AChR clustering and blocking this process with latrunculin A abolishes the clustering *(87)*. This suggests that F-actin assembly is a necessary condition for AChR cluster formation. Thus, local actin polymerization stimulated by synaptogenic signals may lead to the erection of a cytoskeletal scaffold upon which AChR clusters are assembled. It is not clear at this moment how AChR and rapsyn interact with this cytoskeleton, although other proteins within the AChR cluster complex, such as dystrophin and utrophin, are known to interact with F-actin *(88,89)*. A recent study has indicated a novel transmembrane interaction between the ectodomain of MuSK and rapsyn and gives rise to the hypothesis that MuSK is a component of the scaffold for rapsyn and AChR anchorage at the postsynaptic membrane *(90)*. Taken together, the protein complex that serves as an organizer of the AChR cluster seems to consist of ubiquitous cytoskeletal proteins such as actin, specialized sarcolemma components such as rapsyn and signaling molecules such as the tyrosine kinase MuSK.

5. DISPERSAL OF ACHR CLUSTERS

Once assembled, AChR clusters are stable sarcolemma structures that can withstand detergent extraction as a result of their cytoskeletal anchorage *(84)*. However, the dispersal of AChR clusters is observed in vivo in association with synaptic remodeling and competition *(91)*. AChR cluster dispersal is also a prominent feature of cultured muscle cells. In response to nerve innervation or to the treatment of other synaptogenic stimuli such as

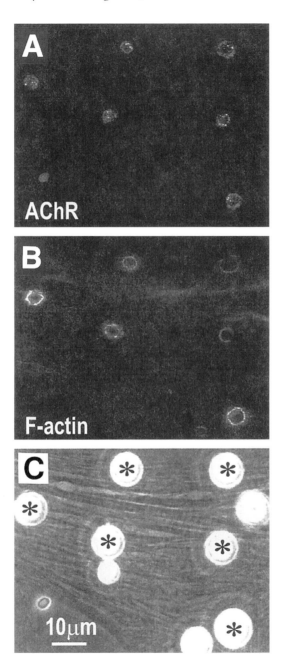

Fig. 8. F-actin and AChR colocalization. HB-GAM-coated beads induce both AChR clustering **(A)** and F-actin assembly visualized with fluorescein-conjugated phalloidin **(B)**. Beads that induce both specializations are marked with asterisks in **(C)**.

beads, agrin, and electric field, pre-existing hot spots are dispersed *(92–94)*. An example of bead-induced hot-spot dispersal is shown in Fig. 9A. Unlike cluster formation, which occurs locally at the site of stimulation, cluster dispersal occurs more globally. Hot spots undergoing dispersal are often far away from sites of new cluster formation. Our recent study has shown that the rate of hot-spot dispersal is inversely related to its distance from the bead stimulus *(93)*. Clusters closest to the beads are the first ones to undergo dispersal.

The role of tyrosine phosphatase in the dispersal of AChR clusters is implicated from our recent study based on two lines of evidence *(93)*. First, cluster dispersal induced by innervation or by beads can be blocked by tyrosine phosphatase inhibitors such as vanadate and phenylarsine oxide. Second, microinjection of the constitutively active form of *Yersinia* tyrosine phosphatase results in hot-spot dispersal in a stimulus-independent fashion. These data suggest that tyrosine phosphatase activity induced by synaptic stimuli is capable of destabilizing AChR clusters globally across the muscle cell to result in their dispersal. Furthermore, we also found that AChR clusters formed in the presence phosphatase inhibitors become more scattered and not strictly confined to contact sites with the neurite or beads (Fig. 9 B and C). This suggests that local tyrosine phosphatase activity at the site of synaptic stimulation may help regulate the spatial discreteness of AChR accumulation. Thus, the phosphatase may exert both a global, action-at-a-distance influence on hot-spot dispersal and a local effect on defining the boundary of newly formed AChR clusters.

6. CONCLUSIONS

The formation of AChR clusters in skeletal muscle as a result of innervation has offered a simple and versatile experimental paradigm for understanding molecular mechanisms of ion-channel clustering. The availability of the highly specific BTX is certainly a key to the rapid advance in cellular, molecular, and biochemical characterization of this receptor. Fluorescently conjugated BTX has provided an extremely powerful tool in this analysis. Recent studies on the signal-transduction process in NMJ formation may lead to an elucidation of the detailed mechanism for the clustering of this prototypical ligand-gated channel. As has been described in this chapter, AChR clustering in cultured muscle cells can be induced by a disparate array of experimental stimuli. It will be of great interest to understand how each type of stimulus impacts on presumably a common signaling cascade.

Studies with fluorescent BTX has not yielded detailed information on the movement of AChRs on the cell surface. Future study with BTX in conjunc-

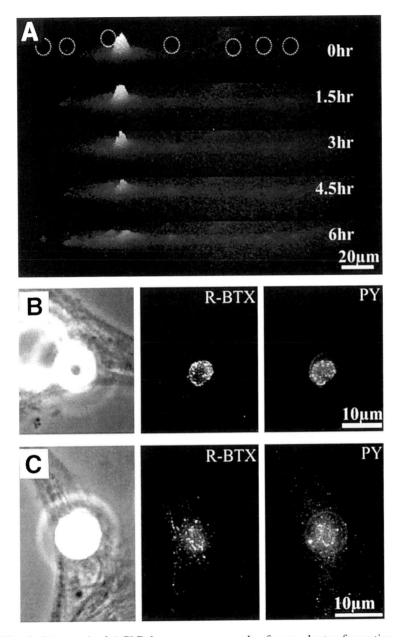

Fig. 9. Dispersal of AChR hot spot as a result of new cluster formation. (**A**) Time course of cluster dispersal after new cluster formation is triggered by beads. A hot spot on the left side of the cell undergoes dispersal as a result of bead-induced new cluster formation. The intensity of R-BTX labeling is represented by height and by shading. (**B**) Discrete localization of AChRs and phosphotyrosine (PY) at the bead-muscle contact. Left, phase contrast; middle, BTX labeling; right, anti-PY antibody labeling. (**C**) Effect of pervanadate, a tyrosine phosphatase inhibitor, in causing a scattering of AChRs and PY clusters at the bead contact.

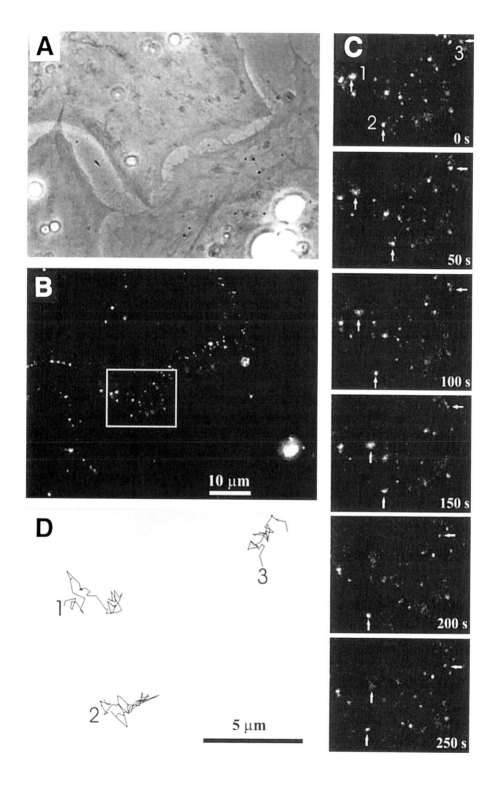

A

B

10 µm

C

3

1

2

0 s

50 s

100 s

150 s

200 s

250 s

D

1

3

2

5 µm

tion with highly fluorescent marker molecule or microspheres may allow detailed mapping of AChR movement on the surface of cultured muscle cells. Toward this goal, we have recently experimented with the use of the highly fluorescent molecule phycoerythrin as a marker for AChR. Muscle cells were first treated with biotinylated BTX followed by labeling with streptavidin-conjugated phycoerythrin (Molecular Probes). As shown in Fig. 10, phycoerythrin specifically labels muscle cells but not fibroblasts in our cultures in a finely punctate manner. With time-lapse recording, these phycoerythrin-BTX puncta are found to undergo movement in the plane of the membrane. This may provide a means for continuous monitoring of AChR movement. Cluster formation, however, has not been observed in these treated cells, presumably owing to the crosslinking of AChRs, as described earlier. Future studies using these highly fluorescent markers in monovalent form may allow unprecedented observation on AChR cluster formation in real time.

ACKNOWLEDGMENTS

Works described in this chapter were supported by NIH grant 23583 and by the Muscular Dystrophy Association. These works were conducted in collaboration with present and previous members of our lab and we gratefully acknowledge their contributions.

REFERENCES

1. Lee, C. Y., Chang, S. L., Kau, S. T., and Luh, S.-H. (1972) Chromatographic separation of the venom of Bungarus multicinctus and characterization of its components. *J. Chromatogr.* **72,** 71–82.
2. McCarthy, M. P., Earnest, J. P., Young, E. F., Choe, S., and Stroud, R. M. (1986) The molecular neurobiology of the acetylcholine receptor. *Ann. Rev. Neurosci.* **9,** 383–413.
3. Schuetze, S. M. and Role, L. W. (1987) Developmental regulation of nicotinic acetylcholine receptors. *Ann. Rev. Neurosci.* **10,** 403–457.
4. Witzemann, V., Brenner, H.-R., and Sakmann, B. (1991) Neural factors regu-

Fig. 10. Tracking AChRs with phycoerythrin. The culture was labeled with biotinylated BTX followed by streptavidin-conjugated phycoerythrin and observed live. Fluorescent puncta are only observed on muscle cells (M) and not on fibroblasts (F) as seen in **(A)** and **(B)**. Thus, these puncta represent small AChR aggregates. These puncta display lateral movement as shown in time lapse in **(C)** and **(D)**. Arrows point to the positions of three spots in (C). Traces of the three particles are shown in (D).

late AChR subunit mRNAs at rat neuromuscular synapses. *J. Cell Biol.* **114,** 125–141.

5. Fertuck, H. C. and Salpeter, M. M. (1974) Localization of acetylcholine receptor by ^{125}I-labeled α-bungarotoxin binding at mouse motor endplates. *Proc. Natl. Acad. Sci. USA* **71,** 1376–1378.

6. Anderson, M. J. and Cohen, M. W. (1974) Fluorescent staining of acetylcholine receptors in vertebrate skeletal muscle. *J. Physiol. (Lond.)* **237,** 385–400.

7. Ravdin, P. and Axelrod, D. (1977) Fluorescent tetramethyl rhodamine derivatives of alpha-bungarotoxin: preparation, separation and characterization. *Anal. Biochem.* **80,** 585–592.

8. Anderson, M. J. and Cohen, M. W. (1977) Nerve-induced and spontaneous redistribution of acetylcholine receptors on cultured muscle cells. *J. Physiol. (Lond.)* **268,** 757–773.

9. Frank, E. and Fischbach, G. D. (1979) Early events in neuromuscular junction formation in vitro. *J. Cell Biol.* **83,** 143–158.

10. Sytkowski, A. J., Vogel, Z., and Nirenberg, M. W. (1973) Development of acetylcholine receptor clusters on cultured muscle cells. *Proc. Natl. Acad. Sci. USA* **70,** 270–274.

11. Bloch, R. J. and Pumplin, D. W. (1988) Molecular events in synaptogenesis: nerve-muscle adhesion and postsynaptic differentiation. *Am. J. Physiol.* **254,** C345-C364.

12. Peng, H. B. (1987) Development of the neuromuscular junction in tissue culture. *CRC Crit. Rev. Anat. Sci.* **1,** 91–131.

13. Weldon, P. R., Moody-Corbett, F., and Cohen, M. W. (1981) Ultrastructure of sites of cholinesterase activity on amphibian embryonic muscle cells cultured without nerve. *Dev. Biol.* **84,** 341–350.

14. Bekoff, A. and Betz, W. J. (1976) Acetylcholine hot spots: development on myotubes cultured from aneural limb buds. *Science* **193,** 915–917.

15. Ko, P. K., Anderson, M. J., and Cohen, M. W. (1977) Denervated skeletal muscle fibers develop discrete patches of high acetylcholine receptor density. *Science* **196,** 540–542.

16. Sohal, G. S. (1988) Development of postsynaptic-like specializations of the neuromuscular synapse in the absence of motor nerve. *Int. J. Dev. Neurosci.* **6,** 553–565.

17. Cohen, I., Rimer, M., Lomo, T., and McMahan, U. J. (1997) Agrin-induced postsynaptic-like apparatus in skeletal muscle fibers in vivo. *Mol. Cell. Neurosci.* **9,** 237–253.

18. Meier, Th., Hauser, D. M., Chiquet, M., Landmann, L., Ruegg, M. A., and Brenner, H. R. (1997) Neural agrin induces ectopic postsynaptic specializations in innervated muscle fibers. *J. Neurosci.* **17,** 6534–6544.

19. Anderson, M. J., Cohen, M. W., and Zorychta, E. (1977) Effects of innervation on the distribution of acetylcholine receptors on cultured muscle cells. *J. Physiol. (Lond.)* **268,** 731–756.

20. Buchanan, J., Sun, Y., and Poo, M.-M. (1989) Studies of nerve-muscle interactions in *Xenopus* cell culture: fine structure of early functional contacts. *J. Neurosci.* **9,** 1540–1554.

21. Nakajima, Y., Kidokoro, Y., and Klier, F. G. (1980) The development of functional neuromuscular junctions in vitro: an ultrastructural and physiological study. *Dev. Biol.* **77,** 52–72.

22. Peng, H. B., Nakajima, Y., and Bridgman, P. C. (1980) Development of the postsynaptic membrane in Xenopus neuromuscular cultures observed by freeze-fracture and thin-section electron microscopy. *Brain Res.* **196,** 11–31.

23. Cohen, M. W. and Weldon, P. R. (1980) Localization of acetylcholine receptors and synaptic ultrastructure at nerve-muscle contacts in culture: dependence on nerve type. *J. Cell Biol.* **86,** 388–401.

24. Role, L. W., Matossian, V. R., O'Brien, R. J., and Fischbach, G. D. (1985) On the mechanism of acetylcholine receptor accumulation at newly formed synapses on chick myotubes. *J. Neurosci.* **5,** 2197–2204.

25. Godfrey, E. W., Nitkin, R. M., Wallace, B. G., Rubin, L. L., and McMahan, U. J. (1984) Components of *Torpedo* electric organ and muscle that cause aggregation of acetylcholine receptors on cultured muscle cells. *J. Cell Biol.* **99,** 615–627.

26. McMahan, U. J., Horton, S. E., Werle, M. J., Honig, L. S., Kroger, S., Ruegg, M. A., and Escher, G. (1992) Agrin isoforms and their role in synaptogenesis. *Curr. Opin. Cell Biol.* **4,** 869–874.

27. Ruegg, M. A. and Bixby, J. L. (1998) Agrin orchestrates synaptic differentiation at the vertebrate neuromuscular junction. *Trends Neurosci.* **21,** 22–27.

28. Tsen, G., Halfter, W., Kroger, S., and Cole, G. J. (1995) Agrin is a heparan sulfate proteoglycan. *J. Biol. Chem.* **270,** 3392–3399.

29. Cole, G. J. and Halfter, W. (1996) Agrin: an extracellular matrix heparan sulfate proteoglycan involved in cell interactions and synaptogenesis. *Persp. Dev. Neurobiol.* **314,** 359–371.

30. Groffen, A. J., Ruegg, M. A., Dijkman, H., van de Velden, T. J., Buskens, C. A., Van den Born, J., et al. (1998) Agrin is a major heparan sulfate proteoglycan in the human glomerular basement membrane. *J. Histochem. Cytochem.* **46,** 19–28.

31. Raats, C. J. I., Bakker, M. A. H., Hoch, W., Tamboer, W. P. M., Groffen, A. J. A., Van den Heuvel, L. P. W. J., et al. (1998) Differential expression of agrin in renal basement membranes as revealed by domain-specific antibodies. *J. Biol. Chem.* **273,** 17,832–17,838.

32. Bowe, M. A. and Fallon, J. R. (1995) The role of agrin in synapse formation. *Ann. Rev. Neurosci.* **18,** 443–462.

33. Hall, Z. W. and Sanes, J. R. (1993) Synaptic structure and development: the neuromuscular junction. *Neuron* **10(Suppl.),** 99–121.

34. Gautam, M., Noakes, P. G., Moscoso, L., Rupp, F., Scheller, R. H., Merlie, J. P., and Sanes, J. R. (1996) Defective neuromuscular synaptogenesis in agrin-deficient mutant mice. *Cell* **85,** 525–535.

35. Sanes, J. R. (1997) Genetic analysis of postsynaptic differentiation at the vertebrate neuromuscular junction. *Curr. Opin. Neurobiol.* **7,** 93–100.

36. Daggett, D. F., Cohen, M. W., Stone, D., Nikolics, K., Rauvala, H., and Peng, H. B. (1996) The role of an agrin-growth factor interaction in ACh receptor clustering. *Mol. Cell. Neurosci.* **8,** 272–285.

37. Nastuk, M. A., Lieth, E., Ma, J., Cardasis, C. A., Moynihan, E. B., McKechnie, B. A., and Fallon, J. R. (1991) The putative agrin receptor binds ligand in a calcium-dependent manner and aggregates during agrin-induced acetylcholine receptor clustering. *Neuron* **7,** 807–818.

38. Baker, L. P. and Peng, H. B. (1995) Induction of acetylcholine receptor cluster formation by local application of growth factors in cultured *Xenopus* muscle cells. *Neurosci. Lett.* **185,** 135–138.

39. Peng, H. B., Ali, A. A., Dai, Z., Daggett, D. F., Raulo, E., and Rauvala, H. (1995) The role of heparin-binding growth-associated molecule (HB-GAM) in the postsynaptic induction in cultured muscle cells. *J. Neurosci.* **15,** 3027–3038.

40. Peng, H. B. and Cheng, P.-C. (1982) Formation of postsynaptic specializations induced by latex beads in cultured muscle cells. *J. Neurosci.* **2,** 1760–1774.

41. Peng, H. B., Cheng, P.-C., and Luther, P. W. (1981) Formation of ACh receptor clusters induced by positively charged latex beads. *Nature* **292,** 831–834.

42. Rauvala, H. and Peng, H. B. (1997) HB-GAM (heparin-binding growth-associated molecule) and heparin-type glycans in the development and plasticity of neuron-target contacts. *Prog. Neurobiol.* **52,** 127–144.

43. Zhou, H., Muramatsu, T., Halfter, W., Tsim, K. W. K., and Peng, H. B. (1997) A role of midkine in the development of the neuromuscular junction. *Mol. Cell. Neurosci.* **10,** 56–70.

44. Luther, P. W. and Peng, H. B. (1985) Membrane-related specializations associated with acetylcholine receptor aggregates induced by electric fields. *J. Cell Biol.* **100,** 235–244.

45. Orida, N. and Poo, M.-M. (1978) Electrophoretic movement and localisation of acetylcholine receptors in the embryonic muscle cell membrane. *Nature* **275,** 31–35.

46. Peng, H. B., Baker, L. P., and Dai, Z. (1993) A role of tyrosine phosphorylation in the formation of acetylcholine receptor clusters induced by electric fields in cultured *Xenopus* muscle cells. *J. Cell Biol.* **120,** 197–204.

47. Fang, K. S., Ionides, E., Oster, G., Nuccitelli, R., and Isseroff, R. R. (1999) Epidermal growth factor receptor relocalization and kinase activity are necessary for directional migration of keratinocytes in DC electric fields. *J. Cell Sci.* **112 (Pt 12),** 1967–1978.

48. Burden, S. J. (1985) The subsynaptic 43kDa protein is concentrated at developing nerve-muscle synapses in vitro. *Proc. Natl. Acad. Sci. USA* **82,** 8270–8273.

49. LaRochelle, W. J. and Froehner, S. C. (1986) Determination of the tissue distributions and relative concentrations of the postsynaptic 43-kDa protein and the acetylcholine receptor in Torpedo. *J. Biol. Chem.* **261,** 5270–5274.

50. Peng, H. B. and Froehner, S. C. (1985) Association of the postsynaptic 43K protein with newly formed acetylcholine receptor clusters. *J. Cell Biol.* **100,** 1698–1705.

51. Sealock, R., Wray, B. E., and Froehner, S. C. (1984) Ultrastructural localization of the M_r 43,000 protein and the acetylcholine receptor in Torpedo postsynaptic membrane using monoclonal antibodies. *J. Cell Biol.* **98,** 2239–2244.

52. Sobel, A., Weber, M., and Changeux, J.-P. (1977) Large-scale purification of the acetylcholine-receptor protein in its membrane-bound and detergent-

extracted forms from Torpedo marmorata electric organ. *Eur. J. Biochem.* **80,** 215–224.

53. Burden, S. J., Depalma, R. L., and Gottesman, G. S. (1983) Crosslinking of proteins in acetylcholine receptor-rich membranes: association between the beta-subunit and the 43 kd subsynaptic protein. *Cell* **35,** 687–692.

54. Maimone, M. M. and Merlie, J. P. (1993) Interaction of the 43 kd postsynaptic protein with all subunits of the muscle nicotinic acetylcholine receptor. *Neuron* **11,** 53–66.

55. Phillips, W. D., Maimone, M. M., and Merlie, J. P. (1991) Mutagenesis of the 43-kD postsynaptic protein defines domains involved in plasma membrane targeting and AChR clustering. *J. Cell Biol.* **115,** 1713–1723.

56. Yu, X.-M. and Hall, Z. W. (1994) The role of the cytoplasmic domains of individual subunits of the acetylcholine receptor in 43 kDa protein-induced clustering in COS cells. *J. Neurosci.* **14,** 785–795.

57. Porter, S. and Froehner, S. C. (1983) Characterization of the Mr 43,000 proteins associated with acetylcholine receptor-rich membranes. *J. Biol. Chem.* **258,** 10034–10040.

58. Gautam, M., Noakes, P. G., Mudd, J., Nichol, M., Chu, G. C., Sanes, J. R., and Merlie, J. P. (1995) Failure of postsynaptic specialization to develop at neuromuscular junctions of rapsyn-deficient mice. *Nature* **377,** 232–236.

59. Dai, Z., Scotland, P. B., Froehner, S. C., and Peng, H. B. (1996) Association of phosphotyrosine with rapsyn expressed in Xenopus embryonic cells. *Neuroreport* **7,** 657–661.

60. Froehner, S. C., Luetje, C. W., Scotland, P. B., and Patrick, J. (1990) The postsynaptic 43K protein clusters muscle nicotinic acetylcholine receptors in *Xenopus* oocytes. *Neuron* **5,** 403–410.

61. Phillips, W. D., Kopta, C., Blount, P., Gardner, P. D., Steinbach, J. H., and Merlie, J. P. (1991) ACh receptor-rich membrane domains organized in fibroblasts by recombinant 43-kilodalton protein. *Science* **251,** 568–570.

62. Musil, L. S., Carr, C., Cohen, J. B., and Merlie, J. P. (1988) Acetylcholine receptor-associated 43K protein contains covalently bound myristate. *J. Cell Biol.* **107,** 1113–1121.

63. Ramarao, M. K. and Cohen, J. B. (1998) Mechanism of nicotinic acetylcholine receptor cluster formation by rapsyn. *Proc. Natl. Acad. Sci. USA* **95,** 4007–4012.

64. Qu, Z., Apel, E. D., Doherty, C. A., Hoffman, P. W., Merlie, J. P., and Huganir, R. L. (1996) The synapse-associated protein rapsyn regulates tyrosine phosphorylation of proteins colocalized at nicotinic acetylcholine receptor clusters. *Mol. Cell. Neurosci.* **8,** 171–184.

65. Axelrod, D. (1980) Crosslinkage and visualization of acetylcholine receptors on myotubes with biotinylated α-bungarotoxin and fluorescent avidin. *Proc. Natl. Acad. Sci. USA* **77,** 4823–4827.

66. Baker, L. P. and Peng, H. B. (1993) Tyrosine phosphorylation and acetylcholine receptor cluster formation in cultured *Xenopus* muscle cells. *J. Cell Biol.* **120,** 185–195.

67. Dai, Z. and Peng, H. B. (1999) The dissociation of ACh receptor and phosphotyrosine cluster formation and dispersal induced by signals for synaptogenesis. *Soc. Neurosci. Abstr.* **25,** 239.

68. Peng, H. B. and Phelan, K. A. (1984) Early cytoplasmic specialization at the presumptive acetylcholine receptor cluster: a meshwork of thin filaments. J. Cell Biol. **99,** 344–349.
69. Axelrod, D., Ravdin, P., Koppel, D. E., Schlessinger, J., Webb, W. W., Elson, E. L., and Podleski, T. R. (1976) Lateral motion of fluorescently labeled acetylcholine receptors in membranes of developing muscle fibers. *Proc. Natl. Acad. Sci. USA* **73,** 4954–4958.
70. Kidokoro, Y. and Brass, B. (1985) Redistribution of acetylcholine receptors during neuromuscular junction formation in *Xenopus* cultures. *J. Physiol. (Paris)* **80,** 212–220.
71. Peng, H. B., Zhao, D.-Y., Xie, M.-Z., Shen, Z., and Jacobson, K. (1989) The role of lateral migration in the formation of acetylcholine receptor clusters induced by basic polypeptide-coated latex beads. *Dev. Biol.* **131,** 197–206.
72. Edwards, C. and Frisch, H. L. (1976) A model for the localization of acetylcholine receptors at the muscle endplate. *J. Neurobiol.* **7,** 377–381.
73. Qu, Z., Moritz, E., and Huganir, R. L. (1990) Regulation of tyrosine phosphorylation of the nicotinic acetylcholine receptor at the rat neuromuscular junction. *Neuron* **4,** 367–378.
74. Wallace, B. G., Qu, Z., and Huganir, R. L. (1991) Agrin induces phosphorylation of the nicotinic acetylcholine receptor. *Neuron* **6,** 869–878.
75. DeChiara, T. M., Bowen, D. C., Valenzuela, D. M., Simmons, M. V., Poueymirou, W. T., Thomas, S., et al. (1996) The receptor tyrosine kinase MuSK is required for neuromuscular junction formation in vivo. *Cell* **85,** 501–512.
76. Glass, D. J., Bowen, D. C., Stitt, T. N., Radziejewski, C., Bruno, J., Ryan, T. E., et al. (1996) Agrin acts via a MuSK receptor complex. *Cell* **85,** 513–523.
77. Besser, J., Zahalka, M. A., and Ullrich, A. (1996) Exclusive expression of the receptor tyrosine kinase MDK4 in skeletal muscle and the decidua. *Mech. Dev.* **59,** 41–52.
78. Fu, A. K. Y., Smith, F. D., Zhou, H., Chu, A. H., Tsim, K. W. K., Peng, B. H., and Ip, N. Y. (1999) Xenopus muscle-specific kinase: molecular cloning and prominent expression in neural tissues during early embryonic development. *Eur. J. Neurosci.* **11,** 373–382.
79. Ganju, P., Walls, E., Brennan, J., and Reith, A. D. (1995) Cloning and developmental expression of Nsk2, a novel receptor tyrosine kinase implicated in skeletal myogenesis. *Oncogene* **11,** 281–290.
80. Valenzuela, D. M., Stitt, T. N., DiStefano, P. S., Rojas, E., Mattsson, K., Compton, D. L., et al. (1995) Receptor tyrosine kinase specific for the skeletal muscle lineage: expression in embryonic muscle, at the neuromuscular junction, and after injury. *Neuron* **15,** 573–584.
81. Sealock, R., Butler, M. H., Kramarcy, N. R., Gao, K.-X., Murnane, A. A., Douville, K., and Froehner, S. C. (1991) Localization of dystrophin relative to acetylcholine receptor domains in electric tissue and adult and cultured skeletal muscle. *J. Cell Biol.* **113,** 1133–1144.
82. Deconinck, A. E., Rafael, J. A., Skinner, J. A., Brown, S. C., Potter, A. C., Metzinger, L., et al. (1997) Utrophin-dystrophin-deficient mice as a model for Duchenne muscular dystrophy. *Cell* **90,** 717–727.

83. Grady, R. M., Teng, H. B., Nichol, M. C., Cunningham, J. C., Wilkinson, R. S., and Sanes, J. R. (1997) Skeletal and cardiac myopathies in mice lacking utrophin and dystrophin: a model for Duchenne muscular dystrophy. *Cell* **90**, 729–738.

84. Bloch, R. J. (1986) Actin at receptor-rich domains of isolated acetylcholine receptor clusters. J. Cell Biol. **102**, 1447–1458.

85. Jasmin, B. J., Changeux, J.-P., and Cartaud, J. (1990) Compartmentalization of cold-stable and acetylated microtubules in the subsynaptic domain of chick skeletal muscle fibre. *Nature* **344**, 673–675.

86. Peng, H. B., Xie, H., and Dai, Z. (1997) The association of cortactin with developing neuromuscular specializations. *J. Neurocytol.* **26**, 637–650.

87. Peng, H. B. and Dai, Z. (1999) The role of actin polymerization in the formation of ACh receptor clusters in muscle cells. *Soc. Neurosci. Abstr.* **25**, 239.

88. Koenig, M., Monaco, A. P., and Kunkel, L. M. (1988) The complete sequence of dystrophin predicts a rod-shaped cytoskeletal protein. *Cell* **53**, 219–228.

89. Rybakova, I. N., Amann, K. J., and Ervasti, J. M. (1996) A new model for the interaction of dystrophin with F-actin. *J. Cell Biol.* **135**, 661–672.

90. Apel, E. D., Glass, D. J., Moscoso, L. M., Yancopoulos, G. D., and Sanes, J. R. (1997) Rapsyn is required for MuSK signaling and recruits synaptic components to a MuSK-containing scaffold. *Neuron* **18**, 623–635.

91. Balice-Gordon, R. J. and Lichtman, J. W. (1994) Long-term synapse loss induced by focal blockade of postsynaptic receptors. *Nature* **372**, 519–524.

92. Daggett, D. F., Stone, D., Peng, H. B., and Nikolics, K. (1996) Full-length agrin isoform activities and binding site distributions on cultured *Xenopus* muscle cells. *Mol. Cell. Neurosci.* **7**, 75–88.

93. Dai, Z. and Peng, H. B. (1998) A role of tyrosine phosphatase in acetylcholine receptor cluster dispersal and formation. *J. Cell Biol.* **141**, 1613–1624.

94. Kuromi, H. and Kidokoro, Y. (1984) Nerve disperses preexisting acetylcholine receptor clusters prior to induction of receptor. *Dev. Biol.* **103**, 53–61.

8

High Affinity Scorpion Toxins for Studying Potassium and Sodium Channels

Lourival D. Possani, Baltazar Becerril, Jan Tytgat, and Muriel Delepierre

1. INTRODUCTION

Snake, scorpion, cone snail, sea anemone, spider, and honeybee venoms contain most of the peptidic natural ligands that recognize ion-channels (for recent reviews, *see* refs. *1–6*). This chapter is focused mainly at peptides isolated from scorpion venoms. Four different families of toxins have been described that specifically interact with ion channels: Na⁺-channels *(2,7,8)*, K⁺-channels *(6,9,10)*, Cl⁻-channels *(11)*, and Ca²⁺-channels *(12)*. There are two classes of peptides that are best studied: K⁺-channel specific toxins (here called K-toxins), represented at this moment by 51 distinct peptides having from 29–42 amino acid residues, closely packed by three or four disulfide bridges *(10,13,14)* and Na⁺-channel specific toxins, simply called Na-toxins, from which 85 different peptides are known *(2)* excluding some for which only the cDNA sequences are published. The Na-toxins contain from 60–76 amino acid residues, closely bound by four disulfide bridges *(2)*. The Cl⁻-channel specific toxins are represented, thus far by chlorotoxin, a 36 amino acid long peptide that affects Cl⁻-channel *(11)*. The Ca²⁺-channel specific toxins refers to the ryanodine sensitive Ca²⁺-channels and a voltage-sensitive Ca²⁺-channel. The first is represented by proteins extracted from the venom of the scorpion *Pandinus imperator*, and were called IpTxi and IpTxa *(12)*, whereas the second is called kurtoxin, with 63 amino acids crosslinked by four disulfide bridges. Kurtoxin affects the function of Ca²⁺-channel of T-type, although not very specific, because it also recognizes

From: *Ion Channel Localization Methods and Protocols*
Edited by: A. Lopatin and C. G. Nichols © Humana Press Inc., Totowa, NJ

Na$^+$-channels at higher concentration *(15)*. IpTxi is a 15 kDa molecular weight heterodimeric protein with phospholipase activity, which inhibits indirectly the binding of ryanodine to its receptor, by a mechanism thought to involve liberation of certain fatty acids from hydrolyzable phospholipids, whereas, IpTxa is a 33 amino acids long peptide, that directly activates ryanodine binding to the Ca^{2+}-channel receptor *(12)*.

Concerning the use of scorpion toxins as markers of ion-channel distribution in various excitable tissues, there is little information in the literature, as it will be discussed later.

In this chapter we will review the state of the art concerning the diversity of K$^+$- and Na$^+$-specific scorpion toxins, their nomenclature, their structures, and sites of action. Genes coding for these toxins will be briefly mentioned. A short review on other natural ligand-peptides from other sources is added at the end of the chapter.

2. ISOLATION AND PRIMARY STRUCTURE DETERMINATION

Hundreds of distinct peptides have been isolated from approx 30 different species of scorpions. Usually, the purification procedure starts with chromatographic separation based on molecular-weight sieving, such as Sephadex G-50, followed by ion-exchange chromatography and a final step using high-performance liquid chromatography (HPLC) (for review, *see* refs. 2,6,8). Recently, most laboratories use direct separation of peptides by HPLC, or use HPLC after a pre-purification of soluble venom by means of gel-filtration chromatography, that resolves families of peptides based on their molecular weights. In the venoms of about 1500 distinct species of scorpions world-wide distributed, a rough calculation close to 100,000 different peptides was estimated to exist, from which less than 200 are really known in terms of their primary sequences and specific functions *(2)*. An important advance has recently been given to this matter, thanks to the development of novel molecular biology techniques, which allow to obtain, in a short time and from small amounts of DNA or mRNA, the primary structure of putative toxic peptides, as will be mentioned later. In the case where direct peptide sequencing and nucleotide sequencing have both been performed, the authenticity of the primary structure found is unequivocal. Sequences deduced from cloned genes or amplified by polymerase chain reaction (PCR) technologies, need further confirmation, owing to peptide maturation and postranslational modifications.

The primary structure is nowadays determined by direct Edman degradation, using automatic machines or by mass spectrometry measurements *(2)*.

Most of the peptides require an enzymatic digestion and separation of peptides by HPLC in order to obtain the overlapping amino acid sequences. Amino acid analysis and mass spectrometry measurements are complementary data necessary to confirm the complete primary structure determination. In special cases, nuclear magnetic resonance (NMR) spectrometry data are used to confirm, for example, amidated residues at the C-terminal position *(16)*. The disulfide bridges are usually obtained by mild enzymatic cleavage of native toxin, followed by HPLC separation and simultaneous sequencing of the pair of peptides maintained together through disulfide bonds *(17,18)*. Exceptional cases, where double cysteine residues are contiguous, require either mass spectrometry analysis or special chemical derivatization for completion of the covalent structure determination of these peptides. But this is a general strategy not restricted to scorpion toxins *(19)*.

3. CLASSIFICATION OF SCORPION TOXINS

Scorpion toxins specific for Na^+-channels were originally divided into alpha and beta-types (for review, *see* refs. *2,8*). The first were initially found in the venom of North African scorpions, from which *Androctonus australis* toxin II was chosen as a prototype. This toxin binds to site 3 of Na^+-channels in a voltage-dependent manner, slowing or blocking the inactivation mechanism of these channels, whereas the beta-type toxins bind to site 4 independently of membrane potential and affect Na^+-channel activation *(2,8,20)*. The model for beta-type was toxin II from the New World scorpion *Centruroides suffusus suffusus*. Additionally several new toxins were isolated and reported to be species specific, that is, they recognize Na^+-channels of nonmammalian tissues, such as excitable membranes of insect and crustaceans *(2)*. Among these newly described types of toxins are those that are excitatory and those that are depressant *(8,21)*. The number of newly investigated toxins is increasing, more than 85 primary sequences are known. They have been functionally subdivided in 10 different subfamilies or groups of peptides, accordingly to differences in structure and function *(2)*. Table 1 exemplifies these different groups. In this figure the amino acid sequence of only representative toxins for each group were selected. Similarly, for the K^+-channel toxins more than 49 sequences are known *(10)*. They all recognize K^+-channels of distinct tissues with different affinities: voltage-dependent K^+-channels; small-conductance, Ca^{2+}-dependent K^+-channels from brain synaptosomes and smooth-muscle membranes; high-conductance, Ca^{2+}-dependent K^+-channels to mention just some of the preparations where these peptides have been assayed (for review, *see* refs. *6,9,10*). In the recent

Table 1
Sodium Channel Scorpion Toxin Repesentatives[a]

Group	Common name	Sequence	Species
1	AaHII	VKDGYIVDDVNCTYFCGRNAYCNEECTKLKGESGYCQWASPYGNACYCYKLPDHVRTKGPGRCH	*A. australis*
2	CssII	KEGYLVSKSTGCKYECLKLGDNDYCLRECKQQYGKSSGGYCYAFACWCTHLYEQAVVWPLPNKTCN	*C. suffussus s*
3	Tsgamma	KEGYLMDHEGCKLSCFIRPSGYCGRECGIKKGSSGYCAWPACYCYGLPNWVKVWDRATNKC	*T. serrulatus*
4	LqhIT2	DGYIKRRDGCKVACLIGNEGCDKECKAYGGSYGYCWTWGLACWCEGLPDDKTWKSETNTCG	*L. quinquestriatus h*
5	LqqIV	GVRDAYIADDKNCVYTCGSNSYCNTECTKNGAESGYCQWLGKYGNACWCIKLPDKVPIRIPGKCR	*L. quinquestriatus q*
6	LqqIII	VRDAYIAKNYNCVYECFRDSYCNDLCTKNGASSGYCQWAGKYGNACWCYALPDNVPIRVPGKCH	*L. quinquestriatus q*
7	AaHIT4	EHGYLLNKYTGCKVWCVINNEECGYLCNKRRGGYYGYCYFWKLACYCOGARKSELWNYKTNKCDL	*A. australis*
8	CsEv3	KEGYLVKKSDGCKYGCLKLGENEGCDTECKAKNQGGSYGYCYAFACWCEGLPESTPTYPLPNKSC	*C. sculpturatus*
9	Cn10	KEGYLVNKSTGCKYNCLILGENKNCDMECKAKNQGGSYGYCYKLACWCEGLPESTPTYPIPGKTCRT	*C. noxius*
10	AaHIT1	KKNGYAVDSSGKAPECLLSNYCNNECTKVHYADKGYCCLLSCYCFGLNDDKKVLEISDTRKSYCDTTIIN	*A. australis*

[a]Adapted with permission from Possani et al., 1999 (2).

148

paper of Tytgat et al. *(10)*, a general nomenclature for these peptides was proposed, which comprises 12 subfamilies of K-channel toxins. In Table 2, an example of each subfamily is shown. As it can be observed they vary from 29 to 41 amino acid long and contain either 3 or 4 disulfide bridges *(10)*. Here not included is another recently found toxin: Ergtoxin, with 42 amino acid residues, that affect HERG-K$^+$-channels *(14)*.

4. THREE-DIMENSIONAL STRUCTURE

Toxins against Na$^+$- and K$^+$-channels differ greatly in the composition and number of amino acids but share a constant structural motif conserved among all toxins and composed of a short segment of alpha-helix and two or three strands of beta-sheet, stabilized by two disulfide bridges *(22,23)*. The only exception to this general rule is the excitatory insect toxin from *Buthotus judaicus* where two short alpha-helix segments are observed instead of one *(24)*.

4.1. Sodium Channel Toxins

The three-dimensional structure of several of these long chain scorpion toxins has been determined by X-ray crystallography *(25,26)* or NMR *(27,28)*, just to mention one of the first and last structure, respectively described. They all display analogous 3D structures based on a triple-stranded antiparallel beta-sheet, a short alpha-helix, and four disulfide bridges. Three of the disulfide bridges are similarly paired of which two contribute to maintain the relative position of the sheet and the helix constituting the cysteine stabilized alpha-helix beta-sheet motif, abbreviated Csab *(29)*. The fourth disulfide bridge is established either between the N- and C-terminal regions via the loop following the first beta-strand or, for the insect-excitatory toxins, between the C-terminal region and the core via the second beta strand *(24,27)*. These different arrangements do not modify the overall folding of the toxins. The numerous and various specificities of all these toxins are based on a conserved scaffold that accommodates different insertions, deletions, and mutations. Insertion fragments are named loops J, M, B, and F and correspond respectively to loop 1 between beta-strand 1 and the alpha-helix, loop-2 between the alpha-helix and the beta-strand 2, loop 3 between beta-strands 2 and 3, and finally the C-terminal end. The Old World toxins, or alpha-toxins, have short J loop and long B loop, whereas the New World toxins, or beta-toxins, have a long J loop and short B loop, excitatory toxins have both short J and B loops. An example of such insertion is the excitatory insect toxin from *B. judaicus* (BjxtrIT) where a five amino acids

Table 2
Subfamily Scorpion K[+]-Toxin Representatives[a]

Sub-family	Toxin systematic name	Common name	Sequence	Species
1	α-KTx1.1	ChTX	ZFTNVSCTTSKECWSVCQRLHNTSRGKCMNKKCRCYS	*L. quinquestriatus hebraeus*
2	α-KTx2.1	NTX	TIINVKCTSPKQCSKPCKELYGSSAGAKCMNGKCKCYNN[b]	*Centruroides noxius*
3	α-KTx3.1	KTX1	GVEINVKCSGSPQCLKPCKDAGMRFGKCMNRKCHCTPK	*A. mauretanicus mauretanicus*
4	α-KTx4.1	TsTXα	VFINAKCRGSPECLPKCKEAIGKAAGKCMNGKCKCYP	*Tityus serrulatus*
5	α-KTx5.1	ScTX	AFCNLRMCQLSCRSLGLLGKCIGDKCECVKH[b]	*L. quinquestriatus hebraeus*
6	α-KTx6.1	Pi1	LVKCRGTSDCGRPCQQQTGCPNSKCINRMCKCYGC[b]	*Pandinus imperator*
7	α-KTx7.1	Pi2	TISCTNPKQCYPHCKKETGYPNAKCMNRKCKCFGR	*Pandinus imperator*
8	α-KTx8.1	PO1	VSCEDCPEHCSTQKAQAKCDNDKCVCEPI	*A. mauretanicus mauretanicus*
9	α-KTx9.1	BmPO2	VGCEECPMHCKGKNAKPTCDDGVCNCNV	*Buthus martensii*
10	α-KTx10.1	CoTX1	AVCVYRTCDKDCKRRGYRSGKCINNACKCYPY[b]	*Centruroides noxius*
11	α-KTx11.1	PBTx1	DEEPKESCSDEMCVIYCKGEEYSTGVCDGPQKCKCSD	*Parabuthus transvaalicus*
12	α-KTx12.1	TsTxIV	WCSTCDDLACGASRECYDPCFKAFGRAHGKCMNNKCRCYTN	*Tityus serrulatus*

[a]Adapted with permission from Tytgat et al., 1999 (*10*).
[b]These toxins are amidated at the COOH terminus.

insertion occurs just before the alpha-helix in loop 1 whereas a short helix is also inserted in the C-terminal part of the molecule *(24)*. Alpha-toxins contain an insertion around residue 42 (part of the B loop), that is believed to play a key role in the modulation of the toxic activity. Thus in the alpha-toxins the B loop is longer than the corresponding loop in beta-toxins *(30)*.

Most of the scorpion toxin structures that have been reported, have been assigned to the alpha-group, or belong to toxins that are relatively nontoxic to mammals. Recently the first structures of two highly toxic anti-mammalian beta-toxins have been reported. The first one was solved by NMR *(28)*. It is toxin Cn 2 from *Centruroides noxius* Hoffmann. The second one was determined by X-ray diffraction and is Ts1, major component of the venom of the Brazilian scorpion *Tityus serrulatus (26)*. The main structural differences between alpha- and beta-toxins active against mammals reside in the structure of the C-terminal end. Indeed, for the two toxins a different orientation of the polypeptide chain is situated around residues 55–59 (Ts1 numbering). In Ts1 there is a turn of helix, whereas in Cn2 there is a proline in cis conformation. An additional factor for the distinction between alpha and beta toxins is related to the distribution of the residues on face B, especially owing to the number of basic residues. Face B is formed by loop 1 or J and the C-terminal end of the molecule the most variable regions in the beta toxins *(26)*. With the increasing number of known toxins, the earlier suggestion that the net charge of the peptide will determine the biological activity does not seem to hold any longer. Finally, the first structure of alpha-like toxins from the scorpion *Buthus martensii* Karsch BmK M1 and BmK M4 have been solved *(31)*. The two toxins possess an overall fold similar to the Na-toxins with a peculiar feature that consist in the presence of a nonproline cis peptide bond for two residues located in the N-terminal part of the molecule (positions 9 and 10). This feature allows to establish contact with the C-terminal fragment 58–64, leading to the exposition of the arginine-58 functional groups, crucial for the interaction with the receptor, whereas these are buried in alpha-toxins. Figure 1 reproduces a three-dimensional picture showing the folding of two typical scorpion toxins: Cn2, a Na-toxin from *Centruroides noxius (28)* and Pi1 a K-toxin, from *Pandinus imperator* scorpion venom *(32)*.

4.2. Potassium Channel Toxins

Potassium channel toxins show a great variability in terms of sequence and specificity, however, the detailed structural basis for this variability is still not very well-understood, in part for the scarcity of material. The structure of K^+-channel toxins like that of Na^+-channel is composed of a

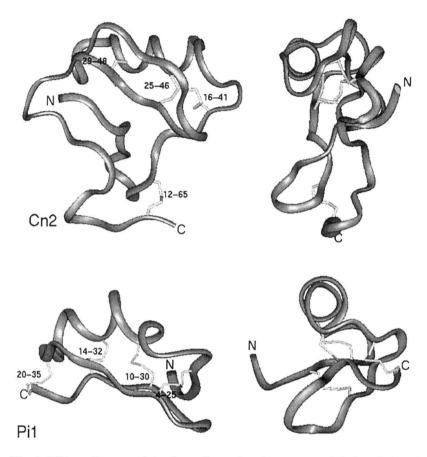

Fig. 1. Ribbon diagram of the three-dimensional structures of Cn2 and Pi1. The left upper figure shows the front view (as defined by Fontecilla-Camps et al. *[25]*) of Cn2, a Na$^+$-channel toxin from *Centruroides noxius (28)*, whereas the left bottom figure is the structure of Pi1, a K$^+$-channel blocking peptide from *Pandinus imperator* scorpion venom *(32)*. The right upper and down figures are from the same structures turned 90° to the right. The NMR coordinates were obtained respectively from Pintar et al. *(28)* and Delepierre et al. *(32)*.

helix and a beta sheet of two or three strands depending on the length of the N-terminal region. Apart from the six common cysteine residues, the only other amino acid absolutely conserved in all these peptides is the lysine at position 24 (27 in Charybdotoxin) shown to be crucial for channel binding and thought to interact directly in the ion-conducting pore *(33)*. There are only two exceptions to this, Pi7 for which this residue is replaced by an arginine and BmPO2, for which it is replaced by a threonine (for review, *see* ref. *10*). For several of these toxins the Gly26-Lys-Cys28 pattern previously proposed as a consensus sequence is not strictly preserved. Indeed, it was suggested that any other residue than a glycine at position 26 would disturb the packing of the helix-sheet interface (*34–36*), however in subfamily 2 a small residue is often inserted between the Gly and the Lys, whereas in subfamily 6, the Gly is replaced by an Ala or a Ser. Finally in subfamily 9 represented by BmPO2, BmPO3, and LpI a proline occupies this position.

In many of these toxins the disulfide pairing is left untouched. However, there are exceptions such as those found in toxins of the subfamily 6, for which five different members were identified, and that are characterized by the presence of an additional disulfide bridge. The fourth disulfide bridge fixes the C-terminus to the turn following the alpha-helix. Toxins from this subfamily display very different toxicity and activity (*9*). Of particular interest is peptide Pi7 for which the molecular target is still unknown, despite the fact that its folding is similar to all K-toxins (*37*). Another toxin containing four disulfide bridges was also purified from *Tityus serrulatus*, where the additional disulfide is located at the N-terminal end, but the 3D-structure is not known yet (*38*).

All toxins but one, HgTx3, active on voltage-dependent potassium channels possess a highly conserved proline at position X3 of the Cys-X1X2X3-Cys helical motif. The presence of proline residues in the highly conserved helical region seems to be a constant for toxins that exhibit a high blockade activity of voltage-dependent K^+-channels compared to the high-conductance Ca^{2+}-activated K^+-channel toxins (*39*).

5. ELECTROPHYSIOLOGICAL STUDIES

5.1. Na-Channels

5.1.1. Alpha-Scorpion Toxins

Because of close pharmacological resemblance to mammalian nerve cells, the first model used to study the effect of alpha-scorpion toxins at the cellular level was the node of Ranvier of frog. In 1966, it was shown that *Leiurus quinquestriatus* venom induced a prolongation of the action potential and that this effect could be abolished by lowering the extracellular Na^+ concentration (*40*). Quickly afterwards and thanks to the development of the voltage-clamp technique, it became clear that some toxins, which we know now as alpha-scorpion toxins, considerably slow down the Na^+-current inactivation process and eventually also induce a maintained current because of a change in the voltage dependence of inactivation of the Na^+-channel (*41,42*).

Based on these electrophysiological observations, several biophysical models have been proposed in which the toxin-induced changes in gating charge and in transitions between the different conformational states (closed, open, and inactive) are being discussed *(43–45)*.

Slowing of the inactivation, the hallmark of this class of toxins, seems to be a general effect as it has been observed in a wide variety of cells, tissues, and species, such as neuroblastoma cells and in crayfish, cockroach, squid axons, frog muscle, and tunicate eggs (for review, *see* ref. *46*).

5.1.2. Beta-Scorpion Toxins

In 1972, Katz and Edwards reported that application of *Centruroides suffusus suffusus* venom on a frog sartorius nerve-muscle preparation was followed by the appearance of repetitive responses in both muscle and nerve *(47)*. Similar to the effect seen with alpha-toxins, the response was also dependent on the external Na^+ concentration. A few years later, Cahalan found that the venom of *Centruroides sculpturatus* induced repetitive firing in frog myelinated nerve under voltage-clamp conditions caused by the appearance of an "abnormal" Na^+ current upon repolarization, which was time- and voltage-dependent *(48)*. These electrophysiological observations led to the definition of beta-toxin-modified currents, of which the following characteristics have been described by several authors: (1) reduced kinetics of activation, (2) requirement of stronger depolarizations for activation, (3) lower maximal macroscopic permeability, and (4) moderate slowing of inactivation process *(49)*. Interestingly, the effect of beta-scorpion toxins was found to be very much dependent on the voltage-clamp protocol used, because a depolarizing "conditioning or prepulse" resulted in beta-toxin-modified currents with opposite features, i.e., faster activation than control currents, shift of the Boltzmann steady-state activation curve to more negative potentials, and a greater peak permeability *(50)*. Although the above is true for *Centruroides* toxins, it was found that *Tityus* toxins can provoke a similar beta-effect without the "requirement" of a depolarizing prepulse *(51)*. Recently, an interesting voltage sensor-trapping model of beta-toxin action in which the IISA voltage sensor of the Na^+-channel is trapped in its outward, activated position by toxin binding has been proposed *(52)*. Beta-scorpion toxins seem to be present predominantly, in the venom of New World scorpions. Finally, it has been shown that alpha- and beta-toxins can exert their modifying effect at the same time on the same type of Na^+-channels *(53)*.

In connection with the new era of molecular biology and cloning of the different types of Na^+-channels from diverse organs and tissues, it will be interesting to find out which Na^+-channel clones are susceptible to alpha- and beta-toxin modification. Currently, 10 different genes (in the human genome) have been identified that are known to encode four-domain alpha-subunits of voltage-gated Na^+-channels: SCN1A to SCN10A. The brain-specific SCN2A gene, the skeletal-muscle specific SCN4A gene, and the heart-specific SCN5A gene are the clones that have been studied most intensively in the presence of alpha- and/or beta-toxins by taking advantage of the latest techniques in heterologous expression systems such as oocytes of *Xenopus laevis* or transfection in mammalian cell lines (e.g., HEK 293), combined with voltage- and patch-clamp techniques. An example of a typical alpha-effect on the human heart Na^+-channel ("hH1," SCN5A) caused by a long-chain toxin purified from *Parabuthus villosus* is shown in Fig. 2A.

5.2. K-Channel Toxins

K^+-channels represent the largest family of ion channels. Generally, K^+-channels can be divided into two major groups, voltage-gated and ligand-gated channels, depending on the stimulus that triggers the conformational changes leading to channel opening. With respect to the inhibitory effect of short-chain toxins from scorpion venom, it can be summarized that several toxins target the group of the voltage-gated K^+-channels, known as Kv-type channels (of which *Drosophila Shaker*-type or Kv1-type channels are most studied thus far) *(54)*; some others, the group of the Slo-type channels (*Drosophila slowpoke* gene product, known as maxi-K-channels because of their high single-channel conductance) *(55)*, and still other toxins the small-conductance Ca^{2+}-activated K^+-channels (for an excellent review, *see* ref. 6). One "exceptional" toxin seems to be the ErgTx, because it is the only one targeting the HERG channel, which is related to the EAG (ether-a-gogo gene) channel *(14)*. Different from Na-toxins, it has to be remembered that K-toxins purified from scorpion venom can be considered as "physical" channel blockers, not channel or gating modifiers. Charybdotoxin (ChTx or alpha-KTx1.1), purified from *Leiurus quinquestriatus* Hebraeus venom and being the most studied short-chain toxin, because it can be produced in large quantities via recombinant techniques, is known to potently block Kv1.2 and 1.3 channels. More importantly, the mechanism by which ChTx blocks *Shaker* channels has been extensively studied electrophysiologically using site-directed mutants on both toxin and channel (leading to the powerful "mutant cycle analysis" to pin-point critical residue interactions). These biophysical investigations allowed to discover that block occurs in a bimolecular fashion, via a simple plugging mechanism driven by electrostatic and hydrophobic interactions, with residue lysine at position 27 of particular importance because of the toxin's voltage- and K-dependent "plug" dip-

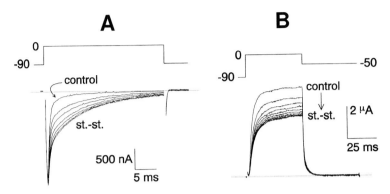

Fig. 2. Examples of electrophysiological effects of Na⁺- and K⁺- channel toxins purified from venom of species belonging to the *Parabuthus* genus. (**A**) The *SCN5A* gene product ("hH1" clone) was expressed in oocytes of *Xenopus laevis* and studied by using the two-microelectrode voltage-clamp technique. Whole-cell Na currents were evoked every 3 s from a holding potential of –90 mV to a test potential of 0 mV. The external [Na] = 96 mM. The effect of approx 2.5×10^{-7} M PBNaTx isolated from the venom of *Parabuthus villosus* is shown. The toxin induces an obvious slowing of the inactivation phase of the Na current, reaching steady-state (st.-st.) conditions after 20 episodes. For clarity, only 7 selected traces of the used protocol are shown. B. Expression of *Kv1.1* ("RCK1" clone) in similar conditions as above. Whole-cell "delayed rectifier-type" K currents were evoked every 5 s from a holding potential of –90 mV to a test potential of 0 mV, followed by a tail potential of –50 mV. The external [K] = 2 mM. The blocking effect of approx 20×10^{-9} M PBTx3 (alpha-KTx1.10) isolated from the venom of *Parabuthus transvaalicus* is shown.

ping into the channel pore. Furthermore, this kind of research has enabled us, in the absence of a crystal structure of Kv-type channels, to deduce the dimensions of the outer and inner pore regions of these channels *(56,57)*. As it is not our aim to mention the biological target of all K-toxins listed here, we only summarize that (1) alpha-KTx1 subfamily toxins can affect Kv-type, as well as the small and large conductance Ca²⁺-activated K⁺-channels; (2) alpha-KTx2 toxins primarily seem to block Kv-type channels; (3) alpha-KTx3 toxins have been studied intensively for their high affinity interaction with Kv1.3 channels; and that (4) alpha-KTx4 subfamily toxins target the small conductance Ca²⁺-activated K⁺-channels. It has also to be kept in mind that for several members of different subfamilies of toxins the precise K⁺-channel type as biological target still needs to be investigated. Experiencing an ever-expanding list of novel K⁺-channel clones (e.g., two-pore background K-channels and G-protein-coupled K-channels), it will be interesting to see if scorpion venom can provide us once again with toxin tools for these channels, enabling their physiological function and pharmacological classification. An example of a typical blocking-effect on the Kv1.1 channel ("RCK1") expressed in oocytes caused by a short-chain toxin purified from *Parabuthus transvaalicus* (PBTx3 or alpha-KTx1.10) is shown in Fig. 2B.

6. CLONING OF cDNAS AND GENES

6.1. Na⁺-Channel Scorpion Toxins

Until now, 53 cDNA and genomic sequences that encode Na⁺-channel toxins, have been reported (for review, *see* refs. *2,38,58*). Analysis of these sequences have revealed that the products of the transcriptional units consist of pre mRNAs of approx 650–950 nucleotides, including an intron of 300–620 bases located at the last third of the region encoding the signal peptide. The processing of these pre mRNAs provides mature mRNAs of approx 300–350 nucleotides, whose translation gives rise to polypeptide precursors of about 82–96 amino acid residues. A conserved sequence, presumably involved in intron processing (branch point), within an ideal distance (47–61 nucleotides) upstream of the splice site *(59)* of the genes encoding Na-toxins, has been observed. A signal peptide of 18–21 residues is released from the toxin precursors, by means of a signal peptidase *(58)*. At the carboxy-terminus (except for the group of excitatory insect toxins, in which there is no postranslational processing), basic residues (Lys and/or Arg), are removed by a carboxypeptidase *(2)*. Several rules of carboxy-end processing have emerged from the analysis of the DNA sequence encoding the precursor and the amino acid sequence of the mature toxin. Typically, one or two basic residues are eliminated and when a glycine residue precedes the basic(s) residue(s), the residue preceding glycine, is amidated *(58)*. If a glycine precedes a group of three basic residues, the basic triad is removed but there is no amidation *(21)*. Although some rules on the carboxy-end processing have been deduced, exceptions might exist *(60)* and new rules might arise when new sequences are determined.

6.2. K⁺-Channel Scorpion Toxins

To date only 14 cDNA and genomic sequences have been reported for K⁺-channel toxins. Genomic and cDNA sequences have been published for KTX₂ from *Androctonus australis* Hector *(61)*; *Bm*PO1, *Bm*PO3, and *Bm*PO5 from *Buthus martensii* Karsch *(62)*; *Ch*Tx-a from *Leiurus quinquestriatus hebraeus (59)*. Only the cDNA sequence has been reported for CoTx1 from *Centruroides noxius* Hoffmann *(63)*; *Bm*PO2 (*Buthus* *martensii* Karsch) *(64)*; *Ch*Tx-b, *Ch*Tx-c and *Ch*Tx-d from *Leiurus quinquestriatus hebraeus (59)*. The cDNA sequences of a new family of long-chain (60–64 amino acid residues), K$^+$ channel-blocking peptides stabilized by three disulfide bridges has been reported: *Aa*TXKβ from *Androctonus australis* Hector *(65)*; *Ts*TXKβ from *Tityus serrulatus (65)*; *Bm*TXKβ and *Bm*TXKβ2 from *Buthus martensii* Karsch *(64)*. The genomic organization of the DNA segments encoding these toxins showed a similarity with sodium channel toxin genes: two exons and one intron interrupting the region that codes for the signal peptide. The analysis of the cDNA and genomic sequences has revealed that the size of the signal peptide is larger (22–28 amino acid residues), but the size of the intron is shorter (78–133 nucleotides), compared to the ones encoding sodium channel toxins *(2)*.

7. PEPTIDES ACTIVE ON ION-CHANNEL FROM OTHER SOURCES

Elapidae and Hydrophidae snakes, specially from the genus *Bungarus* and *Naja*, provided protein-ligands that made possible the identification and isolation of the nicotinic acetylcholine receptor (AchR). To this category of peptides are the family of "three finger" snake peptides that greatly contributed to the study of muscle-type and neuronal AChR *(1)*. Equally important were the venoms from the mamba snakes, that provided several distinct groups of proteins, among which are the dendrotoxins, powerful blockers of Kv1 K$^+$-channels and calcicludines, which are blockers of HVA Ca^{2+} channels with preferred specificity toward L-type Ca^{2+}-channels *(66)*. Also from these snake venoms are the curaremimetic alpha-neurotoxins (short- and long-chain peptides), which are known to act selectively as agonists or antagonists of one or several of the five muscarinic receptors described, thus far *(66)*. Venomous gland extracts of snails of the genus *Conus* provided probably the most widely variable class of peptides that affect not only voltage-dependent Na$^+$-, K$^+$- and Ca^{2+} channels, but also the nicotinic and 5-HT receptors *(3,67)*. Omega-conotoxins GVIA and MVII from *Conus geographus* and *Conus magus* are important pharmacological agents that block the N-type Ca^{2+}-channels *(68)*. Sea anemone extracts provided initially several low molecular-weight peptides capable of binding to the external site on voltage-gated sodium channels and delay the process of inactivation *(69)*. Lately, however, from sea anemone, three peptides ShK, BgK, and ShK were purified and shown to affect K$^+$-channels *(6)*. Owing to the action of these peptides as blockers of K$^+$-channels (Kv1.3 type) in lymphocytes, the role of ShK as a potent immunosuppressant drug was recently discussed *(4)*. From spider venoms, several peptides were purified and reported to affect the function of voltage activated Ca^{2+}-channels, as well as Na^+-channels, among which are the omega-agatoxins and μ-agatoxins, respectively *(5)*. Hanatoxins are 35 amino acid long peptides isolated from a tarantula spider and were shown to modify the gating mechanism of voltage-dependent K^+-channels *(70)*. Another peptide (SNX-482) composed by 41 amino acids, from another tarantula was reported to be an antagonist of the class E Ca^{2+}-channels *(71)*. But not less important are the alpha-latrotoxin proteins, that provoke a massive transmitter release of neuromediators from presynaptic endings *(5)*. Finally, apamin, a honeybee venom short-peptide was also demonstrated to affect small-conductance Ca^{2+}- activated K^+-channel (for review, *see* ref. *6*).

8. PROSPECTS OF USING TOXINS FOR LOCALIZATION STUDIES

As mentioned in the introductory section, the literature information available on the use of scorpion toxins as markers of ion-channel distribution in various excitable tissues, is quite restricted. One of the first publications dealing with this subject used specific antibodies labeled with ferritin to map binding sites of toxic fractions from *Centruroides noxius* venom to rat-brain cortex *(72)*.

It is an open field with plenty of possible applications. There are various positive aspects, such as, the peptides are long enough to allow chemical labeling that do not necessarily modify the function, some of them can easily be expressed using DNA-recombinant techniques *(33,56,57)*, or can be obtained active by chemical synthesis *(73,74)*, where specific modified amino acids can be intercalated (Gurrola, B., Possani, L. D., Menez, A., and Vita, C., unpublished). Labeling of these peptides can be obtained by radio-isotope labeling, fluorescent probes or light-sensitive tags that can attached covalently to the channels or surrounding proteins. The biggest disadvantage of using these peptides for tissue localization of channel distribution, probably could come from the lack of specificity. Some of these toxins bind to more than one type of channel, with highly variable affinities, from p*M* to μ*M* constants.

9. CONCLUDING REMARKS

Venomous animals contain peptidic ligands capable of impairing normal function of excitable membranes of mammals, insects, and crustaceans. From scorpion venoms, peptides specific for ion-channels, such as Na^+, K^+, Cl^-, and Ca^{2+} were found. These peptides have been isolated and characterized, both structurally and functionally. Almost 100 distinct peptides specific for Na^+-channels have been reported. They are 60–76 amino acid residues long, very well compacted by four disulfide bridges, many of which have their three-dimensional structure determined by X-ray crystallography and/or NMR spectroscopy. They show one or two short alpha-helix segments and three anti-parallel beta sheet strands, forming several loops. The Na^+-channel specific peptides affect both the closing and opening mechanisms of ion-channels present in biological membranes. At least 10 different subfamilies of these peptides have been classified. The affinities of the peptides vary greatly, from micromolar to picomolar range depending on the type of tissue and toxin under consideration. They constitute excellent tools to locate the presence and distribution of such channels. Similarly, about 50 different peptides specific for K^+-channels, comprising 12 subfamilies were described. These are shorter peptides (from 29–42 amino acid residues), packed by three or four disulfide bridges. One segment of alpha-helix and two or three beta-strands conform their spatial folding, mainly studied by NMR spectroscopy. These peptides are authentic blockers of the channels, they seat on the mouth of the pore of the channel, impeding passage of potassium. Various peptides, either specific for Na^+- (53 different clones) or K^+-channels (14 clones) have been cloned and some of them were used for site-directed mutagenesis studies, in order to correlate the structure with the function of the channels. For the K^+-channels a section of the C-terminal region comprising a lysine residue was shown to be critical for channel blockage, whereas for the Na^+-channel toxin the active site is still under study, mainly owing to the fact that it is difficult to obtain properly folded mutants generated by molecular biology techniques.

ACKNOWLEDGMENTS

This work was partially supported by grant number 75197-527107 from the Howard Hughes Medical Institute and Dirección General de Asuntos del Personal Académico of the National Autonomous University of Mexico grant IN-217997 to L.D.P; and, grant BIL96/31 from the Flemish Community to J. T. The hH1 clone was kindly provided by R. G. Kallen. The authors wish to thank Dr. Barbara Selisko for support on the modeling of the three-dimensional structures shown.

REFERENCES

1. Tsetlin, V. (1999) Snake a-neurotoxins and other "three finger" proteins. *Eur. J. Biochem.* **264,** 281–286.

2. Possani, L. D., Becerril, B., Delepierre, M., and Tytgat, J. (1999) Scorpion toxins specific for Na⁺-channels. *Eur. J. Biochem.* **264,** 287–300.

3. MacIntosh, J. M., Olivera, B. M., and Cruz, L. J. (1999) *Conus* peptides as probes for ion channels. *Methods Enzymol.* **294,** 605–624.

4. Kem, W., Pennington, M. W., and Norton, R. S. (1999) Sea anemone toxins as templates for the desighn of immunosuppressant drugs. *Perspectives Drug Disc. Design* **15/16,** 111–129.

5. Grishin, E. (1999) Polypeptide neurotoxins from spider venoms. *Eur. J. Biochem.* **264,** 276–280.

6. Garcia, M. L., Hanner, M., Knaus, H. G., Koch, R., Schmalhofer, W., Slaughter, R. S., and Kaczorowski, G. J. (1997) Pharmacology of potassium channels. *Adv. Pharmacol.* **39,** 425–471.

7. Catterall, W. A. (1980) Neurotoxins that act on voltage sensitive sodium channels in excitable membranes. *Annu. Rev. Pharmacol. Toxicol.* **20,** 15–43.

8. Gordon, D., Savarin, P., Gurevitz, M., and Zinn-Justin, S. (1998) Functional anatomy of scorpion toxins affecting sodium channels. *J. Toxicol. Toxin Rev.* **17(2),** 131–159.

9. Possani, L. D., Selisko, B., and Gurrola, G. B. (1999) Structure and function of scorpion toxins affecting K⁺-channel. *Perspectives Drug Disc. Design* **15/16,** 15–40.

10. Tytgat, J., Chandy, G., Garcia, M. L., Gutman, G. A., Martin-Eauclaire, M. F., van der Walt, J. J., and Possani, L. D. (1999) A unified nomenclature for short-chain peptides isolated from scorpion venoms: alpha-KTx molecular subfamilies. *Trends Physiol. Sci.* **20,** 444–447.

11. Debin, J. A., Maggio, J. E., and Strichartz, G. R. (1993) Purification and characterization of chlorotoxin, a chloride channel ligand from the venom of the scorpion. *Am. J. Physiol.* **264** (*Cell Physiol.* **33**) C361–C369.

12. Valdivia, H. H. and Possani, L. D. (1998) Peptide toxins as probes of ryanodine receptor. *Trends Cardiovascular Med.* **8,** 111–118.

13. D´Suze, G., Zamudio, F., Gomez-Lagunas, F., and Possani, L. D. (1999) A novel K⁺ channel blocking toxin from *Tityus discrepans* scorpion venom. *FEBS Lett.* **456,** 146–148.

14. Gurrola, G. B., Rosati, B., Roccheti, M., Pimienta, G., Zaza, A., Arcangeli, A., et al. (1999) A toxin to nervous, cardiac, and endocrine ERG K⁺ channels isolated from *Centruroides noxius* scorpion venom. *FASEB J.* **13,** 953–962.

15. Chuang, R. S. I., Jaffe, H., Cribbe, L., Perez-Reyes, E., and Swartz, K. J. (1998) Inhibition of T-type voltage-gated calcium channels by a new scorpion toxin. *Nature Neurosci.* **1,** 668–674.

16. Vazquez, A., Tapia, J. V., Eliason, W. K., Martin, B. M., Lebreton, F., Delepierre, M., et al. (1995) Cloning and characterization of the cDNAs encoding Na⁺ channel specific toxins 1 and 2 of the scorpion *Centruroides noxius* Hoffmann. *Toxicon* **33,** 1161–1170.

17. Dauplais, M., Gilquin, B., Possani, L. D., Gurrola-Briones, G., Roumestand, C., and Menez, A. (1995) Determination of the three-dimensional solution structure of noxiustoxin: analysis of structural differences with related short-chain scorpion toxins. *Biochemistry* **34,** 16,563–16,573.

18. Lebreton, F., Ramirez, A. N., Balderas, C., Possani L. D., and Delepierre, M. (1994) Primary and NMR three-dimensional structure determination of a novel crustacean toxin from the venom of the scorpion *Centruroides limpidus limpidus* Karsch. *Biochemistry* **33(37)**, 11,135–11,149.

19. Schütte, C. G., Lemm, T., Glombitza, G. J., and Sandhoff, K. (1998) Complete localization of disulfide bonds in GM2 activator protein. *Protein Sci.* **7**, 1039–1045.

20. Jover, E., Couraud, F., and Rochat, H. (1980) Two types of scorpion neurotoxins characterized by their binding to two separate receptor sites on rat brain synaptosomes. *Biochem. Biophys. Res. Comm.* **95(4)**, 1607–1614.

21. Zlotkin, E., Gurevitz, M., Fowler, E., and Adams, M. E. (1993) Depressant insect selective neurotoxins from scorpion venom: chemistry, action and gene cloning. *Arch. Insect Biochem. Physiol* **22**, 55–73.

22. Kobayashi, Y., Takashima, H., Tamaoki, H., Kiogoku, Y., Lambert, P., Kuroda, H., et al. (1991) The cysteine-stabilized alpha-helix: a common structural motif of ion-channel blocking neurotoxic peptides. *Biopolymers* **31**, 1213–1220.

23. Menez, A., Bontems, F., Roumestand, C., Gilquin, B., and Toma, F. (1992) Structural basis for functional diversity of animal toxins. *Proc. Royal Soc. Edinburgh* **99B**, 83–103.

24. Oren, D. A., Froy, O., Amit, E., Kleinberger-Doron, V., Gurevitz, M., and Shaanan, B. (1998) An excitatory scorpion toxin with a distinctive feature: an additional helix at the C-terminus and its implications for interaction with insect sodium channels. *Structure* **6**, 10,995–11,003.

25. Fontecilla-Camps, J. C., Almassy, R. J., Suddath, F. L., Watt, D. D., and Bugg, C. E. (1980) Three-dimensional structure of a protein from scorpion venom: a new structural class of neurotoxins. *Proc. Natl. Acad. Sci. USA* **77(11)**, 6496–6500.

26. Polikarpov, I., Matilde Jr M. S., Marangoni, S., Toyama, M. H., and Teplyakov, A. (1999) Crystal structure of neurotoxin Ts1 from tityus serrulatus provides insights into the specificity and toxicity of scorpion toxins. *J. Mol. Biol.* **290**, 175–184.

27. Darbon, H., Weber, C., and Braun W. (1991) Two-dimensional ^{1}H nuclear magnetic resonance study of AaH IT, an anti-insect toxin from the scorpion *Androctonus australis* Hector. Sequential resonance assignments and folding of the polypeptide chain. *Biochemistry* **30(7)**, 1836–1845.

28. Pintar, A., Possani, L. D., and Delepierre, M. (1999) Solution structure of toxin 2 from *Centruroides noxius* Hoffmann, a β scorpion neurotoxin acting on sodium channel. *J. Mol. Biol.* **287**, 359–365.

29. Fontecilla-Camps, J. C., Almassy, R. J., Suddath, F. L., and Bugg, C. E. (1982) The three-dimensional structure scorpion neurotoxins. *Toxicon* **20**, 1–7.

30. Fontecilla-Camps, J. C, Habersetzer-Rochat, C., and Rochat, H. (1988) Orthorhombic crystals and three-dimensional structure of the potent toxin II from the scorpion *Androctonus australis* Hector. *Proc. Natl. Acad. Sci. USA* **85**, 7443–7447.

31. He, X-L, Li, H. M., Zeng, Z. H., Liu, X-Q, Wang, M., and Wang, D. C. (1999) Crystal structure of two α-like scorpion toxins: non proline cis peptide bonds and implications for new binding site selectivity on the sodium channel. *J. Mol. Biol.* **292**, 125–135.

32. Delepierre, M., Prochnika-Chalufour, A., and Possani, L. D. (1997) A novel potassium channel blocking toxin from the scorpion *Pandinus imperator*: a ^{1}H NMR analysis using a nano-NMR probe. *Biochemistry* **36,** 2649–2658.

33. Park, C. S. and Miller, C. (1992) Mapping function to structure in a channel-blocking peptide: electrostatic mutants of charybdotoxin. *Biochemistry* **31,** 7749–7755.

34. Bontems, F., Roumestand, C., Gilquin, B., Menez, A., and Toma, F. (1991) Refined structure of charybdotoxin: common motifs in scorpion toxins and insect defensins. *Science* **254,** 1521–1523.

35. Bonmatin, J. M., Bonnat, J. L., Gallet, X., Vovelle, F., Ptak, M., Reichhart, J. M., et al. (1992) Two-dimensional ^{1}H NMR study of recombinant insect defensin A in water: resonance assignments, secondary structure and global folding. *J. Biomol. NMR* **2,** 235–256.

36. Krezel, A. M., Kasibhatla, C., Hidalgo, P., MacKinnon, R., and Wagner, G. (1995) Solution structure of the potassium channel inhibitor agitoxin 2: caliper for probing channel geometry. *Protein Sci.* **4,** 1478–1489.

37. Delepierre, M., Prochnika-Chalufour, A., Boisbouvier, J., and Possani, L. D. (1999) Pi7, an orphan peptide from the scorpion *Pandinus imperator*: a ^{1}H NMR analysis using a nano-NMR probe. *Biochemistry* **38,** 16,756–16,765.

38. Becerril, B., Marangoni, S., and Possani, L. D. (1997) Toxins and genes isolated from scorpions of the genus *Tityus*. *Toxicon* **35,** 821–835.

39. Fernandez, I., Romi, R., Szendeffy, S., Martin-Eauclaire, M. F., Rochat, H., Van Rietschoten, J., et al. (1994) Kaliotoxin (1-37) shows structural differences with related potassium channel blockers. *Biochemistry* **33,** 14,256–14,263.

40. Adam, K. R., Schmidt, H., Stampfli, R., and Weiss, C. (1966) The effect of scorpion venom on single myelinated nerve fibers of the frog. *Br. J. Pharmacol.* **26,** 666–677.

41. Koppenhoeffer, E. and Schmidt, H. (1968) Die wirkung von skorpiongift auf die ionenstrome des Ranvierschen schnurrings. II. Unvollstandige natrium inaktivierung. *Pfluegers Arch. Ges. Physiol.* **303,** 150–161.

42. Meves, H., Rubly, N., and Watt, D. D. (1982) Effect of toxins from the venom of the scorpion *Centruroides sculpturatus* on the Na currents of the node of Ranvier. *Pfluegers Arch.* **393,** 56–62.

43. Nonner, W. (1979) Effects of Leiurus scorpion venom on the "gating" current in myelinated nerve. *Adv. Cytopharmacol.* **3,** 345–352.

44. Benoit, E. and Dubois, J. M. (1987) Properties of maintained sodium current induced by a toxin from *Androctonus* scorpion in frog node of Ranvier. *J. Physiol. (Lond.)* **383,** 93–114.

45. Strichartz, G. R. and Wang, G. K. (1986) Rapid voltage-dependent dissociation of scorpion alpha-toxins coupled to Na channel inactivation in amphibian myelinated nerves. *J. Gen. Physiol.* **88,** 413–435.

46. Meves, H., Simard, J. M., and Watt, D. D. (1986) Interactions of scorpion toxins with the sodium channel. *Ann. NY Acad. Sci.* **479,** 113–132.

47. Katz, N. L. and Edwards, C. (1972) The effect of scorpion venom on the neuromuscular junction of the frog. *Toxicon* **10,** 133–137.

48. Cahalan, M. D. (1975) Modification of sodium channel gating in frog myelinated nerve fibers by *Centruroides sculpturatus* scorpion venom. *J. Physiol. (Lond.)* **244,** 511–534.

49. Couraud, F., Jover, E., Dubois, J. M., and Rochat, H. (1982) Two types of scorpion receptor sites, one related to the activation, the other to the inactivation of the action potential sodium channel. *Toxicon* **20(1),** 9–16.

50. Hue, S. L., Meves, H., Rubly, N., and Watt, D. D. (1983) A quantitative study of the action of *Centruroides sculpturatus* toxins III and IV on the Na currents of the node of Ranvier. *Pfluegers Arch.* **397,** 90–99.

51. Vijverberg, H. P., Pauron, D., and Lazdunski, M. (1984) The effect of *Tityus serrulatus* scorpion toxin gamma on Na channels in neuroblastoma cells. *Pfluegers Arch.* **401,** 297–303.

52. Cestele, S., Qu, Y., Rogers, J. C., Rochat, H., Scheuer, T., and Catterall, W. A. (1998) Voltage sensor-trapping: enhanced activation of sodium channels by beta-scorpion toxin bound to the S3-S4 loop domain II. *Neuron* **21,** 919–931.

53. Wang, G. W. and Strichartz, G. (1982) Simultaneous modifications of sodium channel gating by two scorpion toxins. *Biophys. J.* **40,** 174–179.

54. Chandy, K. G. and Gutman, G. A. (1995) Voltage-gated potassium channel genes, in *Ligand- and Voltage-Gated Ion Channels* (North, R. A., ed.), CRC Press, Boca Raton, FL, pp. 1–71.

55. Kaczorowski, G. J., Knaus, H. G., Leonard, R. J., McManus, O. B., and Garcia, M. L. (1996) High conductance calcium-activated potassium channels; structure, pharmacology and function. *J. Biomembr. Bioenerg.* **28,** 253–265.

56. Goldstein, S. A. N. and Miller, C. (1993) Mechanism of charybdotoxin block of a voltage-gated K channel. *Biophys. J.* **65,** 1613–1619.

57. Goldstein, S. A. N., Pheasant, D. J., and Miller, C. (1994) The charybdotoxin receptor of a Shaker K channel: peptide and channel residues mediating molecular recognition. *Neuron* **12,** 1377–1388.

58. Becerril, B., Corona, M., Garcia, C., Bolivar, F., and Possani, L. D. (1995) Cloning of genes encoding scorpion toxins: an interpretative review. *J. Toxicol. Toxin Rev.* **14,** 339–357.

59. Froy, O., Sagiv, T., Poreh, M., Urbach, D., Zilberberg, N., and Gurevitz, M. (1999) Dynamic diversification from a putative common ancestor of scorpion toxins affecting, sodium, potassium and chloride channels. *J. Mol. Evol.* **48,** 187–196.

60. Martin-Eauclaire, M. F., Ceard, B., Ribeiro, A. M., Diniz, C. R., Rochat, H., and Bougis, P. E. (1994) Biochemical, pharmacological and genomic characterization of TsIV, an alpha-toxin from the venom of the South American scorpion *Tityus serrulatus*. *FEBS Lett.* **342,** 181–184.

61. Legros, C., Bougis, P. E. and Martin-Eauclaire, M. F. (1997) Genomic organization of the KTX_2 gene, encoding a "short" scorpion toxin active on K^+ channels. *FEBS Lett.* **402,** 45–49.

62. Wu, J. J., Dai, L., Lan, Z. D., and Chi, C. W. (1999) Genomic organization of three neurotoxins active on small conductance Ca^{2+}-activated potassium channels from the scorpion *Buthus martensii* Karsch. *FEBS Lett.* **452,** 360–364.

63. Selisko, B., Garcia, C., Becerril, B., Gómez-Lagunas, F., Garay, C., and Possani, L. D. (1998) Cobatoxins 1 and 2 from *Centruroides noxius* Hoffmann constitute a subfamily of potassium-channel-blocking scorpion toxins. *Eur. J. Biochem.* **254,** 468–479.

64. Zhu, S., Li, W., Zeng, X., Jiang, D., Mao, X., and Liu, H. (1999) Molecular cloning and sequencing of two "short chain" and two "long chain" K$^+$ channel-blocking peptides from the Chinese scorpion *Buthus martensii* Karsch. *FEBS Lett.* **457,** 509–514.

65. Legros, C., Ceard, B., Bougis, P. E., and Martin-Eauclaire, M. F. (1998) Evidence for a new class of scorpion toxins active against K$^+$ channels. *FEBS Lett.* **431,** 375–380.

66. Schweitz, H. and Moinier, D, (1999) Mamba toxins. *Perspectives Drug Disc. Design* **15/16,** 83–110.

67. Craig, A. G., Bandyopadhyay, P., and Olivera, B. (1999) Post-translationally modified neuropeptides from Conus venoms. *Eur. J. Biochem.* **264,** 271–275.

68. Olivera, B. M., Rivier, J., Clark, C., Ramilo, C. A., Corpuz, G. P., Abogadie, F. C., et al. (1990) Diversity of *Conus* neuropeptide. *Science* **249,** 257–263.

69. Beress, L., Beress, R., and Wunderer, G. (1975) Isolation and characterization of three polypeptides with neurotoxic activity from *Anemonia sulcata*. *FEBS Lett.* **50,** 311–314.

70. Swartz, K. J. and MacKinnon, R. (1997) Hanatoxin modifies the gating of a voltage-dependent K$^+$-channel through multiple binding sites. *Neuron* **18,** 665–673.

71. Newcomb, R., Szoke, B., Palma, A., Wang, G., Chen Xh, Hopkins, W., et al. (1998) Selective peptide antoganist of the class E calcium channel from the venom of the tarantula *Hysterocrates gigas*. *Biochemistry* **37,** 15,353–15,362.

72. Carabez-Trejo, A. and Possani, L. D. (1982) Electron microscopic evidence for scorpion toxin binding to synapses of rat brain cortex. *Neurosci. Lett.* **32,** 103–108.

73. Zamudio, F. Z., Gurrola, G. B., Arévalo, C., Sreekumar, R., Walker, J. W., Valdivia, H. H., and Possani, L. D. (1997) Primary structure and synthesis of Imperatoxin A (IpTxa), a peptide activator of Ca^{2+} release channels/ryanodine receptors. *FEBS Lett.* **405,** 385–389.

74. Gurrola, G. B. and Possani, L. D. (1995) Structural and functional features of noxiustoxin: a K$^+$ channel blocker. *Biochem. Mol. Biol. Int.* **37,** 527–535.

Part II

APPLICATIONS OF GREEN FLUORESCENT PROTEIN (GFP) TECHNOLOGY

9

Bicistronic GFP Expression Vectors as a Tool to Study Ion Channels in Transiently Transfected Cultured Cells

Jan Eggermont, Dominique Trouet, Gunnar Buyse, Rudi Vennekens, Guy Droogmans, and Bernd Nilius

1. INTRODUCTION

The availability of ion-channel cDNAs has greatly increased our insight in the structure, function, pharmacology, and regulation of ion channels at the molecular level. Much of this knowledge has been obtained by expressing wild-type or mutant ion channels in a heterologous host system, thereby facilitating functional approaches and analyses, which are not possible, when the native channel is studied in its *in situ* context *(1)*.

Xenopus oocytes have proven to be a reliable and efficient expression system, especially for voltage-gated cation channels and channels gated by extracellular ligands. However, *Xenopus* oocytes have several drawbacks with respect to the study of ion channels: (1) *Xenopus* oocytes contain several endogenous currents, most notably anion currents, which can interfere with the characterization of expressed channels (for a discussion of endogenous ion currents in *Xenopus* oocytes, *see* refs. *2* and *3*). (2) Because *Xenopus* oocytes are highly specialized nonmammalian cells surrounded by a layer of follicular cells, the processing of the expressed channel protein *(4,5)*, its pharmacological properties *(6,7)* and/or the signal transduction pathways may diverge from those in mammalian cells. (3) Single-channel analysis as well as control of the internal medium are more cumbersome than in mam-

From: *Ion Channel Localization Methods and Protocols*
Edited by: A. Lopatin and C. G. Nichols © Humana Press Inc., Totowa, NJ

malian cells and require specialized techniques *(8)*. Most of these disadvantages can be overcome by expressing ion channels in mammalian cells, although, evidently, mammalian cells are not entirely devoid of endogenous background currents. A specific problem with transfection in mammalian cells is, however, that the transfection efficiency (i.e., the proportion of transfected cells that express the ion channel of interest) varies greatly depending on the cell type, the transfection method, purity of the DNA (contamination with bacterial endotoxins), quality of the cell line, and the biological activity (problem of toxicity). In principle, there are two experimental strategies to overcome the problem of low efficiency. (1) Stable selection of positive cells by drug resistance (e.g., resistance to G418 [an aminoglycoside], puromycin, hygromycin). However, selection and characterization of a monoclonal cell line stably expressing the ion channel under study is a time-consuming process that can take up to several weeks or months. The use of stable cell lines is therefore generally restricted to pharmacological screening experiments or applications that require large amounts of protein (e.g., biochemical characterization of the expressed channel). (2) Identification of transiently transfected cells using a marker that can be detected under patch-clamp conditions without compromising the cellular integrity and function. Ideally, such a marker should not interfere with microfluorescence-based techniques that allow measurement of intracellular Ca^{2+}, intracellular pH, or cell volume. In this chapter, we describe a detection method for transiently transfected cells that uses a variant of green fluorescent protein (GFP) as an in vivo cell marker and an internal ribosomal entry site (IRES)-dependent bicistronic transcription unit to ensure strict coupling between expression of the channel and the GFP marker.

2. METHODOLOGICAL CONSIDERATIONS

2.1. Green Fluorescent Protein

Wild-type GFP is a 26.8 kDa protein (238 amino acids) from the jelly fish *Aequorea victoria* that contains a fluorochrome with two excitation peaks (major at 395 nm; minor at 475 nm) and a single-emission peak at 510 nm *(9)*. Formation of the fluorochrome occurs post-translationally by spontaneous cyclization of a Ser-Tyr-Gly tripeptide (amino acid 65 to 67) followed by oxidation *(10)*. The spectral properties of GFP (excitation and emission wave lengths, fluorescence intensity) can be changed by specific mutations that modify the chromophore structure or promote correct folding of the protein (for a review, *see* ref. *11*). Several properties promoted the use of GFP as an identification tool for cells transfected with ion channels. (1)

GFP fluorescence does not require additional cofactors or substrates *(9)* thereby obviating the need for cell manipulation prior to detection. (2) GFP seems to be non-toxic for mammalian cells as evidenced by the observation that transgenic mice expressing GFP develop normally *(12)*. However, it has been suggested that fluorochrome formation is accompanied by a stoichiometric release of H_2O_2 which could be harmful in case of high level GFP expression *(13)*. (3) Because GFP is a cytosolic protein, it is less likely to interfere with the function of membrane proteins such as ion channels, thereby reducing the possibility of artefacts owing to the expression system. Yet, the application of wild-type GFP as a transfection marker is at least in mammalian cells seriously limited by the weakness of the fluorescent signal and by the background autofluorescence generated by cellular excitation in the UV range *(13)*. Fortunately, these problems have been (partially) resolved by generating mutant GFPs with altered spectral properties *(13)*. One of the first GFP mutants available was enhanced GFP (eGFP), which bears the double mutation F64L and S65T *(14,15)*. When compared to wild-type GFP, eGFP has a red-shifted excitation spectrum with a single excitation peak at 488 nm and a similar emission peak at 510 nm, but the emission light is approx 30-fold more intense. We therefore selected eGFP as an identification tool for transfected cells.

2.1.1. Internal Ribosomal Entry Site

The next question is how to couple the expression of the ion channel to that of eGFP. One possibility is to construct a fusion protein between the ion channel and GFP leading to an ion channel with a fluorescent tag *(16–18)*. Alternatively, mammalian cells can be co-transfected with two vectors, one expressing the ion channel and another GFP *(16)*. We opted for a third possibility in which the ion channel and the eGFP marker are expressed from an IRES-containing, bicistronic mRNA.

IRES is an RNA sequence that allows cap-independent translation of mRNAs in mammalian cells. Translation initiation of the vast majority of cellular mRNAs requires the presence of a methylated cap at the 5' end of the mRNA (Fig. 1). The eukaryotic initiation factor 4F (eIF-4F) binds to the methylated cap and initiates the recruitment of the ribosomal apparatus to the mRNA *(19)*. However, translation initiation of some viral RNAs (e.g., picorna viruses, *see* ref. *20*) and of a small subset of cellular mRNAs *(19)* does not require a 5' cap structure in the mRNA. Instead, cap-independent translation is initiated by binding of the ribosomal apparatus to an internal RNA sequence in the 5' untranslated region (UTR), which is aptly named the internal ribosomal entry site or IRES. The presence of an IRES in the 5' UTR allows cap-independent translation of viral RNA during

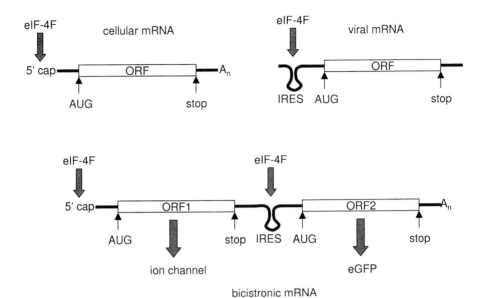

Fig. 1. Cap-dependent vs IRES-dependent translation initiation. Recruitment of the eIF-4F factor is the first step in the translation of cellular mRNAs, picornaviral RNAs and IRES-containing bicistronic RNAs. Both the methylated 5' cap (cellular mRNAs) and the IRES sequence (picornaviral RNAs) function as binding sites for eIF-4F and they can therefore direct ribosomal assembly. The stop codon signals the end of the open reading frame and causes the ribosome to dissociate from the RNA. Thus, translation of the second open reading frame in a bicistronic mRNA requires an eIF-4F binding site upstream of the start codon of the second open reading frame to promote ribosomal assembly.

picornaviral infection when cap-dependent translation of host-cell mRNAs is shut down owing to the virus-mediated cleavage of eIF-4G, a subunit of the eIF-4F complex *(21)*. Intact eIF-4G is required for cap-dependent translation, but cleaved eIF-4G is still capable of sustaining IRES-mediated translation initiation *(22,23)*. Although the naturally occurring viral and cellular IRES sequences are found in the 5' UTR of monocistronic RNAs (i.e., RNAs with a single open reading frame), IRES sequences can be put to work in the context of bicistronic mRNAs *(24–26)*. If positioned between the first and second open reading frame of a bicistronic mRNA, IRES significantly increases the translation of the downstream open reading frame. Structural and functional criteria allow the picornaviral IRESes to be classified in 3 groups with the IRES of cardioviruses (e.g., the Encephalomyocarditis virus or EMCV) and aphtoviruses being the most efficient element for IRES-

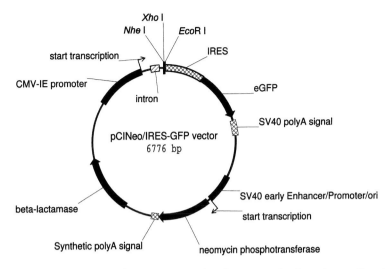

Fig. 2. pCINeo/IRES-GFP vector. The Cytomegalovirus immediate/early enhancer/promoter drives the expression of the bicistronic transcription unit. cDNAs of interest can be inserted in the *Nhe*I, *Xho*I, or *Eco*RI sites. Transcription results in a bicistronic mRNA. The first open reading frame is derived from the inserted cDNA (encoding the protein of interest) and it is translated in a cap-dependent way. The second open reading frame encodes eGFP, which requires the IRES sequence for translation.

dependent translation initiation *(27)*. Thus, owing to their unique property of directing internal translation initiation, IRES elements can be used to couple the expression of two proteins such as GFP and an ion channel on the condition that both are expressed from an IRES-containing bicistronic mRNA.

2.2. pCINeo/IRES-GFP Vector

The pCINeo/IRES-GFP is schematically shown in Fig. 2. The vector was constructed starting from a pCI-neo backbone (Promega), which was modified by inserting an IRES-eGFP cassette in the multiple cloning site *(28)*. The bicistronic transcription unit consists of the following elements: (1) the Cytomegalovirus immediate-early enhancer and promoter for efficient transcription in a broad range of mammalian cells; (2) an artificial intron; (3) a cloning site that consists of unique *Nhe*I, *Xho*I, and *Eco*RI sites and that allows insertion of cDNAs encoding the protein of interest; (4) an IRES sequence corresponding to nucleotides 243–833 of the EMCV RNA (GenBank/EMBL accession number M81861) and containing the essential sequence elements for cap-independent translation; (5) eGFP cDNA encoding the enhanced GFP (F64L/S65T) as described earlier; (6) an SV40 polyA signal for efficient 3' end processing. After transfection in a mammalian cell, a bicistronic mRNA is transcribed: the first open reading frame corresponds to the cDNA inserted in the cloning site upstream of IRES and it is translated in the classical cap-dependent way; the second open reading frame encodes eGFP and is translated via the IRES.

The pCINeo/IRES-GFP vector contains a second transcription unit that allows expression of the neomycin phosphotransferase gene. This transcription unit confers two additional properties: (1) it allows stable selection of transfected cells owing to resistance to neomycin and analogs such as G418; (2) the SV40 enhancer/promoter contains the SV40 origin of replication thereby allowing episomal replication in Large T-antigen expressing hosts such as COS cells.

In addition to the pCINeo/IRES-GFP vector other bicistronic IRES-GFP vectors have been reported, for example pTF-G6/IRES/GFP *(29)*, pCAGGSM2/IRES-GFP *(30)* and commercially available vectors such as pIRES-EGFP and pIRES-EYFP (Clontech, Palo Alto, CA).

2.3. Evaluation of GFP Fluorescence in pCINeo/IRES-GFP Transfected Cells

2.3.1. Patch Clamp Set Up

For current recordings in pCINeo/IRES-GFP transfected cells, a patch clamp set up containing a Zeiss Axiovert 100 microscope, a Xenon light source, and epifluorescence optics (Zeiss, XBO 75 and Zeiss-EPI unit, fluorescence condenser) was used to visualize green fluorescent cells. The excitation light reached the cells via a band-pass filter (Zeiss filter set 9, 487909; BP 450–490) and subsequently a dichroic mirror (Zeiss FT 510). The emitted light passed a 520 nm long-pass filter (Zeiss, LP 520) and was visually detected *(28)*.

2.3.2. FACScan Analysis

Cells transfected with pCINeo/IRES-GFP are trypsinized 24–48 h after transfection and GFP fluorescence is measured with a FACScan (Fluorescence Activated Cell Scan; Becton Dickinson) with FITC settings (excitation at 488 nm; emission detected in FL1-H channel). FACScan of cells transiently transfected with the pCINeo/IRES-GFP vector typically shows an elongated tail which corresponds to the cell population expressing GFP and the protein encoded by the first open reading frame (Fig. 3). In cells stably transfected with pCINeo/IRES-GFP, the entire distribution plot is shifted to higher fluorescence levels (Fig. 4).

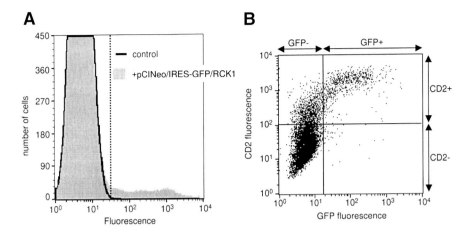

Fig. 3. FACScan of transiently transfected COS cells. **(A)** COS cells were transiently transfected with pCINeo/IRES-GFP/RCK1 and analyzed by FACScan. Nontransfected control cells display background fluorescence as indicated by the black curve (cut off for background fluorescence indicated by the dotted line). The transfected cell population (gray-filled curve) contains a subpopulation (7% of the cells) with increased fluorescence (extended gray-filled tail to the right). Electrophysiological analysis of the transfected population revealed that 100% of the green cells ($n = 32$) expressed a $K_{v1.1}$ delayed rectifier K^+ current typical of RCK1, which was not detected in nonfluorescent COS cells *(28)*. **(B)** COS cells were transfected with pCINeo/IRES-GFP/CD2 and subjected to dual FACScan analysis to simultaneously measure GFP expression (*x*-axis) and CD2 (a lymphocyte surface antigen) expression (*y*-axis). The graph shows that virtually every green fluorescent cell also expresses the CD2 antigen thereby validating the use of the GFP signal as a marker for co-expression.

2.3.3. Fluorescence Microscopy

GFP fluorescence is easily assessed on a classical fluorescence microscope (Nikon Epi-fl microscope) with standard epifluorescence optics (excitation filter: 450 to 490 nm; dichroic mirror at 505 nm and a barrier filter at 520 nm). Transfected cells are seeded on cover slips and turned upside down on a microscope glass.

Imaging of pCINeo/IRES-GFP transfected cells was performed with a Biorad 1024 confocal microscope with a Argon/Krypton laser (488 nm) for excitation and an emission filter (FITC settings) of 522 ± 16 nm. For this purpose, cells were grown in LabTek culture chambers.

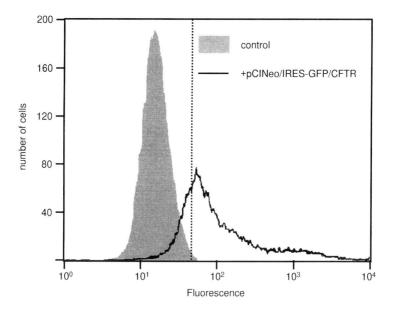

Fig. 4. FACScan of stably transfected CHO cells. CHO cells were transfected with pCINeo/IRES-GFP/CFTR and selected with G418 during 6 wk. The polyclonal G418-resistant cell population was then subjected to FACScan analysis (black curve) and compared to control cells (gray-filled curve). The fluorescence profile of the G418-resistant population is clearly shifted to the right with 76% of the cells being above background fluorescence (cut off for background fluorescence indicated by the dotted line).

3. EVALUATION OF THE BICISTRONIC PCINEO/ IRES-GFP VECTOR

3.1. Indications for Bicistronic IRES-GFP Vectors

In general, the need for a bicistronic IRES-GFP vector to study ion channels after transfection in mammalian cells is inversely correlated with the efficiency of transfection. In some cell lines and under optimal conditions, it is possible to obtain transfection efficiencies of 50% or more. For example, transient transfection of the wild-type $\alpha 1G$ subunit (cloned in a pcDNA3 vector) in HEK cells generated typical T-type Ca^{2+} currents in approx 30% of the patched cells without GFP selection (J. Prenen and B. Nilius, unpublished observations). Efficient "blind patching" also requires that the transfected channel has a characteristic fingerprint that is easily and rapidly recognized after seal formation. However, "blind patching" may cause problems when testing mutant channels of which the expression level and/or the phenotype may drastically differ from those of the wild-type channel. Thus, even if control experiments indicate a high-transfection efficiency for the wild-type channel, a bicistronic IRES-GFP expression system may still facilitate the functional analysis of less-efficiently expressing mutant channels.

A bicistronic IRES-GFP vector is virtually indispensable when working with cell lines with low transfection efficiency irrespective of the transfected ion channel. For example, the transfection efficiency in calf pulmonary artery endothelial cells (CPAE) is generally less than 5%. However, selection of positive cells by means of GFP fluorescence allowed us to efficiently study membrane currents (and cytosolic Ca^{2+} signals) in CPAE cells transfected with the α-subunit of the human large conductance Ca^{2+} activated K^+ channel (hslo), the human trp3 channel *(31,32)*, bovine trp1 and trp4 *(33)*, and human CFTR Cl^- channel *(34)*.

3.2. Alternatives to Bicistronic IRES-GFP Vectors

An interesting question is whether there are alternative strategies for coupled expression of ion channel and GFP and if so, what the respective advantages and disadvantages are. A first alternative is to construct an expression vector encoding a fusion protein between the ion channel and GFP, which results in the expression of an ion channel with a fluorescent tag at its amino or carboxyl terminus *(16)*. The construction of a fusion protein vector is technically more demanding than the insertion of the channel cDNA in the pCINeo/IRES-GFP vector, because synthesis of a full-length fusion protein requires that the ion channel cDNA and GFP cDNA are ligated in frame to preserve the open reading frame. Although the fusion protein approach has been successfully used for several ion channels *(17,18)*, it is impossible to predict *a priori* whether or not the attachment of a 238 amino acid peptide to the NH_2- or COOH-terminus of an ion channel will alter the biosynthesis, localization, stability, or functional properties of the channel. A second alternative is cotransfection of mammalian cells with two vectors, one expressing the ion channel and another GFP *(16)*. This approach has the advantage that it works with any mammalian expression vector because there is no specific need to clone the ion channel cDNA in a bicistronic IRES-GFP vector. However, the fraction of fluorescent cells that will also express the ion channel depends on the efficiency of cotransfection and may therefore vary. Whereas this may not pose problems for cells with a high transfection efficiency, it can seriously slow down experiments on cells with a low transfection efficiency. A third possibility is to couple the expression of fluorescent protein and protein of interest via a bi-directional expression system. Fang et al. *(35)* described a mammalian expression vector in which the eGFP gene and a second gene encoding the protein of interest are transcribed from oppositely oriented CMV promoters controlled by a single tetracycline-regulated element (TRE). Binding of the tetracycline-controlled transactivator (tTA) to TRE simultaneously switches on both CMV promoters resulting in co-expression of the two transcription units *(36,37)*. Moreover, transcription can be shut down by the addition of tetracycline or doxycycline because these antibiotics bind to tTA thereby dissociating it from TRE. Although this method ensures strict coupling, it suffers from the disadvantage that the tTA has to be provided in trans, thus limiting the application of this system to cell lines that have previously been stably transfected with a tTa expression plasmid (a series of tTA positive cell lines is available from Clontech). Finally, one could resort to an expression vector with two independent transcription units (cf pBudCE4; Invitrogen, Carlsbad, CA) with one promoter driving the expression of GFP and the other promoter controlling the expression of a second protein.

In conclusion, in comparison with the aforementioned strategies, the bicistronic IRES-GFP vector offers the following advantages: (1) obligate co-expression of fluorescent marker and ion channel; (2) no structural modification of the ion channel; (3) no requirement for additional trans-activating factors. A technical problem with the pCINeo/IRES-GFP may be the small number of unique restriction sites, which may occasionally complicate subcloning or mutagenesis procedures.

3.3. Effects of GFP Expression on Membrane Currents

Because the purpose of the GFP marker is to identify cells for electrophysiological analysis, one critical question is whether GFP expression affects the functional characteristics of the host cell. The dominant membrane current in nonstimulated CPAE cells is an inwardly rectifying K^+ current *(38)*, which is not affected by the expression of eGFP (e.g., *see* Fig. 2 in ref. *32*). Furthermore, we systematically studied the potential effect of eGFP on $I_{Cl,swell}$, the chloride current through the volume-regulated anion channel (VRAC), which is typically activated by exposing CPAE cells to an extracellular hypotonic solution (for a review of VRAC, *see* ref. *2*). $I_{Cl,swell}$ current densities were not significantly different between control CPAE cells and green fluorescent CPAE cells that had been transfected with an "empty" pCINeo/IRES-GFP vector (*see* Fig. 5 and ref. *34*). Similarly, expression of eGFP alone had no effect on $I_{Cl,swell}$ in Caco-2 cells *(39)*. Smith et al. *(40)* com-

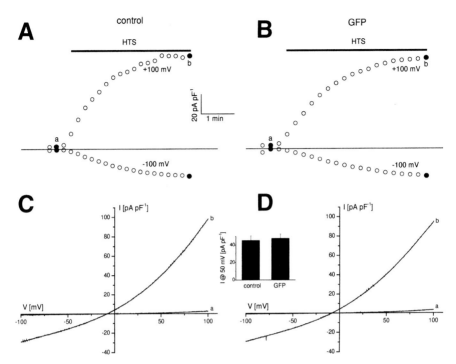

Fig. 5. GFP expression does not interfere with $I_{Cl,swell}$ in CPAE cells. **(A,B)** Time course of $I_{Cl,swell}$ in control (A) and pCINeo/IRES-GFP transfected (B) CPAE cells at +100 mV (upper) and –100 mV (lower). $I_{Cl,swell}$ was triggered by perfusing the cells with a hypotonic solution (HTS; 27% reduction) as indicated. **(C,D)** Current-voltage relationships for control (C) and pCINeo/IRES-GFP transfected (D) CPAE cells. IV plots were reconstructed from ramps at the times *(a,b)* indicated in the time course. The inset shows the mean $I_{Cl,swell}$ (error bar = SEM) at +50 mV for control (*n* = 10) and transfected (*n* = 9) cells. $I_{Cl,swell}$ characteristics are not different between control and GFP-expressing cells.

pared the electrophysiological properties of dorsal root ganglion cells before and after infection with a GFP-expressing adenovirus and found no difference between the two conditions. Finally, agonist-induced Ca^{2+} release as measured by the peak cytosolic Ca^{2+} concentration after application of a Ca^{2+} mobilizing agonist was not significantly different between control cells and GFP-expressing cells, either CPAE *(32)* or COS-7 cells (Fig. 6). To conclude, the available data indicate that expression of GFP does not disturb the electrophysiological properties of the host cell as can be expected from a nontoxic, cytosolic protein.

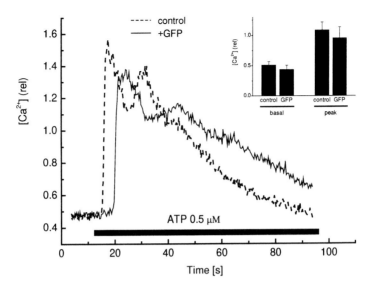

Fig. 6. GFP expression does not interfere with ATP-induced Ca^{2+} transient in COS cells. COS cells were transiently transfected with pCINeo/IRES-GFP and stimulated with 0.5 μM ATP. Free cytosolic Ca^{2+} concentration was ratiometrically measured with indo-1 as a fluorescent indicator. The time course as well as the amplitude of the ATP-triggered $[Ca^{2+}]_{cyt}$ transients were identical in control and GFP-expressing cells. The inset shows no difference between the basal and peak $[Ca^{2+}]_{cyt}$ (mean ± SEM) in control ($n = 25$) and GFP-expressing ($n = 8$) COS cells.

4. APPLICATIONS

4.1. Functional Characterization of Ion Channels in GFP Transfected Cells

Using the bicistronic IRES-GFP vector we have been able to express a wide variety of ion channels in different mammalian cell lines: voltage-dependent K^+ channels RCK1 *(28)*, voltage-dependent ClC-1 Cl^- channels *(41)*, and CFTR Cl^- channels in COS cells *(34,42)*; large conductance Ca^{2+} activated K^+ channels hslo *(32)*, Ca^{2+} permeable trp3 channels *(31)*, bovine trp1 and trp4 *(33)*, and CFTR Cl^- channels *(34)* in CPAE cells; the regulatory β-subunit of the large conductance Ca^{2+} activated K^+ channels hslo in endothelial EA.hy926 cells (Papassotiriou, Nilius; unpublished observations); modulators of VRAC such as caveolin-1 in Caco-2, T47D, and MCF-7 cells *(39)*; ECaC (epithelial Ca^{2+} channel) (Vennekens, Nilius, Bindels; unpublished observations) in HEK cells.

4.2. Ca²⁺ Measurements in GFP Expressing Cells

One interesting application of the bicistronic technology is to measure cytosolic Ca^{2+} in transfected mammalian cells. For example, CPAE cells do not express a large-conductance Ca^{2+}-activated K^+ channel (BK_{Ca}), which provided us with a tool to study the effect of hslo (the human large-conductance Ca^{2+}-activated K^+ channel) on the agonist-induced $[Ca^{2+}]_{cyt}$ in an endothelial cell line. In this study cytosolic Ca^{2+} was measured by using fura-2 as a Ca^{2+} indicator (excitation: 360/380nm; emission > 510 nm) signals with a photomultiplier tube. Stimulation of hslo-transfected CPAE cells with Ca^{2+} mobilizing agonists such as ATP resulted in a significant hyperpolarization and concomitantly an increased Ca^{2+} plateau that depended on Ca^{2+} influx *(32)*. Thus, these experiments allowed us to correlate the effects of BK_{Ca} on membrane potential, membrane currents and $[Ca^{2+}]_{cyt}$ during agonist stimulation. In a similar approach, we were able to show that CPAE cells transfected with htrp3 acquired an agonist-sensitive nonspecific cation current that could be blocked by PLC-β inhibitors and also an increase in the agonist-induced $[Ca^{2+}]_{cyt}$ plateau *(31)*.

4.3. Cell Volume Measurements in GFP Expressing Cells

We have recently developed a method to record simultaneously cell thickness (representing cell volume) and membrane currents *(43)*. Cell thickness is measured using fluorescent beads (Red Neutravidin: excitation peak 580 nm; emission peak 605 nm; Molecular Probes), which are seeded above and below cells plated on coverslips, and which allow to monitor changes in cell height (*see* also ref. *44*). Because there is sufficient difference between the fluorescent properties of eGFP and Red Neutravidin-labeled beads, we have been able to measure cell thickness in pCINeo/IRES-GFP-transfected endothelial cell lines *(34)*. Using this technique, we were able to show that the inhibitory effects of transiently expressed CFTR on the swelling-induced activation of VRAC in CPAE cells cannot be accounted for by altered cell volume responses in CFTR-expressing cells.

4.4. Immunofluorescence of pCINeo/IRES-GFP-Transfected Cells

Usage of the pCINeo/IRES-GFP vector is also compatible with immunofluorescent analysis of transfected cells. In a recent study, we showed that caveolin-1 is required for efficient activation of VRAC and that this effect is isoform-specific: caveolin-1α is completely inactive, whereas caveolin-1β is equipotent with respect to caveolin-1 *(39)*. To find out whether differences in expression or intracellular distribution might account for the isoform-specific effects, we looked at caveolin-1 distribution in transfected Caco-2 cells by immunofluorescence on a

BioRad 1024 confocal fluorescence microscope with the following settings: excitation with Krypton/Argon laser at 488 nm; emission filter for FITC (or GFP): 522 ± 16 nm; emission filter for R-Phycoerythrin: 580 ± 16 nm. Because the cells were transfected with the pCINeo/IRES-GFP vector, we could first identify the transfected cells by their green fluorescent signal and subsequently assess the caveolin-1 expression using a monoclonal antibody (MAb) and R-Phycoerythrin-conjugated secondary antibodies. This revealed that caveolin-1β is expressed in the cell periphery and plasma membrane, whereas expression of caveolin-1α is restricted to the cell interior *(39)*.

The pCINeo/IRES-GFP vector was also used to study the subcellular distribution of transiently transfected ClC-6 isoforms in COS and CHO cells *(41)*. This indicated that transiently expressed ClC-6 co-localized with the endoplasmic reticulum Ca^{2+} pump SERCA2b, which is compatible with an intracellular location of ClC-6.

4.5. Creation of Stable Cell Lines

The pCINeo/IRES-GFP vector allows selection of stably transfected cells with geneticin (G418) owing to the presence of the phosphotransferase gene. We have successfully created CHO cell lines stably transfected with pCINeo/IRES-GFP containing the cDNA for CFTR (data not shown). FACS analysis of the G418-resistant polyclonal cell pool indicated that 70% of the G418-resistant cells showed green fluorescence above background after 6 wk of drug selection (Fig. 4). However, we also observed that the number of GFP-positive cells in the polyclonal population gradually declined during cell culturing. This is probably owing to the fact that the phosphotransferase gene and the bicistronic IRES-GFP unit constitute two different transcription units that can be separated during chromosomal integration of the plasmid DNA. Consequently, only a fraction of the drug-resistant cells will be green fluorescent and express the cDNA that is cloned in the bicistronic IRES-GFP transcription unit.

This problem can be circumvented by using bicistronic vectors in which the resistance gene is placed behind the IRES sequence ensuring that every drug-resistant cell also expresses the cDNA of interest *(45–47)*. Because these vectors do not contain a cDNA for a fluorescent marker, they do not allow visual selection of transfected cells. GFP selection would require the modification of existing vectors. One possibility is to create a tricistronic vector in which the second transcription unit encodes the fluorescent marker and the third transcription unit (also preceded by an IRES) contains the resistance gene. It has indeed been shown that IRES mediates translation of tricistronic RNAs *(24,48)*. An alternative possibility is to construct a bicistronic vector with the second open reading frame encoding a fusion protein between a GFP variant and a resistance marker. Functional GFP-drug resistance fusion proteins have recently been described *(49)* and monocistronic vectors with such fusion proteins are commercially available (Clontech).

4.6. Expression of Heteromeric Channels

An important theme that has emerged from biochemical and molecular biological studies on ion channels is that a functional channel is often composed of a heteromeric complex. Heteromeric channel complexes are found among voltage-dependent cation channels (e.g., Ca^{2+} channels, *see* ref. *50*), ligand-gated channels *(51)*, degenerin/ENaC channels *(52)*, and possibly voltage-dependent Cl^- channels *(53)*. Functional analysis of heteromeric channels requires the simultaneous co-expression of all subunits in a single transfected cell. This has been achieved by co-transfecting the different subunits, but as already mentioned this method suffers from the fact that cotransfection efficiency is never 100% thereby introducing a degree of uncertainty. Kawashima et al. *(54)* have recently described an alternative strategy to study heteromeric channels after transfection in mammalian cells. A tricistronic expression vector encoding the $P2X_2$ subunit, the $P2X_3$ subunits and neomycin phosphotransferase was used to establish stably transfected cells that expressed functional heteromeric ATP-activated channels. It remains to be seen whether such tricistronic constructs will gain more widespread acceptance to study heteromeric channels. Alternatively, one could use two bicistronic vectors containing different versions of green fluorescent protein (e.g., eGFP and BFP or blue fluorescent protein) in a cotransfection procedure followed by identification of cells containing both green and blue fluorescence *(55,56)*. Finally, a growing theme in channel research is the importance of direct protein-protein interactions for channel function and regulation as illustrated by the interaction of PDZ proteins with Drosophila TRP *(57)* or human CFTR *(58)*. Efficient co-expression vectors and/or systems will be extremely useful to study the functional implications of such interactions.

5. CONCLUSION

The bicistronic GFP-expressing vector provides an elegant and efficient tool to identify transiently transfected cells. The main advantages of this technology are: (1) there is a strict coupling between GFP expression and expression of the protein of interest; (2) it does not require covalent modification of the protein of interest; (3) GFP is a nontoxic marker that does not interfere with membrane currents; (4) GFP expression does not interfere with other fluorescent signals such as fluorescent Ca^{2+} indicators or fluorescent beads provided that the appropriate filters are used. As such the pCINeo/IRES-GFP vector is particularly well-suited to study ion channels in cell lines that are transfected with low efficiency.

ACKNOWLEDGMENTS

We thank Diane Hermans for skillful contribution in constructing the parental pCINeo/IRES-GFP vector and derivatives. DT is a Research Assistant and JE is a Research Associate of the Fund for Scientific Research-Flanders. This work has been supported by FWO (G.0214.99), GOA (99/07), IUAP (P4/23) and the "Fonds Alphonse and Jean Forton in the King Boudewijn Foundation, R7115B0, Belgium."

REFERENCES

1. Whiting, P. J., Wafford, K. A., Pribilla, I., and Petri, T. (1995) Channel cloning, mutagenesis and expression, in *Ion channels. A Practical Approach* (Ashley, R. H., ed.), IRL Press, Oxford, pp. 133–169.
2. Nilius, B., Eggermont, J., Voets, T., Buyse, G., Manolopoulos, V., and Droogmans, G. (1997) Properties of volume-regulated anion channels in mammalian cells. *Prog. Biophys. Molec. Biol.* **68,** 69–119.
3. Weber, W. M. (1999) endogenous ion channels in oocytes of Xenopus laevis: recent developments. *J. Membrane Biol.* **170,** 1–12.
4. Pasyk, E. A., Morin, X. K., Zeman, P., Garami, E., Galley, K., Huan, L. J., Wang, Y., and Bear, C. E. (1998) A conserved region of the R domain of cystic fibrosis transmembrane conductance regulator is important in processing and function. *J. Biol. Chem.* **273,** 31759–31764.
5. Smit, L. S., Strong, T. V., Wilkinson, D. J., Macek, M. J., Mansoura, M. K., Wood, D. L., et al. (1995) Missense mutation (G480C) in the CFTR gene associated with protein mislocalization but normal chloride channel activity. *Hum. Molec. Genet.* **4,** 269–273.
6. Madeja, M., Musshoff, U., and Speckmann, E. J. (1997) Follicular tissues reduce drug effects on ion channels in oocytes of Xenopus laevis. *Eur. J. Neurosci.* **9,** 599–604.
7. Krafte, D. S., Davison, K., Dugrenier, N., Estep, K., Josef, K., Barchi, R. L., et al. (1994) Pharmacological modulation of human cardiac Na+ channels. *Eur. J. Pharmacol.* **266,** 245–254.
8. Stefani, E. and Bezanilla, F. (1998) Cut-open oocyte voltage-clamp technique. *Methods Enzymol.* **293,** 300–318.
9. Chalfie, M., Tu, Y., Euskirchen, G., Ward, W. W., and Prasher, D. C. (1994) Green fluorescent protein as a marker for gene expression. *Science* **263,** 802–805.

10. Heim, R., Prasher, D. C., and Tsien, R. Y. (1994) Wavelength mutations and posttranslational autoxidation of green fluorescent protein. *Proc. Natl. Acad. Sci. USA* **91,** 12,501–12,504.

11. Tsien, R. W. (1998) Key clockwork component cloned. *Nature* **391,** 839,840.

12. Okabe, M., Ikawa, M., Kominami, K., Nakanishi, T., and Nishimune, Y. (1997) Green mice as a source of ubiquitous green cells. *FEBS Lett.* **407,** 313–319.

13. Tsien, R. Y. (1998) The green fluorescent protein. *Annu. Rev. Biochem.* **67,** 509–544.

14. Heim, R., Cubitt, A. B., and Tsien, R. Y. (1995) Improved green fluorescence. *Nature* **373,** 664,665.

15. Cormack, B. P., Valvidia, R. H., and Falkow, S. (1996) FACS-optimized mutants of the green fluorescent protein (GFP). *Gene* **173,** 33–38.

16. Marshall, J., Molloy, R., Moss, G. W. J., Howe, J. R., and Hughes, T. E. (1995) The jellyfish green fluorescent protein: a new tool for studying ion channel expression and function. *Neuron* **14,** 211–215.

17. Levitan, E. S. (1999) Tagging potassium ion channels with green fluorescent protein to study mobility and interactions with other proteins. *Methods Enzymol.* **294,** 47–58.

18. Lopatin, A. N., Makhina, E. N., and Nichols, C. G. (1998) Novel tools for localizing ion channels in living cells. *Trends Pharmacol. Sci.* **19,** 395–398.

19. Gray, N. K. and Wickens, M. (1998) Control of translation initiation in animals. *Annu. Rev. Cell Dev. Biol.* **14,** 399–458.

20. Jackson, R. J. and Kaminski, A. (1995) Internal initiation of translation in eukaryotes: the picornavirus paradigm and beyond. *RNA* **1,** 985–1000.

21. Stewart, S. R. and Semler, B. L. (1997) RNA determinants of picornavirus cap-independent translation initiation. *Sem. Virol.* **8,** 242–255.

22. Pestova, T. V., Shatsky, I. N., and Hellen, C. U. (1996) Functional dissection of eukaryotic initiation factor 4F: the 4A subunit and the central domain of the 4G subunit are sufficient to mediate internal entry of 43S preinitiation complexes. *Mol. Cell. Biol.* **16,** 6870–6878.

23. Roberts, L. O., Seamons, R. A., and Belsham, G. J. (1998) Recognition of picornavirus internal ribosome entry sites within cells; influence of cellular and viral proteins. *RNA* **4,** 520–529.

24. Jang, S. K., Davies, M. V., Kaufman, R. J., and Wimmer, E. (1989) Initiation of protein synthesis by internal entry of ribosomes into the 5' nontranslated region of encephalomyocarditis virus RNA in vivo. *J. Virol.* **63,** 1651–1660.

25. Ghattas, I. R., Sanes, J. R., and Majors, J. E. (1991) The encephalomyocarditis virus internal ribosome entry site allows efficient coexpression of two genes from a recombinant provirus in cultured cells and in embryos. *Mol. Cell. Biol.* **11,** 5848–5859.

26. Kim, D. G., Kang, H. M., Jang, S. K., and Shin, H. S. (1992) Construction of a bifunctional mRNA in the mouse by using the internal ribosomal entry site of the encephalomyocarditis virus. *Mol. Cell. Biol.* **12,** 3636–3643.

27. Borman, A. M., Bailly, J. L., Girard, M., and Kean, K. M. (1995) Picornavirus internal ribosome entry segments: comparison of translation efficiency and the

requirements for optimal internal initiation of translation in vitro. *Nucleic Acids Res.* **23**, 3656–3663.

28. Trouet, D., Nilius, B., Voets, T., Droogmans, G., and Eggermont, J. (1997) Use of a bicistronic GFP-expression vector to characterise ion channels after transfection in mammalian cells. *Pflügers Arch. Eur. J. Physiol.* **434**, 632–638.

29. Blair, L. A. C., Bence, K. K., and Marshall, J. (1999) Jellyfish green fluorescent protein: a tool for studying ion channels and second messenger sgnaling in neurons. *Methods Enzymol.* **302**, 213–225.

30. Warnat, J., Philipp, S., Zimmer, S., Flockerzi, V., and Cavalie, A. (1999) Phenotype of a recombinant store-operated channel: highly selective permeation of Ca2+. *J. Physiol. (Lond.)* **518**, 631–638.

31. Kamouchi, M., Philipp, S., Flockerzi, V., Wissenbach, U., Mamin, A., Raeymaekers, L., et al. (1999) Properties of heterologously expressed hTRP3 channels in bovine pulmonary artery endothelial cells. *J. Physiol. (Lond.)* **518**, 345–358.

32. Kamouchi, M., Trouet, D., DeGreef, C., Droogmans, G., Eggermont, J., and Nilius, B. (1997) Functional effects of expression of hslo Ca2+ activated K+ channels in cultured macrovascular endothelial cells. *Cell Calcium* **22 (6)**, 497–506.

33. Vennekens, R., Kamouchi, M., Wissenbach, U., Phillip, S., Eggermont, J., Droogmans, G., et al. (1999) Functional expression of Trp1 and Trp4 in vascular endothelium. *Pflügers Arch. Eur. J. Physiol.* **437**, R42.

34. Vennekens, R., Trouet, D., Vankeerberghen, A., Voets, T., Cuppens, H., Eggermont, J., et al. (1999) Inhibition of volume-regulated anion channels by expression of the cystic fibrosis transmembrane conductance regulator. *J. Physiol. (Lond.)* **515**, 75–85.

35. Fang, Y., Huang, C.-C., Kain, S. R., and Li, X. (1999) Use of coexpressed enhanced green fluorescent protein as a marker for identifying transfected cells. *Methods Enzymol.* **302**, 207–212.

36. Gossen, M., Freundlieb, S., Bender, G., Müller, G., Hillen, W., and Bujard, H. (1995) Transcriptional activation by tetracyclines in mammalian cells. *Science* **268**, 1766–1769.

37. Baron, U., Freundlieb, S., Gossen, M., and Bujard, H. (1995) Co-regulation of two gene activities by tetracycline via a bidirectional promoter. *Nucleic Acids Res.* **23**, 3605–3606.

38. Voets, T., Droogmans, G., and Nilius, B. (1996) Membrane currents and the resting membrane potential in cultured bovine pulmonary artery endothelial cells. *J. Physiol. (Lond.)* **497**, 95–107.

39. Trouet, D., Nilius, B., Jacobs, A., Remacle, C., Droogmans, G., and Eggermont, J. (1999) Caveolin-1 modulates the activity of the volume-regulated chloride channel. *J. Physiol. (Lond.)* **520**, 113–119.

40. Smith, G. M., Berry, R. L., Yang, J., and Tanelian, D. (1997) Electrophysiological analysis of dorsal root ganglion neurons pre- and post-coexpression of green fluorescent protein and functional 5-HT3 receptor. *J. Neurophysiol.* **77**, 3115–3121.

41. Buyse, G., Trouet, D., Voets, T., Missiaen, L., Droogmans, G., Nilius, B., and Eggermont, J. (1998) Evidence for the intracellular location of chloride chan-

nel (ClC)-type proteins: co-localization of ClC-6a and ClC-6c with the sarco/
endoplasmic-reticulum Ca^{2+} pump SERCA2b. *Biochem. J.* **330**, 1015–1021.

42. Wei, L., Vankeerberghen, A., Cuppens, H., Droogmans, G., Cassiman, J.-J., and Nilius, B. (1999) Phosphorylation site independent single R-domain mutations affect CFTR channel activity. *FEBS Lett.* **439**, 121–126.

43. Voets, T., Droogmans, G., Raskin, G., Eggermont, J., and Nilius, B. (1999) Reduced intracellular ionic strength as the initial trigger for activation of endothelial volume-regulated anion channels. *Proc. Natl. Acad. Sci. USA* **96**, 5298–5303.

44. Van Driessche, W., De Smet, P., and Raskin, G. (1993) An automatic monitoring system for epithelial cell height. *Pflügers Arch. Eur. J. Physiol.* **425**, 164–171.

45. Gurtu, V., Yan, G., and Zhang, G. (1996) IRES bicistronic expression vectors for efficient creation of stable mammalian cell lines. *Biochem. Biophys. Res. Commun.* **229**, 295–298.

46. Rees, S., Coote, J., Stables, J., Goodson, S., Harris, S., and Lee, M. G. (1996) Bicistronic vector for the creation of stable mammalian cell lines that predisposes all antibiotic-resistant cells to express recombinant protein. *BioTechniques* **20**, 102–110.

47. Hobbs, S., Jitrapakdee, S., and Wallace, J. C. (1998) Development of a bicistronic vector driven by the human polypeptide chain elongation factor 1alpha promoter for creation of stable mammalian cell lines that express very high levels of recombinant proteins. *Biochem. Biophys. Res. Commun.* **252**, 368–372.

48. Metz, M. Z., Pichler, A., Kuchler, K., and Kane, S. E. (1998) Construction and characterization of single-transcript tricistronic retroviral vectors using two internal ribosome entry sites. *Somatic Cell Mol. Genet.* **24**, 53–69.

49. Lybarger, L., Dempsey, D., Franek, K. J., and Chervenak, R. (1996) Rapid generation and flow cytometric analysis of stable GFP-expressing cells. *Cytometry* **25**, 211–220.

50. Walker, D. and De Waard, M. (1998) Subunit interaction sites in voltage-dependent Ca2+ channels: role in channel function. *Trends Neurosci.* **21**, 148–154.

51. Unwin, N. (1993) Neurotransmitter action: opening of ligand-gated ion channels. *Cell* **72**, 31–41.

52. Fyfe, G. K., Quinn, A., and Canessa, C. M. (1998) Structure and function of the Mec-ENaC family of ion channels. *Sem. Nephrol.* **18**, 138–151.

53. Lorenz, L., Pusch, M., and Jentsch, T. J. (1996) Heteromultimeric CLC chloride channels with novel properties. *Proc. Natl. Acad. Sci. USA* **93**, 13,362–13,366.

54. Kawashima, E., Estoppey, D., Virginio, C., Fahmi, D., Rees, S., Surprenant, A., and North, R. A. (1998) A novel and efficient method for the stable expression of heteromeric ion channels in mammalian cells. *Recept. Channels* **5**, 53–60.

55. Stauber, R. H., Horie, K., Carney, P., Hudson, E. A., Tarasova, N. I., Gaitanaris, G. A., and Pavlakis, G. N. (1998) Development and applications of enhanced green fluorescent protein mutants. *BioTechniques* **24**, 462–466, 468–471.

56. Yang, T. T., Sinai, P., Green, G., Kitts, P. A., Chen, Y. T., Lybarger, L., et al. (1998) Improved fluorescence and dual color detection with enhanced blue

and green variants of the green fluorescent protein. *J. Biol. Chem.* **273,** 8212–8216.

57. Shieh, B. H. and Zhu, M. Y. (1996) Regulation of the TRP Ca2+ channel by INAD in Drosophila photoreceptors. *Neuron* **16,** 991–998.

58. Short, D. B., Trotter, K. W., Reczek, D., Kreda, S. M., Bretscher, A., Boucher, R. C., et al. (1998) An apical PDZ protein anchors the cystic fibrosis trans-membrane conductance regulator to the cytoskeleton. *J. Biol. Chem.* **273,** 19,797–19,801.

10

Confocal Imaging of GFP-Labeled Ion Channels

Bryan D. Moyer and Bruce A. Stanton

1. INTRODUCTION

The generation and maintenance of cell polarity is crucial for vectorial solute and fluid transport in epithelial cells and for the normal function of neurons. Epithelial cells must asymmetrically distribute receptors, transporters, and ion channels between the apical and basolateral membranes in order to establish and maintain polarity and function *(1–4)*. Neurons also must asymmetrically distribute proteins between axons and somatodendritic regions to propagate action potentials from one cell to the next *(5)*. In general, proteins sorted to the apical membrane of epithelia are expressed in the axons of neurons, whereas proteins sorted to the basolateral membrane of epithelia are distributed to the somatodendritic region of neurons *(5)*. To achieve this asymmetry, cells target newly synthesized transport proteins to the appropriate membrane—either apical (axon) or basolateral (dendritic)—and retain them there following their delivery.

Polarization of proteins to apical (axon) and basolateral (somatodendritic) membrane domains is achieved by distinct sorting or retention signals. Basolateral membrane sorting signals are composed of short peptide motifs including tyrosine-dependent signals (i.e., NPXY or YXXØ, where X is any amino acid and Ø is a large hydrophobic amino acid such as leucine, isoleucine, or valine), tyrosine-independent signals and dileucine-based motifs, and generally reside in the cytoplasmic domains of transmembrane proteins *(1,2)*. Some integral membrane proteins such as Na/K ATPase *(6,7)* and β1-integrin *(8)* are not sorted preferentially to either the apical or basolateral

From: *Ion Channel Localization Methods and Protocols*
Edited by: A. Lopatin and C. G. Nichols © Humana Press Inc., Totowa, NJ

membrane from the trans Golgi network (TGN) but are selectively retained and accumulated in the basolateral membrane by interaction with the membrane-associated actin cytoskeleton. By contrast, less is know about the signals that sort and/or retain proteins in the apical (axon) plasma membrane. Three general classes of apical membrane sorting signals have been identified: glycosylphosphatidylinositol membrane anchors, N- and O-linked oligosaccharides, and transmembrane domains *(1,2)*. In addition, PDZ domains, which are named for the three proteins in which this domain was first described (PSD-95, Dlg, and ZO–1), have recently been shown to play a role in determining the polarized distribution of transmembrane proteins *(9–15)*. PDZ domains are modular domains in proteins that bind short peptide sequences at the C-termini of other proteins, termed PDZ interacting domains *(9,16–18)*.

Our laboratory has a long standing interest in the cystic fibrosis transmembrane conductance regulator (CFTR) ion channel, particularly with regard to how it traffics through the secretory pathway and how it becomes polarized to the apical membrane in epithelial cells. CFTR is a member of the ATP-binding cassette family and is a cAMP-activated Cl channel that is polarized to the apical plasma membrane in most epithelial cells *(19–21)*. Mutations in the CFTR gene lead to the autosomal recessive genetic disease cystic fibrosis (CF), which affects ~1 in 2000 live births in Caucasians *(22–24)*. Over 964 different mutations have been identified within the CFTR gene (http://www.genet.sickkids.on.ca/cftr/): however, 70% of individuals with CF are homozygous for the CFTR-ΔF508 mutation, which accounts for nearly 90% of all mutant CFTR alleles *(22)*. CFTR-ΔF508 is trapped in the endoplasmic reticulum (ER) and does not traffic efficiently to the apical plasma membrane *(25,26)*. However, CFTR-ΔF508 retains function as a cAMP-activated Cl channel in the ER *(27)*. Therefore, it is our goal to understand how CFTR traffics through the secretory pathway in order to identify strategies to increase trafficking of CFTR-ΔF508 from the ER to the apical plasma membrane, where CFTR-ΔF508 can function as a cAMP-activated Cl channel. Thus, elucidation of CFTR trafficking has important therapeutic implications for the treatment of CF.

We have used the jellyfish, *Aequoria victoria*, green fluorescent protein (GFP) as a tag to study the trafficking of CFTR in order to identify the determinants that localize CFTR to the apical membrane in polarized epithelial cells. In this chapter, we describe our experimental approach to study the polarized trafficking of CFTR. We describe the advantages and disadvantages of using GFP and laser scanning fluorescence confocal microscopy to monitor CFTR polarization and subcellular localization and we provide details on the experimental approach we have found to work best in our laboratory. Three superb and recent monographs, and a book on confocal microscopy, should also be consulted for additional references and details about GFP and confocal microscopy *(28–31)* and for a list of useful academic and commercial web sites on GFP *(28)*.

2. METHODS AND EXPERIMENTAL APPROACH

2.1. GFP-CFTR Expression Vector

We constructed a GFP-CFTR mammalian expression vector, pGFP-CFTR, by ligating the cDNA for enhanced GFP (eGFP; however, the term GFP will be used in this chapter for simplicity) in frame to the N-terminus of the cDNA for human, wild-type CFTR as described *(32)*. Expression of GFP-CFTR is driven by the constitutively active, immediate early cytomegalovirus (CMV) promoter, which is induced by sodium butyrate and 4-phenyl butyrate *(32,33)*. Proceeding from the N- to the C-terminus, the expressed chimeric protein consists of GFP, which resides in the cytoplasm, followed by a linker sequence of 23 amino acids followed by human wild-type CFTR. We do not know what effect, if any, longer or shorter linker sequences have on GFP-CFTR function and trafficking; however, linker sequences in GFP chimeric proteins have been shown to be important to retain the normal function of the non-GFP protein (personal communication, Dr. Guillermo Romero, University of Pittsburgh). It is prudent to ligate GFP to the N- and C- termini of proteins of interest and then evaluate which chimera functions normally. However, we have not tagged GFP to the C-terminus of CFTR because others and we have shown that the C-terminus contains a PDZ-interacting domain that is required for the polarization of CFTR to the apical plasma membrane *(32,34–37)*. Because PDZ interacting domains are usually at the extreme C-terminus of proteins, tagging GFP to the C-terminus would be expected to prevent CFTR interaction with PDZ proteins, and therefore disrupt the polarized expression of CFTR in the apical membrane.

2.2. MDCK Cell Culture

The cell-culture model used to study trafficking is critical because the polarized expression of many proteins, including CFTR, is dependent on the state of cell polarity, is cell-type specific and depends on the substratum on which cells are grown in culture (*see* ref. *32* and Section 3.5.). For example, CFTR is localized to an intracellular compartment in undifferentiated, unpolarized HT–29A human colonic epithelial cells and is directed to the apical cell membrane subsequent to differentiation and polarization *(38,39)*.

We study CFTR trafficking in human airway and MDCK kidney epithelial cells grown on permeable filter supports because, when grown on filters, the cells polarize and CFTR mediates transepithelial Cl secretion *(32,34)*. MDCK cells are widely used as a model for studies involving epithelial polarity and protein trafficking. MDCK type I cells form a high-resistance epithelium that facilitates measurement of CFTR function in short circuit current experiments, and express low levels of endogenous CFTR Cl channels in the apical membrane *(32,34,40,41)*. We study a homogeneous subclone of MDCK type I cells (clone C7) which expresses low levels of endogenous CFTR *(41–43)*. MDCK type II cells, in contrast, form a low-resistance epithelium, and do not express detectable levels of endogenous CFTR *(40)*. Thus, MDCK type II cells may not express regulatory proteins required for normal CFTR trafficking or function. Cells were seeded on Transwell filter bottom cups (Corning Corp., Corning, NY) at 50,000–75,000 cells/0.33 cm^2 for confocal microscopy or 200,000/4.5 cm^2 for surface biotinylation experiments. Filters were not coated with any collagen or proteinaceous solution. Transwell filters exhibited negligible background green fluorescence. By contrast, Cellagen filter bottom cups (ICN Biomedicals; Aurora, OH) had high levels of green autofluoresence that precluded identification of GFP-CFTR. When cells were grown on glass coverslips for confocal microscopy, 75,000 cells were seeded per 22 × 22 mm coverslip (No. 1.5 thickness). We observed optimal GFP fluorescence in cells grown at 33°C, a temperature that did not affect cell growth or viability, and did not alter GFP-CFTR localization compared to cells grown at 37°C.

2.3. Generation of Stably Transfected MDCK Cell Lines

We generated MDCK cell lines stably transfected with GFP linked to wild-type or mutant forms of CFTR *(32,34)*. Transient transfection efficiency was first optimized with the PerFect Lipid Transfection Kit (Invitrogen, Carlsbad, CA) *(32)*. High transfection efficiency increases the probability of obtaining clonal cell lines. Therefore, we optimized transfection conditions for MDCK type I cells (pFx-2 lipid, a 6:1 lipid:DNA mass ratio, and an 8-h transfection time). Following transfection, cells were selected with 300 µg/mL G-418 (Life Technologies), a concentration of G-418 determined to kill all MDCK cells after 2 wk by a clonogenic assay. Following transfection and selection, single GFP-positive cells were sorted into individual wells of 96 well plates, which contained 300 µg/mL G-418, using a FACStar PLUS flow cytometer (Becton Dickenson; San Jose, CA). Following establishment of clonal cell lines, G-418 was reduced to 150 µg/mL. The purpose of this reduction in G-418 concentration was to increase cell growth rate yet maintain selective pressure on cells. To exclude the possibility that our results were attributable to clonal variation, we studied at least three stable clones for each chimeric GFP-CFTR protein generated.

We treated all cells with 5 m*M* Na-butyrate for 15–18 h prior to experimentation to increase GFP-CFTR expression and removed Na-butyrate 2 h prior to experimentation. The rationale for treating cells with Na-butyrate, which activates transcription from many viral promoters including the CMV promoter used to drive GFP-CFTR expression, was that GFP-CFTR fluorescence was dim and difficult to visualize in noninduced cells. Western blot analyses revealed that Na-butyrate increased GFP-CFTR expression 30-fold *(32)*. Because overexpression of GFP-fusion proteins can cause proteins to mis-localize in subcellular compartments *(44,45)* we were careful to compare the localization of GFP-CFTR before and after Na-butyrate induction. Butyrate treatment did not to affect GFP-CFTR localization *(32)*.

Although efforts were made to generate cells stably transfected with CFTR alone (with no GFP tag), for comparison with GFP-CFTR stable transfectants, these attempts were unsuccessful. This suggests that screening stable transfectants based on GFP fluorescence greatly facilitates the identification of positive clones.

2.4. Processing Cells for Confocal Microscopy

Cells were fixed in paraformaledhyde, methanol, or acetone as described *(32)*. Transwell filters were excised from the plastic holders with a scalpel, placed apical side up on a glass slide, and overlaid with a drop (50 µL) of either n-propyl gallate (Sigma; 10 mg/mL) in 90% glycerol/10% PBS or ProLong Antifade reagent (Molecular Probes, Eugene, OR), followed by a coverslip (No. 1.5 thickness). Keeping a small amount of liquid on top of the filters during excision decreased the tendency of the filters to wrinkle and fold in half. n-propyl gallate and ProLong are an anti-oxidants used to retard fluorophore bleaching in immunofluorescence microscopy. Two strips of scotch tape (~1 cm wide) were placed along the long edges of the glass slides to create a chamber for the excised filter to sit. Because the Transwell filter and monolayer are each approx 10 µm tall, cells would be compressed and cellular morphology would be altered if no spacing was incorporated between the glass slide and coverslip. This small chamber minimizes compression of filter-grown cells when overlaid with the glass coverslip.

For cells grown on glass (No. 1.5 thickness), coverslips were placed cell side down onto a drop (50 µL) of n-propyl gallate/glycerol/PBS antifade cocktail or ProLong antifade reagent. Coverslips containing n-propyl gallate were sealed with liquid Valap heated to 40–50°C. Valap is a wax-based substance made by mixing Vasoline, lanolin, and paraffin in a 1:1:1 ratio. Valap solidifies at room temperature and creates a hardened, air- and water-tight seal around the specimen. Valap has not been reported to affect GFP fluorescence. n-propyl-gallate treated cells can be viewed immediately; however, ProLong treated cells do not require Valap to seal the coverslip. Prolong should be allowed to dry for at least several hours before the cells are visualized by confocal microscopy.

2.5. Confocal Microscopy

Confocal images were acquired using an upright Zeiss (Thornwood, NY) Axioskop microscope equipped with a laser-scanning confocal unit (model MRC-1024, BioRad Labs, Hercules, CA), a 15 mW krypton-argon laser, and a 63X Plan Apochromat/1.4 NA or 40X Plan Neofluor/1.3 NA oil immersion objective. GFP fluorescence was excited using the 488 nm laser line and collected using a FITC filter set (emission filter: 530 ± 30 nm) or a Piston GFP filter set (Chroma Optical, Inc., Brattleboro, VT; excitation filter: HQ470/40, Dichroic: Q495 LP and emission filter HQ515/30). The FITC filter allows longer wavelength background fluorescence to pass to the detector. The Piston GFP filter set reduces background autofluoresence at wavelengths longer than 530 nm. In dual labeling studies to co-localize GFP-chimeric proteins to subcellular compartments, fluorescence associated with subcellular compartments was identified using Texas Red-labeled secondary antibodies, or propidium iodide, a nucleic acid dye used to stain nuclei, and was excited using the 568 nm laser line and collected using a Texas Red filter set (605 ± 32 nm). Using the GFP and Texas Red filter sets, all fluorescent signals were spectrally isolated and negligible signal bleedthrough occurred between channels. To determine signal bleedthrough in a dual labeling GFP experiment, the signal from the green channel was first acquired in a specimen labeled only with a Texas Red fluorophore; then the signal from the red channel was acquired in a specimen expressing only a GFP-CFTR chimera. If Texas Red fluorescence bled into the green channel, then green fluorescence would be observed in the first specimen; similarly, if GFP fluorescence bled into the red channel, then red fluorescence would be observed in the second sample. Signal bleedthrough can generally be avoided by proper selection of fluorophores and filter sets. Acquired images were imported into National Institutes of Health (NIH) Image software (Bethesda, MD; software can be downloaded at no cost at http://shareware.netscape.com/computing/shareware/software_title.tmpl?p=MAC&category_id = 60&subcategory_id = 68&id = 55652) for quantitation and into Adobe Photoshop for image processing and printing.

For semi-quantitative confocal microscopy of GFP-CFTR fluorescence within subcellular compartments, including the distribution of CFTR along

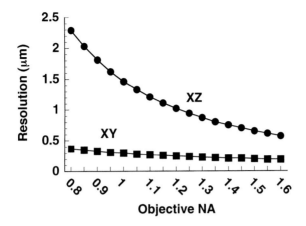

Fig. 1. Resolution in fluorescence confocal laser-scanning microscopy (FCLSM) as a function of the numerical aperature of the objective lens using the 488 nm laser line to view a specimen through a glass coverslip with a refractive index of 1.5. For example, using a 60× objective with a numerical aperature (NA) of 1.4, the optimal resolution in the XY plane is ~0.2 μm and the optimal resolution in the XZ plane is ~0.8 μm. Thus, using these settings and objective two objects will appear to co-localize if they are ≤0.2 μm apart when viewed in the XY plane and ≤0.7 μm apart when viewed in the XZ plane. Thus, co-localization studies using FCLSM should be interpreted cautiously because two objects may appear to co-localize but may, in reality, not be localized within the same compartment *(64)*. For example, although the plasma membrane (10 nm) and endosomal vesicles (10–100 nm) lying <100 nm below the plasma membrane may appear to co-localize by FCLSM, it is not possible to discriminate between these subcellular compartments by FCLSM. (Data in figure supplied by Bio-Rad Laboratories, Hercules, CA). See reference *(31)* for more details on resolution and FCLSM.

the apical to basal axis, all images from the same z-series were collected using the same values for the laser power (range 3–10%), photomultiplier gain (range 1200–1500), iris (range 2.0–3.5), and black level (range –10 to –5). Using these values, we operate close to the theoretical limits of resolution for the confocal microscope (~0.2 μm in the xy plane and ~0.8 μm in the xz plane at 488 nm excitation using an objective lens with a numerical aperture of 1.4: *see* Fig. 1 *(31)*. Typically, three scans were Kalman averaged per z-section and 10 z-sections were collected at 1.0-μm increments beginning at the apical membrane and ending at the basal membrane. Averaging three scans was sufficient to filter out any pixel noise in the detector without causing photobleaching of the GFP fluorophore. Scanning the same section of a cell transfected with GFP 100 times at 3% laser power decreased fluorescence intensity less than 10%, consistent with reports documenting the stability of GFP fluorescence during continuous illumination *(46,47)*. Thus, it is unlikely that appreciable photobleaching of GFP-CFTR occurred during the 30–40 scans required to collect a complete z-series. For accurate quantitation of fluorescent signals, care was taken to set confocal parameters such that pixel saturation was less than 10% and that signal intensities were in the linear range of photomultiplier sensitivity. Because typical MDCK (type I) monolayers are 10 μm tall when grown on filters, and the minimal resolution of the confocal microscope in the xz plane is 0.8 μm, we maximized the amount of data we collected per section "x" without duplicating information contained in sections "x+1" and "x–1" by stepping through the monolayer at 1.0 μm increments. Collecting sections at intervals of 1.0 μm or less will increase the amount of duplicated information between sections without improving resolution.

The fraction of total cell GFP-CFTR fluorescence located in each confocal z-section of the cell was quantitated with NIH Image software. A box was drawn over the section(s) to be measured and mean pixel counts within this area were determined. Box areas were constant for all sections of the same cell and pixel intensity histograms of boxed regions were evaluated to ensure that GFP fluorescence was within the linear range (0–254). Data were exported to Microsoft Excel for assembly of data into spreadsheet form.

The relative distribution of GFP-CFTR fluorescence between apical and lateral membrane regions was quantitated in randomly acquired confocal micrograph xz vertical sections. Using NIH Image software, a box (~2 μm wide and encompassing the length of apical or lateral membranes) was drawn over the region to be measured and pixel counts within the boxed region were determined. The transition between apical and lateral membranes was identified by staining monolayers for the tight junction protein ZO–1. Pixel intensity histograms were evaluated to ensure that GFP fluorescence was within the linear range (0–254). In stable transfectants, apical to basolateral polarity ratios (R) were calculated using the following formula: $R = (a{-}c)/((b_l{-}c)/2 + (b_r{-}c)/2)$ where a corresponds to pixel counts in the apical membrane region, b_l corresponds to pixel counts is the left lateral membrane region, b_r corresponds to pixel counts in the right lateral membrane region, and c corresponds to background pixel counts in the nucleus. Lateral membrane measurements were divided by two when adjacent cells, with opposing lateral surfaces, displayed GFP fluorescence. GFP fluorescence was generally not observed in the basal membrane, which was excluded from analyses. A similar method has been used previously to quantitate the apical to basolateral polarity ratios of Na/K ATPase and H/K ATPase subunits expressed in polarized LLC-PK$_1$ kidney epithelial cells *(48)*. To determine the validity of pixel intensity counts as a measure of apical to basolateral

Table 1
Characteristics of GFP Variants

	Excitation (nm)	Emission (nm)	Extinction coefficient	Quantum yield
RFP[a]	558	583	22,500	0.29[b]
eYFP	514	527	84,000	0.61
eGFP	489	508	55,000	0.60
eCFP	434	477	26,000	0.40
eBFP[c]	380	440	31,000	0.18

[a]RFP is red fluorescent protein *(93)*, YFP is yellow fluorescent protein, CFP is cyan fluorescent protein, and BFP is blue fluorescent protein. e indicates enhanced, which is human codon optimized.

[b]Relative to eGFP. Data adapted from CLONTECHniques, October, 1999 (Clontech, Laboratories, Palo Alto, CA). The extinction coefficient is the light absorbing capacity of the fluorophore and the quantum yield (Q) is a measure of efficiency where Q = photons emitted/photons absorbed. BFP photobleaches rapidly and produces a relatively dim fluorescence signal. CFP and YFP are good FRET pairs. Red fluorescent protein, recently cloned, and GFP may also prove to be a good FRET pair.

[c]eBFP rapidly photobleaches.

polarization using confocal microscopy, we compared the apical/basolateral ratio of GFP-CFTR using this approach to the well-accepted method of biotinylating proteins in the apical and basolateral membranes *(32)*. As presented in Section 3., we obtained similar results with both methods.

3. EXPERIMENTAL OBSERVATIONS

3.1. GFP: An Ideal Reporter for Studying the Polarized Expression and Subcellular Localization of Ion Channels

GFP, a 27 kDa protein, generates striking green fluorescence without the addition of substrates, cofactors, or antibodies. GFP is nontoxic and the fusion of GFP to ion channels and other proteins generally does not alter the function or localization of these proteins *(49–52)*. Several color variants of GFP exist, including cyan, blue, yellow, and red (Table 1), which provide the opportunity to follow the localization of several different fluorescent chimeric proteins simultaneously.

GFP has been used extensively to study the expression and subcellular localization of ion channels by epifluorescence and laser-scanning confocal fluorescence microscopy in living and fixed cells *(45,53–62)*. Although it is possible to study the trafficking of ion channels by an indirect immunofluorescence approach and/or by a selective cell surface biotinylation approach, we have found these techniques to be labor-intensive and have several limitations. First, endogenous expression of ion channels is frequently low; thus, channels are difficult to detect by conventional immunocytochemical techniques, by biotinylation of membrane proteins, and by pulse-chase techniques. Second, antibodies often exhibit nonspecific binding. Third, fixation artifacts may affect localization of proteins *(64)*. We have found that the use of GFP to study the polarized expression of ion channels in living and/or fixed cells overcomes most of these potential limitations.

3.2. GFP Does Not Affect the Function of CFTR Channels

Although others have reported that GFP does not affect the function or subcellular expression of channels or transporters, including voltage-dependent Ca^{2+} channels, ATP-sensitive K^+ channels, and neuronal ligand-gated cation channels *(50,53–55)*, some exceptions exist *(65–68)*. For example, GFP tagged to the N-terminus of GLUT4 disrupts trafficking *(65)*. Fusion of GFP to insulin causes insulin to be misfolded and retained in the ER *(66)*. In addition, we have observed that tagging GFP to the N-terminus of the α, but not the β or γ-subunit of the epithelial sodium channel, ENaC, inhibits the expression of ENaC in the plasma membrane of *Xenopus* oocytes *(67)*. Finally, fusion of GFP to the C-terminus of the aquaporin water channel abolishes AQP2 polarization *(68)*. Thus, it is prudent to confirm that the GFP tag does not affect the function or subcellular distribution of the ion channel of interest. Accordingly, we used a variety of electrophysiological approaches including patch clamp, lipid bilayers, and Ussing chamber analysis to examine the possible effect of GFP on CFTR Cl channel activity. We found that GFP had no effect on CFTR Cl channel function *(32)*. cAMP-activated CFTR Cl currents were similar in COS cells and lipid bilayers expressing GFP-CFTR and CFTR (with no GFP tag). Moreover, GFP-CFTR stably expressed in polarized MDCK cells mediated transepithelial Cl secretion as assessed in Ussing chambers *(32,33)*. Finally, pulse chase studies demonstrated that the half-lives of GFP-CFTR and CFTR were similar *(69)*. Thus, GFP had no effect on the Cl channel function or on the steady-state expression levels or degradation of CFTR. Studies examining the effect of GFP on the subcellular localization of CFTR are described below.

3.3. Transient vs Stable Expression of GFP-CFTR

Transient expression produced very inconsistent results regarding the cellular distribution of GFP-CFTR (Fig. 2). In some cells GFP-CFTR localized to the endoplasmic reticulum and a perinuclear region resembling the Golgi apparatus, whereas in other cells GFP-CFTR localized to the plasma membrane region (Fig. 2). Previous reports have documented

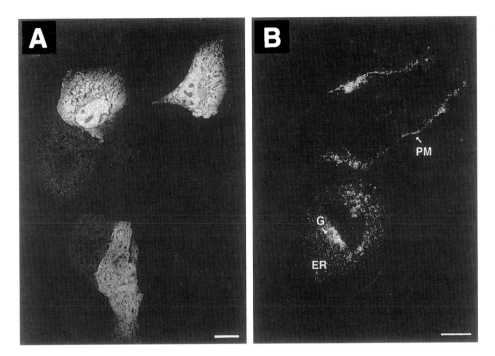

Fig. 2. Localization of GFP and GFP-CFTR in transiently transfected cells. Confocal fluorescence micrographs (xy plane) of MDCK cells grown on glass coverslips and transiently transfected with GFP **(A)** or GFP-CFTR **(B)**. (A) GFP fluorescence (white) is distributed throughout nuclear and cytosolic compartments and is excluded from membrane-bound organelles of the secretory pathway. (B) GFP-CFTR fluorescence (white) is compartmentalized to organelles of the secretory pathway. GFP-CFTR is localized to ER-like tubules (ER) and a perinuclear Golgi-region (G; bottom cell) as well as the plasma membrane region (PM; top cell). Scale bars are 10 μm.

heterogeneous distribution of GFP-fusion proteins in transiently transfected cells, a phenomenon that may be attributable to cell to cell variation in GFP-fusion protein expression level or differences in the stage of the cell cycle *(45,70)*.

3.4. Selecting and Screening Stable Clones of Cells Expressing GFP-CFTR

To obtain a population of cells with a more homogenous pattern of GFP-CFTR distribution, MDCK cells were stably transfected with GFP-CFTR. In stable transfectants grown to confluence on filters, we observed a very consistent expression of GFP-CFTR, primarily in the apical plasma membrane (Fig. 3). Although stable cell lines were clonally derived from single cells, all cells did not display detectable levels of GFP-CFTR fluorescence and GFP-CFTR fluorescence intensity was variable among cells and varied with each pass (*see* ref. *32* and personal communication J. Pier, Harvard Medical School). Similar results have been reported for other cell lines stably expressing GFP-chimeras *(44,46,71,72)* and other non-GFP chimeric proteins *(48,73)*. This variation may be owing to differences in the stage of the cell cycle among cells in the population, although no supporting datum has been provided to validate this claim *(46)*.

For all stable cell lines expressing GFP-CFTR chimeric proteins produced in our laboratory, including wild-type and mutant forms of CFTR, we routinely performed Western blot analysis of the expressed chimeric protein and compared the subcellular localization of the GFP-CFTR chimera with untagged CFTR. Because GFP was fused to the N-terminus of CFTR, it was important to demonstrate that full-length GFP-CFTR protein was produced in stable transfectants and that the tagged mutant trafficked like the untagged CFTR. If the GFP-CFTR plasmid was linearized within the CFTR cDNA upon genomic integration, the GFP cDNA would remain intact but the CFTR cDNA would be disrupted. Upon expression, a truncated GFP-CFTR fusion protein would be generated that retains GFP fluorescence but lacks portions of the C-terminus of CFTR. To this end, we performed Western blot analyses on total cell lysates from all GFP-CFTR stable transfectants grown on permeable filter supports using antibodies that recognize GFP and the C-terminus of CFTR. Both antibodies routinely recognized two bands on Western blots with relative molecular masses of 210 (core glycosylated band B) and 240 (mature glycosylated band C) kDa in stably transfected, but not in parental MDCK cells *(32)*. In addition, using confocal microscopy, GFP fluorescence co-localized with GFP-CFTR immunoreactivity using both R domain and C-terminal CFTR antibodies. Because the epitope for the CFTR C-terminal antibody comprises the last 4 amino acids of the CFTR protein sequence (DTRL; amino acids 1477–1480) *(74)*, these studies demonstrated that stable transfectants express full-length GFP-CFTR fusion protein.

To our surprise, in one clone *(G1)* the apparent molecular mass of GFP-CFTR was ~40 kDa smaller than all of the other clonal lines and GFP-CFTR was polarized to the lateral, vs the apical, plasma membrane. Because the antibody that recognizes the C-terminal motif did not recognize GFP-CFTR in the G1 cells, we concluded that, during stable integration into the genome the GFP-CFTR chimera broke within the cDNA for CFTR, resulting in a truncated GFP-CFTR chimeric protein. By contrast, in every other clone studied in which GFP-CFTR was full length as determined by Western blot

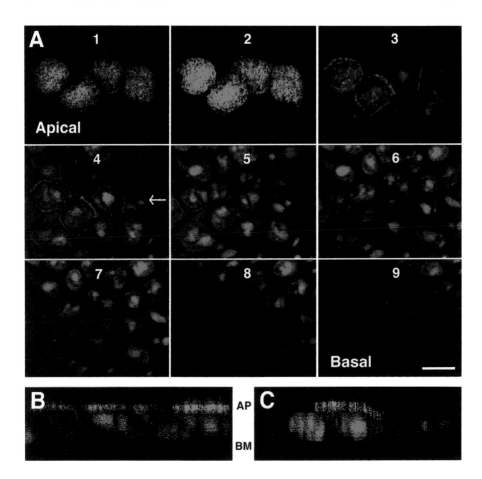

Fig. 3. Localization of GFP-CFTR in cells grown on permeable filter supports.
(A) Series of confocal fluorescence micrographs (xy plane) beginning at the apical
membrane (section 1, upper left) and ending at the basal membrane (section 9,
lower right) were acquired in 1.0 μm increments. GFP-CFTR fluorescence is green
and double-stranded nucleic acids, stained with propidium iodide, are red.
Propidium iodide was detected using the 568 nm laser line and a Texas Red filter
set along the apical-basal axis. GFP-CFTR is predominantly localized to the apical
plasma membrane (first three sections) above cell nuclei. **(B)** Confocal fluorescence micrograph (xz plane) showing distribution of GFP-CFTR in green, as
detected using the 488 nm laser line and a GFP filter set. **(C)** Confocal fluorescence
micrograph (xz plane) showing distribution of CFTR, as detected using the 488 nm
laser line, a GFP filter set and the anti-R domain CFTR antibody. CFTR was
pseudocolored blue to illustrate that GFP-CFTR was detected in the apical membrane by the anti-R domain antibody. Thus, using two different detection methods,
CFTR expression was observed in the apical and subapical membrane regions.
Arrow in section #4 of panel (A) indicates plane of vertical section in panel (B).
AP, apical membrane; BM, basal membrane. Scale bar is 10 μm.

analysis, GFP-CFTR was polarized to the apical membrane *(32)*. We also observed that GFP-CFTR was expressed in the apical membrane of human airway epithelial cells *(34)*. Thus, apical membrane expression of GFP-CFTR was similar in kidney (MDCK) and human airway epithelial cells lines, an expression pattern observed in vivo *(21)*. These observations underscore the importance of evaluating several stable clones expressing GFP-chimeric proteins to avoid artifacts induce during the generation of stable cell lines.

3.5. GFP-CFTR Expression is Substratum and Cell Type Dependent

The cellular distribution of GFP-CFTR was substratum dependent in MDCK I cells. As described earlier (Fig. 3) GFP-CFTR was localized to the apical and subapical plasma membrane regions of stably transfected, fully polarized MDCK I cells cultured on permeable filter supports. By contrast, in MDCK I cells stably expressing GFP-CFTR and grown to confluency on glass coverslips, GFP-CFTR was localized to a perinuclear Golgi-like region, punctate endosomal-like structures, and surprisingly to the lateral plasma membrane region (Fig. 4). The localization of GFP-CFTR to these organelles was confirmed by co-localization studies using markers for each compartment.

3.6. Activation of CFTR Does Not Involve Trafficking of CFTR from an Intracellular Pool to the Apical Plasma Membrane

Stimulation of wild-type CFTR-mediated Cl secretion by cAMP has been reported to occur by two mechanisms that are not mutually exclusive: first, cAMP stimulates protein kinase A-mediated phosphorylation and activation of CFTR Cl channels resident in the plasma membrane, and second, cAMP increases the number of CFTR molecules resident in the plasma membrane *(25,32,75–80)*. Agonist-stimulated trafficking of transport proteins from intracellular storage pools to the plasma membrane, or vice versa, is a well-established mechanism for regulating solute transport rates *(81,82)*. However, the hypothesis that cell Cl permeability is acutely controlled by regulated budding of CFTR-containing vesicles from organelles of the secretory pathway and/or regulated insertion of CFTR-containing vesicles into the plasma membrane is controversial. Accordingly, we conducted studies to test the hypothesis that cAMP activates CFTR by stimulating CFTR trafficking from an intracellular pool to the apical plasma membrane. Confluent monolayers of MDCK cells stably expressing GFP-CFTR

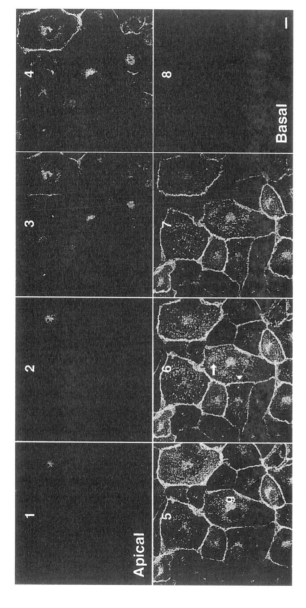

Fig. 4. Localization of GFP-CFTR in stably transfected cells grown on glass coverslips. Confocal fluorescence microgr (xy plane) beginning at the apical membrane (section 1, upper left) and ending at the basal membrane (section 8, lower right) acquired in 0.5 μm increments. GFP-CFTR fluorescence, in white, is localized to a perinuclear Golgi-like region (g, sectio punctate and vesicular endosomal-like structures (arrow, section 6), and the lateral plasma membrane region (arrowhead, se 6). GFP-CFTR fluorescence is also visible in the ER when higher laser power settings are used. Scale bar is 10 μm.

and grown on permeable filter supports were treated with a cAMP-stimulating cocktail and the distribution of GFP-CFTR fluorescence along the apical to basal axis was quantitated in optical sections using confocal
fluorescence microscopy. As shown in Fig. 5, cAMP did not affect GFP-
CFTR distribution. Approximately 70% of GFP-CFTR fluorescence localized to the apical membrane and subapical membrane regions, which
comprise the first three optical sections in Fig. 5, in vehicle and cAMP-
treated monolayers. Similar results were obtained using confocal microscopy to localize GFP-CFTR in longitudinal cryosections of polarized
MDCK cell monolayers sectioned along the apical-basal axis. GFP-CFTR
was predominantly localized to the apical membrane region under basal conditions and detectable translocation of GFP-CFTR to the apical membrane
was not observed following cAMP treatment *(32)*. By contrast, we could
observe a shift of GFP-CFTR from the TGN to the plasma membrane by
increasing the temperature. MDCK cells stably expressing GFP-CFTR were
grown at 20°C, a temperature at which newly synthesized proteins, including GFP-CFTR, are retained in the TGN (Fig. 6) *(83)*. Increasing the temperature to 37°C caused GFP-CFTR fluorescence to redistribute from the
cell interior to the apical membrane (Fig. 6). These experiments independently verified that the semiquantitative confocal microscopy technique was
capable of detecting changes in the subcellular location of GFP-CFTR. A
similar quantitative approach has been used to quantitate the distribution of
CFTR along the apical to basal axis of polarized shark rectal glands *(84)*.
This study reported a shift in CFTR immunoreactivity toward the apical
plasma membrane following treatment with cAMP-stimulating agents, demonstrating that the technique was sensitive enough to detect alterations in
CFTR localization.

   Because of the limited resolution of the confocal microscope in the vertical dimension (which corresponds to 0.8 μm in the xz plane under optimal
scanning conditions using an objective with a numerical aperature of 1.4)
(31), it is possible that cAMP stimulates GFP-CFTR trafficking from subapical vesicles, less than 0.8 μm from the apical surface, to the apical plasma
membrane. To address this possibility, apical cell-surface GFP-CFTR molecules were biotinylated following treatment of cells with vehicle or cAMP-
stimulating cocktail. The amount of surface biotinylated GFP-CFTR in
apical plasma membranes did not change following 10 or 60 min of cAMP
treatment *(32)*. Similar results were obtained in stable clones expressing 20–
30-fold less GFP-CFTR and in cells not induced with sodium butyrate,
indicating that results were independent of GFP-CFTR expression level over

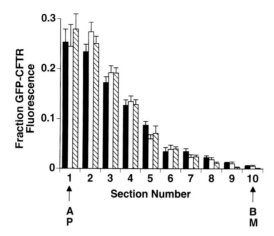

Fig. 5. cAMP has no effect of GFP-CFTR localization in cells grown on permeable filter supports: semiquantitative confocal microscopy. Distribution of GFP-CFTR fluorescence along the apical-basal axis in MDCK cells grown on permeable filters and treated with cAMP-stimulating cocktail (10 min, black bars or 60 min, white bars) or vehicle (60 min, hatched bars). GFP-CFTR fluorescence in fixed cells was quantitated in 1 μm confocal optical sections along the apical (section 1) to basal (section 10) axis. GFP-CFTR distribution did not change following cAMP treatment. For each treatment, 3 z-series, each with 15–25 cells per field, were analyzed from each of four separate monolayers. $p > 0.05$ for vehicle compared to 10-min or 60-min cAMP treatment for each section. AP, apical membrane; BM, basal membrane.

the range examined. Thus, two independent experimental approaches, laser-scanning confocal fluorescence microscopy and cell-surface biotinylation, gave similar results and support our conclusion that cAMP does not measurably stimulate trafficking of GFP-CFTR to the apical membrane in MDCK type I cells.

3.7. The C-Terminal PDZ Interacting Domain Is an Apical Polarization Signal for CFTR

Recent studies have demonstrated that PDZ interacting domains are required for the localization of some proteins to the basolateral and apical plasma membrane *(9,11–15,34,85)*. To determine if the C-terminal PDZ interacting domain (i.e., the three C-terminal amino acids in CFTR are T-R-L, using the single letter code for amino acids) is important for the polarization of CFTR to the apical membrane of epithelial cells we stably expressed either GFP-wt-CFTR or GFP-CFTR-ΔTRL (which lacks the 3 C-terminal

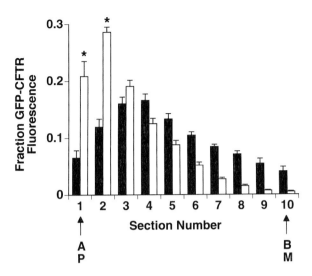

Fig. 6. Semi-quantitative confocal microscopy can detect alterations in GFP-CFTR localization. Distribution of GFP-CFTR fluorescence along the apical-basal axis in MDCK cells grown on permeable filters and incubated at 20°C for 24 h (black bars) or maintained at 33°C (white bars). MDCK cells stably expressing GFP-CFTR were grown at 20°C, a temperature at which newly synthesized GFP-CFTR is retained in the TGN *(83)*. Increasing the temperature to 37°C redistributed GFP-CFTR fluorescence from the cell interior to the apical plasma membrane. For each temperature, 2 z-series, each with 15–25 cells per field, were examined from two separate monolayers. AP, apical membrane; BM, basal membrane. * indicates significantly different from 20°C.

amino acids) in MDCK cells. Examination of GFP-wt-CFTR localization by confocal microscopy demonstrated that GFP-wt-CFTR was polarized to the apical plasma membrane region (Fig. 7). By contrast, GFP-CFTR-ΔTRL was nonpolarized and roughly equally expressed at apical and basolateral plasma membrane regions *(34)*. Semi-quantitative confocal fluorescence microscopy demonstrated that GFP-wt-CFTR exhibited an apical to basolateral ratio of 3.0, whereas GFP-CFTR-ΔTRL exhibited an apical to basolateral ratio of 0.6. These results were independently corroborated by domain-selective cell surface biotinylation experiments *(34)*, demonstrating the utility of the semiquantitative approach in determining the polarized distribution of CFTR Cl channels on apical and basolateral surfaces. Similar results were also obtained in polarized human airway epithelial cells (16HBE14o-) *(34)*. Thus, the C-terminal PDZ interacting domain (T-R-L) is required for CFTR apical polarization in kidney (MDCK) and human airway epithelial cells (16HBE14o-) *(34)*.

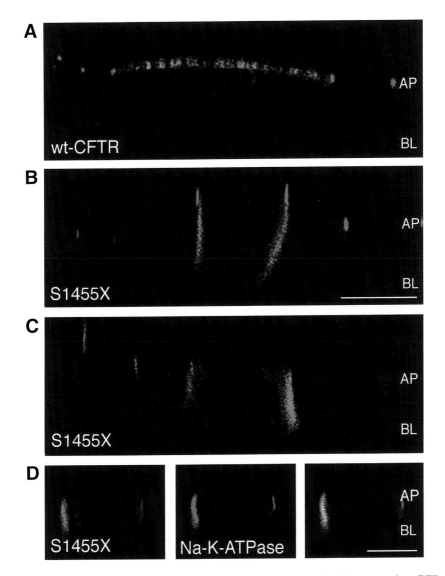

Fig. 7. Confocal fluorescence micrographs (xz plane) of cells expressing GFP-wt-CFTR or GFP-CFTR-S1455X. GFP fluorescence is green and ZO–1, a protein in tight junctions that separates apical and basolateral membrane domains, is red. **(A)** GFP-wt-CFTR is localized in the apical membrane of MDCK cells. **(B)** GFP-CFTR-S1455X is localized in the lateral membrane of MDCK cells. **(C)** GFP-CFTR-S1455X is located in the lateral membrane of 16HBE14o- cells. **(D)** GFP-CFTR-S1455X (left panel in green) co-localizes with Na/K-ATPase (middle panel in red) in the lateral membrane of MDCK cells (right panel is a merge of red and green channels, yellow-orange indicates co-localization). GFP-wt-CFTR is expressed in the apical membrane of 16HBE14o- cells (image not shown). Scale bars, 10 μm; AP, location of apical membrane; BL, location of basal membrane. Reproduced from ref. *34* with permission.

Nearly 10% of all CFTR mutations result in the deletion of the C-terminal region including the PDZ interacting domain. Because deletion of 61 or fewer C-terminal amino acids of CFTR does not alter cAMP-stimulated Cl permeability in nonpolarized cells *(86,87)*, the mechanism(s) whereby these mutations cause CF is unknown. Therefore, we examined the polarized distribution of a naturally occurring C-terminal truncation mutant, S1455X, which lacks the C-terminal 26 amino acids including the PDZ interacting domain *(88)*. Examination of GFP-CFTR-S1455X localization by confocal microscopy demonstrated that CFTR-S1455X was polarized to the lateral plasma membrane region and co-localized with the lateral membrane protein Na/K ATPase (Fig. 7) *(34)*. GFP-CFTR-S1455X exhibited an apical to basolateral ratio of 0.1–0.2 by both semiquantitative confocal fluorescence microscopy and cell surface biotinylation *(34)*. These results confirmed that the C-terminus of CFTR is required for the apical polarization of CFTR in polarized epithelial cells. The fact that CFTR-S1455X was expressed primarily in the basolateral membrane, whereas CFTR-ΔTRL was equally distributed in the apical and basolateral plasma membranes suggests that some basolateral targeting information is suppressed or inactive in CFTR-ΔTRL or that cryptic basolateral targeting signals are activated in CFTR-S1455X.

4. CONCLUSIONS

4.1. GFP as a Reporter for Studying the Polarized Distribution of Ion Channels

The studies summarized here demonstrate the feasibility of using GFP to study the polarized expression and trafficking of ion channels in epithelial cells by laser-scanning confocal fluorescence microscopy. Fusion of GFP to the N-terminus of CFTR did not interfere with CFTR Cl channel function, expression levels, and degradation or with the polarized expression of CFTR in the apical membrane. The polarized expression of GFP-CFTR, however, was cell-type and substratum dependent. Thus, we stress the importance of using fully polarized monolayers grown on permeable filter supports when examining the trafficking of ion channels. Our studies demonstrated that: 1) cAMP does not stimulate trafficking of CFTR from a submembranous pool to the apical surface and 2) the C-terminal PDZ interacting domain of CFTR comprises an apical polarization determinant, which when deleted results in a loss of CFTR polarization to the apical plasma membrane. Studies underway in our laboratory are focused on elucidating the mechanism whereby the PDZ interacting domain localizes CFTR to the apical plasma membrane in epithelial cells.

4.2. Confocal Microscopy as a Tool to Monitor Channel Polarity and Trafficking

The confocal microscope and GFP are useful tools for determining the polarity and trafficking of ion channels. The ability of the confocal microscope to section through cells in the vertical dimension (i.e., z axis) and to obtain xz vertical sections along the apical-basal axis make it a superior tool to the epifluorescence microscope. However, the confocal microscope has limitations. We stress the need to confirm semiquantitative measurements obtained by the confocal microscope using a second, independent technique such as cell-surface biotinylation, or electron microscopy which has a resolution of 0.2 nm. Confocal analysis of the polarized distribution of ion channels can assess the relative levels of protein in the apical vs the basolateral membrane regions. However, confocal analysis cannot accurately differentiate between channels localized in the plasma membrane and channels localized beneath the plasma membrane in endosomal vesicles or other organelles such as the ER, which is diffusely distributed throughout the entire cell. Thus, confocal microscopy cannot specifically be used to determine whether a membrane protein is localized in the plasma membrane. Because the limit of resolution of the confocal microscope in the xy plane is 0.2 μm and cellular membranes are ~10-nm thick, confocal microscopy also cannot be used to accurately determine if two proteins co-localize in the same cell membrane, or even the same organelle if the compartment is relatively small. The more labor-intensive technique of electron microscopy is required to conclusively demonstrate co-localization. However, using FRET (Fluorescence Resonance Energy Transfer), it is possible to use confocal microscopy to localize GFP-chimeric proteins to well-defined subcellular regions with a resolution of <100Å.

FRET is a phenomenon that occurs when two fluorophores (e.g., CYP and YFP) are in close proximity (<100 Å) and an appropriate orientation such that an excited fluorophore (donor) transfers its energy to a second, longer wavelength fluorophore in a nonradiative way *(89–92)*. Thus, when the donor and acceptor are <100Å apart excitation of the donor (i.e., CFP) elicits light emission from the acceptor (i.e., YFP), with a loss of emission from the donor. However, when the two fluorophores are >100Å apart excitation of donor does not elicit excitation of acceptor. Because FRET is a nondestructive method to monitor molecular interactions, it can be used in living cells to determine if two proteins associate in well-defined cellular compartments. For example, to determine if an ion channel is expressed in the plasma membrane, the channel could be tagged with YFP and a plasma membrane resident protein could be tagged with CFP. When the YFP-chimeric channel is inserted into the plasma membrane and YFP and CFP interact (<100Å apart), excitation of CFP would cause YFP to emit yellow light. By contrast, when the YFP-chimeric channel is not in the membrane, excitation of CFP would not cause YFP to emit light. Accordingly, by monitoring the emission of cyan vs yellow light the location of the YFP-chimera in the membrane can be determined.

ACKNOWLEDGMENTS

We thank Alice Givan, Ken Orndorff, and Gary Ward for assistance with confocal microscopy and flow cytometry and our colleagues in the Stanton laboratory for helpful discussions. B. D. Moyer was supported by a predoctoral grant from the Dolores Zohrab Liebmann Foundation. This work was supported by the Cystic Fibrosis Foundation (STANTO98), and the National Institutes of Health (DK–45881 and DK–51067. to B.A.S.).

REFERENCES

1. Caplan, M. J. (1997) Ion pumps in epithelial cells: sorting, stabilization, and polarity. *Am. J. Physiol. Gastrointest. Liver Physiol.* **272,** G1304–G1313.
2. Brown, D. and Stow, J. L. (1996) Protein trafficking and polarity in kidney epithelium: from cell biology to physiology. *Physiol. Rev.* **76,** 245–297.
3. Mays, R. W., Nelson, W. J., and Marrs, J. A. (1995) Generation of epithelial cell polarity: roles for protein trafficking, membrane-cytoskeleton, and E-Cadherin-mediated cell adhesion. *Cold Spring Harbor Symp. Quant. Biol.* **LX,** 763–773.
4. Aroeti, B., Okhrimenko, H., Reich, V., and Orzech, E. (1998) Polarized trafficking of plasma membrane proteins: emerging roles for coats, SNAREs, GTPases and their link to the cytoskeleton. *Biochim. Biophys. Acta Rev. Biomembr.* **1376,** 57–90.
5. Bradke, F. and Dotti, C. G. (1998) Membrane traffic in polarized neurons. *Biochim. Biophys. Acta Mol. Cell Res.* **1404,** 245–258.
6. Hammerton, R. W., Krzeminski, K. A., Mays, R. W., Ryan, T. A., Wollner, D. A., and Nelson, W. J. (1991) Mechanism for regulating cell surface distribution of Na^+, K^+-ATPase in polarized epithelial cells. *Science* **254,** 847–850.
7. Morrow, J. S., Cianci, C. D., Ardito, T., Mann, A. S., and Kashgarian, M. (1989) Ankyrin links fodrin to the alpha subunit of Na,K-ATPase in Madin-Darby canine kidney cells and in intact renal tubule cells. *J. Cell Biol.* **108,** 455–465.
8. Gut, A., Balda, M. S., and Matter, K. (1998) The cytoplasmic domains of a β_1 integrin mediate polarization in Madin-Darby canine kidney cells by selective basolateral stabilization. *J. Biol. Chem.* **273,** 29,381–29,388.
9. Fanning, A. S. and Anderson, J. M. (1999) PDZ domains: fundamental building blocks in the organization of protein complexes at the plasma membrane. *J. Clin. Invest.* **103,** 767–772.

10. Perego, C., Vanoni, C., Villa, A., Longhi, R., Kaech, S. M., Fröhli, E., et al. (1999) PDZ-mediated interactions retain the epithelial GABA transporter on the basolateral surface of polarized epithelial cells. *EMBO J.* **18,** 2384–2393.

11. Rongo, C., Whitfield, C. W., Rodal, A., Kim, S. K., and Kaplan, J. M. (1998) LIN-10 is a shared component of the polarized protein localization pathways in neurons and epithelia. *Cell* **94,** 751–759.

12. Simske, J. S., Kaech, S. M., Harp, S. A., and Kim, S. K. (1996) LET-23 receptor localization by the cell junction protein LIN-7 during C. elegans vulval induction. *Cell* **85,** 195–204.

13. Kaech, S. M., Whitfield, C. W., and Kim, S. K. (1998) The LIN–2/LIN–7/ LIN–10 complex mediates basolateral membrane localization of the C. elegans EGF receptor LET–23 in vulval epithelial cells. *Cell* **94,** 761–771.

14. Ponce, A., Vega-Saenz de Miera, E., Kentros, C., Moreno, H., Thornhill, B., and Rudy, B. (1997) K+ channel subunit isoforms with divergent carboxy-terminal sequences carry distinct membrane targeting signals. *J. Memb. Biol.* **159,** 149–159.

15. Muth, T. R., Ahn, J., and Caplan, M. J. (1998) Identification of sorting determinants in the C-terminal cytoplasmic tails of the gamma-aminobutyric acid transporters GAT–2 and GAT–3. *J. Biol. Chem.* **273,** 25,616–25,627.

16. Kornau, H. C., Seeburg, P. H., and Kennedy, M. B. (1997) Interaction of ion channels and receptors with PDZ domain proteins. *Curr. Opin. Neurobiol.* **7,** 368–373.

17. Saras, J. and Heldin, C. H. (1996) PDZ domains bind carboxy-terminal sequences of target proteins. *Trends Biochem. Sci.* **21,** 455–458.

18. Tsunoda, S., Sierralta, J., Sun, Y., Bodner, R., Suzuki, E., Becker, A., et al. (1997) A multivalent PDZ-domain protein assembles signalling complexes in a G- protein-coupled cascade. *Nature* **388,** 243–249.

19. Crawford, I., Maloney, P. C., Zeitlin, P. L., Guggino, W. B., Hyde, S. C., Turley, H., et al. (1991) Immunocytochemical localization of the cystic fibrosis gene product CFTR. *Proc. Natl. Acad. Sci. USA* **88,** 9262–9266.

20. Denning, G. M., Ostedgaard, L. S., Cheng, S. H., Smith, A. E., and Welsh, M. J. (1992) Localization of cystic fibrosis transmembrane conductance regulator in chloride secretory epithelia. *J. Clin. Invest.* **89,** 339–349.

21. Stanton, B. A. (1997) Cystic fibrosis transmembrane conductance regulator (CFTR) and renal function. *Wien Klin Wochenschr* **109,** 457–464.

22. Mickle, J. E. and Cutting, G. R. (1998) Clinical implications of cystic fibrosis transmembrane conductance regulator mutations. *Clin, in Chest Med.* **19,** 2/1–2/16.

23. Davis, P. B., Drumm, M., and Konstan, M. W. (1996) Cystic fibrosis. *Am. J. Respir. Crit. Care Med.* **154,** 1229–1256.

24. Riordan, J. R., Rommens, J. M., Kerem, B., Alon, N., Rozmahel, R., Grzelczak, Z., et al. (1989) Identification of the cystic fibrosis gene: Cloning and characterization of complementary DNA. *Science* **245,** 1066–1073.

25. Jilling, T. and Kirk, K. L. (1997) The biogenesis, traffic, and function of the cystic fibrosis transmembrane conductance regulator. *Int. Rev. Cytol.* **172,** 193–241.

26. Cheng, S. H., Gregory, R. J., Marshall, J., Paul, S., Souza, D. W., White, G. A., et al. (1990) Defective intracellular transport and processing of CFTR is the molecular basis of most cystic fibrosis. *Cell* **63,** 827–834.

27. Pasyk, E. A. and Foskett, J. K. (1997) Cystic fibrosis transmembrane conductance regulator-associated ATP and adenosine 3'-phosphate 5'-phosphosulfate channels in endoplasmic reticulum and plasma membranes. *J. Biol. Chem.* **272,** 7746–7751.

28. Chalfie, M. and Kain, S. (1998) *Green Flourescent Protein: Properties, Applications and Protocols*, Wiley-Liss & Sons, Inc., New York.

29. Conn, P. M. (1999) *Methods In Enzymology: Green Fluorescent Protein*, Academic, San Diego.

30. Sullivan, K. F. and Kay, S. A. (1999) *Methods In Cell Biology: Green Fluorescent Proteins*, Academic, San Diego.

31. Sandison, D. R., Williams, R. M., Wells, K. S., Strickler, J., and Webb, W. W. (1995) Quantitative fluorescence confocal laser scanning microscopy (CLSM), in *Handbook of Biological Confocal Microscopy* (Pawley, J. B., ed.), Plenum, New York, pp. 39–54.

32. Moyer, B. D., Loffing, J., Schwiebert, E. M., Loffing-Cueni, D., Halpin, P. A., Karlson, K. H., et al. (1998) Membrane trafficking of the cystic fibrosis gene product, cystic fibrosis transmembrane conductance regulator, tagged with green fluorescent protein in Madin-Darby canine kidney cells. *J. Biol. Chem.* **273,** 21,759–21,768.

33. Moyer, B. D., Loffing-Cueni, D., Loffing, J., Reynolds, D., and Stanton, B. A. (1999) Butyrate increases apical membrane CFTR but reduces chloride secretion in MDCK cells. *Am. J. Physiol (Renal Physiol.)* **277,** F271–F276.

34. Moyer, B. D., Denton, J., Karlson, K. H., Reynolds, D., Wang, S., Mickle, J. E., et al. (1999) A PDZ-interacting domain in CFTR is an apical membrane polarization signal. *J. Clin. Invest.* **104,** 1363–1374.

35. Wang, S. S., Raab, R. W., Schatz, P. J., Guggino, W. B., and Li, M. (1998) Peptide binding consensus of the NHE-RF-PDZ1 domain matches the C-terminal sequence of cystic fibrosis transmembrane conductance regulator (CFTR). *FEBS Lett.* **427,** 103–108.

36. Short, D. B., Trotter, K. W., Reczek, D., Kreda, S. M., Bretscher, A., Boucher, R. C., et al. (1998) An apical PDZ protein anchors the cystic fibrosis transmembrane conductance regulator to the cytoskeleton. *J. Biol. Chem.* **273,** 19,797–19,801.

37. Hall, R. A., Ostedgaard, L. S., Premont, R. T., Blitzer, J. T., Rahman, N., Welsh, M. J., and Lefkowitz, R. J. (1998) A C-terminal motif found in the β_2-adrenergic receptor, P2Y1 receptor and cystic fibrosis transmembrane conductance regulator determines binding to the Na^+/H^+ exchanger regulatory factor family of PDZ proteins. *Proc. Natl. Acad. Sci. USA* **95,** 8496–8501.

38. Morris, A. P., Cunningham, S. A., Benos, D. J., and Frizzell, R. A. (1992) Cellular differentiation is required for cAMP but not Ca^{2+}-dependent Cl^- secretion in colonic epithelial cells expressing high levels of cystic fibrosis transmembrane conductance regulator. *J. Biol. Chem.* **267,** 5575–5583.

39. Morris, A. P., Cunningham, S. A., Tousson, A., Benos, D. J., and Frizzell, R. A. (1994) Polarization-dependent apical membrane CFTR targeting underlies cAMP-stimulated Cl⁻ secretion in epithelial cells. *Am. J. Physiol. Cell Physiol.* **266,** C254-C268.

40. Mohamed, A., Ferguson, D., Seibert, F. S., Cai, H. M., Kartner, N., Grinstein, S., et al. (1997) Functional expression and apical localization of the cystic fibrosis transmembrane conductance regulator in MDCK I cells. *Biochem. J.* **322,** 259–265.

41. Gekle, M., Wunsch, S., Oberleithner, H., and Silbernagl, S. (1994) Characterization of two MDCK-cell subtypes as a model system to study prinicpal cell and intercalated cell properties. *Pflügers Arch.* **428,** 157–162.

42. Blazer-Yost, B. L., Record, R. D., and Oberleithner, H. (1996) Characterization of hormone stimulated Na⁺ transport in a high-resistance clone of the MDCK cell line. *Pflugers Arch.* **432,** 685–691.

43. Blazer-Yost, B. L., Record, R. D., and Lahr, T. (1997) cAMP stimulation of ion transport in a high resistance subclone of the MDCK cell line. *Physiologist* **40(5),** A4 (Abstract).

44. Girotti, M. and Banting, G. (1996) TGN38-green fluorescent protein hybrid proteins expressed in stably transfected eukaryotic cells provide a tool for the real-time, in vivo study of membrane traffic pathways and suggest a possible role for ratTGN38. *J. Cell Sci.* **109,** 2915–2926.

45. Tarasova, N. I., Stauber, R. H., Choi, J. K., Hudson, E. A., Czerwinski, G., Miller, J. L., et al. (1997) Visualization of G protein-coupled receptor trafficking with the aid of the green fluorescent protein: endocytosis and recycling of cholecystokinin receptor type A. *J. Biol. Chem.* **272,** 14,817–14,824.

46. Olson, K. R., McIntosh, J. R., and Olmsted, J. B. (1995) Analysis of MAP 4 function in living cells using green fluorescent protein (GFP) chimeras. *J. Cell Biol.* **130,** 639–650.

47. Rizzuto, R., Brini, M., Pizzo, P., Murgia, M., and Pozzan, T. (1995) Chimeric green fluorescent protein as a tool for visualizing subcellular organelles in living cells. *Curr. Biol.* **5(6),** 635–642.

48. Gottardi, C. J. and Caplan, M. J. (1993) An ion-transporting ATPase encodes multiple apical localization signals. *J. Cell Biol.* **121,** 283–293.

49. Cubitt, A. B., Heim, R., Adams, S. R., Boyd, A. E., Gross, L. A., and Tsien, R. Y. (1995) Understanding, improving and using green fluorescent proteins. *Trends Biochem. Sci.* **20,** 448–455.

50. Marshall, J., Molloy, R., Moss, G. W. J., Howe, J. R., and Hughes, T. E. (1995) The jellyfish green fluorescent protein: a new tool for studying ion channel expression and function. *Neuron* **14,** 211–215.

51. Prasher, D. C., Eckenrode, V. K., Ward, W. W., Prendergast, F. G., and Cormier, M. J. (1992) Primary structure of the *Aequorea victoria* green fluorescent protein. *Gene* **111,** 229–233.

52. Chalfie, M., Tu, Y., Euskirchen, G., Ward, W. W., and Prasher, D. C. (1994) Green fluorescent protein as a marker for gene expression. *Science* **263,** 802–805.

53. Makhina, E. N. and Nichols, C. G. (1998) Independent trafficking of KATP channel subunits to the plasma membrane. *J. Biol. Chem.* **273,** 3369–3374.

54. Grabner, M., Dirksen, R. T., and Beam, K. G. (1998) Tagging with green fluorescent protein reveals a distinct subcellular distribution of L-type and non-L-type Ca^{2+} channels expressed in dysgenic myotubes. *Proc. Natl. Acad. Sci. USA* **95**, 1903–1908.

55. John, S. A., Monck, J. R., Weiss, J. N., and Ribalet, B. (1998) The sulphonylurea receptor SUR1 regulates ATP-sensitive mouse Kir6. 2 K^+ channels linked to the green fluorescent protein in human embryonic kidney cells (HEK 293). *J. Physiol. (Lond.)* **510**, 333–345.

56. Meyer, E. and Fromherz, P. (1999) Ca^{2+} activation of hSlo K+ channel is suppressed by N-terminal GFP tag. *Eur. J. Neurosci.* **11**, 1105–1108.

57. Johns, D. C., Nuss, H. B., and Marban, E. (1997) Suppression of neuronal and cardiac transient outward currents by viral gene transfer of dominant-negative Kv4. 2 constructs. *J. Biol. Chem.* **272**, 31,598–31,603.

58. Rae, J. L. and Shepard, A. R. (1998) Inwardly rectifying potassium channels in lens epithelium are from the IRK1 (Kir 2. 1) family. *Exp. Eye Res.* **66**, 347–359.

59. Rae, J. L. and Shepard, A. R. (1998) Molecular biology and electrophysiology of calcium-activated potassium channels from lens epithelium. *Curr. Eye Res.* **17**, 264–275.

60. Neuhuber, B., Gerster, U., Doring, F., Glossmann, H., Tanabe, T., and Flucher, B. E. (1998) Association of calcium channel α1S and β1a subunits is required for the targeting of β1a but not of α1S into skeletal muscle triads. *Proc. Natl. Acad. Sci. USA* **95**, 5015–5020.

61. Park, K., Arreola, J., Begenisich, T., and Melvin, J. E. (1998) Comparison of voltage-activated Cl⁻ channels in rat parotid acinar cells with ClC-2 in a mammalian expression system. *J. Membrane Biol.* **163**, 87–95.

62. Petrecca, K., Atanasiu, R., Akhavan, A., and Shrier, A. (1999) N-linked glycosylation sites determine HERG channel surface membrane expression. *J. Physiol. (Lond.)* **515**, 41–48.

63. Mall, M., Bleich, M., Kuehr, J., Brandis, M., Greger, R., and Kunzelmann, K. (1999) CFTR-mediated inhibition of epithelial Na^+ conductance in human colon is defective in cystic fibrosis. *Am. J. Physiol. Gastrointest. Liver Physiol.* **277**, G709–G716.

64. Griffiths, G., Parton, R. G., Lucocq, J., Van Deurs, B., Brown, D., Slot, J. W., and Geuze, H. J. (1993) The immunofluorescent era of membrane traffic. *Trends Cell Biol.* **3**, 214–219.

65. Dobson, S. P., Livingstone, C., Gould, G. W., and Tavare, J. M. (1996) Dynamics of insulin-stimulated translocation of GLUT4 in single living cells visualised using green fluorescent protein. *FEBS Lett.* **393**, 179–184.

66. Pouli, A. E., Kennedy, H. J., Schofield, J. G., and Rutter, G. A. (1998) Insulin targeting to the regulated secretory pathway after fusion with green fluorescent protein and firefly luciferase. *Biochem. J.* **331**, 669–675.

67. Chalfant, M. L., Denton, J. S., Langlogh, A. L., Karlson, K. H., Loffing, J., Benos, D. J., and Stanton, B. A. (1999) The NH_2-terminus of the epithelial sodium channel contains an endocytic motif. *J. Biol. Chem.* **274(12)**, 32,889–32,896.

68. Gustafson, C. E., Levine, S., Katsura, T., McLaughlin, M., Aleixo, M. D., Tamarappoo, B. K., et al. (1998) Vasopressin regulated trafficking of a green fluorescent protein-aquaporin 2 chimera in LLC-PK1 cells. *Histochem. Cell Biol.* **110,** 377–386.

69. Johnston, J. A., Ward, C. L., and Kopito, R. R. (1998) Aggresomes: a cellular response to misfolded proteins. *J. Cell Biol.* **143,** 1883–1898.

70. Carey, K. L., Richards, S. A., Lounsbury, K. M., and Macara, I. G. (1996) Evidence using a green fluorescent protein-glucocorticoid receptor chimera that the RAN/TC4 GTPase mediates an essential function independent of nuclear protein import. *J. Cell Biol.* **133,** 985–996.

71. Lybarger, L., Dempsey, D., Franek, K. J., and Chervenak, R. (1996) Rapid generation and flow cytometric analysis of stable GFP-expressing cells. *Cytometry* **25,** 211–220.

72. Muldoon, R. R., Levy, J. P., Kain, S. R., Kitts, P. A., and Link, C. J., Jr. (1997) Tracking and quantitation of retroviral-mediated transfer using a completely humanized, red-shifted green fluorescent protein gene. *BioTechniques* **22,** 162–167.

73. Evers, R., Kool, M., van Deemter, L., Janssen, H., Calafat, J., Oomen, L. C., et al. (1998) Drug export activity of the human canalicular multispecific organic anion transporter in polarized kidney MDCK cells expressing cMOAT (MRP2) cDNA. *J. Clin. Invest.* **101,** 1310–1319.

74. Marshall, J., Fang, S., Ostegaard, L. S., O'Riordan, C. R., Ferrara, D., Amara, J. F., et al. (1994) Stoichiometry of recombinant cystic fibrosis transmembrane conductance regulator in epithelial cells and its functional reconstitution into cells *in vitro*. *J. Biol. Chem.* **269,** 2987–2995.

75. Cheng, S. H., Rich, D. P., Marshall, J., Gregory, R. J., Welsh, M. J., and Smith, A. E. (1991) Phosphorylation of the R domain by cAMP-dependent protein kinase regulates the CFTR chloride channel. *Cell* **66,** 1027–1036.

76. Tabcharani, J. A., Chang, X.-B., Riordan, J. R., and Hanrahan, J. W. (1991) Phosphorylation-regulated Cl⁻ channel in CHO cells stably expressing the cystic fibrosis gene. *Nature* **352,** 628–631.

77. Lidofsky, S. D., Sostman, A., and Fitz, J. G. (1997) Regulation of cation-selective channels in liver cells. *J. Membr. Biol.* **157,** 231–236.

78. Loffing, J., Moyer, B. D., McCoy, D., and Stanton, B. A. (1998) Exocytosis is not involved in activation of Cl⁻ secretion via CFTR in Calu–3 airway epithelial cells. *Am. J. Physiol. Cell Physiol.* **275,** C913–C920.

79. Howard, M., Jilling, T., DuVall, M., and Frizzell, R. A. (1996) cAMP-regulated trafficking of epitope-tagged CFTR. *Kidney Int.* **49,** 1642–1648.

80. Bradbury, N. A. (1999) Intracellular CFTR: localization and function. *Physiol. Rev.* **79,** S175–S191.

81. Bradbury, N. A. and Bridges, R. J. (1994) Role of membrane trafficking in plasma membrane solute transport. *Am. J. Physiol. Cell Physiol.* **267,** C1–C24.

82. Morris, A. P. and Frizzell, R. A. (1994) Vesicle targeting and ion secretion in epithelial cells: implications for cystic fibrosis. *Ann. Rev. Physiol.* **56,** 371–397.

83. Matlin, K. S. and Simons, K. (1983) Reduced temperature prevents transfer of a membrane glycoprotein to the cell surface but does not prevent terminal glycosylation. *Cell* **34,** 233–243.

84. Lehrich, R. W., Aller, S. G., Webster, P., Marino, C. R., and Forrest, J. N., Jr. (1998) Vasoactive intestinal peptide, forskolin, and genistein increase apical CFTR trafficking in the rectal galnd of the spiny dogfish. Acute regulation of CFTR trafficking of CFTR in an intact epithelium. *J. Clin. Invest.* **101,** 737–747.

85. Perego, C., Vanoni, C., Villa, A., Longhi, R., Kaech, S. M., Frohli, E., et al. (1999) PDZ-mediated interactions retain the epithelial GABA transporter on the basolateral surface of polarized epithelial cells. *EMBO J.* **18,** 2384–2393.

86. Rich, D. P., Gregory, R. J., Cheng, S. H., Smith, A. E., and Welsh, M. J. (1993) Effect of deletion mutations on the function of CFTR chloride channels. *Receptors Channels* **1,** 221–232.

87. Zhang, L., Wang, D. H., Fischer, H., Fan, P. D., Widdicombe, J. H., Kan, Y. W., and Dong, J. Y. (1998) Efficient expression of CFTR function with adeno-associated virus vectors that carry shortened CFTR genes. *Proc. Natl. Acad. Sci. USA* **95,** 10,158–10,163.

88. Mickle, J. E., Macek, M., Jr., Fulmer-Smentek, S. B., Egan, M. M., Schwiebert, E., Guggino, W., et al. (1998) A mutation in the cystic fibrosis transmembrane conductance regulator gene associated with elevated sweat chloride concentrations in the absence of cystic fibrosis. *Hum. Mol. Genet.* **7,** 729–735.

89. Rizzuto, R., Brini, M., De Giorgi, F., Rossi, R., Heim, R., Tsien, R. Y., and Pozzan, T. (1996) Double labelling of subcellular structures with organelle-targeted GFP mutants *in vivo. Curr. Biol.* **6,** 183–188.

90. Heim, R. and Tsien, R. Y. (1996) Engineering green fluorescent protein for improved brightness, longer wavelengths and fluorescence resonance energy transfer. *Curr. Biol.* **6(2),** 178–182.

91. Tsien, R. Y. (1998) The green fluorescent protein. *Annu. Rev. Biochem.* **67,** 509–544.

92. Gonzalez, J. E. and Negulescu, P. A. (1998) Intracellular detection assays for high-throughput screening. *Curr. Opin. Biotechnol.* **9,** 624–631.

93. Matz, M. V., Fradkov, A. F., Labas, Y. A., Savitsky, A. P., Zaraisky, A. G., Markelov, M. L., and Lukyanov, S. A. (1999) Fluorescent proteins from nonbioluminescent Anthozoa species. *Nat. Biotechnol.* **17,** 969–973.

11

Localization and Quantification of GFP-Tagged Ion Channels Expressed in *Xenopus* Oocytes

Tooraj Mirshahi, Diomedes E. Logothetis, and Massimo Sassaroli

1. INTRODUCTION

The green fluorescent protein (GFP) from the jellyfish *Aequorea victoria* has recently emerged as a very powerful tool in cell biology. Fused to the protein of interest, GFP serves as a marker for gene expression as well as protein localization in living cells. We have used GFP as a marker for ion-channel localization and expression in *Xenopus* oocytes. As with any study using heterologous expression of proteins, these studies should be interpreted in the biological context in which they are presented, considering the cell biology and physiology of the protein under study. Furthermore, there are potential artifacts using these techniques necessitating the use of stringent control experiments. Nevertheless, in our studies, this approach has proven extremely useful, as we hope to convey in the current chapter.

2. GFP

2.1. Green Fluorescent Protein

GFP from the jellyfish *Aequorea victoria* is a protein of 238 amino acids. Although the protein was discovered some 40 years ago *(1)*, cloning of the GFP gene was accomplished only recently *(2)*. The crystal structure of GFP revealed a single α-helix positioned along the axis of a surrounding 11-stranded β-barrel. The GFP fluorophore is attached to the α-helix and consists of a 4-(*p*-hydroxybenzylidene)-imidazolidin-5-one formed by

From: *Ion Channel Localization Methods and Protocols*
Edited by: A. Lopatin and C. G. Nichols © Humana Press Inc., Totowa, NJ

cyclization of residues 65-67, Ser-Thr-Gly, followed by dehydration and oxidation of the intermediate by molecular oxygen. The protection provided to the fluorophore by the surrounding β-barrel probably contributes to the relative resistance of GFP fluorescence to chemical quenchers as well as to photobleaching. The fact that no additional factor(s) are required to form its chromophore *(3)* confers GFP its unique qualities as a marker for gene expression in a variety of tissues and cells from different species (for a review, *see* ref. *4*).

The fluorescence excitation spectrum of wild-type GFP is characterized by a major peak at ~395 nm, ~2.6 times higher than a minor peak at ~475 nm. These two peaks correspond to absorption by the neutral and anionic form of the fluorophore, respectively. The fluorescence emission spectrum is characterized by a main peak centered at ~504 nm. The photophysical properties of the GFP fluorophore are quite complex, including a reversible excited state deprotonation of the phenol group and a photoisomerization process which, under prolonged illumination, leads to photoconversion of the fluorophore from the neutral to the anionic form, with loss of absorbance at 395 nm and gain at 495 nm. Because spectroscopic and photoconversion measurements have shown that the extinction coefficient of the anionic form of the chromophore is about two times that of the neutral form, it has been deduced that ~15% of the wild-type GFP molecules in the ground state contain anionic fluorophores *(5)*.

For the purpose of localization, the sensitivity with which a fluorescent marker can be detected depends on several factors. The first is its intrinsic brightness, defined as the product of the extinction coefficient at the wavelength of excitation, ε, times the fluorescence quantum yield, Q. In addition, the photobleaching quantum yield, defined as the probability of each excitation event resulting in the photochemical destruction of the fluorophore, is also important because it limits the total number of fluorescence photons that can be emitted by an individual molecule. In this respect, all GFP variants tested have been shown to photobleach much more slowly than fluorescein. When imaging is performed using laser-scanning confocal microscopy, the fluorescent marker should also have an optical absorption peak as close as possible to one of the strong lines of the available lasers. This will maximize the specific excitation of the marker relative to the endogenous fluorophores, such as NADH and flavins. Finally, the excitation and emission spectra of the fluorescent marker should be well-separated from that of the endogenous fluorophores, in order to minimize the background autofluorescence. In general, this is achieved by selecting markers with long wavelength or red-shifted excitation peaks.

A number of GFP mutants have been characterized with a range of useful properties, such as modified excitation and/or emission spectra, higher extinction coefficients and emission quantum yields, as well as improved photostability and expression in mammalian systems *(6)*. For example, mutation of serine-65 to threonine yields a protein with a single excitation peak at ~489 nm, which coincides with one of the strong lines of argon/krypton lasers commonly used in confocal microscopes, while its emission maximum remains at ~510 nm. Consequently, this mutant is several folds brighter than the wild-type protein. The additional mutation F64L, introduced in the background of the S65T mutant, resulted in the protein called Enhanced GFP, or EGFP, which has been the marker of choice in our laboratory for ion channel localization in *Xenopus* oocytes, owing to its brightness, spectral properties, and stability. EGFP is commercially available from Clontech.

Mutation Y66H results in a protein with a blue-shifted excitation peak at ~384 nm and emission at ~450 nm, hence the name blue fluorescent protein, or BFP. Because of the overlap between the BFP emission and the EGFP excitation spectra, these probes can be used in Fluorescence Resonance Energy Transfer (FRET) studies of protein-protein interactions and oligomerization, in which they serve as energy donor and acceptor, respectively. As a marker for protein localization and expression, however, BFP is of limited value, owing to its lower brightness and photostability, as well as to the increased autofluorescence excited at the shorter wavelengths.

Two relatively new variants of GFP, called Enhanced Cyan (ECFP) and Enhanced Yellow (EYFP) Fluorescent Protein, with excitation and emission spectra blue- and red-shifted relative to EGFP, respectively, have recently been used in FRET studies. In addition, Clontech has recently introduced a red fluorescent protein from a sea anemone under the name of DsRed. This protein exhibits excitation and emission maxima at 558 nm and 583 nm, respectively, well above any of the previous GPP variants. We have not tested these proteins in localization studies of ion channels in *Xenopus* oocytes.

2.2. Tagging Channels with GFP

To study ion channel localization in living cells as well as fixed tissue, the channel of interest must be tagged with GFP. Obvious locations for tagging are the N- or the C-terminus of the channel. The choice of where to tag the channel depends on the structure of the channel in question. Because in G protein-sensitive inwardly rectifying K^+ (GIRK) channels both termini are intracellular, we have tagged either the N- or the C-terminus with no apparent difference in the cellular localization of the two constructs. In many other ion channels, either one or both of the termini are extracellular. In a recent study, Bueno and colleagues *(7)* tagged GFP to the C-terminus of GABA-A receptors. They showed that the GFP-tagged channel retains its normal functional properties. Furthermore, they showed, using a GFP antibody in nonpermeablized oocytes, that the GFP is extracellular and they could observe the GFP signal using either epifluorescence or confocal microscopy.

Another important issue in tagging channels is that GFP may interfere with N- or the C-terminal sequences of certain channels important for membrane targeting or for interacting with clustering proteins. For instance, several channels, such as the Shaker potassium channels and NMDA receptors, have been shown to require a free C-terminus to interact with clustering proteins containing PDZ domains *(8,9)*. Therefore, disruption of these signals may affect the clustering of these channels or their cellular localization. Such considerations should be kept in mind when choosing the placement of the GFP tag. It is noteworthy that there are studies where GFP was inserted within the channel protein sequence. In an elegant study, Siegel and Isacoff *(10)* found that such placement of GFP in the Shaker potassium channel yielded a spectrophotometric probe for the inactivation process of the channel.

Placing GFP at the beginning or end of a sequence is accomplished using standard molecular biological methods. The commercially available vectors for GFP are provided in a series of constructs that allow subcloning of ion channels using common restriction sites. For in-frame subcloning, the EGFP vectors from Clontech are available in three different frame-shifts, from which one may be chosen to fit the desired insert. These vectors are available in two sets that are suited for either N- or C-terminal tagging. The vectors designed for N-terminal tagging have the stop codon removed from the EGFP sequence. However, in order to place GFP at the C-terminus, the stop codon must be removed from the channel cDNA using standard PCR techniques. In our work, we use vectors that have been specifically modified to give optimal protein expression in oocytes. These are derived from popular vectors, such as pGEM3Z or pBluescript, by addition of untranslated regions from the *Xenopus* β-globin gene flanking both the 5' and 3' ends of the multiple cloning sequences *(11)*. For oocyte work, because cRNA made from some of the GFP vectors may not give sufficient levels of expression, we recommend subcloning the channel-GFP construct into an oocyte-optimized vector. Alternatively, cDNA can be directly injected into the nuclei of oocytes. Vectors containing a CMV promoter are suitable for this purpose and the EGFP vectors from Clontech are all driven by CMV promoters. Whereas injection of cDNA into oocytes works well for some investigators and simplifies some of the experimental procedures, we have found that in our hands cRNA injection yields reproducible results.

We use polymerase chain reaction (PCR) strategies in tagging the channel with GFP in order to minimize the number of extra amino acids placed between the channel sequence and GFP. All the normal precautions to avoid introducing mutations while using PCR techniques are applicable here.

Regardless of the approach for tagging ion channels with GFP, it is always crucial to determine whether the modifications lead to functional changes in the channel of interest. For this purpose, we use whole-cell recordings to examine some of the macroscopic properties of our GFP-tagged GIRK channels, including inward rectification and G protein sensitivity. At the single-channel level we measure unitary conductance as well as mean open and closed times of the GFP-tagged channels and compare them to the wild-type channels. All these studies have shown that addition of GFP to the C-terminus of GIRK channels does not alter their functional properties *(12)*.

3. LOCALIZATION OF CHANNELS IN OOCYTES

3.1. Xenopus *Oocytes*

The oocytes of *Xenopus laevis* frogs have been an invaluable tool in electrophysiological studies of ion channels (for reviews, *see* ref. *13*). Expression of ion channels in oocytes has been the subject of many studies. We utilize oocytes for recording whole-cell currents, using double electrode voltage clamp, as well as for single channels and macro-patch recordings, using the patch-clamp technique. We often use the same oocyte from which we record, to study channel localization. The techniques for oocyte isolation, cRNA synthesis, oocyte injection and maintenance have been described elsewhere and are beyond the scope of this review (e.g., refs. *13,14*). However, there are a few details worth reviewing about preparing oocytes for localization studies. Oocytes have an unusually high level of background autofluorescence (which will be discussed later). For this reason, it is critical that the fluorescence from the GFP-tagged channel be strong enough to be easily distinguished from the background. In order to achieve this, it is crucial to have sufficient GFP expression. To this end, we recommend using oocyte-optimized vectors for expression and using EGFP for a brighter signal. These are two important choices for increasing the sensitivity and signal-to-noise ratio in localization studies. In addition, electrophysiological recordings from the same oocytes used for the localization studies are good indicators of the level of expression of the particular channel in oocytes. Correlation of functional expression with adequate fluorescence signal can help determine whether sufficient levels of expression for imaging studies have been achieved. Because two-electrode voltage clamp measurements are relatively straightforward and can be accomplished in little time, they may actually save the experimenter time and effort by demonstrating insufficient levels of expression before undertaking the more laborious channel localization experiments. Occasionally, oocytes that morphologically appear healthy may in fact show little or no expression. Using such oocytes may mislead the experimenter in localization studies. In dealing with this issue, electrophysiological recording is perhaps the most efficient indicator of the health of the oocytes under study.

3.2. Use of Albino Oocytes for Channel Expression

Oocytes are large cells with diameters of ~1.2 mm. Normal frogs produce oocytes with an animal pole that is pigmented and a vegetal pole that lacks pigment. Albino frogs, however, produce oocytes with no pigment. These oocytes are lightly colored all around and the animal and vegetal poles cannot be distinguished based on differences in appearance. Studies by others, using methods including recordings from agarose-embedded oocytes, have shown that the density of potassium channels expressed on the surface of oocytes is maximal near the point of mRNA injection *(15)*. We have confirmed these results with our GFP-tagged K^+ channels in normal oocytes. Owing to their lack of pigment, albino oocytes are more easily examined using an epifluorescence microscope. An albino oocyte expressing a GFP-tagged protein at the plasma membrane shows a rim of bright green that is easily detected by epifluorescence. This is a relatively simple yet powerful way of identifying specific areas on the surface of the oocyte in which channels are expressed. However, as mentioned above, because it is difficult to distinguish the two poles in these oocytes, one cannot easily use this method to track the expression of ion channels on different parts of the membrane. However, we must stress here that, at least in our hands, albino oocytes are more difficult to manipulate than normal oocytes, because they are more fragile.

Development of more advanced and affordable confocal microscopes has played a significant role in the progress of imaging microscopy. However, because whole oocytes are very large and opaque, confocal microscopes with even the most powerful lasers cannot image deeper than ~100 µm from the surface of the oocyte. Furthermore, this can only be accomplished in albino oocytes because normal oocytes are pigmented.

Multi-photon microscopy is an emerging technology that holds great promise for imaging intact oocytes expressing GFP-tagged channels. In a multi-photon microscope, excitation of visible light-absorbing fluorophores by the infrared laser radiation is confined to a small volume around the focal point, which allows high-resolution, three-dimensional imaging of living samples with higher sensitivity, less photodamage and at greater depths than standard confocal microscopes.

3.3. Preparation of Oocytes for Confocal Imaging

3.3.1. Fixing Oocytes

Since, as discussed earlier, oocytes are thick and opaque, they must be sectioned for imaging by a confocal or a wide-field epifluorescence microscope. Once it has been determined that oocytes are expressing adequate levels of the channel of interest and that the channel is functioning normally, we fix the oocytes using a fresh 4% paraformaldehyde (PFA) solution in phosphate-buffered saline (PBS). Paraformaldehyde is a carcinogen and must be handled properly. Some of the steps should be done under a chemical hood to avoid noxious fumes. To prepare the solution, preheat two-thirds the final volume of ddH$_2$O to 60°C, add the required amount of PFA and stir on a hot plate at low heat. Boiling of the solution must be avoided. In order for the PFA to go into solution, add a few drops of 5 N NaOH. After a few minutes, when the PFA is completely dissolved, add 1/10 the volume of 10X PBS and then adjust the pH to 7.2 using 5 N HCl. The amount of HCl required may be large if excess NaOH was added in the beginning. Adjust the volume and store at 4°C. Although freshly prepared PFA is preferable, we have used solutions for 1 wk after preparation without problems. To fix the oocytes, remove them from the storage medium (we use ND96 supplemented with calcium, sodium pyruvate, and antibiotics), wash once in 4% PFA, and then place them in 4% PFA overnight, either at room temperature or at 4°C. However, fixing at 4°C sometimes leads to the undesirable appearance of an invagination in the animal pole of the oocytes. Because oocytes have large diameters and their yolk is viscous, penetration of PFA is much more difficult than in most cells. We usually fix cultured mammalian cells for 5–10 min with PFA as compared with overnight incubation for oocytes. Although prolonged fixation increases the background autofluorescence in oocytes, under-fixed oocytes are difficult to section and, once sectioned, their yolk tends to spread and obstruct the clarity of the sections. For these reasons, we have settled on the compromise fixation time of 10–16 h. This time is long enough to fix the oocyte thoroughly while keeping the autofluorescence to a manageable level. In order to overcome the background autofluorescence, we have always used the brightest GFP as well as the highest levels of channel expression.

3.3.2. Embedding Oocytes in Agarose

Once the oocytes are fixed, they are washed 2–3 times; 10 min each time with 1X PBS to remove any excess PFA and embedded in agarose for sectioning. For this purpose, 2.5–3% agarose in 1X PBS is prepared by heating (in a microwave oven or on a hot plate). Once the agarose is melted, it is kept on a hot plate to prevent it from solidifying. The agarose should be warm enough to transfer using a 1 mL pipet. In the meantime, oocytes are placed into plastic base molds, which are available from many manufacturers. We use $7 \times 7 \times 5$ mm Fisher Scientific base molds (cat. no. 22-038216). The choice of this size mold is for convenience in sectioning using the Vibratome. Once the oocytes are placed in the base mold, the excess PBS is removed. We usually place between 5 and 20 oocytes in a mold so that a large number of sections can be obtained from each agarose block. However, if too many oocytes are placed in a single block, they may not be embedded as strongly and they may come out of the block during sectioning. After removing the excess PBS, the appropriate amount of agarose is poured into the mold (300–500 µL for our molding blocks) on the oocytes. There are several issues to keep in mind in embedding oocytes. To the best of our experience and from our communications with others who use agarose-embedded oocytes, pouring relatively warm agarose onto fixed oocytes does not exert adverse effects on them. Additionally, after pouring the agarose onto the oocytes, the blocks are placed at 4°C for a few minutes so that the agarose solidifies. At this stage, the block is ready for sectioning. Additional considerations in making the agarose blocks will be presented below.

3.3.3. Sectioning Oocytes and Preparing for Imaging

For confocal microscopy, we cut 50 µm thick oocyte sections using a Vibratome. Figure 1 shows the Vibratome that we use and some of the materials needed for sectioning and mounting oocytes as well as some agarose-embedded oocytes and sections mounted on a microscope slide. For sectioning with a Vibratome, we glue the agarose block to the sectioning plate of the Vibratome using a drop of water resistant glue. During the embedding procedure, the oocytes have a tendency to sink to the bottom of the agarose. Therefore, once the agarose block is solidified and removed from the mold, the oocytes are found at one end of the block. We normally glue this end to the Vibratome stage because gluing the other end places the oocytes on top of the block and immediately subjects them to be cut by the Vibratome. When the oocytes are on the top, they tend to be dislodged from the agarose block rather than remain in the block to be sectioned. Thus, gluing the oocyte end of the agarose block ensures that more of the oocytes will remain intact and will be properly cut in the sectioning procedure. However, consequently the very bottom of the agarose block becomes inaccessible. Therefore, one must keep this sectioning strategy in mind while embedding the oocytes. In order to obtain sections from a desired pole of the oocyte (either animal or vegetal) it must face up in the molding block. Using this strategy, it is possible to determine whether channels localize preferentially at the animal or vegetal pole. For the purpose of determining the extent of membrane localization of expressed GFP-tagged channels, sections from the middle three quarters of the oocyte are most useful, because the resulting rim images allow the best measurement of the distribution of fluorescence intensity perpendicular to the membrane surface.

For sectioning, add ice-cold PBS to the Vibratome stage plate covering the agarose block and proceed by sectioning through the block, cutting large pieces of agarose from the top until the blade reaches the oocytes, then proceed with 50-μm sections. Most sections will separate from the surrounding agarose, however some will remain stuck to the agarose. These can be removed from the agarose section by using a fine brush made by trimming an inexpensive small watercolor brush to leave only a few bristles. The sections can be left to accumulate in the Vibratome before they are picked up with the brush or they can be removed as they are cut. Each section is picked up with the brush (probably the most tedious part of this entire procedure) and transferred to the mounting medium on a microscope slide. Many commercially available mounting media suffice for this purpose. Because fading is a potential problem one must remember to obtain media with good fluorescence preservation properties. Most of these media are glycerol based with an added agent to prevent fading. Several chemicals have been reported to preserve the fluorescence including sodium azide, polyvinyl pyrrolidone (PVP), and DABCO among others. We use DABCO as it has been reported to be very stable and a good retarding agent *(14)*. For mounting oocyte sections, we use DTG, which contains 2.5% DABCO and 50 m*M* Tris, pH 8.6, in 90% Glycerol. A stock of DTG can be made and stored in aliquots at –20°C indefinitely. Sections are mounted by transferring them with the brush into a drop of mounting medium placed on a microscope slide. The sections are then covered with a No. 1^1/$_2$ coverslip and sealed with quick-drying nail polish. It is important to determine the appropriate coverslip for the particular objective and microscope in use in order to obtain the best imaging results.

3.3.4. Viewing the Oocyte Sections

Once the nail polish is completely dry, the sections are ready for viewing by conventional epifluorescence or confocal microscopy. Because the spectral properties of wild-type GFP and several of its variants are very similar

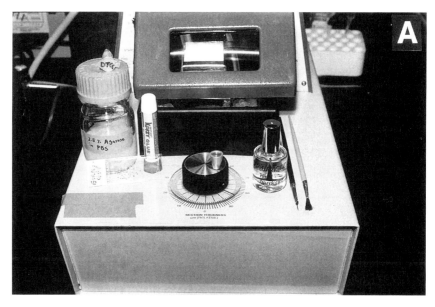

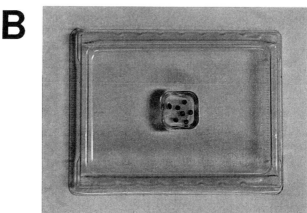

Fig. 1. (A) The Vibratome and some of the materials needed for sectioning and mounting fixed *Xenopus* oocytes. **(B)** The agarose block with oocytes in the base mold.

to those of fluorescein, the microscope needs only to be equipped with a standard FITC filter set, which is readily available from the microscope manufacturer or from a number of vendors. Epifluorescence microscopy is used in many electrophysiology laboratories that use GFP co-transfection to select transfected cells in patch clamp studies. Conventional wide-field microscopes are useful for quickly determining whether the oocyte sections

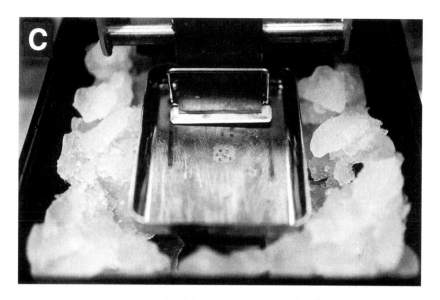

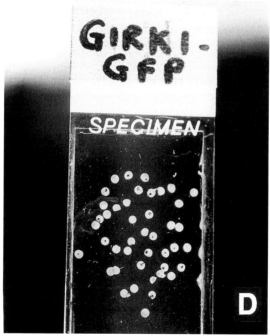

Fig. 1. (C) The agarose block glued to the Vibratome sectioning plate. The block is submerged in ice-cold PBS. **(D)** A microscope slide with oocytes sections mounted and covered with a coverslip. The hole in the middle of some of the sections is the nucleus.

are GFP-positive and how strong the signal is. However, to carefully characterize the localization of GFP-tagged ion channels, a confocal microscope is highly recommended. In examining oocyte sections with the confocal microscope, we usually first use a 10× objective to obtain a general survey of the distribution of channel protein and then switch to a 40× oil objective to carry out a more detailed analysis of channel localization. For a quantitative comparison of channel localization between different constructs and sections, it is necessary to keep parameters such as laser intensity, pinhole size, and detector settings constant.

4. LOCALIZATION OF GIRK CHANNELS IN *XENOPUS* OOCYTES: A CASE STUDY

GIRK channels are multimeric ion channels expressed in the heart and brain (for reviews, *see* ref. *12*). They are composed of four different subunits (GIRK1-GIRK4) that are thought to form heteromultimers to give rise to functional channels. GIRK2-GIRK4 subunits exhibit low activity as homomultimers in oocytes and other expression systems, whereas GIRK1 subunits are completely nonfunctional when expressed by themselves in mammalian cells. In oocytes, a *Xenopus* specific subunit of GIRK channels, XIR, interacts with GIRK1 subunits and give rise to low GIRK channel activity *(17)*. One possible reason for this behavior may be a deficiency in localization of GIRK1 channels to the plasma membrane. This represents an interesting case suited for using GFP-tagged channels to assess their localization. We have constructed GIRK1 and GIRK4 subunits tagged with the S65T variant of GFP at the C-terminus and expressed them in oocytes. Figure 2A,B shows sections from oocytes expressing GIRK1-GFP and GIRK4-GFP, respectively. It is clear from these pictures that GIRK4 is strongly localized to the membrane, whereas GIRK1 shows little or no membrane localization. However, when non-GFP tagged GIRK4 is co-expressed with GIRK1-GFP, GIRK1 becomes strongly localized to the membrane (Fig. 2C). Images acquired using the 40× objective give a similar but higher resolution view of the GIRK channels subunit localization (Fig. 2D–F). This demonstrates that assembly of GIRK1 and GIRK4 is necessary for translocation of GIRK1 to the membrane. Similar studies from Flag-tagged channels expressed in Cos-1 cells are presented for comparison (Fig. 2G–I). These results show that GIRK channel localization is similar in oocytes and mammalian cells. However, the oocyte data show a level of clarity that is seldom obtained in cells.

The level of expression of GFP-tagged channels in oocytes can also be measured by a standard spectrofluorometric assay. We have used this method

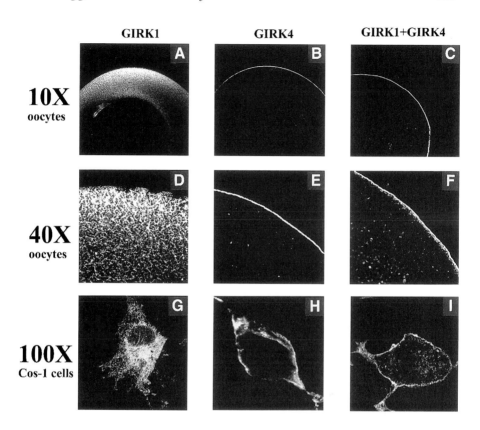

Fig. 2. Confocal images from GFP-tagged as well as flag-tagged GIRK channels subunits. **(A)** GIRK1-GFP alone, 10×. It is clear that only a small portion of the signal resides in the membrane. The dark region in the middle represents the nucleus that has been cut through. **(B)** GIRK4-GFP,10×. Almost all of the GFP signal is localized to the membrane. **(C)** GIRK1-GFP co-expressed with non-tagged GIRK4, 10×. Co-expression of GIRK4 enables GIRK1-GFP to localize mostly to the plasma membrane (for comparison see Fig. 2A). **(D–F)** Images from the same oocytes as above obtained using a 40× oil immersion objective. The localization in different cellular compartments is well-appreciated at the higher magnification. **(G)** Antibody staining of flag-tagged GIRK1 transfected in Cos-1 cells. Permeablized cells were used for antibody staining using a primary anti-flag antibody and a Texas-Red conjugated secondary antibody. Again, GIRK1 shows a mainly cytoplasmic distribution with little membrane expression. **(H)** Same as (G), but with flag-tagged GIRK4. **(I)** Same as (G), except for co-expression of non-tagged GIRK4.

to assess the amount of GIRK1 and GIRK4 subunits tagged with the S65T GFP variant expressed in oocytes. In order to isolate the total membrane fraction, oocytes are homogenized in lysis buffer (5 mM Tris, 1 mM ethylene glycol-bis β-aminoethylether N,N,N',N'-tetraacetic acid [EGTA], 1 mM ethylenediaminetetracetic acid [EDTA], pH 8.0) containing a protease inhibitor cocktail, using a Dounce homogenizer. The homogenate, kept at 4°C, is spun at 5,000 rpm for 5 min in an Eppendorf tabletop centrifuge. The supernatant is removed (the pellet consists mainly of the yolk) and spun for 30 min at 100,000g. The resulting pellet, containing the packed membranes, is solubilized in 250 µL of an equal volume mixture of 2% Triton X-100 and sodium dodecyl sulfate (SDS)-deficient RIPA buffer (150 mM NaCl, 1% NP-40 and 50 mM Tris, pH 8.0) transferred to a 3-mm pathlength fluorescence cuvet. In our laboratory the fluorescence intensity is measured with a computer-interfaced SLM spectrofluorometer equipped with a double-grating excitation monochromator, which lowers the background contribution owing to stray light scattered by the sample. In order to convert fluorescence intensity into GFP concentration, a standard curve must be produced using serial dilutions of a solution of purified recombinant GFP. To simplify the procedure, the same variant used for tagging the channels should be used as standard. However, this is not absolutely essential, as demonstrated by the data in Fig. 3, in which the standard curve was generated using recombinant wild-type GFP (rGFP; Clontech, Palo Alto, CA) while the GIRK subunits were tagged with the S65T variant. In this case, the calculation of the unknown concentration must take into account the differences between the spectroscopic properties of the two GFP proteins. Neglecting common terms, the fluorescence intensity, F, integrated over the entire corrected emission spectrum, of a fluorophore in solution is given by $F = c \, \varepsilon \, Q$, where c is its concentration and ε and Q are the extinction coefficient at the wavelength of excitation and the fluorescence quantum yield, respectively. Thus, the general relationship between the fluorescence intensity, F, of a fluorophore of unknown concentration and that of a standard, F_{std}, is given by

$$F/F_{std} = ce \, Q/c_{std} \, \varepsilon_{std} \, Q_{std}$$

where c_{std}, ε_{std}, and Q_{std} represent the same parameters for the standard as defined above for the fluorophore. In the case where the fluorophore of unknown concentration and that used as a standard are the same, the equation reduces to the simple form $c = F/B$, where $B = F_{std}/c_{std}$ is the slope of the standard calibration line. However, when the two molecules are different, the correction term $K = (\varepsilon \, Q)/(\varepsilon_{std} \, Q_{std})$ must be applied, so that $c = F/(K \, B)$. The peak intensity can be used instead of the integrated intensity over the entire corrected emission spectrum if the fluorophore and the standard have similar spectra, as in the case of rGFP and S65T-GFP. Based on published values *(18)*, the extinction coefficients at the wavelength of excitation, $\lambda =$

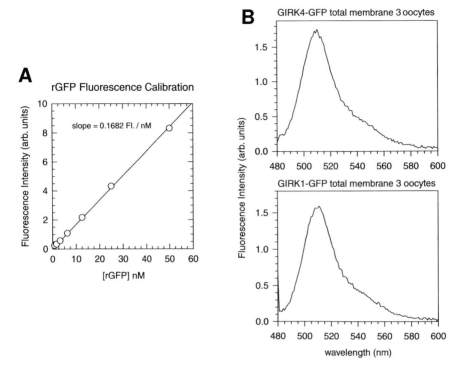

Fig. 3. (A) Standard curve obtained by measuring the fluorescence intensity, in arbitrary units, of serial twofold dilutions of rGFP (Clontech), using a 3-mm square fluorescence cuvet and 470 nm excitation light. The line represents the least-squares fit to the data, with a slope of 0.1682 arbitrary fluorescence units per nanomolar rGFP concentration. **(B)** The emission spectra of S65T GFP-tagged GIRK4 (top) and GIRK1 (bottom) subunits in the detergent-solubilized membrane fractions from two groups of three *Xenopus* oocytes transfected with the respective subunits.

470 nm, were calculated to be $\varepsilon_{rGFP} = 9100\ M^{-1}\ cm^{-1}$ and $\varepsilon_{S65T} = 42{,}700\ M^{-1}\ cm^{-1}$ whereas $Q_{rGFP} = 0.79$ and $Q_{S65T} = 0.64$. Therefore, given the value of the slope of the standard curve shown in Fig. 2, $K = 3.8$ and $c_{S65T} = F_{S65T}/(3.8 \times 0.1682)$. Based on this equation, the concentration in the lysates of three oocytes expressing GIRK4-GFP and GIRK1-GFP shown in Fig. 2 were 2.7 and 2.4 nM, respectively.

Once the concentration of GFP in the lysate is known, the average number of molecules per oocyte can be calculated as (Lysate Conc.) $\times$ (Lysate Vol.) $\times$ (Avogadro Number). Thus, each of the oocytes injected with GIRK4-GFP cRNA expressed $(2.7 \times 10^{-9}) \times (250 \times 10^{-6}) \times (6.022 \times 10^{23}) / 3 = 1.4 \times 10^{11}$ molecules of GIRK4-GFP.

5. TROUBLESHOOTING, RANDOM OBSERVATIONS

In some instances, there appears to be a gap between the membrane-localized GFP signal and the cytoplasm. This gap is owing to the oocyte pigment on the animal pole. Sections from albino oocytes or from the vegetal pole of the oocyte do not display this gap. The presence of this gap can be used to assess the localization of the channel to specific regions of the oocyte. Additionally, the presence of fluorescent signal on the outer rim of this dark region is perhaps the most definitive indicator of membrane localization of the particular channel.

We have performed experiments in which we have removed both the follicular and vitelline membranes of the oocytes and no difference in the appearance of membrane-targeted channels was observed. This indicates that removal of these membranes may not be required for imaging experiments. As discussed earlier, these membranes are likely to come off during sectioning. Nevertheless, removal of the follicular membrane may allow more efficient fixation of the oocyte.

6. FINAL REMARKS

Xenopus oocytes have been an important tool in electrophysiological studies of ion channels in the past 20 years. Recent advances in imaging techniques as well as the use of GFP as a molecular marker have opened new avenues for the study of protein localization and expression. We have combined the oocyte-expression system and imaging techniques that use GFP to answer questions about the processing and localization of potassium channels as well as their levels of expression. This has been a powerful tool in our hands and we hope readers find the methods described here useful in their own studies.

REFERENCES

1. Shimomura, O., Johnson, F. H., and Saiga, Y. (1962) Extraction, purification and properties of aequorin, a bioluminescent protein from the luminous hydromedusan, *Aequorea. J. Cell. Comp. Physiol.* **59,** 223–239.
2. Prasher, D. C., Eckenrode, V. K., Ward, W. W., Prendergast, F. G., and Cormier, M. J. (1992) Primary structure of the Aequorea victoria green-fluorescent protein. *Gene* **111(2),** 229–233.
3. Chalfie, M., Tu, Y., Euskirchen, G., Ward, W. W., and Prasher, D. C. (1994) Green fluorescent protein as a marker for gene expression. *Science* **263(5148),** 802–805.

4. Tsien, R. Y. (1998) The green fluorescent protein. *Annu. Rev. Biochem.* **67**, 509–544.
5. Chattoraj, M., King, B. A., Bublitz, G. U., and Boxer, S. G. (1996) Ultra-fast excited state dynamics in green fluorescent protein: multiple states and proton transfer. *Proc. Natl. Acad. Sci. USA* **93 (16)**, 8362–8367.
6. Heim, R., Cubitt, A. B., and Tsien, R. Y. (1995) Improved green fluorescence. *Nature* **373 (6516)**, 663,664.
7. Bueno, O. F., Robinson, L. C., Alvarez-Hernandez, X., and Leidenheimer, N. J. (1998) Functional characterization and visualization of a GABA-A receptor-GFP chimera expressed in *Xenopus* oocytes. *Brain Res. Mol. Brain Res.* **59(2)**, 165–177.
8. Kim, E., Niethammer, M., Rothschild, A., Jan, Y. N., and Sheng, M. (1995) Clustering of Shaker-type K⁺ channels by interaction with a family of membrane-associated guanylate kinases. *Nature* **378(6552)**, 85–88.
9. Kornau, H. C., Schenker, L. T., Kennedy, M. B. and Seeburg, P. H. (1995) Domain interaction between NMDA receptor subunits and the postsynaptic density protein PSD-95. *Science* **269(5231)**, 1737–1740.
10. Siegel, M. S. and Isacoff, E. Y. (1997) A genetically encoded optical probe of membrane voltage. *Neuron* **19(4)**, 735–741.
11. Liman, E. R., Tytgat, J., and Hess, P. (1992) Subunit stoichiometry of a mammalian K⁺ channel determined by construction of multimeric cDNAs. *Neuron* **9(5)**, 861–871.
12. Sui, J. L., Chan, K., Langan, M. N., Vivaudou, M., and Logothetis, D. E. (1999) G protein gated potassium channels. *Adv. Second Messenger Phosphoprotein Res.* **33**, 179–201.
13. Stühmer, W. (1992) Electrophysiological recording from *Xenopus* oocytes. *Methods Enzymol.* **207**, 319–339.
14. Chan, K. W., Langan, M. N., Sui, J., Kozak, J. A., Pabon, A., Ladias, J. A. A., and Logothetis, D. E. (1996) A recombinant inwardly rectifying potassium channel coupled to GTP-binding proteins. *J. Gen. Physiol.* **107**, 381–397.
15. Lopatin, A. N., Makhina, E. N., and Nichols, C. G. (1998) A novel crystallization method for visualizing the membrane localization of potassium channels. *Biophys. J.* **74(5)**, 2159–2170.
16. Johnson, G. D., Davidson, R. S., McNamee. K. C., Russell, G., Goodwin, D., and Holborow, E. J. (1982) Fading of immunofluorescence during microscopy: a study of the phenomenon and its remedy. *J. Immunol. Methods.* **55(2)**, 231–242.
17. Hedin, K. E., Lim, N. F., and Clapham, D. E. (1996) Cloning of a *Xenopus laevis* inwardly rectifying K⁺ channel subunit that permits GIRK1 expression of IKACh currents in oocytes. *Neuron* **16(2)**, 423–429.
18. Patterson, G. H., Knobel, S. M., Sharif, W. D., Kain, S. R., and Piston, D. W. (1997) Use of the green fluorescent protein and its mutants in quantitative fluorescence microscopy. *Biophys. J.* **73**, 2782–2790.

12

Applications of Green Fluorescent Protein (GFP) Technology

Watching Ion Channel Biogenesis in Living Cells Using GFP Fusion Constructs

Scott A. John and James N. Weiss

1. INTRODUCTION

Things that go flash in the night are usually deep in the sea. Autofluorescent and bioluminescent proteins are found almost exclusively in the salt-water world. One notable exception is the glow-in-the-dark firefly—a result of bioluminescence from the protein called luciferase—in which a chemical reaction drives the process, unlike autofluorescence, which is driven by photons. The spectral characteristics of sea water, with its almost complete absorption of longer wavelength light >479 nm, has resulted in a preponderance of light-making proteins that fluoresce or bioluminesce in wavelengths of blue or blue green (450–480 nm)

One member of this family of light emitting proteins that has recently garnered much attention is called "green fluorescent protein" (GFP), which "captures" light from the bioluminescent protein aequorin and emits it at longer wavelengths by a process called fluorescence resonance energy transfer.

GFP, as it is almost universally known, was originally cloned by Prasher in 1992 *(1)* from *Aequorea victoria*. It is composed of 238 amino acids. The crystal structure, solved independently by two groups *(2,3)*, shows that GFP is a beta barrel composed of 11 strands threaded by an alpha helix running up the axis of the cylinder, with the chromophore buried centrally within the barrel. Its spectral characteristics are such that its peak absorption is ~395 nm and peak emission ~504 nm *(4)*.

From: *Ion Channel Localization Methods and Protocols*
Edited by: A. Lopatin and C. G. Nichols © Humana Press Inc., Totowa, NJ

Table 1
Spectral Characteristics of Autofluorescent Proteins[a]

Autofluorescent protein variant	Excitation λ (nm)	Emission λ (nm)	Extinction coefficient	Quantum yield
Wild-type (GFP)	395–397	504	25000	0.79
UV	360	442		
Blue				
BFP	384	448	21000	0.24
EBFP	380	440	31000	0.18
H9	399	511	20000	0.6
Cyan				
W7	434	476	24000	0.42
ECFP	452	505	26000	0.4
Green				
Emerald	487	509	57500	0.68
EGFP	55000	0.6		
Yellow				
10C	514	527	83400	0.61
Topaz	514	527	95000	0.6
EYFP	514	527	84000	0.61
Red Fluorescent Protein	558	583	22500	0.29

[a]The table lists mutants of the wild-type GFP from *A. victoria* and the most recent cloned autofluorescent protein from *D. striata* (RFP). Emission and excitation peak values are given in nanometers. Extinction coefficients in units of 10^3 $M^{-1}cm^{-1}$ Quantum yield is dimensionless. *See* Tsien *(5)* for more mutants and their descriptions.

Extensive mutational studies have generated seven different classes of GFP, reviewed by Tsien 1998 *(5)* and *see* Table 1. These mutants show improved light-emitting characteristics (absorbance extinction coefficients and quantal yield), changes in excitation/emission wavelengths (blue and red shifted) and improved folding characteristics at elevated temperatures, i.e., 37°C. These variants of GFP cover the excitation range from 360–514 nm and emission range from 442–529 nm. Most recently a red fluorescent protein has been cloned from the IndoPacific sea anemone *Discosoma striata* that extends the range of autofluorescent protein emission spectra quite dramatically to 583 nm *(6)*. This is also the first report of an autofluorescent protein cloned from a species other that *A. victoria* and may provoke another round of mutational analysis to further broaden the excitation and emission spectral range of these class of proteins.

Commercialization of GFP and its variants has also led to the generation of constructs that have multiple cloning sites both upstream and downstream of the coding region of GFP. Thus, fusion constructs can be made to either the N or C- terminus of ion channels by simple restriction enzyme subcloning while ensuring that the ion channel coding sequence is in the same frame as the GFP and has no intervening stop codons.

Polymerase chain reaction (PCR) techniques have the added advantage that not only can N or C terminal fusions be constructed, but GFP can be inserted into the coding sequence of the ion channel to create "internal chimeras." An additional advantage to using PCR is that linker or intervening amino acids of user defined length and composition can be placed between the GFP and ion channel coding regions, which may assist in the functional expression of the chimera.

GFP is unique in its ability to monitor protein expression patterns in living cells. Because its cDNA sequence is known, it can be subjected to a large battery of molecular biological techniques with the following advantages:

1. Fusion proteins can be made to specific proteins or pieces of proteins in specific locations with specific linkages *(7)*.
2. The subsequent fusion proteins require no secondary co-factors or substrates. Of course, if the wild-type channel requires subunits or co-factors then the fusion protein will likewise. For example, fusion of the GFP to the beta subunit of the Ca channel when expressed alone showed diffuse distribution in the cytoplasm. Upon coexpression with the alpha 1S subunit, the beta-GFP fusion distribution became clustered at the T-tubule/sarcoplasmic reticulum junctions *(8)*.
3. GFP is stable with regard to high pH, temperature, detergents, and proteolytic breakdown. Some newer variants have been made, which are more pH-sensitive and therefore are capable of monitoring synaptic-vesicle generation *(9)*.
4. The GFP variant can be chosen so that the spectral characteristics match the methods of visualization. Epifluorescence microscopy with Mercury or Xenon lamps can excite nearly all the variants and with the appropriate excitation, dichroic emission filter sets, fluorescent light from the fusion construct can be readily visualized. To help distinguish between GFP and autofluorescence, use a short pass emission, because the GFP has a shorter wavelength than typically yellow autofluorescence. Autofluorescence is less of a problem when using confocal microscopy but the laser light can be more limiting in its excitation of the various autofluorecent chromophores (*see* Table 1).
5. The expressed fusion protein can be monitored in living cells in real time without the need for fixation or cell permeabilization. As such, GFP is a window into the living cell. However, tissue can also be fixed for subsequent analysis using antibody staining or to compare the images pre- and post-fixation. For example, Meyer's group *(7)* has shown that there is a difference between unfixed cells expressing a PKC-GFP fusion protein and one obtained after fixation and antibody staining. High-grade paraformaldehyde or glutaraldehyde should be used and care taken to avoid organic solvents, e.g., nail polish can inhibit the GFP signal *(10)*.

6. GFP or GFP fusion proteins have been expressed in a multitude of organisms from prokaryotes to eukaryotes and from plants to animals *(11,12)*.
7. GFP fusion proteins have been used in a multitude of mammalian cell types, allowing the selection of cell type to be optimized for the protein under study *(12)*.

One potential restriction for GFP expression is the obligate need for oxygen in the generation of the chromophore *(13)*. Thus anaerobes are precluded from forming fluorescent GFP. However if they can tolerate aerobic conditions for a brief time, sufficient for chromophore generation, and then returned to anaerobic conditions, GFP can still be used. Indeed, this requisite for oxygen has the potential advantage of enabling "pulse " or On/Off switching of fluorescent GFP fusion proteins in anaerobic cells.

We have seen from the previous brief introduction that GFP and its variants can be used to determine ion-channel localization by fusing the open reading frames of the ion channel and the fluorescent protein. Below we will discuss the practical approaches that have been taken to accomplish this. We will examine how some of the fusion proteins have been made and how they have been expressed.

2. METHODS

2.1. What Color Do You Want Your Protein to Be?

Table 1 lists the currently available colors in increasing wavelength: blue, cyan, green, yellow, and red. These are all commercially available. How to choose the color of your protein may be as pragmatic as to what filters you have in the microscope, e.g., FITC filters work adequately with GFP. Filters are now available from a variety of sources, which can visualize each of the colors just mentioned.

Other considerations are: how many different proteins make up your channel and do you want to monitor them all? In this case it may be desirable to choose two or even more colors. Choose the spectra which give the best separation *(14,15)*.

Another more recent point to consider is the availability of commercial and noncommercial markers of the biological pathway of ion channel synthesis, namely ER, Golgi and the plasma-membrane *(16)*. Each of these subcellular compartments has been labeled with autofluorescent proteins. Thus, one can monitor the progress of the fusion protein as it traverses the biosynthetic pathway by co-transfecting these subcellular markers and the ion-channel construct. These markers also make it possible to detect where mutant channels fail in their progression through the biosynthetic pathway.

In addition to the marking of the biosynthetic pathway, this approach can be combined with classical cell biological approaches to monitor the pattern of expression, i.e., use of the drugs monensin and brefeldin to examine the effects of inhibiting the ER and Golgi transport, respectively. With the advent of GFP, it is now possible to examine the different components of the ER and Golgi networks, e.g., the trans golgi network *(17)*.

2.2. Choosing the Expression System to Study the Location of the Ion Channel

Having chosen the color, where do you want your protein to be? With ion channels, this is almost exclusively a mammalian expression or *Xenopus* expression system, although the pattern of expression of ion channels can be monitored in almost any model system. Each expression system has its own peculiarities. For example, in *Caenhorhabititis elegans*, it has been shown that GFP expression is enhanced by the insertion of multiple introns into the coding region of GFP *(18)*. The same laboratory has also demonstrated that it is not possible to use the expression pattern of GFP fusion proteins as the sole means to determine the physiological expression pattern of an endogenous gene in *C. elegans*, a note of caution that maybe applicable to other "model" systems.

2.2.1. Xenopus *Oocyte*

This expression system has been used extensively to biophysically characterize ion channels.

Ion-channel expression in *Xenopus* oocytes can be improved by a variety of techniques. Firstly, vectors with either T3 or T7 as the RNA polymerase promoter have higher yields of cRNA than those with the SP6 promoter. Engineer the construct to have either the 5' and 3' *Xenopus* globin sequences, or place the start codon as close as possible to the promoter and try to ensure a "Kozak" initiation sequence with "A" at −3 and "G" at +4 relative to the ATG initiating methionine *(19)*.

The insertion of a "Kozak" sequence is probably a ubiquitous advantage to all GFP fusion constructs and is worth employing in most model systems.

Oocytes expressing GFP can be observed with low power optics.

2.2.2. Mammalian Expression

Mammalian cells have two distinct advantages over *Xenopus* oocytes: they have a low profile and are transparent enabling biosynthetic pathways of ion-channel chimeras to be followed visually. Mammalian expression can be either transient or stable. The former appears to give higher levels of expression, which maybe further enhanced by incubating the cells in 2 m*M* sodium butyrate for approx 24 h. In our hands, we routinely use one of three techniques to transfect the DNA into the cells: Calcium phosphate precipitation, Lipofectamine (Life Technologies) or Geneporter (Gene Therapy Systems). For electrophysiological studies the efficiency of transfection is not of practical concern as there always more than enough cells to study.

Some serums have autofluorescence, which can be eliminated by rinsing and imaging for short periods of time in balanced serum-free salt solutions.

Tissue-culture cells are grown either on the plastic tissue-culture dishes, cover slips, or tissue-culture dishes that have glass coverslips incorporated into their bases. The choice depends on the type of microscope used to visualize the cells. We have had success with all three approaches using HEK293 and COS7 cells. In the case of the glass coverslips or the glass-bottomed dishes we usually treat the glass with either polylysine or "Cell-tak" (Collaborative Biomedical Products) to increase cellular adhesion. The HEK293 cells become more rounded in our hands when cultivated on untreated glass.

The choice of substratum can also be important. In Madin-Darby canine kidney type I cells expressing a cystic fibrosis transmembrane conductance regulator (CFTR) fused with GFP at the N-terminus, it was shown that the expression pattern was substratum dependent (*see* also Stanton et al. in this book). Cells grown on glass coverslips showed basolateral expression, whereas those grown on permeable supports demonstrated apical expression. In either case the fusion protein demonstrated a normal phenotype as judged by whole cell patch-clamping and planar lipid bilayer experiments *(20)*.

2.3. Vectors for GFP Fusion Proteins

All of our constructs are under the control of the constitutively active early viral promoter from cytomegalovirus (CMV). We are unaware of inducible promoters being used for ion-channel GFP constructs, but in principle they might prove useful for generating pulses of fluorescent protein, i.e., monitoring the biosynthetic pathway of ion channels. In addition to the CMV promoter, several GFP constructs have been used with the HIV LTR promoter (Quantum Biotechnologies). The strength of the promoter can play an important role in how the GFP fusion construct is expressed inside the cell, but we are unaware of any comparative studies examining the pattern of expression of ion-channel GFP chimeras with different promoters.

2.4. Adenoviral Constructs

The major advantages of adenoviral constructs is they can be used to transform a wide variety of cell types independent of cell division and they

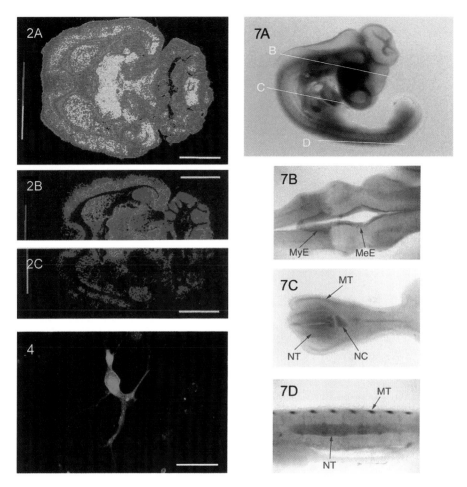

Plate 1, Figures 2, 4, 7. (*See* discussion and full captions on p. 62 in Chapter 4).

Figure 2: Pseudocolor images of autoradiograph of [^{3}H]α,β-methyleneATP binding sites in rat brain.

Figure 4: Immunostaining of recombinant P2X$_4$ receptors in 1321N1 cells with a mouse monoclonal antibody.

Figure 7: Whole mount *in situ* hybridization of chick embryos (Day 4) with digoxigenin-labeled cP2X$_8$ RNA probe.

A Control

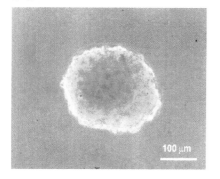

B Kir6.2-GFP Tg. (line C)

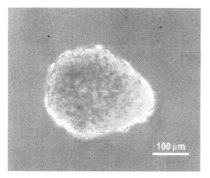

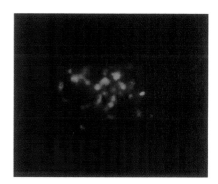

C Kir6.2-GFP Tg. (line F)

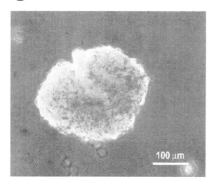

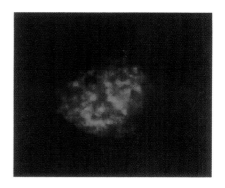

Plate 2, Figure 2 (*See* full caption on p. 255, and discussion in Chapter 13).
Fluorescence of GFP-tagged K_{ATP} channels in isolated islets from transgenic mice.

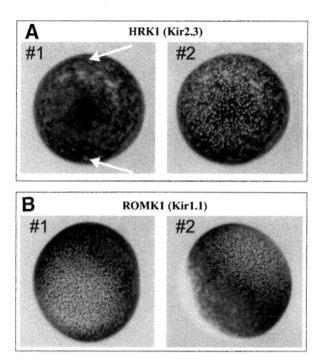

Plate 3, Figure 3 (*See* full caption on p. 318 and discussion in Chapter 17).
Crystal growth is determined by the flow of T1+ ions through K+ channels.

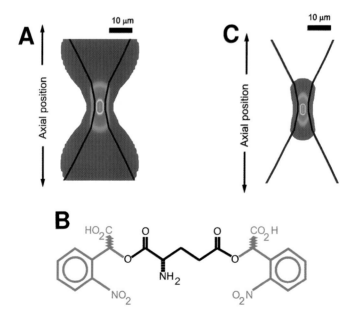

Plate 4, Figure 2 (*See* full caption on p. 353 and discussion in Chapter 19).
Theoretical improvement in axial resolution with double-caged glutamate.

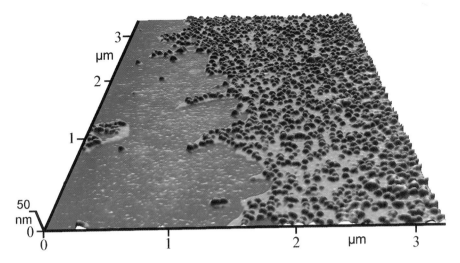

Plate 5, Figure 4 (*See* full caption on p. 418 and discussion in Chapter 22). Plasma membrane of *Xenopus laevis* oocyte spread on glass and studied by AFM in air.

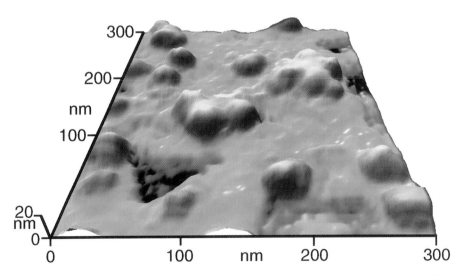

Plate 6, Figure 8 (*See* full caption on p. 422 and discussion in Chapter 22). Plasma membrane patch of *Xenopus laevis* oocyte imaged by AFM in air (size: 0.09 µm²).

express high levels of the ion-channel chimeras. The major disadvantage of using adenoviral constructs is one of time, as homologous recombination is usually carried out within mammalian cells capable of complementing the defective adenoviruses (i.e., using packaging cell lines). However, recently Vogelstein's group *(21)* have constructed a system for generating recombinant adenoviruses that relies on homologous recombination in bacteria. This obviates the need for plaque purification and thereby shortens the time required for generating adenoviral ion-channel GFP fusion constructs.

2.5. Other Means of Getting Fusion Proteins Into Cells

Plasmid DNA is probably the most common way of introducing GFP constructs into cells, but Teurel and Meyer *(22)* have shown that RNA synthesized in vitro, can be electroporated into adherent cells. This particular technique has the advantage that the expressed protein is usually observed much quicker than with plasmid DNA transfections.

Another way for getting ion-channel GFP constructs into postmitotic cells is to use the biolistic technique. Gold particles are coated with ion channel fusion plasmids and fired into cells using a helium pulse of gas (biolistic particle delivery system [Bio-Rad]). Arnold and Clapham *(23)* used this approach to express Kv1.4 in rat brain slices. The technique was also novel because they linked the GFP to PSD-95 rather than Kv 1.4. They showed that in co-transfection experiments, Kv1.4 was expressed in axons with GFP-PSD-95 while in the absence of Kv 1.4 the GFP-PSD-95 was only present in dendrites.

2.5. Where to Put GFP in the Channel

GFP has been placed at a variety of locations within ion channels. Two reports show that GFP attached to extracellular regions of the protein fluoresce. GFP fusion to the C-terminus of the GABAA receptor, a chloride channel belonging to the ligand-gated ion channel superfamily of which nACh receptor is prototypic, showed that the C-tail was located not only extracellularly, but it was restricted to the animal pole when expressed in *Xenopus* oocytes *(24)*. The external location of the GFP marker was shown by antibodies to GFP in nonpermeabilized oocytes. Similarly, antibodies applied to nonpermeabilized HEK293 cells expressing an N-terminal GFP fusion to the alpha subunit of the human slow poke K^+ channel demonstrated an extracellular location of GFP *(25)*. This fusion was notable because the phenotype of the channel changed: the voltage dependence of gating and the left-shift of gating induced by intracellular binding of calcium were both reduced.

This example demonstrates an important point about GFP chimeras: not all fusion proteins are inocuous as to their effects on channel phenotype. In addition, GFP can sometimes affect the targeting of the channel. For example, GFP was linked to the aquaporin 2 vasopressin regulated water channel at both the N terminus and the C- terminus and both chimeras appeared to be functional. The N-terminal GFP fusion showed normal cycling from intracellular vesicles to the basolateral plasma membrane in response to vaspopressin. However, the C terminal GFP fusion was localized constitutively at both the apical and basolateral plasma membranes and was refractory to vasopressin application *(26)*.

Most of ion-channel fusion proteins are designed to place GFP on the cytoplasmic side of the membrane. In this location it has been used as a marker of conformational change *(27)*. Siegel and Isacoff fused a truncated functional *(28)* into an internal region of *Shaker,* just proximal to the sixth transmembrane domain with the C- tail extending beyond GFP. Upon depolarization, there was a change in the emitted fluorescence of GFP. Not only was this use for GFP as a marker for dynamic conformational changes novel, but it is the only reported ion-channel chimera in which the GFP fusion was internal, i.e., with ion channel sequences on both sides of GFP. Biondi et al. *(29)* have placed a paired concantemer of GFP used for FRET analysis within a variety of locations of the cAMP regulatory subunit. They showed that some "internal chimeras" were both fluorescent and retained cAMP regulatory activity. Thus, in principal it maybe possible to make "internal chimeras" within ion channels. However, given the paucity of data, this will have to be determined empirically with special consideration given to the size of loops and known functional domains such as phosphorylation, etc.

To decide whether to place the GFP at the N or C terminus of the ion channel depends on how much is known about the channel. For example Grabner et al. *(30)* linked GFP to the N-terminus of the alpha 1 subunit of the skeletal Ca channel to avoid the potential loss of GFP because of the known, physiological truncation of the C terminus of various Ca channel alpha 1 subunits.

We have found that linking GFP to the Kir 6.2 subunit at the C-terminus gave functional channels when expressed in HEK293 cells *(31)* (Fig. 1F). However, linking the same Kir 6.2 subunit to GFP via the N-terminus gave nonfunctional channels with a dramatically different morphological pattern (*see* Fig. 1E). When co-transfected with the sulphonylurea receptor (SUR) plasmalemmal expression of the C-terminal fusion construct was markedly enhanced, and was associated with an increased number of channels recorded in the excised patch configuration. In contrast, SUR did not affect expression pattern of the N-terminal fusion construct.

There may also be a question as to the type of cells expressing the various constructs. For example, Makhina et al. *(32)* using a GFP chimera to SUR C-terminus showed plasma membrane labeling in COSm6 cells following treatment with a brief exposure to trypsin. The same construct when expressed in our laboratory in HEK293 cells failed to give any plasma membrane labeling.

2.6. How to Put It Where You Want It

There is a multitude of ways of making GFP-fusion proteins. To illustrate we will describe two techniques we have relied upon: subcloning with available restriction enzyme sites and polymerase chain reaction (PCR).

2.6.1. Subcloning

For example, to insert GFP at the C-terminus of Kir2.1 we adopted the following two approaches using restriction enzyme cloning. Sequence analysis showed that within the last 22 amino acids of Kir2.1 there were four unique restriction enzyme sites: *Bgl*II, *Afl*II, *Bgl*I, and *Mse*I. Previous studies within the laboratory had shown that it was possible to delete up to 75 amino acids from the C-tail of Kir2.1 without changing the electrophysiological phenotype of the channel. Therefore a small deletion of the C-tail before linkage to GFP appeared to be a rational approach in generating the fusion protein.

Sequence analysis of pEGFP N–1, purchased from Clontech, showed that it was possible to ligate the *Bgl*II site of Kir2.1 to the *Bam*HI or *Bgl*II site of pEGFP within the multiple cloning site and still retain the same open reading frame for GFP as Kir2.1. A compatible restriction site between the vector carrying Kir2.1 and the multiple cloning site of pEGFP upstream of the *Bam*H1 or *Bgl*II sites was *Hin*dIII. Therefore a *Hin*dIII and *Bgl*II digest of Kir2.1 was made and ligated into: (1) an *Hin*dIII/*Bam*HI digest of pEGFP or, (2) an *Hin*dIII/*Bgl*II digest of pEGFP.

The constructs were transfected into HEK293 cells with the calcium-phosphate method and examined on either an upright or inverted microscope with a FITC filter cube. The *Bgl*II-*Bgl*II ligated product gave cells that were diffusely green but produced no current, as judged by excised patch analysis (Fig. 1C). However the *Bgl*II- *Bam*HI construct gave plasmalemmal labeling (Fig. 1D) and strong inwardly rectifying currents in excised patches. We have not compared these constructs in Xenopus oocytes to see whether there is a difference in the expression capabilities of oocytes and HEK293 cells, but the *Bgl*II-*Bam*HI fusion protein did give strong inward rectifying

GFP

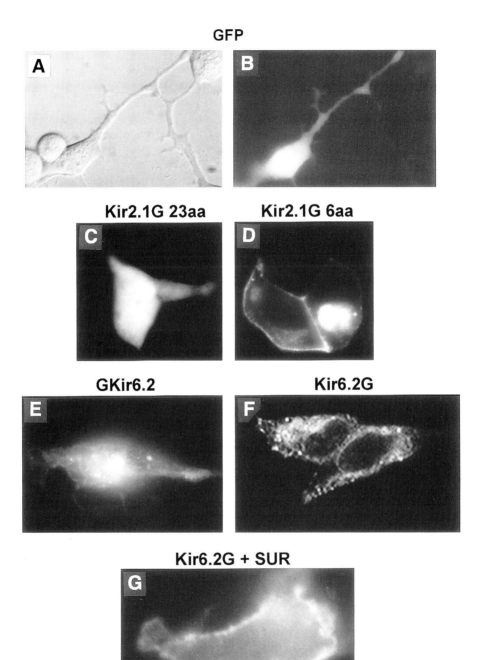

Kir2.1G 23aa   **Kir2.1G 6aa**

GKir6.2   **Kir6.2G**

Kir6.2G + SUR

currents in oocytes. The only difference between the two constructs was the linker region:

*Bgl*II-*Bgl*II   Kir2.1 coding   DLELKLRILQSTVPRAR DPPVAT GFP coding
*Bgl*II- *Bam*HI   Kir2.1 coding   DPPVAT GFP coding

Sequence analysis also shows that there is a third way to make a fusion protein between Kir2.1 and pEGFP N-1 using restriction sites. We did not make this particular fusion but we describe it as a potential alternative procedure. As mentioned earlier, there are four unique restriction sites present in the last 22 amino acids of Kir2.1. It is possible to cut Kir2.1 with *Afl*II and then "polish" the ends with Mung Bean Nuclease. Similarly pEGFP is cut with *Sal*I and polished with Mung Bean Nuclease. After removal of Mung Bean Nuclease (phenol/chloroform) both DNAs are digested with *Hind*III and the Kir2.1 fragment is ligated into pEGFP.

2.6.2. PCR

The polymerase chain reaction (PCR) has revolutionized molecular biology. It enables nonmolecular biology laboratories to create biological constructs at minimal expense.

Using PCR, one can insert GFP into the coding region of any protein at any location. As mentioned earlier, most chimeras have been made either to

---

Fig. 1. Cellular location of Kir GFP fusion constructs in HEK293 cells. HEK293 cells were transiently transfected with various GFP constructs. (**A**) and (**B**) phase and fluorescent images, respectively, of cells transfected with GFP alone. The GFP diffuses throughout the cytoplasm of the cell (B). (**C**) Cells transfected with Kir2.1G 23 aa, which has 23 amino acids between the Kir2.1 coding region and the GFP start codon. The pattern of distribution looks similar to that in (B). No currents were detectable in these cells when examined in the excised patch configuration. (**D**) Transfection with Kir2.1G 6 aa, which has six amino acids between the Kir2.1 coding region and the GFP start codon. This construct gave plasmalemmal labeling and strong inwardly rectifying currents as judged by excised patch analysis. (**E**) Cells transfected with GKir6.2 where the GFP moiety is at the N-terminus of the KATP subunit. Intramembranous structures are labeled and are presumably parts of the ER and Golgi complexes. No currents could be detected with this construct. In contrast, (**F**) shows cells transfected with Kir6.2G, where the GFP is fused to the C-terminus of the channel subunit. There is both punctate and intramembranous labeling. These cells gave ATP sensitive current when examined in the excised patch configuration. (**G**) Using the same construct as in (F) the cells were co-transfected with SUR. The morphological pattern changed to a more intense plasmalemmal distribution and increased the number of channels recorded in the excised patch configuration. *See* John et al. *(31)* for details.

the C- or N- terminus of ion channels. To use PCR, the sequence of the channel must be known, therefore, only cloned channels can be made "green." To illustrate the PCR technique we have adopted within the laboratory, we describe how we linked GFP to the KATP channel. KATP channels are comprised of two subunits: the inward rectifier Kir6.x, and the ABC family binding protein, SUR.

There are two ways to link the proteins to GFP: Either make an oligonucleotide promoter that has GFP, linker, and ion-channel sequences within it *(33)*, or engineer unique restriction enzyme sites into either GFP, the ion channel, or both using oligonucleotide primers.

Primers are designed that have as many as three parts:

1. The hybridizing region which is composed of the ion-channel sequence N or C terminus. To calculate the length of the ion-channel hybridization region we try and make this region have a Tm of 50–54° based on the formula (Tm = 2(A + T)+ 4(G + C)). This usually works out as 17–19 nucleotides.
2. The linker region, coding for amino acids between the ion channel and the autofluorescent protein. The linker region is experimentor dependent. Some people have used three to six glycines *(23,32,34)* for linking proteins together, whereas others have used glutamates for making tandem ion-channel constructs *(35)*. There appears to be no systematic studies on the linker region. Our experience with the Kir2.1 GFP fusion and the above studies suggest that the shorter linkers are preferred, but this needs to be determined empirically for each individual fusion construct.
3. Either the GFP hybridization region or the restriction enzyme region. Similar to the ion channel hybridization region, we design the GFP hybridization region to have a Tm of around 50–54. If one decides to insert a restriction site instead of a GFP hybridization region, then at that site put at least four extra nucleotides at the end, e.g., ACGT. This ensures that when directly subcloning the PCR fragment into GFP or the ion channel, the restriction enzymes will have a good chance to fully digest the DNA. New England Biolabs have a table in the Appendix section of their catalog that describes the efficiency of digestion of various restriction enzymes at the end of DNA oligonucleotides. If possible, use a site that digests fully in under 2 h.

In our laboratory we routinely directly subclone the PCR products into a cassette vector, which has two advantages *(36)*. The first is that the PCR-generated sequence can easily be sequenced for misincorporated nucleotides during the PCR reaction, which we limit by using high-fidelity PCR polymerases. The second is that we now have an unlimited supply of product for the final subcloning step of placing the GFP or ion channel into the chimeric construct. The ion-channel cassette is also useful for making mutations to examine the function of the ion channel.

2.7. When You Have It How Do You See It

A major advantage of GFP is that it can be visualized without fixing the cells. Depending on how the cells have been plated, visualization can be achieved with standard epifluorescent upright or inverted microscopes *(12)*. Confocal microscopes can also be used. An Argon laser emitting at 488 nm is particularly good for exciting GFP *(12)*.

3. CONCLUSIONS

The GFP ion channel field is rapidly expanding, and this short chapter can only give a glimpse at some of the "tips and tricks" possible with GFP. For those interested in more detailed accounts of GFP, several highly recommended sources for additional details include: a recent review by Rodger Tsien in the Annual review Biochemistry 1998 *(5)*, the book *Methods in Cell Biology: Green Fluorescent Proteins* by Kevin Sullivan and Steve Kay (eds.) *(12)*, and the internet website www.pantheon.cis.yale.edu/~wfm5/gfp_gateway.html. Another useful source for help and hints with regard to GFP and its applications is the newsgroup: bionet.molbio.proteins.fluorescent.

Given the rapid progress in the GFP field, GFP fusion proteins will increasingly be able to address the dynamics of ion channels both at the single molecule level (as already discussed with Siegal and Iscacoff's *[27]* data on the *Shaker*-GFP chimera) and the macro-structural level as illustrated by Jordan et al. *(37)*, who followed a connexin43-GFP fusion and the dynamics of formation and movement of whole gap-junction plaques (www.molbiolcell.org for movies).

In summary, the future's so bright, you gotta wear shades (corrupted from Timbuk3).

ACKNOWLEDGMENTS

We would like to thank our colleagues Drs. Jonathon Monck and Bernard Ribalet for allowing us to incorporate some previously unpublished images. We also would like to thank Dr. Yujuan Lu for technical help in making the ion-channel fusion proteins and Dr. Michela Ottolia for constructive criticism of the manuscript. This work was supported by NIH grants P50HL52319, R37HL60025, RO1HL36729, the Laubish and Kawata endowments, and AHA Western Affiliate 9960053Y.

REFERENCES

1. Prasher, D. C., Eckenrode, V. K., Ward, W. W., Prendergast, F. G., and Cormier, M. J. (1992) Primary structure of the Aequorea victoria green-fluorescent protein. *Gene* **111,** 229–233.
2. Ormo, M., Cubitt, A. B., Kallio, K., Gross, L. A., and Tsien, R. Y. (1996) Crystal structure of the *Aequorea Victoria* green fluorescent protein. *Science* **273,** 1392–1395.
3. Yang, F., Moss, L. G., and Phillips, G. N. J. (1996) The molecular structure of green fluorescent protein. *Nat. Biotechno.* **14,** 1246–1251.
4. Patterson, G. H., Knobel, S. M., Sharif, W. D., Kain, S. R., and Piston, D. W. (1997) Use of the green fluorescent protein and its mutants in quantitative fluorescence microscopy. *Biophys. J* **73,** 2782–2790.
5. Tsien, R. Y. (1998) The green fluorescent protein. *Ann. Rev. Biochem.* **67,** 509–544.
6. Matz, M. V., Frakov, A. F., Labas, Y. A., Savitsky, A. P., Zaraisky, A. G., Markelov, M. L., et al. (1999) Fluorescent proteins from non-bioluminescent anthoza species. *Nat. Biotechnol.* **17,** 969–973.
7. Oancea, E., Teruel, M. N., Quest, A. F., and Meyer, T. (1998) Green fluorescent protein (GFP)-tagged cysteine-rich domains from protein kinase C as fluorescent indicators for diacylglycerol signaling in living cells. *J. Cell Biol.* **140,** 485–498.
8. Neuhuber, B., Gerster, U., Doring, F., Glossmann, H., Tanabe, T., and Flucher, B. E. (1998) Association of calcium channel alpha1S and beta1a subunits is required for the targeting of beta1a but not alpha1S into skeletal muscle triads. *Proc. Natl. Acad. Sci. USA* **95,** 5015–5020.
9. Miesenbock, G., De Angelis, D. A., and Rothman, J. E. (1998) Visualizing secretion and synaptic transmission with pH-sensitive green flourescent proteins. *Nature* **394,** 192–195.
10. Brock, R., Hamelers, I. H., and Jovin, T. M. (1999) Comparison of fixation protocols for adherent cultured cells applied to a GFP fusion protein of the epidermal growth factor receptor. *Cytometry* **35,** 353–362.
11. Satiat-Jeunemaitre, B., Boevink, P., and Hawes, C. (1999) Membrane trafficking in higher plant cells: GFP and antibodies, partners for probing the secretory pathway. *Biochimie* **81,** 597–605.
12. Sullivan, K. F. and Kay, S. A. (1999) Green fluorescent proteins, in *Methods in Cell Biology,* vol. 58. (Sullivan, K. F. and Kay, S. A., eds.), Academic, San Diego, CA, pp. xvii, 386.
13. Heim, R., Prasher, D. C., and Tsien, R. Y. (1994) Wavelength mutations and posttranslational autoxidation of green fluorescent protein. *Proc. Natl. Acad. Sci. USA* **91,** 12,501–12,504.
14. Ellenberg, J., Lippincott-Schwartz, J., and Presley, J. F. (1998) Two-color green fluorescent protein time-lapse imaging. *Biotechniques* **25,** 838–842, 844–846.
15. Ellenberg, J., Lippincott-Schwartz, J., and Presley, J. F. (1999) Dual-colour imaging with GFP variants. *Trends Cell Biol.* **9,** 52–56.

16. De Giorgi, F., Ahmed, Z., Bastianutto, C., Brini, M., Jouaville, L. S., Marsault, R., et al. (1999) Targeting GFP to organelles. *Methods Cell Biol.* **58,** 75–85.

17. Girotti, M. and Banting, G. (1996) TGN38-green fluorescent protein hybrid proteins expressed in stably transfected eukaryotic cells provide a tool for the real-time, in vivo study of membrane traffic pathways and suggest a possible role for rattGN38. *J. Cell Sci.* **109,** 2915–2926.

18. Miller, D. M., III, Desai, N. S., Hardin, D. C., Piston, D. W., Patterson, G. H., Fleenor, J., Xu, S., and Fire, A. (1999) Two-color GFP expression system for C. elegans. *Biotechniques* **26,** 914–921.

19. Kozak, M. (1989) The scanning model for translation: an update. *J. Cell Biol.* **108,** 229–241.

20. Moyer, B. D., Loffing, J., Schwiebert, E. M., Loffing-Cueni, D., Halpin, P. A., Karlson, K. H., et al. (1998) Membrane trafficking of the cystic fibrosis gene product, cystic fibrosis transmembrane conductance regulator, tagged with green fluorescent protein in madin-darby canine kidney cells. *J. Biol. Chem.* **273,** 21,759–21,768.

21. He, T.-C., Zhou, S., Da Costa, L. T., Yu, J., Kinzler, K. W., and Vogelstein, B. (1998) A simplified system for genearating recombinat adenoviruses. *Proc. Natl. Acad. Sci. USA* **95,** 2509–2514.

22. Teruel, M. N. and Meyer, T. (1997) Electroporation-induced formation of individual calcium entry sites in the cell body and processes of adherent cells. *Biophys. J.* **73,** 1785–1796.

23. Arnold, D. B. and Clapham, D. E. (1999) Molecular determinants for subcellular localization of PSD-95 with an interacting K^+ channel. *Neuron* **23,** 149–157.

24. Bueno, O. F., Robinson, L. C., Alvarez-Hernandez, X., and Leidenheimer, N. J. (1998) Functional characterization and visualization of a $GABA_A$ receptor-GFP chimera expressed in *Xenopus* oocytes. *Mol. Brain Res.* **59,** 165–177.

25. Meyer, E. and Fromherz, P. (1999) Ca2+ activation of hSlo K^+ channel is suppressed by N-terminal GFP tag. *Eur. J. Neurosci.* **11,** 1105–1108.

26. Gustafson, C. E., Levine, S., Katsura, T., McLaughlin, M., Alexio, M. D., Tamarappoo, B. K., et al. (1998) Vasopressin regulated trafficking of a green flourescent protein-aquaporin 2 chimera in LLC-PK1 cells. *Histochem. Cell Biol.* **110,** 377–386.

27. Siegel, M. S. and Isacoff, E. Y. (1997) A genetically encoded optical probe of membrane voltage. *Neuron* **19,** 735–741.

28. Dopf, J. and Horiagon, T. M. (1996) Deletion mapping of the *Aequorea victoria* green fluorescent protein. *Gene* **173,** 39–44.

29. Biondi, R. M., Baehler, P. J., Reymond, C. D., and Véron, M. (1998). Random insertion of GFP into the cAMP-dependent protein kinase regulatory subunit from Dictyostelium discoideum. *Nucleic Acids Res.* **26,** 4946–4952.

30. Grabner, M., Dirksen, R. T., and Beam, K. G. (1998) Tagging with the green flourecent protein reveals a distinct subcellular distribution of L-type and non L-type Ca^{2+} channels expressed in dysgenic myotubes. *Proc. Natl. Acad. Sci. USA* **95,** 1903–1908.

31. John, S. A., Monck, J. R., Weiss, J. N., and Ribalet, B. (1998) The sulphonylurea receptor SUR1 regulates ATP-sensitive mouse Kir6. 2 K^+ chan-

nels linked to the green fluorescent protein in human embryonic kidney cells (HEK 293). *J. Physiol.* **510,** 333–345.

32. Makhina, E. N., and Nichols, C. G. (1998) Independent trafficking of KATP channel subunits to the plasma membrane. *J. Biol. Chem.* **273,** 3369–3374.

33. Horton, R. M., Hunt, H. D., Ho, S. N., Pullen, J. K., and Pease, L. R. (1989) Engineering hybrid genes without the use of restriction enzymes: gene splicing by overlap extension. *Gene* **77,** 61–68.

34. Zerangue, N., Schwappach, B., Jan, Y. N., and Jan, L. Y. (1999) A new ER trafficking signal regulates the subunit stoichiometry of plasma membrane K(ATP) channels. *Neuron* **22,** 537–548.

35. Lu, T., Nguyen, B., Zhang, X., and Yang, J. (1999) Architecture of a K^+ channel inner pore revealed by stoichiometric covalent modification. *Neuron* **22,** 571–580.

36. Costa, G. L. and Weiner, M. P. (1994) Protocols for cloning and analysis of blunt ended PCR-generated DNA fragments. *PCR Methods Appl.* **3,** S95—S106.

37. Jordan, K., Solan, J. L., Dominguez, M., Sia, M., Hand, A., Lampe, P. D., and Laird, D. W. (1999) Trafficking, assembly, and function of a connexin43-green fluorescent protein chimera in live mammalian cells. *Mol. Biol. Cell* **10,** 2033–2050.

13

Tagging Ion Channels with the Green Fluorescent Protein (GFP) as a Method for Studying Ion Channel Function in Transgenic Mouse Models

Joseph C. Koster and Colin G. Nichols

1. INTRODUCTION

In the past ten years, a multitude of cDNAs encoding ion channels have been cloned and have led to a greater understanding of the biological aspects of ion-channel function. Relevant information on structure, function, and pharmacology has come primarily from expressing reconstituted wild-type or mutant ion channels in heterologous expression systems and assaying channel activity using standard biochemical and electrophysiological techniques. In particular, *Xenopus* oocytes have proven to be a useful expression system owing to the high level of expression of functional ion channels at the cell surface and the large size of the oocyte, which makes it particularly amenable to ion channel analysis using various electrophysiological techniques. However, interpretation of the functional data can be complicated by the presence of several endogenous oocyte currents that can be induced upon exogenous channel expression *(1,2)*. Expressing cloned ion channels in cultured mammalian cells using the transfection technique can often overcome the problem of superimposed endogenous currents while providing an appropriate model of the mammalian cell. This is especially important when addressing questions of channel protein-processing, pharmacology, and roles of ion channels in signal transduction. Ultimately, however, questions of ion-channel physiology and a potential role of altered channel activity in

From: *Ion Channel Localization Methods and Protocols*
Edited by: A. Lopatin and C. G. Nichols © Humana Press Inc., Totowa, NJ

the disease state requires expression in the whole animal model. Numerous ion channels have now been expressed in a tissue-specific fashion in genetically defined strains of mice using the transgenic expression system *(3–8)*. With a rise in the number of core facilities at most research institutions to generate and house transgenic mouse colonies, as well the increased affordability, the transgenic mouse model has become an increasingly important and informative tool for many researchers. In brief, a linearized DNA construct containing the ion-channel cDNA under control of a tissue-specific promoter, the "transgene," is microinjected into the pronuclei of mouse zygotes. Generally, the transgene integrates into the mouse chromosomal DNA at the one cell-stage, so it is present in every cell of the animal and is capable of being transmitted through the germ line of the adult mouse. Although integration of the transgene usually occurs at a single site in the genome, the site itself is usually random and may contain several copies of the transgene. Theoretically, each founder mouse may express the transgene differently based on the number of transgene copies present and the site of the integration event (however, copy number in itself is not an adequate predictor of the level of transgene expression *[9]*). Moreover, analysis of the transgene can be further complicated owing to intrafamily variation of expression *(10)* within a founder line as well as variegated expression within the target tissue itself *(11)* (i.e., not every cell within the target tissue expresses the transgene or expression levels vary from cell to cell despite the fact that every cell contains the transgene, *see* Figs. 2 and 3). For these reasons, determining the level of transgene expression is critical when comparing phenotypes of different transgenic mouse lines and analyzing the physiology of individual cells within the target tissue. In this regard, we now describe a detection method for transgenic mice that uses variant of the green fluorescent protein (GFP) to tag a transgenically expressed ion channel. As demonstrated below, addition of the GFP-tag has no deleterious effect on channel activity and allows for easy and efficient detection of the GFP-tagged ion channels in individual cells of the transgenic animal using UV illumination. Moreover, as fluorescence intensity is related to the level of transgene expression, this method allows for a quick and qualitative assessment of transgene expression on a cell to cell basis.

2. METHODOLOGICAL CONSIDERATIONS

2.1. Green Fluorescent Protein

The green fluorescent protein, or GFP, is a fluorochrome containing cytosolic protein approx 27 kDa in size that was originally cloned from the jellyfish *Aequorea victoria (12,13)* The wild-type GFP is characterized by a maximal absorption peak at approx 395 nm, a minor peak at 475 nm, and a maximal emission peak at 504 nm *(14)*. Because of its high stability with regards to pH and temperature, its species independence, and autofluorescent properties that are independent of cofactors, the GFP has become an ideal marker for gene expression and as a tag to study protein localization patterns in the living cell in real time. In this chapter we have utilized a commercially available variant of GFP, EGFP (available from Clontech, Pal Alto, CA), which has a single, red-shifted excitation peak at 488 nm and fluoresces about 35 times more intensely than GFP when excited at 488 nm.

ATP-sensitive K^+-channels (K_{ATP}) couple cellular metabolism to electrical activity in multiple cell types, most notably in pancreatic β-cells and cardiac myocytes (for review, *see* ref. *15*). The K_{ATP} channel complex is comprised of two distinct subunits, the regulatory subunit, the sulfonylurea receptor, or SUR1, and the pore-forming subunit, Kir6.2, a member of the inward rectifying family of K^+-channels *(16–18)*. The hallmark of the K_{ATP} channel is its sensitivity to intracellular nucleotides: a rising [ATP]/[ADP] ratio inhibits the channel, whereas a falling [ATP]/[ADP] ratio activates channel activity (reviewed in ref. *15*). To follow the activity of K_{ATP} channels in living cells, EGFP was first directly fused to the C-terminus of the pore-forming subunit, Kir 6.2 (with no additional linker sequence added), and the fusion construct, Kir6.2wt-GFP, was subsequently co-expressed with the regulatory SUR1 subunit in transfected COSm6 cells. Characterization of GFP-tagged channel activity was performed using the inside-out patch-clamp technique. As shown in Fig. 1A, the C-terminally tagged construct generated channels that were inhibited by ATP with wild-type sensitivity ([ATP] causing half-maximal inhibition; (K_i) = 8.6 μM for Kir6.2-GFP + SUR1 compared to 11.1 μM for wild-type channels). Moreover, the single channel behavior with respect to open probability and cation conductance was unaltered in the Kir6.2 tagged channels *(25)*. Similarly, addition of the GFP tag to the N-terminus of Kir6.2 did not alter channel activity (data not shown), although functional expression of other ion channels may depend on positioning of the GFP and this should be considered when generating the transgene construct. Previously, we have demonstrated that an N-terminal truncation of the Kir6.2 subunit, termed Kir6.2[ΔN2–30], results in an approx 10-fold decrease in sensitivity of reconstituted K_{ATP} channels to inhibitory ATP *(19)*. As shown in Fig. 1A, addition of the GFP tag to the C-terminus of Kir6.2[ΔN2–30] did not further alter the ATP-sensitivity of reconstituted channels.

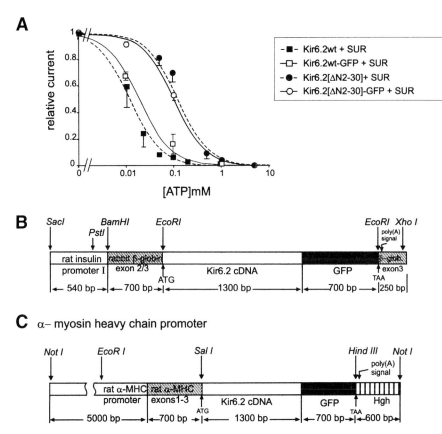

Fig. 1. ATP sensitivity of K_{ATP} currents from COSm6 cells co-expressing wild-type Kir6.2-GFP or Kir6.2[ΔN2-30]-GFP subunit and SUR1. (**A**) Steady-state dependence of membrane current on [ATP] (mean + SEM, relative to current in zero ATP [I_{rel}]) for wild-type and mutant channels. Data points represent the mean ± SEM (n = 3–8 patches). The fitted lines correspond to least squares fits of the Hill equation (relative current = $100/(1 + ([ATP]/K_{i})^{H})$, with H fixed at 1.3, and K_{i} = 12 μM (Kir6.2wt +SUR1, dashed), 9 μM (Kir6.2wt-GFP+SUR1), 123.8 μM (Kir6.2[ΔN2-30] + SUR1, dashed), and 107 μM (Kir6.2[ΔN2-30]-GFP + SUR1. (**B**) the insulin promoter transgene construct. The cDNA is cloned as an *Eco*RI/*Eco*RI fragment within 5'-non-coding exons of the rabbit β-globin gene. (**C**) the α-myosin heavy chain (α-MHC) promoter transgene construct. The cDNA is cloned as a *Sal*I/*Hind*III fragment downstream of 5'-noncoding exons of the rat α-MHC gene and upstream of the human growth hormone (Hgh) polyadenylation signal sequence.

To date, numerous studies have utilized GFP as a tag to follow ion channels expression in various heterologous expression systems *(20–25)*. In only one report, with the human slow poke (hSlo) K⁺-channel, was addition of the GFP tag shown to alter channel properties, specifically with respect to the voltage dependence of gating *(26)*. Thus, GFP represents a viable and simple method to tag exogenously expressed proteins without significantly perturbing channel function.

2.2. Selection of Transgenic Promoter

In transgenic mice, a transgene utilizing its own promoter will normally be expressed in all the tissues where the gene is normally expressed, while it can be targeted to widespread tissues by choice of a promiscuous promoter *(27)* (e.g., cytomegalovirus and ROSA26 promoters). More commonly, choice of an appropriate promoter can be used to drive tissue-specific expression of the transgene when the role of the channel in a specific tissue is addressed. In our studies, the rat α-myosin heavy chain *(28)* and rat insulin *(29)* promoters are used to specifically direct expression of the GFP-tagged mutant Kir6.2 transgene in mouse cardiac myocytes and pancreatic β-cells, respectively. Both promoters have been used extensively to successfully direct expression of numerous transgenes with high specificity *(4–8)*. As shown in Fig. 1B, for pancreatic-directed expression, the Kir6.2 cDNA was cloned downstream of the rat insulin promoter (540 b.p.) as an *Eco*RI/*Eco*RI restriction fragment. Flanking the cloning site are noncoding rabbit β-globin sequences, which are believed to stabilize the transcript and result in higher level of transgene expression. The entire transgene is released from the parent plasmid as a *Sac*I/*Xho*I fragment (~2200 b.p., excluding the cDNA insert) and used in microinjection of mouse zygotes.

In the cardiac transgenic construct (Fig. 1C), the α-myosin heavy chain promoter segment, in addition to containing proximal *cis*-acting regulatory regions necessary for high-level transgene expression, includes extensive upstream intergenomic sequence (5000 b.p.) that is important to drive cardiac-specific expression in a developmentally appropriate fashion. The cDNA is cloned in as either a *Sal*I/*Sal*I fragment or a *Sal*I/*Hin*dIII fragment downstream of noncoding exons I-III of the α-myosin heavy-chain gene in order to facilitate the splicing event in which the normal nascent RNA participates. Downstream of the the cloning site is human growth hormone (hGH) polyadenylation site. The transgene construct is excised as a *Not*I/*Not*I fragment (~7000 b.p., excluding the cDNA insert).

3. ANALYSIS OF TRANSGENE EXPRESSION

3.1. Expression of Transgene in the Pancreas

Although the following summary describes our specific transgenic expression of GFP-tagged K_{ATP}, similar results are likely to be obtained with directed expression of other GFP-tagged ion channels.

To express a mutant Kir6.2-GFP subunit with reduced ATP-sensitivity in mouse pancreatic β-cells, the insulin-promoter driven Kir6.2-GFP transgene (Fig. 1B) was microinjected in to zygotes derived from a C57B16 × CBA mouse strain, and six founder mice were generated (lines A–F). To demonstrate expression of the mutant Kir6.2-GFP transgene, pancreatic islets were isolated from two of these lines (lines E and F; for protocol on islet isolation, refer to ref. *30*) and level of fluorescence was determined under UV illumination (excitation 450–490 nm) using a mercury short arc lamp source attached to a standard patch-clamp rig. As can be seen in Fig. 2A, islets from control littermate mice showed no significant green fluorescence in the 515–555 nm emission range. By way of contrast, isolated islets from both the Kir6.2-GFP transgenic (Tg.) C and F lines, displayed significant levels of β-cell specific fluorescence of the GFP-tagged channel, although, qualitatively, the level in line F was significantly higher (Fig. 2B,C). The fluorescence level in positively expressing cells is qualitatively similar in both lines. As described earlier, variegated expression of the transgene in the target tissue is common and is likely to underlie the differential level of expression observed between the founder lines *(11)*.

To establish functional activity of the transgenic mutant Kir6.2-GFP transgene, isolated pancreatic β-cells were analyzed using the inside-out patch-clamp technique. Representative traces showing K_{ATP} channel activity in varying concentrations of inhibitory ATP is shown in Fig 3A. In transgenic mice, patches from green fluorescing β-cells invariably expressed K_{ATP} channels with reduced ATP sensitivity, consistent with high level of transgene expression. On average, nonfluorescing β-cell patches exhibited an ATP-sensitivity consistent with native pancreatic K_{ATP} channels; however, occasionally, nonfluorescing cells contained K_{ATP} channels with reduced sensitivity, which may reflect a low level of transgene expression below the limit of UV detection.

3.2. Expression of Transgene in the Heart

Similarly, variegated expression was also observed when the α-MHC promoter was used to drive expression of mutant K_{ATP} channels in heart. In three of the four founder lines analyzed (e.g., line II; Fig. 4A), differential fluorescence was observed in isolated cardiac myocytes. Similar to expression in pancreatic β-cells, inside-out patch clamp analysis revealed a high level of transgenic channels in green fluorescing β-cells (based on reduced ATP-sensitivity of the channels) and only native K_{ATP} channels in nonfluorescing myocytes (Fig. 4C). Interestingly, in one transgenic line (Line IV; Fig. 4B) complete expression of the transgene was observed, with

A Control

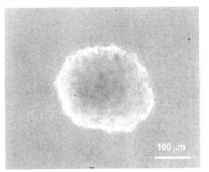 

B Kir6.2-GFP Tg. (line C)

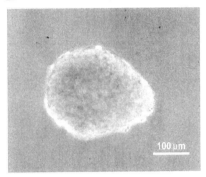 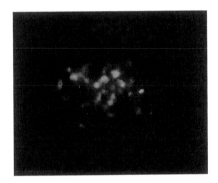

C Kir6.2-GFP Tg. (line F)

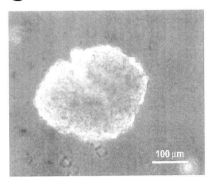 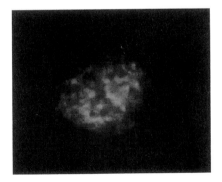

Fig. 2. Fluorescence of GFP-tagged K_{ATP} channels in isolated islets from transgenic mice. Clear field and fluorescent images (shown in grayscale) of isolated islets from a control mouse (**A**), the C-line mouse expressing the Kir6.2-GFP transgene (**B**), and the F-line mouse (**C**).

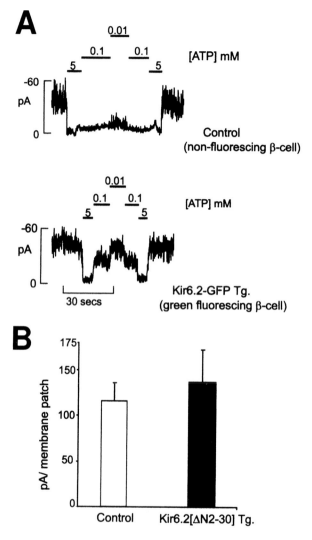

Fig. 3. ATP-sensitive K⁺-currents in pancreatic β-cells from both Kir6.2wt transgenic and control littermate mice. (**A**) Representative K⁺ current recorded from inside-out membrane patches from either GFP-fluorescing, pancreatic β-cells from Kir6.2[ΔN2-30] transgenic mice or nonfluorescing, pancreatic β-cells from a control littermate. K_{ATP} currents were measured at –50 mV in K_{int} solution and patches were exposed to differing [ATP] as shown. (**B**) Averaged maximal ATP-sensitive K⁺ currents from membrane patches. Micropipet size for each patch was assumed similar and corresponded to pipet resistance of ≈1 MΩ. Mean currents in the absence of ATP were as follows: Kir6.2-GFP Tg = 137 ± 35 (sem) pA ($n = 15$); control = 116 ± 20 pA ($n = 15$).

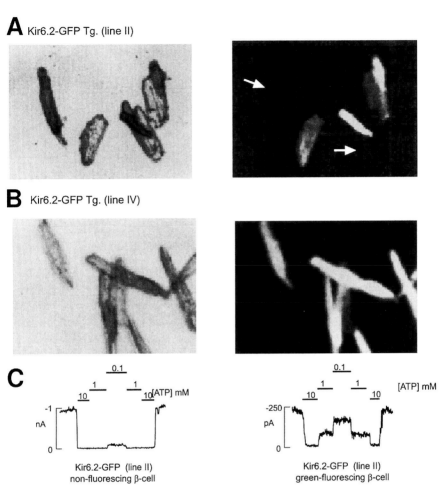

Fig. 4. Fluorescence of GFP-tagged K_{ATP} channels in isolated cardiac myocytes from transgenic mice. Clear field and fluorescent images (shown in grayscale) of isolated cardiac myocytes from a line II transgenic mouse (**A**), or a line IV transgenic mouse (**B**). Arrows in *A* indicate nonfluorescing cells with native K_{ATP} channels. (**C**) Representative K^+ current recorded from inside-out membrane patches from either GFP-fluorescing cardiac myocytes from line II transgenic mice or nonfluorescing cardiac myocytes from line II mice. K_{ATP} currents were measured at –50 mV in K_{int} solution and patches were exposed to differing [ATP] as shown.

all cells fluorescing and containing K_{ATP} channels with reduced ATP-sensitivity that approximates the ATP-sensitivity of the reconstituted mutant channels. This suggests complete replacement, or "knock-in," of the endogenous K_{ATP} with the transgene derived K_{ATP} subunit.

Finally, K_{ATP} channel density, as estimated by average ATP-sensitive current per patch, was not significantly altered (Fig. 3B) in pancreatic K_{ATP} channels. As numerous transgenic studies have demonstrated overexpression of the transgene protein, the lack of an increase in K_{ATP} channel density suggests the existence of a limiting factor that restricts overexpression of K_{ATP} channels in this tissue. We suggest that this may be the SUR1 subunit, which is also required for reconstitution of channel activity. Whether similar factors exist to tightly regulate expression of other ion channels transgenes is not known.

5. CONCLUSION

The GFP provides a quick and efficient method to identify target cells within a transgenic animal expressing the GFP-tagged ion channel. The major advantages of this method are: (1) coupling of GFP moiety to the ion channel is unlikely to alter channel activity with respect to single channel behavior and sensitivity to regulatory ligands; (2) expression of the transgene within the target tissue can be easily assessed under UV illumination; (3) differences in expression levels from cell to cell can be easily assessed when incomplete penetrance of the transgene occurs (i.e., variegated expression) because fluorescence intensity is directly related to the level of transgene expression; and (4) differences in expression levels of the transgene between founder lines, which is particularly important when comparing phenotypes among the founder lines, can be readily determined.

ACKNOWLEDGMENTS

The work described in this chapter was done in collaboration with Bess Marshall, Nancy Ensor, and John Corbett, primarily supported under the NIH grant DK55282 to Colin Nichols. We thank Rebecca Dunlap for technical assistance with these experiments. We are grateful to Carina Ämmälä for expert assistance in β-cell isolation and Anatoli Lopatin for assistance in cardiac myocyte isolation.

REFERENCES

1. Weber, W. M. (1999) Endogenous ion channels in oocytes of Xenopus laevis: recent developments. *J. Membrane Biol.* **170,** 1–12.
2. Attali, B., Guillemare, E., Lesage, F., Honoré, E., Romey, G., Lazdunski, M., and Barhanin, J. (1993) The protein IsK is a dual activator of K+ and Cl channels. *Nature* **365,** 850–852.

3. Sutherland, M. L., Williams, S. H., Abedi, R., Overbeek, P. A., Pfaffinger, P. J., and Noebels, J. L. (1999) Overexpression of a Shaker-type potassium channel in mammalian central nervous system dysregulates native potassium channel gene. *Proc. Natl. Acad. Sci. USA* **96**, 2451–2455.

4. Xu, H. and Nerbonne, J. M. (1999) Elimination of the transient outward current and action potential prolongation in mouse atrial myocytes expressing a dominant negative Kv4 alpha subunit. *J. Physiol.* **519**, 11–21.

5. Philipson, L. H., Rosenberg, M. P., Kuznetsov, A., Lancaster, M. E., Worley, J. F. III, Roe, M. W., and Dukes, I. D. (1994) Delayed rectifier K$^+$ channel overexpression in transgenic islets and β-cells associated with impaired glucose responsiveness. *J. Biol. Chem.* **269**, 27,787–27,790.

6. Miki, T., Tashiro, F., Iwanaga, T., Nagashima, K., Yoshitomi, H., Aihara, H., et al. (1997) Abnormalities of pancreatic islets by targeted expression of a dominant-negative K$_{ATP}$ channel. *Proc. Natl. Acad. Sci. USA* **91**, 11,969–11,973.

7. Babij, P., Askew, G. R., Nieuwenhuijsen, B., Su, C. M., Bridal, T. R., Jow, B., et al. (1998) Inhibition of cardiac delayed rectifier K$^+$-current by overexpression of the long-QT syndrome HERG G628S mutation in transgenic mice. *Circ. Res.* **83**, 668–678.

8. Muth J. N., Yamaguchi, H., Mikala, G., Grupp, I. L., Lewis, W., Cheng, H., et al. (1999) Cardiac-specific overexpression of the alpha(1) subunit of the L-type voltage-dependent Ca(2+) channel in transgenic mice. Loss of isoproterenol-induced contraction. *J. Biol. Chem.* **274**, 21,503–21,506.

9. Bieberich, C. J., Utset, M. F., Awgulewitsch, A., and Ruddle, F. H. (1990) Evidence for positive and negative regulation of the Hox–3. 1 gene. *Proc. Natl. Acad. Sci. USA* **87**, 8462–8466.

10. Overbeek, P. (1994) Factors affecting transgenic animal production, in *Transgenic Animal Technology: A Laboratory Handbook* (Pinkert, C. A., ed.), Academic, New York, pp. 96–107.

11. Dobie, K. W., Lee, M., Fantes, J. A., Graham, E., Clark, A. J., Springbett, A., et al. (1996) Variegated transgene expression in mouse mammary gland is determined by the transgenic integration locus. *Proc. Natl. Acad. Sci. USA* **93**, 6659–6664.

12. Prasher, D. C., Eckenrode, V. K., Ward, W. W., Prendergast, F. G., and Cormier, M. J. (1992) Primary structure of the Aequorea victoria green-fluorescent protein. *Gene* **111**, 229–233.

13. Chalfie, M., Tu, Y., Euskirchen, G., Ward, W. W., Prasher, D. C. (1994) Green fluorescent protein as a marker for gene expression. *Science* **263(5148)**, 802–805.

14. Patterson, G. H., Knobel, S. M., Sharif, W. D., Kain, S. R., and Piston, D. W. (1997) Use of the green fluorescent protein and its mutants in quantitative fluorescence microscopy. *Biophys. J.* **73**, 2782–2790.

15. Ashcroft, F. M. (1988) Adenosine 5'-triphosphate-sensitive potassium channels. *Annu. Rev. Neurosci.* **11**, 97–118.

16. Inagaki, N., Gonoi, T., Clement, J. P. IV, Namba, N., Inazawa, J., Gonzales, G., et al. (1995) Reconstitution of IK$_{ATP}$: an inward rectifier subunit plus the sulfonylurea receptor. *Science* **270**, 1166–1170.

17. Inagaki, N., Gonoi, T., and Seino, S. (1997) Subunit stoichiometry of the pancreatic b-cell ATP-sensitive K⁺ channel. *FEBS Lett.* **409**, 232–236.

18. Clement, J. P. IV, Kunjilwar, K., Gonzalez, G., Schwanstecher, M., Panten, U., Aguilar Bryan, L., and Bryan, J. (1997) Association and stoichiometry of K_{ATP} channel subunits. *Neuron* **18**, 827–838.

19. Koster, J. C., Sha, Q., Shyng, S.-L., and Nichols, C. G. (1999a) ATP Inhibition of K_{ATP} Channels: Control of nucleotide sensitivity by the N-terminal domain of the Kir6. 2 subunit. *J. Physiol.* **515**, 19–30.

20. Kupper, J. (1998) Functional expression of GFP-tagged Kv1. 3 and Kv1. 4 channels in HEK 293 cells. *Eur. J. Neurosci.* **10**, 3908–3912.

21. Bueno, O. F., Robinson, L. C., Alvarez-Hernandez, X., and Leidenheimer, N. J. (1998) Functional characterization and visualization of a GABAA receptor-GFP chimera expressed in Xenopus oocytes. *Brain Res. Mol. Brain Res.* **59**, 165–177.

22. John, S. A., Monck, J. R., Weiss, J. N., and Ribalet, B. (1998) The sulphonylurea receptor SUR1 regulates ATP-sensitive mouse Kir6. 2 K+ channels linked to the green fluorescent protein in human embryonic kidney cells (HEK 293). *J. Physiol.* **510**, 333–345.

23. Moyer, B. D., Loffing, J., Schwiebert, E. M., Loffing-Cueni, D., Halpin, P. A., Karlson, K. H., et al. (1998) Membrane trafficking of the cystic fibrosis gene product, cystic fibrosis transmembrane conductance regulator, tagged with green fluorescent protein in madin-darby canine kidney cells. *J. Biol. Chem.* **273**, 21,759–21,768.

24. Grabner, M., Dirksen, R. T., and Beam, K. G. (1998) Tagging with green fluorescent protein reveals a distinct subcellular distribution of L-type and non-L-type Ca^{2+} channels expressed in dysgenic myotubes. *Proc. Natl. Acad. Sci. USA* **95**, 1903–1908.

25. Makhina, E. N. and Nichols, C. G. (1998) Independent trafficking of KATP channel subunits to the plasma membrane. *J. Biol. Chem.* **273**, 3369–3374.

26. Meyer, E. and Fromherz, P. (1999) Ca2+ activation of hSlo K+ channel is suppressed by N-terminal GFP tag. *Euro. J. Neurosci.* **11**, 1105–1108.

27. Kisseberth, W. C., Brettingen, N. T., Lohse, J. K., and Sandgren, E. P. (1999) Ubiquitous expression of marker transgenes in mice and rats. *Develop. Biol.* **214**, 128–138.

28. Palermo, J., Gulick, J., Ng, W., Grupp, I. L., Grupp, G., and Robbins J. (1995) Remodeling the mammalian heart using transgenesis. *Cell. Mol. Biol. Res.* **41**, 501–509.

29. Dandoy-Dron, F., Monthioux, E., Jami, J., and Bucchini, D. (1991) Regulatory regions of rat insulin I gene necessary for expression in transgenic mice. *Nucleic Acids Res.* **19**, 4925–4930.

30. Sakura, H., Ashcroft, S. J., Terauchi, Y., Kadowaki, T., and Ashcroft, F. M. (1998) Glucose modulation of ATP-sensitive K-currents in wild-type, homozygous and heterozygous glucokinase knock-out mice. *Diabetologia* **41**, 654–659.

14

Mutant GFP-Based FRET Analysis of K⁺ Channel Organization

Elena N. Makhina and Colin G. Nichols

1. INTRODUCTION

The fact that genetic incorporation of the green fluorescent protein GFP *(1)* into an ion channel does not usually abolish function of either protein (*see* Part 2 of this book) enables a researcher to localize an ion channel in a living cell at almost every step of its biogenesis. Indeed, by means of light and confocal microscopy ion channels have been observed through the major steps of the secretory pathway: ER-Golgi- TGN- plasma membrane *(2–4)*. Single GFP tagging can be used to sort out various trafficking mutants *(5)* and to demonstrate ion channel interaction with other proteins *(3,6–8)*. Potentially this approach allows the monitoring of ion channel trafficking and turnover in real time. The advantage of such in vivo localization is partly compromised by the necessity of labeling and detecting a control protein specific for a given compartment—usually achieved by immunostaining followed by cell fixation. This complication was bypassed by the development of blue, cyan, yellow, red, and other mutant fluorescent proteins (BFP, CFP, YFP, and RFP, respectively), that make it possible to monitor two proteins labeled with optically distinguishable fluorescent tags almost simultaneously in vivo and localize one protein relative to another. Ion channel examples are absent for the moment, application for other proteins is reviewed in ref. *9*. Such co-coloring allows attributing two proteins roughly to the same compartment but does not reveal their closer association owing to the limited spatial resolution of light microscopy.

Fluorescence resonance energy transfer (FRET) between two appropriate Gfps provides a method to reveal closer association of two co-localized

From: *Ion Channel Localization Methods and Protocols*
Edited by: A. Lopatin and C. G. Nichols © Humana Press Inc., Totowa, NJ

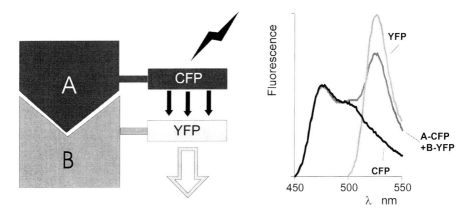

Fig. 1. Principles of the mutant GFP-based FRET assay. When two proteins or domains tagged with donor and acceptor GFPs are in a close proximity, inter-GFP FRET can occur and is registered as the acceptor emission spectrum at a donor excitation wave length (top). Absence of protein-protein interaction is characterized by an emission spectrum lacking an acceptor emission peak.

proteins. FRET is a process by which an excited fluorescent molecule (donor) transfers its energy in a nonradiative mode to another molecule (acceptor) causing the latter to emit light. Because FRET efficacy is proportional to the donor-acceptor proximity, FRET between chemical fluorescent markers has become a standard method to measure distances within, or between, biological molecules *(10)*. GFP mutants with shifted wavelengths of excitation and emission have been created to form donor-acceptor couples producing FRET *(11,12)*. Figure 1 shows the general principle of FRET between two mutant GFPs. A sample containing two proteins tagged with donor and acceptor GFP molecules is illuminated by light that specifically excites the donor but does not affect the acceptor. When the donor-acceptor proximity and orientation are favorable, nonradiative energy transfer from the donor can excite the acceptor GFP. When donor and acceptor GFPs are incorporated in the same molecule, changes in FRET reflect conformational changes in the protein. There are two main constraints for FRET occurrence: the fluorophores have to be in a permissive relative orientation and lie within 100 Å. Thus, in principle, mutant GFP-based FRET assays should permit: (1) ion channels to be localized by an optical event in a live cell or in dispersed cellular fraction; (2) conformation to be monitored through biogenesis; and (3) association with a second GFP-labeled protein to be detected in different cellular compartments.

Information on the physics of inter-GFP FRET can be found in recent reviews *(12,13)*. Potential advantages of GFP FRET assays in testing conformation dynamics and protein–protein interaction have been considered in other recent reviews *(14–16)*, but experimental applications are limited so far to the following examples, none of which involves ion channels. BFP fused to red shifted GFP via a short peptide with a X_a cleavage site displayed FRET, which disappeared after X_a separated the two fluorescent proteins *(17)*. Placing calmodulin between two GFPs resulted in a FRET-producing chimera, where calcium binding changed its conformation and FRET efficacy, with sufficient resolution to measure calcium concentrations in various cellular compartments *(18,19)*. Mutant GFP-based FRET has been used to monitor dimerization in vivo of the apoptotic proteins Bcl and Bax *(20)* and G-protein coupled receptors *(21)*. Changes in metallothionein conformation owing to metal release have also been detected using GFP-based FRET *(22)*. Here we describe potential benefits and considerations for the use of the approach in the study of K_{ATP} channels, an ion-channel complex that poses a number of questions that may be addressed by FRET assay.

K_{ATP} channels couple cell metabolism to electric activity in multiple cell types. In pancreatic beta-cells, loss of K_{ATP} function is associated with persistent hyperinsulinemia *(23–25)*, and alternatively, expression of K_{ATP} mutant with high open probability results in neonatal diabetes in transgenic mice *(26)*. In contrast to the well-developed electrophysiology of the K_{ATP} complex, relatively few papers address its cell biology *(2,3,27,28)*. However the heterologous composition of K_{ATP} complex and its relevance to disease call for a better understanding of its assembly and trafficking, which basically means localization of K_{ATP} subunits. The K_{ATP} complex includes 4 pore forming subunits (Kir6.1 or Kir6.2) and 4 regulatory subunits of sulfonylurea receptor (SUR1, SUR2A, or SUR2B) *(29,30)*. Neither sulfonylurea receptor, nor Kir6.2, subunits are normally capable of channel activity when expressed alone in mammalian cells or in *Xenopus* oocytes *(31,32)*, however deletion of the 36 C-terminal amino acids, which removes an endoplasmic reticulum retention signal *(27)* enables Kir6.2 to reach the plasma membrane and exhibit channel activity without SUR1 *(33)*. We have introduced donor-acceptor couples of two mutants GFPs into the K_{ATP} complex. Here we describe the methodologies involved, and the analysis of FRET signals from such complexes.

2. INTRODUCING MULTIPLE GFP MOIETIES INTO AN ION CHANNEL

GFP is a 238 amino acid protein packed in a dense cylinder, 48 Å high and 24 Å in diameter *(34)*. GFP can be fused to cytoplasmic N- and C-

Table 1
GFP-Tagged K$_{ATP}$ Subunits

Construct	No. FPs per complex	Functional with SUR1 or Kir6.2?
CFP-Kir6.2	4	+
YFP-Kir6.2	4	+
Kir6.2-CFP	4	+
Kir6.2-YFP	4	+
CFP-Kir6.2-YFP	8	+
SUR1-CFP	4 expected	+
Kir6.2-YFP/SUR1-CFP	8 expected	+
YFP-Kir6.2/SUR1-CFP	8 expected	−

termini of ion channels Kir6.2, Kir2.1, Kir2.3, Kir1.1 without compromising channel function *(2,3)*. We found essentially no differences between the properties of channels attached to GFP in direct fusion of GFP to C-terminus of Kir2.3 or via 6-glycine linker *(2)*. However, C-terminal tagging of SUR1 with GFP resulted in a functional chimera only when we placed 6 alanines between the two proteins. Even if the high rate of success in creating GFP-channel chimeras may be to some degree explained by the lack of reports of unsuccessful fusion, cytoplasmic termini of ion channels seem to be a suitable domain for GFP-tagging. Placing GFP into a coding sequence remains a challenge, however a clever design may result in a functional chimera, as shown for a voltage-gated Kv channel with GFP introduced just beyond the membrane-spanning S6 domain *(35)*. For our FRET experiments we attached mutant GFPs to K$_{ATP}$-termini in several configurations (Table 1).

Almost all constructs were functional (Table 1), and expressed ATP-sensitive potassium currents in transfected COSm6 cells. Clearly, ion channels are quite tolerant to GFP incorporation. Does GFP fusion to an ion channel affect GFP fluorescence? When GFP was utilized as an optical sensor for conformational changes in a Shaker-GFP chimera, the intensity of GFP fluorescence correlated with voltage-dependent gating of the channel *(35)*. In another report, close physical proximity of two GFP molecules shifted the ratio of their excitation peaks (from 395 nm to 475 nm). This effect results from structural interaction between two fluorophores and is not connected with spectral energy transfer *(36)*. So far, there is no evidence that attachment of GFP to a second protein changes the GFP spectral properties, although we cannot exclude the possibility that a certain peptide context may change fluorescence intensity. In numerous chimeras of CFP, GFP, and

Table 2
Mutant FPs and Spectral Properties

Name	Mutations	Excitation maxima (nm)	Emission maxima (nm)
CFP	F64L, S65T, Y66W,	434	478
	M153T, N164I, V163A,	452	505 (minor)
	N212K		
YFP	S65G, S72A, T203Y	480	525

YFP with Kir channels and their cytoplasmic or transmembrane fragments that we have made, the excitation and emission characteristics of the fluorescent proteins did not change.

Relevant criteria for selection of a FRET producing pair of GFP mutants based on their spectral properties and quantum yield are listed elsewhere *(11,12)*. We used cyan-shifted (CFP) and yellow-shifted (YFP) mutants *(21)* (*see* Table 2). The emission spectrum of the CFP donor overlaps the excitation spectrum of the YFP acceptor, and major emission peaks of CFP and YFP are well separated and distinguishable. Of practical importance: YFP emission at the CFP excitation maximum (cross-talk) is low and CFP is the brightest donor available so far.

The usual technique to make fusion constructs is polymerase chain reaction (PCR). Because GFP fluorescence can be destroyed by random mutations generated in PCR, GFP amplification should be avoided whenever possible. Even with a high-fidelity PCR-polymerase, a reasonably short cassette should be generated by PCR and cloned. All PCR-originated fragments are verified by sequencing. Vectors that allow cloning of a protein of interest in frame with the N- or C-terminus of wild-type and mutant GFP, are available from Clontech, Invitrogen, Pharmigen, and other companies. At the present time there are no commercially available vectors like those constructed by Miyawaki et al. *(19)*, widely referred to as "chameleons," for FRET constructs. When initiating a GFP-FRET project, it may be reasonable to begin by creating such a vector and then cloning a variety of fragments into a multiple cloning site between two fluorescent proteins. However, the nature of FRET may require varying channel-GFP junctions and individual construction of plasmids. In this case a hybrid primer connecting GFP and an ion channel is designed according to a desired structure (flexible, rigid, or other) of the protein junction. We have achieved relative orientation of CFP and YFP that permits FRET by their direct fusion with N- and C-termini of Kir6.2.

3. EXPRESSION OF FRET CONSTRUCTS IN MAMMALIAN CELLS

GFP-channel chimeras are bright enough to be monitored in transfected mammalian cells. The choice of transfection method for FRET constructs is dictated by the necessity to test many constructs. We performed FRET measurements on transiently transfected COSm6 cells. A DEAE-dextran-chloroquine transfection protocol was applied when GFP-K_{ATP} constructs were tested for channel activity; for morphological and spectral analyses, cells were transfected using lipofectamine reagent (chloroquine causes swelling of acidic compartments and changes the cell morphology).

The presence of a functional chimeric protein should be confirmed prior to fluorescence measurements and we have used direct patch-clamping of our K_{ATP} channel chameleons. If a construct in question is devoid of electrical activity, it may be recognized by Western blot with anti-GFP or anti-channel antibodies and visualized in cells by microscopy. The major fraction of GFP-tagged channels are located in inner membranes, and it is primarily the state of this fraction that is tested in fluorescent measurements performed on untreated live cultures. A certain cellular compartment could be enriched in chimeric protein by cytostatic agents or isolated by fractionation, in order to assay channel constructs located in specific compartments.

We tagged K_{ATP} subunits with one or two mutant GFPs and expressed them under the control of the cytomegalovirus promoter in the pCMV6 vector. COSm6 cells were plated on 100 mm Petri dishes at a density of 10^6 cells per plate 24 h before transfection using lipofectamine reagent (Life Technologies, Inc.) or a DEAE-dextran/chloroquine method *(2)*. Measurements were made on the second day after transfection when the fraction of fluorescent transfectants was from 10–70% depending on the construct. Cells collected from a single plate generated robust fluorescence, easily detected by spectroscopic measurements in vivo and in vitro. In the constructs with covalently linked CFP and YFP, the donor:acceptor molar ratio is constrained to 1:1 and provides conditions suitable for FRET. When Kir 6.2 subunits tagged individually with CFP and YFP were cotransfected appropriate donor-acceptor ratios may be easily obtained by mixing DNA. However we were unable to achieve ~1:1 ratio when Kir6.2-YFP was coexpressed with SUR-CFP. The level of SUR-CFP and SUR-GFP fluorescence remained invariantly low even when SUR-GFP was expressed alone, and despite the fact that SUR-GFP with Kir6.2 formed active K_{ATP} channels and was visible *(2)*. One possible explanation is that folding of this particular protein "damages" the fluorophore and weakens its fluorescence. When the SUR-GFP construct was shortened by deletions of various length the fluorescence dramatically increased (unpublished observations).

When culturing cells expressing GFP fusion one might consider incubating them at 33°C, which is reported to improve GFP folding and to enhance fluorescence, or using a mutant whose folding is insensitive to high (37°C) temperature *(37,38)*.

4. DATA ACQUISITION AND ANALYSIS

Screening for a FRET-producing combination requires rapid fluorescence measurements of many cultures. This can be done by an easily available spectrofluorometer, where an emission scan takes 1–2 min. Later the population measurements can be followed by FRET microscopy (reviewed in ref. *13*). We resuspended transfected and untransfected COSm6 cells in 3 mL of K solution (140 mM KCl, 10 mM HEPES, 1 mM ethylenglycoltetraacetic acid [EGTA], pH 7.3) and measured fluorescence in a stirred cuvet in a FluoroMax fluorometer. CFP and YFP were excited at 430 nm and 480 nm, respectively, and emission scans were performed. Excitation and emission slit widths were 5 mm, fluorescence points were acquired in 1 nm increments. Spectroscopic scans were transferred to Microsoft Excel for analysis, during which autofluorescence of the cells was subtracted from CFP- or YFP-associated fluorescence after normalizing the spectra by cell density.

Figure 2 illustrates FRET between CFP and YFP flanking Kir6.2 and the Kir6.2 N-terminal cytoplasmic domain. In each case, prominent 525 nm emission peaks with excitation at 430 nm are much greater than the emission of YFP caused by 430 nm excitation. A simple qualitative way to test whether the acceptor emission is owing to FRET is to cleave the link between the two GFPs by protease and observe gradual decrease of acceptor emission and increase of donor emission. In K_{ATP} channels, trypsin cleaves cytoplasmic regions of Kir6.2 *(39,40)*, and we have demonstrated inversion of emission spectra (FRET disappearance) after cytoplasmic trypsin cleavage (Fig. 2). Once FRET is proven it has to be characterized quantitatively. The following practical formula may be suggested for FRET measurements (Fig. 3):

$$FRET\% = (F_{430} - C_{430}) / F_{480} \qquad (1)$$

where F_{430} and F_{480} is emission of the FRET producing sample at 430 nm and 480 nm excitation, and C_{430} is emission of the donor (CFP) at 430 nm excitation. It can be applied to FRET between covalently linked GFPs in one construct or to compare different samples. FRET values obtained this way for Kir6.2 constructs are presented in Fig. 3B.

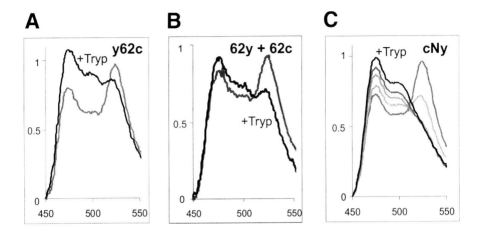

Fig. 2. Emission scans of CFP and YFP-tagged K_{ATP} at 430 nm excitation. In this and following figures, emission (ordinate, arbitrary units) is plotted vs wavelength (abscissa, nm). **(A)** Kir6.2 is tagged with YFP at the N-terminus and CFP at the C-terminus (y62c construct). **(B)** Kir6.2 subunits were tagged with CFP and YFP at their C-termini (62c, 62y) and co-expressed. **(C)** The N-terminal domain of Kir6.2 was flanked by CFP and YFP (cNy). Emission scans were performed on disrupted cells before and after trypsin treatment. Panel (C) shows scans performed at 3-min intervals after treatment with 0.1 mg/mL trypsin at room temperature.

5. INTERPRETATION OF FRET DATA

Can FRET values obtained above be converted into physical distances? The Forster Equation 2 relates the distance (r) between donor (D) and acceptor (A) fluorophores and the spectroscopic properties of each:

$$K_T = (1/\tau_D) \ (R_0/r)^6 \tag{2}$$

where K_T is the rate of energy transfer from D to A, τ_D is the fluorescence lifetime of D in the absence of A, R_0 (the Forster distance) is the distance at which the average efficiency of transfer is 50%. Because K_T is proportional $1/r^6$, FRET efficiency becomes negligible above ~1.5 R_0. Critically, the definition of the Forster distance includes an (inherently in this context) unknown parameter, the relative fluorophore orientations. The main limitation of the FRET assay in testing protein-protein interactions is a requirement of proper fluorophore alignment. GFP molecules are not point sources, and placing two GFPs in the correct relative orientation may be a problem even if the crystal structure of a hosting protein were known. Figure 4 shows how FRET results can depend on fluorophore orientation in K_{ATP} channels.

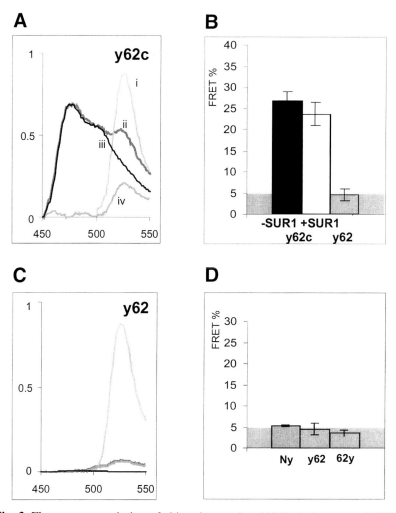

Fig. 3. Fluorescence emission of chimeric proteins. (**A**) Emission scan of COSm6 cells transfected with y62c, excited at 480 nm (i) or 430 nm (ii), and of cells transfected with 62c, excited at 430 nm, normalized to the y62c emission at 476 nm (iii). Subtraction of the 62c cyan emission spectrum from the y62c emission spectrum yields the apparent FRET in the spectrum (iv). In this and all subsequent figures, the abscissa is the emission wavelength (nm), and the ordinate is the emission intensity in instrument fluorescence units. (**B**) FRET efficiency expressed by 525 nm emission (430 nm excitation) as a percentage of 525 nm emission at 480 nm excitation, for y62c (expressed with or without SUR1) and for y62 constructs. Bars show mean ± SEM, n = 7–10 independent transfections. (**C**) Emission scan of COSm6 cells transfected with y62, excited at 480 nm or 430 nm, together with normalized CFP scan, and subtracted scan, as in (A). (**D**) FRET efficiency expressed by 525 nm emission (excited at 430 nm) as a percentage of 525 nm emission with 480 nm excitation, for YFP-containing constructs as indicated. Bars show mean ± SEM, n = 6–10 independent transfections.

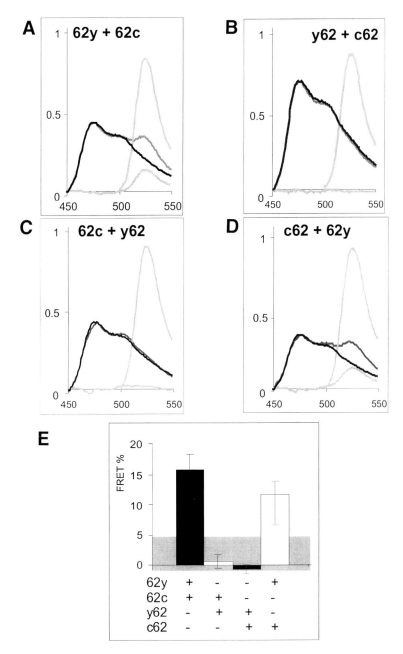

Fig. 4. Fluorescence emission of combinations of mutant GFP-tagged Kir6.2 proteins. (**A–D**) Emission scans of COSm6 cells transfected with mixtures of YFP and CFP tagged full-length Kir6.2 constructs as indicated. (**E**) FRET efficiency expressed by 525 nm emission (excited at 430 nm) as a percentage of 525 nm emission with 480 nm excitation, for YFP-containing constructs as indicated. Bars show mean ± SEM, n = 5–10 independent transfections. Note that otherwise identical pairs of combinations give large FRET signals, or no FRET signal, depending on fluorophore orientation.

When CFP and YFP are attached to the N- and C-terminus respectively, or to C-termini of Kir6.2, FRET occurs. In two other configurations FRET does not occur. We cannot formally distinguish between orientation or distance factor in the interpretation of these results. However, because pairs of constructs are structurally identical with the exception of the point mutations to generate CFP or YFP fluorophores, the simplest interpretation is that the orientations of each fluorophore are critical.

Thus, for practical purposes, because R_0 for GFP based FRET pairs is probably about 40 Å *(11)*, FRET is not typically observed between GFP pairs that are separated by > ~60 Å, and observed FRET may be taken to indicate that the fluorophores are within this distance. However, a change of FRET signal may indicate that either fluorophore distance, or orientation, is changing. Separating these possibilities may be impractical.

In our experiments the background fluorescence of YFP attached to Kir6.2, Kir1.1, Kir2.1, and SUR1 at 430 nm excitation did not exceed 5%. Is any level of "background FRET" possible owing to nonspecific closeness of the tested proteins in overexpressing cells? When different Kir subunits with single CFP or YFP tags were co-expressed the FRET peaks were above the background 5% but below the FRET amplitude observed between homologous subunits (unpublished observations). Moreover, Kir6.2 reduced to its transmembrane domains and tagged with CFP/YFP displayed FRET. Although this may reflect appropriate assembly of truncated channels, artefactual clustering remains an alternate possibility.

6. CONCLUSIONS

At the present time (early 2000), experimental data obtained with inter-GFP FRET on ion channels are very limited and do not allow serious conclusions about its usefulness. Our experience shows that FRET between two GFPs can be achieved relatively easily in a functional ion channel. However, we could not demonstrate physiologically reversible modulation of FRET by channel-specific agents. Unlike the two-hybrid system, the FRET based protein–protein interaction assay does not provide a means of cloning new proteins, because it does not provide an easy selection of positive interactants. Nevertheless it may be useful in a limited screen of prospective candidates for protein-protein interaction. It also permits a quantitative evaluation of any such interaction and spatial "sketching" of the resulting complex. The main attraction of this approach remains in the possibility of encoding a fluorescent marker genetically and watching the life of a channel in real time.

REFERENCES

1. Chalfie, M., Tu, Y., Euskirchen, G., Ward, W. W., and Prasher, D. C. (1994) Green fluorescent protein as a marker of gene expression. *Science* **263,** 802–805.
2. Makhina, E. N. and Nichols, C. G. (1998) Independent trafficking of K_{ATP} channel subunits to the plasma membrane. *J. Biol. Chem.* **273,** 3369–3374.
3. John, S. A., Monck, J. R., Weiss, J. N., and Ribalet, B. (1998) The sulphonylurea receptor SUR1 regulates ATP-sensitive mouse Kir6. 2 K^+ channels linked to the green fluorescent protein in human embryonic kidney cells (HEK 293). *J. Physiol.* **510,** 333–345.
4. Moyer, B. D., Loffing, J., Schwiebert, E. M., Loffing-Cueni, D, Halpin, P. A., Karlson, K. H., et al. (1998) Membrane trafficking of the cystic fibrosis gene product, cystic fibrosis transmembrane conductance regulator, tagged with green fluorescent protein in madin-darby canine kidney cells. *J. Biol. Chem.* **273,** 21,759–21,768.
5. Moyer, B. D., Loffing-Cueni, D., Loffing, J., Reynolds, D., and Stanton, B. A. (1999) Butyrate increases apical membrane CFTR but reduces chloridesecretion in MDCK cells. *Am. J. Physiol.* **277,** F271–F276.
6. Burke, N. A., Takimoto, K., Li, D., Han, W., Watkins, S. C., and Levitan, E. S. (1999) Distinct structural requirements for clustering and immobilization of K^+ channels by PSD-95. *J. Gen. Physiol.* **113,** 71–80.
7. Chan, K. W., Sui, J. L., Vivaudou, M., and Logothetis, D. E. (1997) Specific regions of heteromeric subunits involved in enhancement of G protein-gated K+ channel activity. *J. Biol. Chem.* **272,** 6548–6555.
8. Arnold, D. B. and Clapham, D. E. (1999) Molecular determinants for subcellular localization of PSD-95 with an interacting K^+ channel. *Neuron* **23,** 149–157.
9. Ellenberg, J., Lippincott-Schwartz, J., and Presley, J. F. (1999) Dual-colour imaging with GFP variants. *Trends Cell Biol.* **9,** 52–56.
10. Lakowicz, J. R. (1983) *Principles of Fluorescence Spectroscopy*. Plenum, New York, p. 0-496, monograph.
11. Heim, R. and Tsien, R. (1996) Engineering green fluorescent protein for improved brightness, longer wavelengths and fluorescence resonance energy transfer. *Curr. Biol.* **6,** 178–182.
12. Tsien, R. Y. (1998) The green fluorescent protein. *Ann. Rev. Biochem.* **67,** 509–544.
13. Periasamy, A. and Day, R. N. (1999) Vizualizing protein interactions in living cells using digitized GFP imaging and FRET microscopy. *Methods Cell Biol.* **58,** 293–314.
14. Pollok, B. A. and Heim, R. (1999) Using GFP in FRET-based applications. *Trends Cell Biol.* **9,** 57–60.
15. Bastiaens, P. I. and Squire, A. (1999) Fluorescence lifetime imaging microscopy: spatial resolution of biochemical processes in the cell. *Trends Cell Biol.* **9,** 48–52.
16. Weiss, S. (1999) Fluorescence spectroscopy of single biomolecules. *Science* **283,** 1676–1682.

17. Mitra, R. D., Silva, C. M., and Youvan, D. C. (1996) Fluorescence resonance energy transfer between blue-emitting and red-shifted excitation derivatives of the green fluorescent protein. *Gene* **173,** 13–17.

18. Romoser, V. A., Hinkle, P. M., and Persechini, A. (1997) Detection in living cells of Ca²⁺-dependent changes in the fluorescence emission of an indicator composed of two green fluorescent protein variants linked by a calmodulin-binding sequence. A new class of fluorescent indicators. *J. Biol. Chem.* **272,** 13,270–13,274.

19. Miyawaki, A., Llopis, J., Heim, R., McCaffery, J. M., Adams, J. A., Ikura, M., and Tsien, R. Y. (1997) Fluorescent indicators for Ca²⁺ based on green fluorescent proteins and calmodulin. *Nature* **388,** 882–887.

20. Mahajan, N. P., Linder, K., Berry, G., Gordon, G. W., Heim, R., and Herman, B. (1998) Bcl-2 and Bax interactions in mitochondria probed with green fluorescent protein and fluorescence resonance energy transfer. *Nature Biotech.* **16,** 547–552.

21. Overton, M. C. and Blumer, K. J. (2000) G protein coupled receptors function as oligomers in vivo. *Curr. Biol.* **10,** 341–344.

22. Pearce, LL, Gandley, R. E., Han, W., Wasserloos, K., Stitt, M., Kanai, A. J., et al. (2000) Role of metallothionein in nitric oxide signaling as revealed by a green fluorescent fusion protein. *Proc. Natl. Acad. Sci. USA* **97,** 477–482.

23. Nichols, C. G., Shyng, S.-L., Nestorowicz, A., Glaser, B., Clement, J. P. IV, Gonzales, G., et al. (1996) Adenosine diphosphate as an intracellular regulator of insulin secretion. *Science* **272,** 1785–1787.

24. Nestorowicz, A., Wilson, B. A., Schoor, K. P., Inoue, H., Glaser, B., Landau, H., et al. (1996) Mutations in the sulonylurea receptor gene are associated with familial hyperinsulinism in Ashkenazi Jews. *Hum. Mol. Genetics* **5,** 1813–1822.

25. Dunne, M. J., Kane, C., Shepherd, R. M., Sanchez, J. A., James, R. F., Johnson, P. R., et al. (1997) Familial persistent hyperinsulinemic hypoglycemia of infancy and mutations in the sulfonylurea receptor. *N. Engl. J. Med.* **336,** 703–706.

26. Koster, J. C., Marshall, B. A., Ensor, N., Corbett, J. A., and Nichols, C. G. (2000) Targeted overactivity of beta cell K$_{ATP}$ channels induces profound neonatal diabetes. *Cell* **100,** 645–654.

27. Zerangue, N., Schwappach, B., Jan, Y. N., and Jan, L. Y. (1999) A new ER trafficking signal regulates the subunit stoichiometry of plasma membrane K(ATP) channels. *Neuron.* **22,** 537–548.

28. Sharma, N., Crane, A., Clement, J. P. IV, Gonzalez, G., Babenko, A. P., Bryan, J., and Aguilar-Bryan, L. (1999) The C terminus of SUR1 is required for trafficking of K$_{ATP}$ channels. *J. Biol. Chem.* **274,** 20,628–20,632.

29. Shyng, S.-L. and Nichols, C. G. (1997) Octameric stoichiometry of the K$_{ATP}$ channel complex. *J. Gen. Physiol.* **110,** 655–664.

30. Clement, J. P., Kunjilwar, K., Gonzalez, G., Schwanstecher, M., Panten, U., Aguilar-Bryan, L., and Bryan, J. (1997) Association and stoichiometry of K(ATP) channel subunits. *Neuron* **18,** 827–838.

31. Aguilar-Bryan, L., Nichols, C. G., Wechsler, S. W., Clement, J. P. IV, Boyd, A. E. III, et al. (1995) Cloning of the beta cell high-affinity sulfonylurea receptor: a regulator of insulin secretion. *Science* **268,** 423–426.

32. Inagaki, N., Gonoi, T., Clement, J. P. IV, Namba, N., Inazawa, J., Gonzalez, G., et al. (1995) Reconstitution of IK$_{ATP}$: an inward rectifier subunit plus the sulfonylurea receptor. *Science* **270,** 1166–1170.

33. Tucker, S. J., Gribble, F. M., Zhao, C., Trapp, S., and Ashcroft, F. M. (1997) Truncation of Kir6. 2 produces ATP-sensitive K+ channels in the absence of the sulphonylurea receptor. *Nature* **387,** 179–183.

34. Ormo, M., Cubitt, A. B., Kallio, K., Gross, L. A., Tsien, R. Y., and Remington, S. J. (1996) Crystal structure of the Aequorea victoria green fluorescent protein *Science* **273,** 1392–1395.

35. Siegel, M. S. and Isacoff, E. Y. (1997) A genetically encoded optical probe of membrane voltage. *Neuron* **19,** 735–741.

36. De Angelis, D. A., Miesenbock, G., Zemelman, B. V., and Rothman, J. E. (1998) PRIM: proximity imaging of green fluorescent protein-tagged, polypeptides. *Proc. Natl. Acad. Sci. USA* **95,** 12,312–12,316.

37. Siemering, K. R., Golbik, R., Sever, R., and Haseloff, J. (1996) Mutations that suppress the thermosensitivity of green fluorescent protein. *Curr. Biol.* **6,** 1653–1663.

38. Kimata, Y., Iwaki, M., Lim, C. R., and Kohno, K. (1997) A novel mutation which enhances the fluorescence of green fluorescent protein at high temperatures. *Biochem. Biophys. Res. Comm.* **232,** 69–73.

39. Nichols, C. G. and Lopatin, A. N. (1993) Trypsin and alpha-chymotrypsin treatment abolishes glibenclamide sensitivity of K$_{ATP}$ channels in rat ventricular myocytes. *Pflugers Arch.* **422,** 617–619.

40. Proks, P. and Ashcroft, F. M. (1993) Modification of K-ATP channels in pancreatic beta-cells by trypsin. *Pflugers Arch..* **424,** 63–72.

15

Delivering Ion Channels to Mammalian Cells by Membrane Fusion

David C. Johns, Uta C. Hoppe, Eduardo Marbán, and Brian O'Rourke

1. INTRODUCTION

Ion channels in the plasma membrane play a critical role in cellular function. These proteins are the gatekeepers that control ion homeostasis and shape excitability. Excitable cells use a variety of different ion channels to fashion their hallmark electrical signal, the action potential. Advances in molecular electrophysiology have led to the identification of more ion-channel genes than there are identified membrane currents. This excess is particularly striking with potassium channels, where a wide diversity of genes is compounded by variable levels of hetero-multimerization, alternative splicing, and post-translational modification. The classical methods of studying the roles of each gene rely either on exogenous expression in frog oocytes or pharmacological manipulation of native currents (1). Although these techniques have yielded a wealth of information concerning ion channel structure and function, they have come up short in linking individual genes and their products to physiology and disease.

Defects in ion channels have been linked to a number of inherited diseases including epilepsy, periodic paralysis, cystic fibrosis, and long QT syndrome (2). In addition, changes in cellular excitability are associated with several common disease states including drug addiction, depression, and heart failure (3–5). An enormous number of pharmaceutical agents affect cellular excitability either directly or indirectly. This may be by design, as in the case of local anaesthetic block of sodium channels, or as an unwanted

From: *Ion Channel Localization Methods and Protocols*
Edited by: A. Lopatin and C. G. Nichols © Humana Press Inc., Totowa, NJ

side effect that limits the potential usefulness of the agent, such as erythro-mycin-induced block of cardiac potassium channels leading to fatal arrhythmias *(6)*. The study of the role ion channels play in various patho-logical states has been greatly advanced by the application of molecular genetics. The study of germ line mutations affecting ion channels in an organism, and somatic cell gene transfer, have become two powerful ways by which investigators have unraveled the role of specific ion channels in normal physiology.

As previously stated, one of the first techniques used to study cloned ion-channel genes involved injection of in vitro transcribed cRNA into oocytes isolated from *Xenopus laevis.* This technique has several advantages and is still widely used today. Channels expressed in this way are generally expressed robustly and, because each cell is individually injected, the expression efficiency is near 100%. Some downfalls to this approach include the high number of exogenous channels expressed in the oocyte cell mem-brane, the large size of the oocyte makes it difficult to obtain a complete clamp of the cell, and differences in the biophysical properties of expressed channels presumably owing to lack of endogenous modulators of channel function *(7–9)*. The ideal situation would enable examination of the behav-ior of the expressed ion channel in its native environment to determine not only its native biophysical, but also its physiological function.

Improvements in the ability to transfect cloned DNA into cultured mam-malian cells along with the creation of mammalian expression vectors has led to the technique of transient transfection as another way of expressing ion-channel proteins. The cDNA of interest is cloned into a plasmid vector between a mammalian (or avian) promoter and poly-adenylation sequence (both often of viral origin). The DNA is then transfected into cultured cells by anyone of several techniques with a resulting transfection efficiency any-where between 2 and 80% depending on the transfection technique and the cell line used. Although this technique obviates, to some extent, the prob-lems listed for the oocyte technique, it also lacked the ease with which posi-tive cells could be identified. In addition, in some cases clones that could be expressed in the oocyte system were more difficult to express in this system. To eliminate the problems in identifying positive cells, a selectable marker, usually an antibiotic resistance gene, can be included in the transfection. Cells that integrate and stably express the resistance gene can then be selected for and then screened for the expression of the gene of interest. This technique has been used extensively with a number of different proteins to create stable cell lines that express the protein of interest. Results with ion-channel genes were more varied and seemed to depend on the channel of interest as well as the cell line used. In some cases the use of an inducible promoter driving the ion channel made obtaining positive expressers easier *(10,11)*. More recently the advent of auto-fluorescent reporter proteins such as the green fluorescent protein (GFP) has greatly simplified both of forms of transfection *(12–17)*. The inclusion a GFP expression cassette makes it possible to visualize, on an epi-fluorescence equipped microscope, positive cells. This technique has now become a standard way of expressing ion-channel proteins in cultured cells with the only drawback being that many primary cells are refractory to transfection.

More recently, refinements in viral vectors that have accompanied the surge of interest in gene therapy have resulted in a third way of expressing ion channels. Recombinant viral vectors are engineered to express the desired protein and these vectors can then be used to efficiently infect not only cultured cells but also primary cells either in vitro or in vivo *(16–22)*. The advantages of this technique are numerous and the continued refinement in vector design promise to make this a widely used technique in the future. One potential drawback with this technique is the potential for adaptive responses in the target cell from the time of infection until the time of functional expression and analysis.

Another potential way to deliver exogenous proteins or macromolecules is through cell fusion. The creation of heterokaryons was first used to demonstrate rapid mixing of membrane components *(23–25)*. Further applications have included delivery of macromolecules to mammalian cells, inhibition of ouabain-induced arrhythmias in embryonic myocytes, investigation of the dynamics of organelle turnover and processing, and studies of a dominant regulator of skeletal muscle differentiation *(26–31)*. From these previous studies it appeared that this technique would be a useful way to deliver ion-channel proteins to target cells. Several techniques have been employed to facilitate the fusion of two cells. The most straightforward of these is to use polyethylene glycol (PEG) to dehydrate the cells, which upon re-hydration results not only in the fusion of the cell membranes but an opening of a pore that connects the cytosolic compartments *(32)*. Proteins in the cytosol then diffuse freely between the two cells and proteins in the different membrane compartments begin to mix at somewhat slower rates dependent on the protein in question *(30,33–35)*. The opening of the pore can be readily observed by the loading of one of the cell types with a viable marker (either a dye or auto-fluorescent protein). There are several advantages of this technique; first, premade functional proteins are rapidly delivered to the cell of interest, preventing the potential for adaptive changes. Second, the vectors used are standard plasmid vectors that are readily manipulated in most laboratories. Lastly, it allows a before and after picture of the channel's properties to be elucidated (for example, one could for look for an endogenous factor in the native cell that modulates channel function).

This chapter is intended to provide an introduction into the use of GFP and cell fusion in studying ion-channel function. This work, in part, has been previously published *(36)*.

2. MATERIALS AND METHODS

2.1. Plasmid Constructs

The expression plasmid for Kv4.3 (pCGI-Kv4.3) was generated by cloning the coding sequence from rat Kv4.3 (kindly supplied by Dr. Bernardo Rudy, New York University, New York) into the vector pCGI (formerly pGFP-IRES *[37]*). The vector pEGFP-N3 (Clontech, Palo Alto, CA) was used for control transfections. The coding sequence for the human CD8 was PCR-amplified from the plasmid pEBO-CD-Leu2 (ATCC #59564, American Type Culture Collection, Manassas, VA 20110-2209) and cloned into pCGI in place of the EGFP sequence (pC8I). All vectors were purified by alkaline lysis followed by cesium chloride gradient centrifugation *(38)*.

2.2. Transient Transfections

CHO-K1 cells (ATCC CCL 61, American Type Culture Collection, Manassas, VA 20110–2209) were cultured in Ham's F12 medium (Cellgro, Mediatech, Washington, DC) supplemented with 10% fetal bovine serum (FBS) (Life Technologies, Gaithersburg, MD), 2 mM glutamine, 100 U/mL penicillin, and 100 µg/mL streptomycin (Life Technologies, Gaithersburg, MD) in a 5% CO_2 incubator at 37°C. Twenty four hours prior to transfection, cells were plated at a density of 2.0×10^5 per 35 mm plate. Cells were transfected using 9 µL of lipofectamine (LifeTechnologies) and 0.75 µg of the respective plasmid mixed as directed by the manufacturer. All transfections were done for 6 h, after which cells were washed once with growth media and returned to the incubator in growth media.

2.3. Stable Cell Lines

Stable cell lines were generated by first linearizing the desired plasmid at the *Ase*I site. Linearized DNA was transfected into CHO-K1 cells using lipofectamine. Forty-eight hours after transfection, cells were placed in growth media containing geneticin sulfate (500 µg/mL; G 418, Life Technologies). Following selection cells were sorted on a fluorescence activated cell sorter (FACS). Cells exhibiting fluorescence levels above background were plated at low density and allowed to grow until single colonies could be picked for further analysis. Expanded colonies were analyzed by flow cytometry and patch clamp analysis.

2.4. Flow Cytometrical Analysis

Flow cytometry was performed using a Becton Dickinson Facstar and analyzed using CellQuest (Becton Dickinson) or Win MDI software (Scripps Institute). Forward and side scatter was used to gate single cells, and excitation at 488 nm and collection at 530 nm measured GFP fluorescence. Cells transfected with a plasmid expressing LacZ were used as nonfluorescent controls. GFP-positive cells were selected as those whose fluorescence intensity exceeded the fluorescence of 99.9% of the control cells.

2.5. Ventricular Myocyte Isolation

Guinea pig ventricular myocytes were isolated using Langendorff perfusion as previously described *(39)*. Adult guinea pigs (300–350 g) were sacrificed by pentobarbital (50 mg/kg i.p.). The heart was extracted and retrogradely perfused via the ascending aorta with nominally Ca^{2+}-free modified Tyrode's solution (140 mM NaCl, 5 mM KCl, 10 mM glucose, 1 mM $MgCl_2$, 10 mM HEPES; pH was adjusted to 7.4 with NaOH, 37°C) for 6 min, followed by 9 min in the same solution with added collagenase (type II, 200 IU/mL; Worthington Biochemical Corp., Freehold, NJ) and protease (type XIV, 0.3 IU/mL; Sigma Chemical Co, St Louis, MO). Finally, the enzyme was washed out for 5 min with modified Tyrode's solution that contained 200 μM Ca^{2+}. After digestion, cells from the left ventricular myocardial wall were disaggregated by mechanical agitation, strained through a nylon mesh filter, and stored at room temperature in a high potassium solution (120 mM K-glutamate, 25 mM KCl, 1 mM $MgCl_2$, 10 mM glucose, 10 mM HEPES, 1 mM EGTA; pH was adjusted to 7.4 with KOH) for 30 min. Myocytes were then placed on laminin-coated (20 μL/mL culture medium; Becton Dickinson Labware, Bedford, MA) cover slips in 6-well plates in medium 199 (Cellgro, Mediatech, Washington DC) supplemented with 2% FBS (Life Technologies) and maintained at 37°C in a 5% CO_2 humidified incubator for 1 h.

2.6. Cell Fusion

Control (CHO) or test (CHO-Kv4.3) cells were grown to 70% confluency in 75 cm^2 flasks in normal growth media. Before fusion, CHO cells were loaded with calcein-AM (2 μL/mL growth medium; 1 mM stock solution in dimethyl sulfoxide (DMSO); Molecular Probes, Eugene, OR) and incubated in the presence of the dye for 30 min. Following staining, cells were twice washed with phosphate-buffered saline (PBS), trypsinized, centrifuged, and resuspended in 6 mL medium 199 supplemented with leucoagglutinin 40 μg/mL (Sigma Chemical Co., St. Louis, MO). The myocyte growth medium was exchanged with this CHO cell suspension at 0.5 mL/well. One hour after co-plating, myocytes and CHO cells were fused with prewarmed (37°C) polyethylene glycol 1500 40% (PEG) (Boehringer Mannheim, Mannheim, Germany). After 2–4 min exposure to PEG cells were rehydrated with high potassium solution.

2.7. Electrophysiology

Experiments were carried out using standard microelectrode whole-cell patch-clamp technique *(40)* with an Axopatch 1D amplifier (Axon instruments, Foster City, CA) while sampling at 10 kHz and filtering at 2 kHz. Data were digitized and stored on personal computer for off-line analysis using custom software. All experiments were performed at a temperature of 37°C.

Cells were superfused with a physiological saline solution containing: 138 mM NaCl, 5 mM KCl, 2 mM CaCl$_2$, 10 mM glucose, 0.5 mM MgCl$_2$, 10 mM HEPES; pH was adjusted to 7.4 with NaOH. The micropipet electrode solution was composed of: 130 mM K-glutamate, 9 mM KCl, 8 mM NaCl, 0.5 mM MgCl$_2$, 10 mM HEPES, 2 mM ethyleneglycol-bis(β-aminoethyl ether)-N,N,N',N'-tetraacetic acid (EGTA), and 5 mM Mg-ATP; pH was adjusted to 7.2 with KOH. Borosilicate microelectrodes had tip resistances of 1–5 MΩ when filled with the internal recording solution.

Currents were normalized to membrane capacitance to calculate current densities when indicated. Action potentials were initiated by short depolarizing current pulses (2–3 ms, 500–800 pA). Action potential duration was measured as the time from the overshoot to 50% or 90% repolarization (APD$_{50}$, APD$_{90}$).

Membrane capacitance was established by applying 10 mV depolarization test pulses from a holding potential of –80 mV. Mean cell capacitance determined by integrating the area under the capacity current transient was not different between myocytes fused with CHO-Kv4.3 cells (99.1 ± 10.5 pF; n = 19), myocytes fused with nontransfected CHO cells (84.5 ± 9.2 pF; n = 5) and nonfused myocytes (86.2 ± 9.8 pA/pF; n = 6). Data were corrected posthoc for the measured liquid junction potential between the pipet and bath solution *(41)*. A xenon arc lamp was used to view calcein fluorescence at 488/530 nm (excitation/emission).

2.8. Confocal Imaging

For confocal imaging guinea-pig myocytes were fused with CHO-K1 cells transiently cotransfected with pEGFP-N3 and pC8I (0.4 μg each per

2.0×10^5 cells). Following PEG exposure and rehydration cells were fixed with 3% paraformaldehyde and stained with R-phycoerythrin conjugated monoclonal CD8 antibodies (Sigma). Until cells were fixed, they were kept at 37°C. Images were taken on a laser confocal microscope (*PCM* 2000, Nikon Inc. Melville, NY) with a 60× water immersion objective lens.

2.9. Statistical Analysis

Pooled data are presented as mean ± standard error of the mean (SEM) when appropriate. Regression analysis was used to test for a relationship between I_{to1} density and repolarization velocity, plateau height, and action potential duration. Comparisons between groups were made using unpaired Student's *t*-tests. Values of $p < 0.05$ were considered significant.

3. RESULTS

3.1. Stable Cell Lines

Figure 1A shows a schematic of the plasmid, pCGI, that was used to generate the stable cell lines. The use of an internal ribosome entry site allowed easy identification and analysis of the different stable cell lines. There were some interesting differences between HEK293 and CHO-K1 stable cell lines. The first and most dramatic difference was in the number of positive cells within a pooled population of G418 resistant cells with the 76% of the HEK cells expressing GFP levels above background and only 32% of the CHO-K1 cells (Fig. 1B). These positive CHO-K1 cells could be readily selected for by FACS with the resulting population resembling the HEK293 cells both in the percentage of positive cells (Fig. 1B) and the mean fluorescence (Fig. 1D). The reason for this initially lower number of positive cells did not seem to stem from the development of spontaneous resistance as no CHO-K1 cells survived selection following a mock transfection. The inclusion of the ion-channel gene caused a decrease in the average level of expression that was more subtle but consistent no matter which cell line was used (Fig. 1C). CHO-K1 and Hek293 cells also responded differently to cell-to-cell contact. Figure 1D shows that upon reaching confluence, there is no change in the level of fluorescence in HEK293 cells but CHO-K1 cells have a dramatic decrease in the level of expression. Upon splitting the cells, the level of fluorescence returns to the original level suggesting that this decrease is a transient response to contact inhibition.

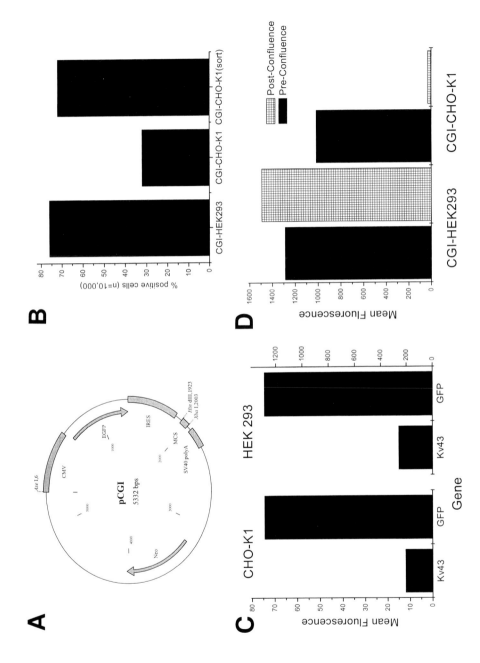

3.2. CHO Cell Line Stably Expressing Kv4.3

The CHO cell line stably expressing Kv4.3 depicted in Fig. 1C was further subcloned by one round of FACS followed by picking individual colonies. As shown in Fig. 2A, mean fluorescence measured by FACS analysis of the three stable CHO-Kv4.3 clones (A-C) clearly exceeded background autofluorescence of nontransfected CHO cells. Clone A was examined by patch-clamp analysis and shown to express robust transient outward currents upon step depolarizations from −100 mV to +40 mV. Figure 2B shows a representative fully inactivating outward current that could be recorded in all cells of the clone used in these experiments ($n = 12$). Mean peak current density at +40 mV, obtained by subtracting the prepulse inactivated current (0 mV prepulse) from the fully primed current (−100 mV prepulse), was 39.9 ± 16.6 pA/pF ($n = 12$) (Fig. 2C).

3.3. Confocal Imaging of Myocytes Fused with CHO Cells Expressing GFP and CD8

To test whether cell fusion of guinea-pig myocytes with CHO cells led only to cytosolic exchange between fused cells or also to a mixture of cell-membrane proteins, myocytes were fused with CHO cells transiently transfected with GFP and CD8. Figure 3A depicts a confocal green-fluorescence image of a typical heterokaryon of a guinea-pig myocyte and CHO cell membrane (cell fixed 5 min after cell fusion). Green fluorescence of the myocyte verified a transfer of cytosolic GFP from the CHO cell to the fused myocyte. Following CD8 visualization using phycoerthyrin labeled anti-CD8 antibodies, red fluorescence of the surface membrane and of t-tubular structures of the myocytes indicated that CD8 from the CHO cell membranes mixed with the surface membranes of the myocytes (cell fixed 2 h after cell fusion) (Fig. 3B). Cell fusion had no obvious effects on myocyte morphology, except at the site of fusion itself.

Fig. 1. Stable cell lines made with pCGI. Map of the plasmid, pCGI (**A**), CMV, cytomegalovirus immediate early promoter; EGFP, coding sequence of the enhanced green fluorescent protein; IRES, polio virus internal ribosome entry site; MCS, multiple cloning site; Neo, the neomycin resistance gene under the control of the SV40 early promoter. Flow cytometrical analysis of cells stably expressing pCGI (**B**), CGI-CHO-K1-S represent the population after sorting for cells exhibiting fluorescence above background. Inclusion of the Kv4.3 coding sequence reduces the level of expression in both cell backgrounds (**C**). Cell-to-cell contact does not affect GFP expression levels from HEK293s but does decrease expression levels form CHO-K1 cells (**D**).

A

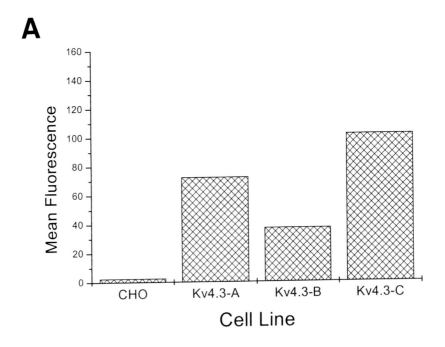

B

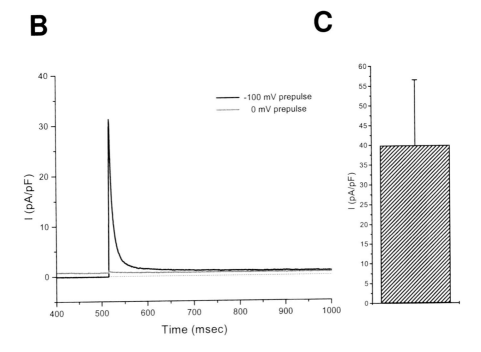

C

3.4. Cell Fusion of Myocytes with Noninfected CHO Cells Has No Effect on Action Potential Morphology

To test the role of I_{to1} on repolarization of cardiomyocytes, freshly isolated guinea-pig myocytes were chosen for cell-fusion experiments, as guinea-pig myocytes physiologically lack transient outward potassium currents. Before attempting to modify the electrophysiology of guinea-pig cells, we needed to confirm that myocytes could be fused with CHO cells without altering the basic electrophysiology. Because GFP fluorescence of stable CHO-Kv4.3 cells was too light to lead to a reliable fluorescence of fused myocytes, stable CHO cells were additionally loaded with calcein-AM. Cell fusion was verified by the obvious transfer of calcein or cytosolic GFP from CHO cells to the cardiomyocytes. Fused myocytes were readily distinguishable from the background autofluorescence of nonfused cells. To test for nonspecific effects of cell fusion on the electrophysiology of guinea-pig myocytes, action potentials were recorded in nonfused cells that had not undergone PEG exposure and compared with recordings obtained in myocytes fused with nontransfected CHO cells. Cell fusion did not produce any appreciable effects on the waveform or duration of action potentials. As shown in Fig. 4, action potential durations measured at 50% and 90% repolarization did not differ significantly in myocytes that had not undergone PEG exposure ($n = 6$) and myocytes fused with nonexpressing CHO cells ($n = 5$).

3.5. Effect of Myocyte/CHO-Kv4.3 Cell Fusion on Action Potential Plateau and Duration

Myocytes fused with CHO-Kv4.3 cells exhibited robust transient outward currents. The density of I_{to1} introduced into guinea-pig myocytes by cell fusion ranged from 1.9 pA/pF to 44.2 pA/pF at +40 mV. Figure 5C,E,G show transient outward currents recorded in three different myocytes fused with CHO-Kv4.3 cells that exhibited different I_{to1} current amplitudes. Mean peak current density was 16.5 ± 2.6 pA/pF at +40 mV ($n = 19$). In myocytes

---

Fig. 2. CHO cell clones stably expressing Kv4.3. Mean fluorescence measured by FACS analysis of four different clones stably expressing Kv4.3 (**A–C**) clearly exceeded background autofluorescence of noninfected CHO cells (A). In CHO-Kv4.3 cells of clone (A) (clone used in these experiments) depolarization to +40 mV from a holding potential of –100 mV elicited a fully inactivating transient outward current (B). Mean peak current density was obtained by subtracting the prepulse inactivated current (0 mV prepulse) from the fully primed current (–100 mV prepulse) ($n = 12$) (C). Reprinted by permission from ref. *36*.

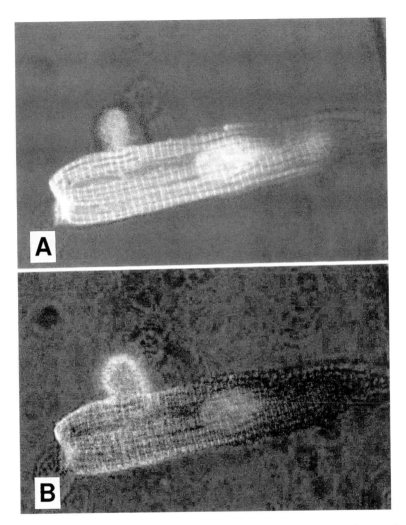

Fig. 3. Confocal images of heterokaryons. CHO cells were transiently transfected with GFP and CD8. After cell fusion cells were fixed and CD8 was visualized with R-phycoerythrin conjugated monoclonal CD8 antibodies. **(A)** Green fluorescence image: green fluorescence of the myocyte indicates transfer of cytosolic GFP from the fused CHO cell. **(B)** Red fluorescence image: red staining of the surface membrane and of t-tubular structures of the myocyte verifies that CD8 from the CHO cell membrane mixed with the membranes of the myocyte. Cell fusion had no obvious effects on myocyte morphology. **(H)** Reprinted by permission from ref. *36.*

fused with nontransfected CHO cells no transient outward currents were recorded (*n* = 5) (Fig. 5A).

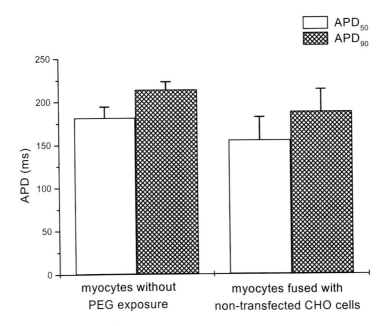

Fig. 4. Action potential duration in control heterokaryons. Action potential durations measured at 50% (APD$_{50}$) and 90% (APD$_{90}$) repolarization were not altered in guinea-pig myocytes fused with nontransfected CHO cells ($n = 5$) compared to myocytes that had not undergone PEG exposure ($n = 6$). Reprinted by permission from ref. *36*.

In all fused myocytes action potentials were obtained. The resting membrane potential in myocytes fused with CHO-Kv4.3 cells (-89.9 ± 1.2 mV; $n = 19$) and nontransfected CHO cells (-88.3 ± 3.0 mV; $n = 5$) were not different. Figure 5D,F,H demonstrate the effect of I$_{to1}$ on repolarization of guinea-pig cardiomyocytes. The introduction of I$_{to1}$ substantially changed the action potential waveform compared with myocytes fused with control CHO cells (Fig. 5B). The modification of the action potential became more pronounced as the amount of I$_{to1}$ increased. Extremely large I$_{to1}$ densities resulted in a spike-like configuration of the action potential reminiscent of that recorded in normal rat ventricular myocytes (Fig. 5H).

The most prominent effect of introduction of I$_{to1}$ into guinea-pig myocytes was depression (hyperpolarization) of the action potential plateau. In most fused myocytes, the whole plateau phase was suppressed; only in one fused myocyte was a small notch and dome obtained (Fig. 5G). To assess the plateau height of the action potential, the voltage during the plateau phase at $d^2V/dt^2 = 0$, i.e., at the transition from phase 1 to phase 2 repolarization was

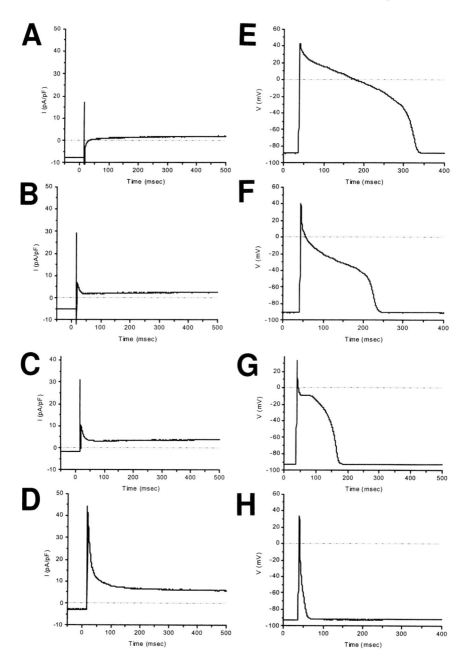

measured as previously reported for human ventricular subendocardial myocytes *(42)*. For the fused myocyte that exhibited the small notch and dome, the maximum plateau voltage after the notch at phase 1 was obtained.

As shown in Fig. 6A, the suppression of the voltage level of the early plateau phase correlated well with the introduced I_{to1} density ($r = -0.90$; $p < 0.0001$).

I_{to1} also decreased the overall action potential duration. As shown in Fig. 6B, the reduction of the action potential duration at 90% repolarization (APD_{90}; $r = -0.65$; $p = 0.0006$) became more pronounced with the amount of the introduced transient outward current. I_{to1} density was not correlated to the maintained outward current measured at the end of a 500 ms depolarization pulse to +20 mV ($r = 0.43$; $p = 0.03$) or +40 mV ($r = 0.39$; $p = 0.11$). Indeed, these were insignificant differences in maintained current between myocytes fused with nonexpressing CHO cells and myocytes fused with CHO-Kv4.3 cells; e.g., mean maintained outward current densities at the end of a 500 ms depolarization pulse to +40 mV equaled 7.6 ± 2.3 pA/pF vs 7.4 ± 0.7 pA/pF, respectively.

4. DISCUSSION

Stable expression of ion-channel genes in a mammalian cell background devoid of most ionic currents makes detailed analysis of the resulting ionic currents straightforward. The use of a dual selection process, G418 resistance and green fluorescence simplified the selection of a clone with the desired characteristic. The reason for the much lower initial expression level in CHO-K1 cells vs HEK293 cells is unclear as is the mechanism by which cell-to-cell contact decreases expression from the CMV promoter. The decreased expression levels obtained with constructs containing ion channels genes may represent decreased mRNA stability owing to the increased size of the transcript or a deleterious effect of the ion-channel protein on cell survival. Owing to the relative ease and efficiency with which CHO-K1 cells can be transfected, it may not be worth the trouble of creating a stable cell

---

Fig. 5. Kv4.3 currents in guinea-pig myocytes. Transient outward currents and action potentials of myocytes fused with CHO-Kv4.3 cells and nontransfected CHO cells ($I_{to1} = 0$ pA/pF). In myocytes fused with nontransfected CHO cells no I_{to1} could be recorded (**A**). Introduction of I_{to1} into guinea-pig myocytes (**C,E,G**) substantially changed the action potential waveform (**D,F,H**) compared to myocytes fused with nontransfected CHO cells (**B**). These changes became more pronounced with increasing densities of transient outward currents, resulting in a suppression of the plateau potential and abbreviation of the overall action potential duration. Introduction of very large I_{to1} densities (G) caused a spike-like action potential. Reprinted by permission from ref. *36*.

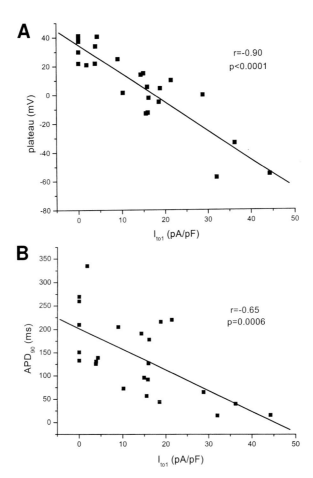

Fig. 6. Effect of I_{to1} on the action potential plateau. The suppression of the voltage of the early plateau phase measured at $d^2V/dt^2 = 0$ (at the transition from early repolarization to final repolarization) correlated well with the introduced I_{to1} density. The action potential duration at 90% repolarization (APD_{90}) **(B)** is plotted vs I_{to1} current density at +40 mV. Reduction of APD_{90} correlated well with I_{to1} density evaluated by regression analysis. Reprinted by permission from ref. *36*.

line vs doing transient transfections. On the other hand, in these experiments, having a stable cell line made for more consistent results.

The preliminary results in cell fusions as well as a review of the literature pointed out a couple of areas where the technique could be modified to suit the cell type of interest. These included the time of PEG treatment, the concentration of PEG used, the density of cells, the temperature of the fusion, inclusion of agents to enhance cell-to-cell contact and the speed with which the PEG is removed. The conditions given in the methods provided the most consistent results in our experiments. As might be expected the process of dehydrating and rehydrating can cause the cell to become refractory to patch clamping experiments. Therefore, the ideal fusion conditions will depend both on fusion efficiency and the quality of the fused cells.

With this technique we have demonstrated that I_{to1} substantially changes the early repolarization phase and leads to an abbreviation of the action potential duration. Previously, the role of I_{to1} in shaping the action potential waveform has been assessed indirectly by either by comparison of I_{to1} densities and action potentials throughout the layers of the myocardial wall (i.e., humans [42,43], dogs [44–46], cats [47], rats [48], and rabbits [49]) or in disease states such as hypertrophy and heart failure (50–52). To further elucidate the role of I_{to1}, I_{to1} has been blocked pharmacologically, knocked out by dominant-negative constructs or artificially introduced into heart failure cells with brief repolarizing current pulses (48,51,53,54). However, K$^+$ channel blockers such as 4-aminopyridine also exhibit nonspecific effects (48), current pulses lack physiological current kinetics, and previous knockout studies were limited by action potential changes during cell culture (53) or adaptive upregulation of other outward currents in transgenic mice (54). Using cell fusion to introduce Kv4.3 in freshly isolated guinea-pig cardiomyocytes to probe the role of I_{to1} on repolarization, we obviated culture-related alterations of the action potential and nonspecific drug effects in the present study.

I_{to1} accelerated the early repolarization velocity and suppressed the voltage level of the plateau phase in guinea-pig myocytes. Both effects became more pronounced as I_{to1} density increased. Therefore, these results support the conclusion that I_{to1} exerts significant effects on early repolarization and plays an important role in setting the voltage of the plateau phase. Previously, reduction of I_{to1} density in tachycardia-induced heart failure of dogs has also been related to observed changes in the plateau height, i.e., an elevation of the plateau voltage in failing canine ventricular myocytes compared to nonfailing control cells (51). In human subendocardial myocytes that exhibit small I_{to1} sizes, the plateau voltage tended to be higher than in subepicardial cells, which have significantly larger I_{to1} densities (42).

The introduction of I_{to1} into guinea-pig myocytes shortened the action potential duration in a dose-dependent manner. Although the rapid inactivation of Kv4.3 makes a direct contribution to the late phase of repolarization unlikely, the observed changes in the action potential duration may be owing to indirect effects on other currents secondary to changes in the early plateau potential (42,55).

Cell fusion has previously been used in embryonic cardiomyocytes and skeletal muscle cells *(26,28–30)*. In the present study we could demonstrate, that heterologous cell fusion is also possible with adult cardiomyocytes without any appreciable effect on cell morphology or viability. Because the space constant of myocardial tissue is much larger (~10×) than the length of an isolated myocyte *(56)*, punctate delivery of current into a myocyte will electrically affect the entire cell. Thus, the observed changes of the action potential waveform of guinea-pig myocytes fused to CHO-Kv4.3 cells would be readily explained even if the Kv4.3 channels remained localized in the CHO cell membrane. Nevertheless, fusion of myocytes with CHO cells transiently expressing GFP and CD8 demonstrated that there is not only prompt cytosolic exchange, but also eventual redistribution of membrane proteins between fused cells. Thus, this technique provides further applications to introduce premade proteins into cardiomyocytes and to study their interaction with the endogenous myocyte membrane.

In summary, the use of GFP greatly simplifies the isolation and characterization of cell lines stably expressing ion-channel genes. These lines are useful both for direct analysis of the expressed protein as well as provide a vector for the delivery of the ion-channel protein. Upon transfer to a primary cell the direct electrical effects can be readily observed. In addition, the rapid mixing of both cytosolic and membrane components may prove useful in assessing downstream modification of the primary cell by the donated protein. With the increasing array of fluorescent proteins, which emit different wavelengths of light, this technique may also be useful in determining spatial relationships between proteins.

ACKNOWLEDGMENTS

This study was supported by grants from the NIH (HL61711 to B.O'R.; P50 HL52370 to E.M.), a Research Career Development Award from the CARE Foundation (to D.C.J.), and a fellowship from the Deutsche Forschungsgemeinschaft (to U.C.H.). E.M. was the recipient of the Michel Mirowski, M.D. Professorship in Cardiology of The Johns Hopkins University.

REFERENCES

1. Hille, B. (1992) *Ionic Channels of Excitable Membranes*, 2nd ed. Sinauer Associates, Sunderland, Mass.
2. Ackerman, M. J. and Clapham, D. E. (1997) Ion channels — basic science and clinical disease. *N Engl J Med* **336(22),** 1575–1586.

3. Hoffman, P. L. and Tabakoff, B. (1994) The role of the NMDA receptor in ethanol withdrawal. *EXS* **71**, 61–70.
4. Nestler, E. J., Berhow, M. T., and Brodkin, E. S. (1996) Molecular mechanisms of drug addiction: adaptations in signal transduction pathways. *Mol. Psychiatry* **1(3)**, 190–199.
5. Sanguinetti, M. C., Jiang, C., Curran, M. E., and Keating, M. T. (1995) A mechanistic link between an inherited and an acquired cardiac arrhythmia: HERG encodes the IKr potassium channel. *Cell* **81(2)**, 299–307.
6. Honig, P. K., Woosley, R. L., Zamani, K., Conner, D. P., and Cantilena, L. R., Jr. (1992) Changes in the pharmacokinetics and electrocardiographic pharmacodynamics of terfenadine with concomitant administration of erythromycin. *Clin. Pharmacol. Ther.* **52(3)**, 231–238.
7. Zhou, J. Y., Potts, J. F., Trimmer, J. S., Agnew, W. S., and Sigworth, F. J. (1991) Multiple gating modes and the effect of modulating factors on the microI sodium channel. *Neuron* **7(5)**, 775–785.
8. Ukomadu, C., Zhou, J., Sigworth, F. J., and Agnew, W. S. (1992) muI Na+ channels expressed transiently in human embryonic kidney cells: biochemical and biophysical properties. *Neuron* **8(4)**, 663–676.
9. Chang, S. Y., Satin, J., and Fozzard, H. A. (1996) Modal behavior of the mu 1 Na+ channel and effects of coexpression of the beta 1-subunit. *Biophys. J.* **70(6)**, 2581–2592.
10. Snyders, D. J., Tamkun, M. M., and Bennett, P. B. (1993) A rapidly activating and slowly inactivating potassium channel cloned from human heart. Functional analysis after stable mammalian cell culture expression. *J. Gen. Physiol.* **101(4)**, 513–543.
11. Ashen, M. D., O'Rourke, B., Kluge, K. A., Johns, D. C., and Tomaselli, G. F. (1995) Inward rectifier K+ channel from human heart and brain: cloning and stable expression in a human cell line. *Am. J. Physiol.* **268(1 Pt 2)**, H506–H511.
12. Chalfie, M., Tu, Y., Euskirchen, G., Ward, W. W., and Prasher, D. C. (1994) Green fluorescent protein as a marker for gene expression. *Science* **263(5148)**, 802–805.
13. Marshall, J., Molloy, R., Moss, G. W., Howe, J. R., and Hughes, T. E. (1995) The jellyfish green fluorescent protein: a new tool for studying ion channel expression and function. *Neuron* **14(2)**, 211–215.
14. Trouet, D., Nilius, B., Voets, T., Droogmans, G., and Eggermont, J. (1997) Use of a bicistronic Gfp-expression vector to characterise ion channels after transfection in mammalian cells. *Pflugers Arch. Eur. J. Physiol.* **434(5)**, 632–638.
15. Kawashima, E., Estoppey, D., Virginio, C., Fahmi, D., Rees, S., Surprenant, A., and North, R. A. (1998) A novel and efficient method for the stable expression of heteromeric ion channels in mammalian cells. *Receptors Channels* **5(2)**, 53–60.
16. Johns, D. C., Marx, R., Mains, R. E., O'Rourke, B., and Marban, E. (1999) Inducible genetic suppression of neuronal excitability. *J. Neurosci.* **19(5)**, 1691–1697.

17. Johns, D. C., Nuss, H. B., and Marban, E. (1997) Suppression of neuronal and cardiac transient outward currents by viral gene transfer of dominant-negative Kv4. 2 constructs. *J. Biol. Chem.* **272(50),** 31,598–31,3603.

18. Johns, D. C., Nuss, H. B., Chiamvimonvat, N., Ramza, B. M., Marban, E., and Lawrence, J. H. (1995) Adenovirus-mediated expression of a voltage-gated potassium channel in vitro (rat cardiac myocytes) and in vivo (rat liver). *J. Clin. Invest.* **95,** 1152–1158.

19. Nuss, H. B., Johns, D. C., Kaab, S., Tomaselli, G. F., Kass, D., Lawrence, J. H., and Marban, E. (1996) Reversal of potassium channel deficiency in cells from failing hearts by adenoviral gene transfer: a prototype for gene therapy for disorders of cardiac excitability and contractility. *Gene Ther.* **3(10),** 900–912.

20. Holt, J. R., Johns, D. C., Wang, S., Chen, Z. Y., Dunn, R. J., Marban, E., and Corey, D. P. (1999) Functional expression of exogenous proteins in mammalian sensory hair cells infected with adenoviral vectors [In Process Citation]. *J. Neurophysiol.* **81(4),** 1881–1888.

21. Ehrengruber, M. U., Lanzrein, M., Xu, Y., Jasek, M. C., Kantor, D. B., Schuman, E. M., et al. (1998) Recombinant adenovirus-mediated expression in nervous system of genes coding for ion channels and other molecules involved in synaptic function. *Methods Enzymol.* **293,** 483–503.

22. Ehrengruber, M. U., Doupnik, C. A., Xu, Y., Garvey, J., Jasek, M. C., Lester, H. A., and Davidson, N. (1997) Activation of heteromeric G protein-gated inward rectifier channels overexpressed by adenovirus gene transfer inhibits the excitability of hippocampal neurons. *Proc. Natl. Acad. Sci. USA* **94,** 7070–7075.

23. Harris, H., Sidebottom, E., Grace, D. M., and Bramwell, M. E. (1969) The expression of genetic information: a study with hybrid animal cells. *J. Cell Sci.* **4(2),** 499–525.

24. Frye, L. D. and Edidin, M. (1970) The rapid intermixing of cell surface antigens after formation of mouse- human heterokaryons. *J. Cell Sci.* **7(2),** 319–335.

25. Okada, Y. (1993) Sendai virus-induced cell fusion. *Methods Enzymol.* **221,** 18–41.

26. Matsuda, R., Noro, N., and Ichimura, T. (1988) Myoblast-mediated fusion-injection: a new technique for introduction of macromolecules specifically into living skeletal muscle cells. *Exp. Cell. Res.* **176(2),** 366–370.

27. Uchida, T. (1988) Introduction of macromolecules into mammalian cells by cell fusion. *Exp. Cell. Res.* **178(1),** 1–17.

28. Goshima, K. and Wakabayashi, S. (1981) Inhibition of ouabain-induced arrhythmias of ouabain-sensitive myocardial cells (quail) by contact with ouabain-resistant cells (mouse) and its mechanism. *J. Mol. Cell Cardiol.* **13(1),** 75–92.

29. Goshima, K., Kaneko, H., Wakabayashi, S., Masuda, A., and Matsui, Y. (1984) Beating activity of heterokaryons between myocardial and non-myocardial cells in culture. *Exp. Cell. Res.* **151(1),** 148–159.

30. Kaprielian, Z., Robinson, S. W., Fambrough, D. M., and Kessler, P. D. (1996) Movement of Ca(2+)-ATPase molecules within the sarcoplasmic/endoplasmic reticulum in skeletal muscle. *J. Cell Sci.* **109(Pt 10),** 2529–2537.

31. Evans, S. M., Tai, L. J., Tan, V. P., Newton, C. B., and Chien, K. R. (1994) Heterokaryons of cardiac myocytes and fibroblasts reveal the lack of dominance of the cardiac muscle phenotype. *Mol. Cell Biol.* **14(6)**, 4269–4279.

32. Ahkong, Q. F., Desmazes, J. P., Georgescauld, D., and Lucy, J. A. (1987) Movements of fluorescent probes in the mechanism of cell fusion induced by poly(ethylene glycol). *J. Cell Sci.* **88(Pt 3)**, 389–398.

33. Deng, Y. P. and Storrie, B. (1988) Animal cell lysosomes rapidly exchange membrane proteins [published erratum appears in *Proc. Natl. Acad. Sci. USA* **86(9)**, 3214]. *Proc. Natl. Acad. Sci. USA* **85(11)**, 3860–3864.

34. Deng, Y. P., Griffiths, G., and Storrie, B. (1991) Comparative behavior of lysosomes and the pre-lysosome compartment (PLC) in in vivo cell fusion experiments. *J. Cell Sci.* **99(Pt 3)**, 571–582.

35. Deng, Y., DeCourcy, K., and Storrie, B. (1992) Intermixing of resident Golgi membrane proteins in rat-hamster polykaryons appears to depend on organelle coalescence. *Eur. J. Cell Biol.* **57(1)**, 1–11.

36. Hoppe, U. C., Johns, D. C., Marban, E., and O'Rourke, B. (1999) Manipulation of cellular excitability by cell fusion: effects of rapid introduction of transient outward K+ current on the guinea pig action potential. *Circ. Res.* **84(8)**, 964–972.

37. Johns, D. C., Nuss, H. B., and Marban, E. (1997) Suppression of neuronal and cardiac transient outward currents by viral gene transfer of dominant-negative Kv4. 2 constructs. *J. Biol. Chem.* **272(50)**, 31,598–31,603.

38. Maniatis, T., Fritsch, E. F., and Sambrook, J. (1989) *Molecular Cloning: A Laboratory Manual*, 2nd ed., Cold Spring Harbor Laboratory, Cold Spring Harbor, NY.

39. Mitra, R. and Morad, M. (1986) Two types of calcium channels in guinea pig ventricular myocytes. *Proc. Natl. Acad. Sci. USA* **83(14)**, 5340–5344.

40. Hamill, O. P., Marty, A., Neher, E., Sakmann, B., and Sigworth, F. J. (1981) Improved patch-clamp techniques for high-resolution current recording from cells and cell-free membrane patches. *Pflügers Arch.* **391(2)**, 85–100.

41. Neher, E. (1992) Correction for liquid junction potentials in patch clamp experiments. *Methods Enzymol.* **207**, 123–131.

42. Näbauer, M., Beuckelmann, D. J., Uberfuhr, P., and Steinbeck, G. (1996) Regional differences in current density and rate-dependent properties of the transient outward current in subepicardial and subendocardial myocytes of human left ventricle. *Circulation* **93(1)**, 168–177.

43. Wettwer, E., Amos, G. J., Posival, H., and Ravens, U. (1994) Transient outward current in human ventricular myocytes of subepicardial and subendocardial origin. *Circ. Res.* **75(3)**, 473–482.

44. Anyukhovsky, E. P., Sosunov, E. A., and Rosen, M. R. (1996) Regional differences in electrophysiological properties of epicardium, midmyocardium, and endocardium, in vitro and in vivo correlations. *Circulation* **94(8)**, 1981–1988.

45. Liu, D. W., Gintant, G. A., and Antzelevitch, C. (1993) Ionic bases for electrophysiological distinctions among epicardial, midmyocardial, and endocardial myocytes from the free wall of the canine left ventricle. *Circ. Res.* **72(3)**, 671–687.

46. Lukas, A. and Antzelevitch, C. (1993) Differences in the electrophysiological response of canine ventricular epicardium and endocardium to ischemia. Role of the transient outward current. *Circulation* **88(6)**, 2903–2915.

47. Furukawa, T., Myerburg, R. J., Furukawa, N., Bassett, A. L., and Kimura, S. (1990) Differences in transient outward currents of feline endocardial and epicardial myocytes. *Circ. Res.* **67(5)**, 1287–1291.

48. Clark, R. B., Bouchard, R. A., Salinas-Stefanon, E., Sanchez-Chapula, J., and Giles, W. R. (1993) Heterogeneity of action potential waveforms and potassium currents in rat ventricle. *Cardiovasc. Res.* **27(10)**, 1795–1799.

49. Fedida, D., Braun, A. P., and Giles, W. R. (1991) Alpha 1-adrenoceptors reduce background K+ current in rabbit ventricular myocytes. *J. Physiol. (Lond.)* **441**, 673–684.

50. Beuckelmann, D. J., Näbauer, M., and Erdmann, E. (1993) Alterations of K+ currents in isolated human ventricular myocytes from patients with terminal heart failure. *Circ. Res.* **73**, 379–385.

51. Kääb, S., Nuss, H. B., Chiamvimonvat, N., O. Rourke, B., Pak, P. H., Kass, D. A., et al. (1996) Ionic mechanism of action potential prolongation in ventricular myocytes from dogs with pacing-induced heart failure. *Circ. Res.* **78(2)**, 262–273.

52. Rozanski, G. J., Xu, Z., Zhang, K., and Patel, K. P. (1998) Altered K+ current of ventricular myocytes in rats with chronic myocardial infarction. *Am. J. Physiol.* **274(1 Pt 2)**, H259–H265.

53. Johns, D. C., Nuss, H. B., and Marban, E. (1997) Suppression of neuronal and cardiac transient outward currents by viral gene transfer of dominant-negative Kv4. 2 constructs. *J. Biol. Chem.* **272**, 31,598–31,603.

54. Barry, D. M., Xu, H., Schuessler, R. B., and Nerbonne, J. M. (1998) Functional knockout of the transient outward current, long-QT syndrome, and cardiac remodeling in mice expressing a dominant-negative Kv4 alpha subunit. *Circ. Res.* **83(5)**, 560–567.

55. Antzelevitch, C., Sicouri, S., Litovsky, S. H., Lukas, A., Krishnan, S. C., Di Diego, J. M., et al. (1991) Heterogeneity within the ventricular wall. Electrophysiology and pharmacology of epicardial, endocardial, and M cells. *Circ. Res.* **69(6)**, 1427–1449.

56. Weidmann, S. (1970) Electrical constants of trabecular muscle from mammalian heart. *J. Physiol. (Lond.)* **210(4)**, 1041–1054.

Part III

FUNCTIONAL ASSAYS IN ION CHANNEL LOCALIZATION

16

Detection of Neurons Expressing Calcium-Permeable AMPA Receptors Using Kainate-Induced Cobalt Uptake

Cristóvão Albuquerque, Holly S. Engelman,
C. Justin Lee, and Amy B. MacDermott

1. INTRODUCTION

α-Amino-3-hydroxy-5-methyl-4-isoxaxole propionic acid (AMPA) receptors are a family of ligand-gated ion channels sensitive to the excitatory neurotransmitter glutamate. Many of these receptors are localized postsynaptically along with other glutamate-sensitive receptors such as N-methyl-D-aspartate (NMDA) receptors. Some AMPA receptors are permeable to Ca^{2+}, whereas all molecular configurations of NMDA receptors studied thus far are permeable to Ca^{2+}. Postsynaptic Ca^{2+} influx through both NMDA receptors and the less well-known Ca^{2+}-permeable AMPA receptors has been shown to mediate long term changes in synaptic strength *(1,2)*. Thus efforts have intensified in recent years to identify which neurons express Ca^{2+}-permeable AMPA receptors to help understand the role of these receptors in nervous system function.

There are four subunits, GluR1–4 or GluRA-D, that contribute to the final configuration of the multimeric AMPA receptors. The GluR2 subunit is subject to RNA editing such that a glutamine within the membrane loop that lines the pore of the channel is replaced by an arginine. This RNA editing happens for over 99% of GluR2 mRNA. When one or more edited GluR2 subunits is included in the AMPA receptor multimeric assembly, that receptor has low permeability to Ca^{2+} *(3)*. When GluR2 is not present, such as

From: *Ion Channel Localization Methods and Protocols*
Edited by: A. Lopatin and C. G. Nichols © Humana Press Inc., Totowa, NJ

when an AMPA receptor is assembled from GluR1 alone, for example, the receptor has comparatively high permeability to Ca^{2+}.

Because the absence, rather than the presence, of a subunit determines the Ca^{2+} permeability of AMPA receptors, it is difficult to use immunocytochemistry or mRNA detection methods to determine when Ca^{2+}-permeable AMPA receptors are expressed by a neuron. This is true because GluR2 protein or mRNA may be expressed by a neuron yet the GluR2 subunit may not incorporate into all of the AMPA receptors functionally expressed on the cell surface. Such a GluR2-expressing neuron would have some AMPA receptors with high Ca^{2+} permeability and some with low Ca^{2+} permeability. A functional assay is the most reliable method for detecting whether Ca^{2+}-permeable AMPA receptors are present on a neuronal surface membrane.

Two channel properties that may be used to functionally identify Ca^{2+}-permeable AMPA receptors are selective ion permeability and channel rectification. Receptor identification sensitivity is improved when one or both of these properties are studied together with specific combinations of receptor agonists and antagonists. Ca^{2+}-permeable AMPA receptors are not only permeable to Ca^{2+}, they are also permeable to Na^+, K^+, Mg^{2+}, and Co^{2+}, among other ions. Although strong permeability to Co^{2+} is not entirely unique among known ligand-gated or voltage-gated Ca^{2+} permeable ion channels, neither is it common. Thus, Co^{2+} entry through agonist-activated Ca^{2+}-permeable AMPA receptors has proved to be a relatively selective way of identifying neurons expressing Ca^{2+}-permeable AMPA receptors when performed together with careful receptor pharmacology. This technique was first demonstrated by Pruss et al. *(4)* and has been subsequently widely applied. We will provide details of the technique here, for application with cultured neurons and with brain or spinal cord slices.

2. MATERIALS AND METHODS

2.1. Overview of the Technique with General Considerations

2.1.1. Summary of Methods

Neurons expressing Ca^{2+}-permeable AMPA receptors are loaded with Co^{2+} by exposing them for a few minutes to a nondesensitizing agonist, such as kainate, while bathing in a Co^{2+}-containing solution. Following this Co^{2+} loading procedure, the cells are washed in the presence of the divalent cation chelator, ethylenediaminetetraacetic acid (EDTA), to help remove extracellular Co^{2+}. After removing the extracellular Co^{2+}, the cells are briefly exposed to ammonium sulfide to precipitate the intracellular Co^{2+} by forming CoS. After this step, the cells are fixed and, if required, the appropriate procedure for immuno-identification of desired neuronal epitopes is performed. Afterwards, the CoS precipitate is enhanced with silver intensification *(5)*.

2.1.2. Pharmacology

Extensive pharmacological testing should be used to make certain that the route by which Co^{2+} enters the neurons under study is through Ca^{2+}-permeable AMPA receptors. In addition, we have found that it is important to include at least one control with receptor antagonists in each set of agonist-induced Co^{2+} uptake experiments to monitor whether Co^{2+} loading is receptor-mediated for each experiment and not owing to some technical or conflicting biological problem. Alternative possible causes for Co^{2+} loading that would not be blocked by non-NMDA receptor antagonists include heavy-metal ion transporters *(6)* and poor cell health allowing nonselective Co^{2+} leak. Including CNQX or another non-NMDA receptor antagonist together with kainate in a parallel preparation helps ensure that the Co^{2+} loading induced by kainate is blockable.

Other useful control pharmacology to show that the route of Co^{2+} entry is via Ca^{2+}-permeable AMPA receptors includes use of AMPA receptor selective antagonists such as GYKI 52466 *(7)* and Ca^{2+} permeable non-NMDA receptor blockers such as Joro spider toxin (JsTx) or other polyamines *(8)*. Block of kainate-induced agonist loading by GYKI 52466 rules out kainate receptors as a possible route of Co^{2+} entry and good block with JsTx means that only the Ca^{2+} permeable form of the AMPA receptor is involved in Co^{2+} loading. Because JsTx and the other polyamines block Ca^{2+}-permeable AMPA receptors in a use-dependent manner, we apply JsTx together with kainate prior to the kainate-induced Co^{2+} loading step (*see* Section 2.2.2. for details). Other useful controls include agonists for other Ca^{2+} permeable receptors that might be present including NMDA for NMDA receptors, nicotine for nicotinic ACh receptors, m-chlorophenylbiguanide for $5HT_3$ receptors, and ATP or ATPγS for P2X receptors. Lack of Co^{2+} loading in the presence of these agonists helps exclude the possibility that the kainate effect was indirect owing to kainate-induced release of transmitters that in turn acted on these receptors to induce Co^{2+} loading. None of these receptors have been shown to mediate Co^{2+} loading (but not all have been tested).

2.1.3. Considerations for Cobalt-Loading Bath Solutions

Kainate is well known as an excitotoxin for neurons. Thus, bath conditions should be chosen that minimize the negative impact of prolonged exposure to kainate. Use of a low Na^+, low Ca^{2+} bath helps minimize both Na^+ and Ca^{2+} loading of neurons in kainate *(4)*. We recommend a HEPES-buffered salt solution for use with cultured neurons and a bicarbonate-buffered Krebs solution for use with acutely prepared slices of brain or spinal cord tissue. It should be noted that the salt of bicarbonate and Co^{2+} is insoluble, and care must be taken, therefore, to prevent the precipitation of the Co^{2+}. It is possible to dissolve 1.5 mM Co^{2+} together with 0.5 mM Ca^{2+} in a bicarbonate buffered solution.

2.2. Specific Methods for Kainate-Induced Cobalt Loading with Slices of Brain and Spinal Cord

2.2.1. Solutions for Cobalt Loading of Slices

Bicarbonate-buffered Krebs solution is used for allowing slices to recover after their initial preparation and for recovery from periods of prolonged drug application. The Krebs solution is: 125 mM NaCl, 2.5 mM KCl, 26 mM NaHCO$_3$, 1.25 mM NaH$_2$PO$_4$, 25 mM glucose, 2 mM CaCl$_2$, 1 mM MgCl$_2$ bubbled with 95% O$_2$/5% CO$_2$.

The solution in which the Co^{2+} uptake experiments are performed is called the uptake Krebs. As described earlier, uptake Krebs is a low sodium, low calcium Krebs with: 50 mM NaCl, 2.5 mM KCl, 26 mM NaHCO$_3$, 1.25 mM NaH$_2$PO$_4$, 25 mM glucose, 0.5 mM CaCl$_2$, 2 mM MgCl$_2$, and 0.5 μM TTX bubbled at room temperature with 95% O$_2$/5% CO$_2$. Either 135 mM sucrose or 80 mM NMDG (pH adjusted with HCl) is added to adjust for the low sodium *(9)*. CoCl$_2$ is added to well-bubbled uptake Krebs immediately before use to prevent Co^{2+} precipitation with bicarbonate.

The wash solution is divalent cation-free Krebs: 125 mM NaCl, 2.5 mM KCl, 26 mM NaHCO$_3$, 1.25 mM NaH$_2$PO$_4$, 25 mM glucose, and 5 mM EDTA (pH adjusted with NaOH).

The ammonium sulfide solution is 0.12% (NH$_4$)$_2$S in uptake Krebs. This is diluted immediately before use from a 20% stock solution. We purchase the stock solution in small (25-mL) bottles (Aldrich), as (NH$_4$)$_2$S oxidizes in contact with air. This solution should be used in a chemical fume hood.

The blocking solution for silver intensification is 2% sodium tungstate in distilled water.

The developer for silver intensification consists of 1 part 5% sodium tungstate, 8 parts AgNO$_3$ solution, and 1 part 0.25% ascorbic acid. The AgNO$_3$ solution is 355 mL distilled water, 15 mL 1% Triton X-100, 1.5 g sodium acetate·3H$_2$O, 30 mL glacial acetic acid, and 0.5 g silver nitrate *(10)*. The tungstate and AgNO$_3$ solutions are stable for weeks to months. The AgNO$_3$ solution is light-sensitive, and should be kept in a dark bottle. The ascorbic acid solution should be prepared within 30 min of use. The three components of the developer should be mixed immediately before use.

2.2.2. Agonist-Induced Cobalt Loading

Slices of brain *(4)* or spinal cord *(9)* are prepared in the usual way and allowed to recover at 37°C in Krebs bubbled with 95% O$_2$/5% CO$_2$. Following a recovery period of at least 1 h, slices are transferred into the uptake Krebs for 15 min at room temperature. For subsequent stimulation of Co^{2+} loading, the above solutions are replaced with bubbled uptake Krebs containing 250 μM kainate and 1.5 mM $CoCl_2$. For antagonist controls, the uptake Krebs may also contain 50 μM CNQX, 100 μM GYKI 52466, or 100 μM APV. Note that CNQX and APV are competitive antagonists of non-NMDA and NMDA receptors, respectively, so if the concentration of kainate is increased, the concentration of antagonist must be increased. When using JsTx, the slices are pretreated with 5–10 μM JsTx together with 250 μM kainate in uptake Krebs for 15 min and then exposed to the uptake Krebs containing kainate and Co^{2+}. Parallel control slices are also pretreated with 250 μM kainate in uptake Krebs before the Co^{2+} loading. The slices are incubated in these solutions at room temperature for 20 min following which the stimulation solution is replaced with divalent-free Krebs for 10 min. The slices are then rinsed in normal Krebs and incubated in a 0.12% solution of $(NH_4)_2S$ in normal Krebs for 5–6 min. After another rinse in normal Krebs, the slices are fixed in cold 4% paraformaldehyde in 0.1 M phosphate buffer overnight at 4°C. The slices are rinsed the next day in 0.1 M phosphate buffer, then put into to a solution of 30% sucrose in 0.1 M phosphate buffer until they sink. They may then be mounted with OCT for cryostat sectioning.

The sections made from the slices are exposed to the silver intensification process to darken the CoS reaction product using the method of Davis *(10)*. After the sections have dried, they are incubated in a 2% solution of sodium tungstate for 10 min, followed by 15–20 min in developer. Control and experimental sections are incubated in parallel for the same amounts of time. They are rinsed one last time in 2% sodium tungstate and then mounted in either 50% glycerol/50% PBS, Gel/Mount, or 2.5% DABCO in 90% glycerol/10% PBS for slides containing Cy3 labeled fluorescent antibodies, or ProLong Antifade for slides containing Alexa-488 conjugated secondary antibodies *(see* below). An example of two spinal-cord sections prepared in this manner are shown in Fig. 1. In this example, the section on the left was prepared in uptake Krebs with 1.5 mM $CoCl_2$ and 250 μM kainate while the one on the right in uptake Krebs with 1.5 mM $CoCl_2$, 250 μM kainate and 100 μM GYKI 53655, an AMPA receptor antagonist.

2.3. Specific Methods for Kainate-Induced Cobalt Loading for Neurons in Tissue Culture

2.3.1. Solutions for Cobalt Loading of Cultured Neurons

The HEPES uptake solution is used to wash and stimulate cells. It is HEPES based and has low Na^+ and low Ca^{2+} to minimize kainate-induced

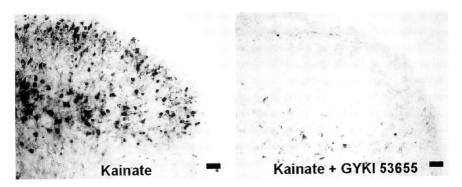

Fig. 1. Kainate-induced cobalt loading of neurons in the dorsal horn of a P10 rat spinal cord slice is shown. Slices were treated with 1.5 mM Co^{2+} and 250 µM kainate (left) or 250 µM kainate plus 100 mM GYKI 53655 (right). Scale bars are 40 µm. (Adapted with permission from ref. 9).

Na^+ and Ca^{2+} uptake. The HEPES uptake solution contains: 139 mM sucrose, 57 mM NaCl, 5 mM KCl, 2 mM $MgCl_2$, 1 mM $CaCl_2$, 12 mM glucose, 10 mM HEPES, pH 7.6 with NaOH.

The EDTA wash solution is the HEPES uptake solution without divalents and with 5 mM EDTA added.

2.3.2. Agonist-Induced Cobalt Loading of Neurons in Tissue Culture

Cultures should be washed once with the HEPES uptake solution, then incubated at room temperature with 250 µM kainate and 5 mM $CoCl_2$ in HEPES uptake solution for 20 min. This is followed by wash with EDTA wash solution, then with HEPES uptake solution. Thereafter, the preparation of cells is incubated in a 0.12% solution of ammonium sulfide in HEPES uptake solution for 5 min. The cells are then washed and fixed for 10–30 min in 4% paraformaldehyde in PBS. If necessary, 4% sucrose may be added to the fixative to help preserve morphology. Finally, the CoS precipitate is silver-intensified according to Davis *(10)*, as described for slices. The progress of the silver intensification should be followed under the microscope in order to optimize the time of development. Again, it must be stressed that the ascorbic acid solution must be made within 30 min, and the developer mixed immediately before use. After stopping the development by washing with the 2% sodium tungstate solution, the coverslips with cells are dipped in double-distilled water to remove excess salts, then mounted in Aquamount (Lerner Laboratories, Pittsburgh, PA) plus 50% glycerol. After removing the excess of mounting solution, they are sealed with nail polish.

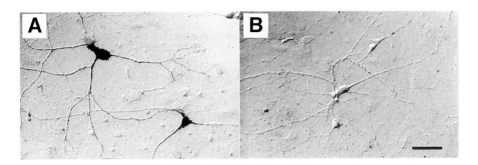

Fig. 2. GYKI 53655 (100 μ*M*) potently blocks kainate-induced cobalt loading in these cultured dorsal horn neurons indicating AMPA receptor involvement. Methods as in text. Scalebar, 50 μm.

Pharmacological controls for kainate-induced Co^{2+} loading with cultured neurons are similar to those used for slices. Figure 2 shows kainate-induced Co^{2+} loading in dissociated rat dorsal horn neurons in the left panel and good block of that loading when it was performed in the presence of 100 μ*M* GYKI 53655, a selective AMPA receptor antagonist, in the right panel. When using JsTx with cultured neurons, either uptake solution or a 0 Na^+, 0 Ca^{2+} solution: 155 m*M* NMDG, 144 m*M* HCl, 20 m*M* CsCl, 0.02 m*M* $CaCl_2$, 10 m*M* HEPES, 5.5 m*M* glucose, pH 7.3, 317 mOsm, adjusted with sucrose *(11)*; may be used for the pretreatment with JsTx and kainate. Specifically, the cultures are preincubated with 5–10 μ*M* JsTx plus 100–250 μ*M* kainate for 4–5 min, immediately followed by the kainate-induced Co^{2+} loading. Parallel control cultures without JsTx are incubated in 0 Na^+ 0 Ca^{2+} solution with kainate prior to Co^{2+} uptake *(5)*. The 0 Na^+ 0 Ca^{2+} solution helps to prevent the neuritic blebbing that is observed in Ca^{2+}-permeable AMPA receptor-positive cells subjected to this protocol. However, while using low Ca^{2+} solutions prevents neuritic blebbing, it also causes retraction of the underlying astrocytic layer.

3. LABELING FOR OTHER NEURONAL CHARACTERISTICS

3.1. Double Labeling Using Immunocytochemistry and Co^{2+} Staining

When combining immunocytochemistry with Co^{2+} staining, the preparation is stimulated in the presence of Co^{2+}, then washed and treated with ammonium sulfide, then fixed. After that, immunocytochemistry can be per-

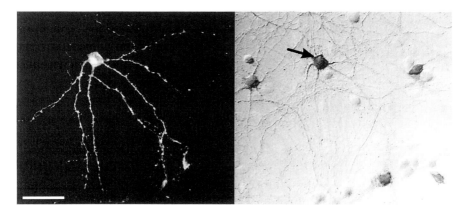

Fig. 3. Ca^{2+}-permeable AMPA receptors are expressed by some dorsal horn neurons also expressing the substance P-sensitive, NK1 receptor. On the left is a microscopic field from a dorsal horn culture showing a neuron expressing NK1-like immunoreactivity. On the right is a differential interference contrast picture of the same field after silver enhancement of cobalt uptake. Arrow indicates cell positive for both NK1-LI and cobalt. Scalebar, 50 µm.

formed either before *(5,9)* or after *(4)* silver intensification of the Co^{2+} staining. The problem with the second choice is that the silver deposits tend to obscure the signal from the immunocytochemistry if the antigen is intracellular, making it more difficult to distinguish double-positive cells. Therefore, we perform the complete immunocytochemical assay, using either fluorophore- or enzyme-coupled secondary antibodies, record images of random fields, and then perform the silver intensification, and re-record images of the previously examined fields (Fig. 3). Our protocols are detailed below (after refs. *5,9*).

3.1.1. Immunocytochemistry in Slices

Primary antibodies are diluted in PBS with 0.1% Triton X-100, required if intracellular epitope is involved, and 1% normal serum. All serum is from the same species as the host that generated the secondary antibody. Sections are first incubated in a blocking solution of 10% normal serum in PBS with 0.1% Triton X-100. Primary antibody solution is applied overnight at 4°C or for 2 h at room temperature. For negative controls, parallel sections are incubated in the same solutions lacking primary antibody. Sections are rinsed, then incubated in fluorophore-coupled secondary antisera appropriately diluted in PBS plus Triton X-100 and 1% normal serum. For sequential immunofluorescence and Co^{2+} staining, sections are coverslipped with a temporary mounting medium, consisting of 50% glycerol in PBS, before silver intensification. The slides are then taken to the microscope for image acquisition. After that, the coverslips are removed, by immersing the slides in PBS, and the sections are then treated for silver intensification as described. The previously imaged fields are then located and imaged again.

3.1.2. Immunocytochemistry of Cell Cultures

Cultured neurons are fixed for 15 min with 4% paraformaldehyde in PBS plus 4% sucrose. In some instances, such as for the monoclonal antibody (MAb) anti-GABA MAB316 *(12)*, 0.0025–0.005% glutaraldehyde must be added to the fixative, in order to make the epitope recognizable by the antibody. These glutaraldehyde concentrations are enough to provide good antigenicity without eliciting significant autofluorescence. However, it should be noted that even low concentrations of glutaraldehyde might produce false-positives with the silver intensification. Therefore, we do not recommend that antibodies requiring glutaraldehyde fixation be used together with Co^{2+} staining. After fixation, the cultures are incubated for 30 min to 2 h with the appropriate concentration of primary antibody, in PBS plus 0.1% (or 0.5%) Triton X-100, at room temperature. After careful wash, the cells are treated either with the LSAB peroxidase kit (DAKO, Carpinteria, CA), or with fluorophore-coupled secondary antibodies. The LSAB kit is used according to the instructions of the manufacturer (a 20-min development time was usually required for optimum staining), except that the hydrogen peroxide incubation must be eliminated, because it interferes with the Co^{2+} staining. No increased background was observed in the absence of primary antibody because of this modification of the original protocol. Fluorophore-coupled secondary antisera are added for 30 min at room temperature and then the cells are washed.

After this step, the coverslips are mounted in a perfusion chamber with PBS to maintain a constant orientation. Images of sequentially located fields may be acquired with videomicroscopy or with standard photographic techniques, using a water-immersion objective. The coordinates of each field are recorded from the stage verniers. The Co^{2+} staining is then silver-enhanced as described, the fields previously recorded are found again from the coordinates, and new pictures of the same fields are taken for comparison.

4. TROUBLESHOOTING

The Co^{2+} staining technique we present here is fairly straightforward. Problems, if they arise, will usually be owing to the use of solutions that are not fresh enough. First and foremost, one must remember to always mix the developer immediately before use, and to prepare the ascorbic acid solution within about 30 min of use. If the technique stops working, the $AgNO_3$ solution is the prime suspect, and should be made fresh again. The $(NH_4)_2S$ stock solution might also be to blame for lack of staining; $(NH_4)_2S$ oxidizes in contact with air and eventually the concentration in the stock solution might be too low to produce significant amounts of CoS. One way to tell whether this solution is the culprit is to look at the preparation immediately after the $(NH_4)_2S$ treatment. Usually the CoS deposit can be detected as a yellow-gray coloring. Alternatively, the color or the stock solution itself provides a rough indication of aging. When new, the 20% $(NH_4)_2S$ solution we purchase from Aldrich is almost clear; months after being removed from its sealed package, it becomes strongly yellow.

Another potential problem is the false-positive staining, or staining that is observed in the absence of agonist or in the presence of antagonist. In this case, the problem tends to be that the washing step after incubation with Co^{2+} was insufficient. Using an EDTA-containing solution for washing usually helps solving this problem.

5. POSITIVE CONTROL FOR COBALT STAINING

The multispecific ionophore lasalocid (X537A, Sigma, St. Louis, MO) provides a pathway for Co^{2+} to enter a cell *(13)* and, therefore, can be used as a positive control for the Co^{2+} staining techniques. We used lasalocid to control for the possibility that calretinin or calbindin, by chelating Co^{2+}, made it undetectable by our staining techniques *(5)*. We compared cultures stimulated with kainate in the presence of 5 m*M* $CoCl_2$ with sister cultures treated for the same time with 40 μ*M* lasalocid and 5 m*M* $CoCl_2$. In the kainate-treated cultures, only a subpopulation of neurons was stained while in the lasalocid-treated cultures, all cells, including the underlying glia, were stained. Although the degree of staining, or darkness, varied among kainate-treated neurons, lasalocid treatment caused all cells to be comparably stained.

6. TWO-COLOR METHOD
FOR THE SIMULTANEOUS DETECTION
OF COBALT AND NICKEL UPTAKE

An alternative to the Co^{2+} detection method just presented is the rubeanic acid method, first described by Quicke and Brace *(14)*. This method employs the spot-test reagent rubeanic acid (dithio-oxamide) and has the advantage of allowing the simultaneous detection of two, or even three different heavy-metal entry pathways, with each metal forming a precipitate of different color. In order to use it to detect multiple heavy-metal-permeable pathways, the preparation must be sequentially incubated with the appropriate metal-agonist combination, with careful washes between successive incubations. This is necessary, because a pathway permeable to one heavy-metal ion is frequently permeable to others as well. A saturated solution of rubeanic acid in 70% ethanol is then applied to the preparation immediately after washing the stimulation solution. In a matter of seconds to minutes, depending on the thickness of the preparation, a colored precipitate will form. This precipitate will be yellow to orange for Co^{2+}; gray to blue-black for Ni^{2+}; and bright red to purple when those two ions are co-precipitated. Cupric ion (Cu^{2+}) will form a green precipitate. Another advantage of this method is that it dispenses with the highly toxic $(NH_4)_2S$ solution *(14)*. This method has been reported to be amenable to silver intensification using hydroquinone as the reducing agent *(15)* but, to our knowledge, the Davis technique *(10)* has not been successfully employed with it.

7. FLUORESCENT INDICATORS FOR COBALT UPTAKE

Co^{2+} uptake can be studied on a cell-by-cell basis with the use of Ca^{2+}-sensitive fluorescent dyes, such as fura-2 *(4)*. Co^{2+} quenches the fluorescence of fura-2 *(16)*, and the rate of quenching can be used as a comparative measure of the permeability of each cell to Co^{2+}. In our experiments, this method is a more sensitive measure of Co^{2+} entry than cobalt staining, but is considerably more time-consuming for performing population screens. Furthermore, some fluorescent dye quenching can be obtained with agonists that cause no detectable Co^{2+} staining with the cobalt staining method presented earlier.

8. CONCLUSIONS

Co^{2+} uptake provides an useful method for the functional detection of some Ca^{2+}-permeable pathways. In particular, it is especially useful for detecting the presence of Ca^{2+}-permeable AMPA receptors in populations of neurons where Ca^{2+}-permeable AMPA receptors might be co-expressed with Ca^{2+}-impermeable AMPA receptors. This technique has the power of allowing the analysis of entire populations of cells at one time, and of being amenable to simultaneous use with other staining techniques, such as immunocytochemistry.

ACKNOWLEDGMENTS

The development of these techniques and some of the work described were supported by NIH-NS29797 and the Christopher Reeve Paralysis Foundation. We thank Dr. John Koester for suggesting the rubeanic acid two-color method.

REFERENCES

1. Bliss T. V. and Collingridge G. L. (1993) A synaptic model of memory: long-term potentiation in the hippocampus. *Nature* **361,** 31–39.
2. Mahanty, N. K. and Sah, P. (1998) Calcium-permeable AMPA receptors mediate long-term potentiation in interneurons in the amygdala. *Nature* **394,** 683–687.
3. Jonas, P. and Burnashev, N. (1995) Molecular mechanisms controlling calcium entry through AMPA-type glutamate receptor channels. *Neuron* **15,** 987–990.
4. Pruss, R. M., Akeson, R. L., Racke, M. M., and Wilburn, J. L. (1991) Agonist-activated cobalt uptake identifies divalent cation-permeable kainate receptors on neurons and glial cells. *Neuron* **7,** 509–518.
5. Albuquerque, C., Lee, C. J., Jackson, A. C., and MacDermott, A. B. (1999) Subpopulations of GABAergic and non-GABAergic rat dorsal horn neurons express Ca2+-permeable AMPA receptors. *Eur. J. Neurosci.* **11,** 2758–2766.
6. Gunshin, H., Mackenzie, B., Berger, U. V., Gunshin, Y., Romero, M. F., Boron, W. F., Nussberger, S., Gollan, J. L., and Hediger, M. A. (1997) Cloning and characterization of a mammalian proton-coupled metal-ion transporter. *Nature* **388,** 482–488.
7. Wilding, T. J. and Huettner, J. E. (1995) Differential antagonism of alpha-amino-3-hydroxy-5-methyl-4-isoxazolepropionic acid-preferring and kainate-preferring receptors by 2,3-benzodiazepines. *Mol. Pharmacol.* **47,** 582–587.
8. Washburn, M. S. and Dingledine, R. (1996) Block of alpha-amino-3-hydroxy-5-methyl-4-isoxazolepropionic acid (AMPA) receptors by polyamines and polyamine toxins. *J. Pharmacol. Exp. Ther.* **278,** 669–678.
9. Engelman, H. S., Allen, T. B., and MacDermott, A. B. (1999) The distribution of neurons expressing calcium-permeable AMPA receptors in the superficial laminae of the spinal cord dorsal horn. *J. Neurosci.* **19,** 2081–2089.
10. Davis, N. T. (1982) Improved methods for cobalt filling and silver intensification of insect motor neurons. *Stain Technol.* **57,** 239–244.
11. Gu, J. G., Albuquerque, C., Lee, C. J., and MacDermott, A. B. (1996) Synaptic strengthening through activation of Ca^{2+}-permeable AMPA receptors. *Nature* **381,** 793–796.
12. Szabat, E., Soinila, S., Häppölä, O., Linnala, A., and Virtanen, I. (1992) A new monoclonal antibody against the GABA-protein conjugate shows immunoreactivity in sensory neurons of the rat. *Neuroscience* **47,** 409–420.

13. Homan, R. and Eisenberg, M. (1985) A fluorescence quenching technique for the measurement of paramagnetic ion concentrations at the membrane/water interface. Intrinsic and X537A-mediated cobalt fluxes across lipid bilayer membranes. *Biochim. Biophys. Acta* **812,** 485–492.
14. Quicke, D. L. J. and Brace, R. C. (1979) Differential staining of cobalt- and nickel-filled neurones using rubeanic acid. *J. Microsc.* **115,** 161–163.
15. Quicke, D. L. J., Brace, R. C., and Kirby, P. (1980) Intensification of nickel- and cobalt-filled neurone profiles following differential staining by rubeanic acid. *J. Microsc.* **119,** 267–272.
16. Kwan, C. Y. and Putney, J. W., Jr. (1990) Uptake and intracellular sequestration of divalent cations in resting and methacholine-stimulated mouse lacrimal acinar cells: Dissociation by Sr^{2+} and Ba^{2+} of agonist-stimulated divalent cation entry from the refilling of the agonist-sensitive intracellular pool. *J. Biol. Chem.* **265,** 678–684.

17

Crystallization Technique for Localizing Ion Channels in Living Cells

Anatoli N. Lopatin, Elena N. Makhina, and Colin G. Nichols

1. INTRODUCTION

A detailed mechanistic understanding of ion-channel function has been achieved over the last 40 years, propelled in the last 15 years by advances in patch-clamp technology and most recently by determination of channel structures and their manipulation. From the pharmacological perspective, perhaps as important as knowing how channels work, is knowing where they are—both where in tissues, and ultimately, where in individual cells. Because ion channels are integral membrane proteins, their localization can be studied using established general approaches. Immunofluorescent labeling has been widely used to map cloned Ca^{2+} *(1)*, Na^+*(2)*, and K^+ *(3)* channels, for which antibodies have been raised against the channel protein. Different variations of channel immunolabeling, including immunogold *(4)* (Na^+ channels) or radiolabel staining are available in this arsenal. A less general but specific technique commonly used with ion channels is to use high-affinity toxins, either fluorescently or radioactively labeled, that specifically bind to the channel pore or regulatory subunits. Among these are scorpion toxins to map Na^+ channels *(5)*, Ω-conotoxin to map Ca^{2+} channels *(6)*, α-dendrotoxin to map voltage-gated channels *(7)* and α-bungarotoxin *(8)* to map nicotinic ACh receptors. Such techniques, in addition to being expensive and time consuming, generally require tissue fixation, and are not amenable to living cells. Green fluorescent protein (GFP) *(9)* based technology is now revolutionizing the localization of proteins, including ion chan-

From: *Ion Channel Localization Methods and Protocols*
Edited by: A. Lopatin and C. G. Nichols © Humana Press Inc., Totowa, NJ

nels (*see* Part 2 of this book). Attaching GFP to N or C termini of the protein of interest permits visualization in living or fixed preparations, generally without significantly affecting channel function.

All the above techniques, including GFP-tagging, label proteins, not functional channels. Given that nonfunctional channel proteins may be the most abundant species in many cases, if it is the localization of channel function that is desired, other techniques are required. To localize channel function we must obtain an indication of ion flow through channels. The most direct way to localize channels on cell membranes is by analyzing currents in membrane patches, and scanning the surface of the cell. "Tight-seal" patch-clamp scanning is a particularly laborious means of detecting surface localization *(10)*, and in many cases, the cell is destroyed after the first seal has been made.

To circumvent these problems, we are developing a novel "crystallization method" to localize ion-channel function on the surface of individual cells as well as identifying cells carrying specific ion channels in multicellular preparations. The general idea of this approach has already been successfully implemented in the past to localize cells expressing kainate receptors *(11)* (*see* also Chapter 16 in this book). In our particular approach, thallium ions flowing through potassium channels meet specific anions on the other side of the membrane with which they generate an insoluble precipitate, forming visible crystals. In principle, by appropriate choice of ion combinations, this method may be applicable to other ion-selective channels, and to any cell type.

2. MATERIALS AND METHODS

2.1. Expression of K^+ Channels in Xenopus Oocytes

Stage V-VI oocytes were surgically isolated from adult female *Xenopus* using tricaine anesthesia (1 g/L). Oocytes were defolliculated by 1–1.5 h treatment with 1–2 mg/mL collagenase (Sigma Type 1A, Sigma Chemical, St. Louis, MO) in zero Ca^{2+} ND96 (below), with slow continuous rocking in a 50 mL tube with ~20 mL ND96 solution. Two to 24 h after defolliculation, oocytes were pressure-injected with ~50 nl of 1–100 ng/µL in vitro transcribed cRNA encoding for a specific K^+ channel. Oocytes were kept in ND96 supplemented with 1.8 mM Ca^{2+}, penicillin (100 U/mL) and streptomycin (100 µg/mL) for 1–2 d prior to experimentation.

2.2. Loading Xenopus Oocytes with Bromide

Xenopus oocytes expressing K^+ channels (IRK1 = Kir2.1, HRK1 = Kir2.3, ROMK1 = Kir1.1 and DRK1 = Kv2.1) were pressure injected (about 10% of oocyte volume; ~100 nL) with 30 or 300 mM potassium bromide (KBr dissolved in water) to give a final internal concentration of ~3 or 30 mM at least 10 min prior to exposure to thallium containing solution. Oocytes were then kept in ND96 solution containing 3 or 30 mM KBr to compensate for diffusion of Br$^-$ ions out of oocytes if they were to be used later than 10 min after Br$^-$ injection.

2.3. Electrophysiology

Ionic currents were studied by standard two-microelectrode voltage-clamp technique using an OC-725 voltage-clamp amplifier (Warner Instruments). Microelectrodes were pulled from thin-walled capillary glass (WPI Inc., New Haven, CT) on a horizontal puller (Sutter Instrument, Co., Novato, CA). Tips were mechanically broken against a small bead of glass under microscope control, to bring electrode resistance to 0.5–2 MΩ when filled with 3 M KCl solution. PClamp software and a Digidata 1200 converter were used to generate voltage pulses and collect data. Oocytes expressing Kir channels and having resting potential less then –80 mV in low K$^+$ ND96 solution were discarded.

When working with thallium, bromide, and chloride ions were excluded from the bath solution to prevent extracellular precipitation of TlBr or TlCl. KD98 (Cl$^-$ containing) bath solution was completely exchanged for KN98 (NO$_3^-$ containing) solution before applying thallium containing solution (NT100). Standard Ag/AgCl grounding electrodes were bathed first in 3 M KCl and then connected to the bath using 3 M KCl agar bridge followed by 3 M NaNO$_3$ agar bridge. Glass microelectrodes were filled with 3 M NaNO$_3$.

2.4. Image Handling

Photo images of oocytes were obtained using an Olympus OM-2 camera attached to a dissecting microscope (Nikon SMZ–1B, Japan). Photo-prints were then digitized and imported to CorelDraw 5.0–6.0 graphics package for presentation. Confocal images of oocytes were obtained using a Biorad MR 1000 confocal microscope by illuminating oocytes with 548 nm yellow light from an argon laser and capturing reflection from TlBr crystals. Details of the chamber used for imaging can be found in Fig. 4. Image Tool (UTHSCSA, V-1.27) and CorelDraw PhotoPaint software were used for image analysis and presentation.

2.5. Solutions

NT100: 100 mM TlNO$_3$, 1 mM Mg(OH)$_2$, 5 mM Na·HEPES, pH ~7.4, with NaOH. This is standard solution for application of thallium.

KN 98: 98 m*M* KNO$_3$, 1 m*M* Mg(OH)$_2$, 5 m*M* K·HEPES, pH ~7.4 with KOH. Before application of NT100 Cl⁻ or traces of Br⁻ ions are carefully washed out with KN98 solution.

ND 96: 96 m*M* NaCl, 2 m*M* KCl, 1 m*M* MgCl$_2$, 5 m*M* Na·HEPES, pH~7.5. This is standard solution for oocytes incubation.

3. CRYSTALIZATION METHOD FOR K⁺ CHANNEL LOCALIZATION

3.1. General Approach

Only one picoamp (pA) of ionic current corresponds to a flow of a monovalent cation of about 6 million/s. One can imagine the potential for a channel labeling method if a fraction of these ions could be used to visualize the ion channel. We have exploited the high permeability of K⁺ channels to monovalent thallium (Tl[I]⁺) ions and the weak solubility of thallium halide salts to develop a simple, yet very sensitive, method to study membrane localization of potassium channels (Fig. 1A; *12*). When thallium ions are applied to one side of the membrane, they will pass through the channel pore(s), create a local increase in thallium concentration, and eventually crystallize with, for example, Br⁻ ions applied to other side of the membrane. Crystals will rapidly grow to visible size, thus marking the location of ion channels on the membrane.

3.2. Theoretical Background

The low solubility of Tl halides will ensure that, if thallium ions can pass the membrane into the cell, then [Tl⁺] concentration will eventually rise to a value high enough to crystallize with an appropriate counter ion. At equilibrium, thallium ions will be evenly distributed inside the cell, and this would make ion channel localization, by crystal formation, impossible. However, equilibrium crystal distribution could be used to differentiate between cells expressing a significant thallium permeability from nonpermeable (i.e., non-K⁺ channel expressing) cells. To apply the "crystallization technique" to really localize ion channels, some specific conditions have to be met: the flow of thallium ions through channels should create (1) a local increase of concentration, which should be (2) big enough to cause crystallization processes. Although numerical calculation of Tl*halide crystallization conditions is not practically possible because of the undefined intracellular environment and complexity of crystallization *per se*, some major characteristics of this process are worth considering.

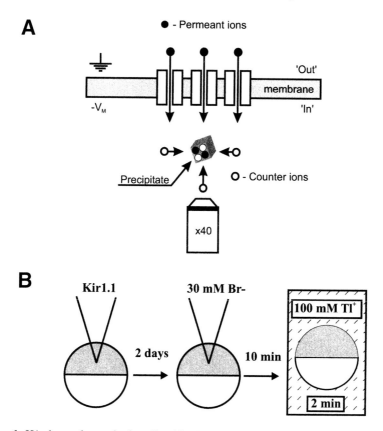

Fig. 1. K^+ channels can be localized in the membrane by crystallization method. **(A)** When extracellularly applied monovalent thallium ions, Tl^+, are driven through open K^+ channels into the cell, either by diffusion and/or applied negative membrane potential, they create a local concentration increase which can then be visualized by observing crystallization of Tl^+ ions with intracellularly loaded bromide (Br^-) anions. Tl^+ and Br^- ions represent a preferred ion pair compared to K^+ and Cl^-, because Tl^+ is more conductive for some inward rectifier channels and TlBr salt is less soluble than TlCl. TlBr crystals can only grow where potassium channels are located and can be easily visualized in *Xenopus* oocytes because of their "macrosize" using low power microscopy. **(B)** Practically, oocytes are first injected with cRNA encoding a specific potassium channel, additionally injected with appropriate amount of Br^- ions and after a short time exposed to high concentration of monovalent thallium.

The concentration of Tl^+ ions at the exit from the pore can be estimated assuming steady-state current flow. Integrating the diffusion Equation 1 where J is ion flux, $S(r)$ is the surface area of hemisphere of radius r, D is the diffusion coefficient, and r is the distance from the center of the pore exit,

$$J = D \cdot S(r) \, dC(r)/dr = const \qquad (1)$$

$$C_O = J/2\pi Dr_O \qquad (2)$$

gives the following (2) estimation of Tl$^+$ concentration (Co) at a distance r_O from the pore exit. Assuming an inner pore vestibule of $r_O = 5$ A, 1 pA current, and $\sim 2*10^{-5}$ cm^2/s diffusion coefficient for Tl$^+$ (*see* ref. *13*; Chapter 10), the concentration of [Tl] = 1.65 mM can be estimated. The precipitating concentration of bromide can be estimated from the solubility product of TlBr salt at room temperature, 0.05 g/100 mL ~ 1.8 mM, as referenced in Handbook of Chemistry and Physics (72nd ed., 1991–1992): [Br$^-$] = [1.8 mM]^2/[Tl] = 1.96 mM. Thus loading oocytes with Br$^-$ ions at a higher concentration, or using less soluble salts (TlI, Tl$_2$Se) would suffice to form a microcrystal by ion flow originating from a single channel. More detailed analysis of the crystallization process (*12*) suggests that many other parameters including temperature and type of halide counter ion will also be important. Having in mind the complexity of this process practical experimentation is the only way of proving the applicability of the crystallization technique.

3.3. Ionic Currents in Thallium-Containing Solutions

3.3.1. Some Practical Notes

When working with thallium salts, some simple but essential precautions should be observed. First, thallium is a poisonous compound and should be handled with care at all times (premature baldness is one unfortunate effect!). Because most physiological solutions contain Cl$^-$ as the major anion, and TlCl is rather insoluble salt, Cl$^-$ should be excluded from any solutions that will contact thallium. In practical terms, this means that standard bath KCl agar salt bridges should be replaced with, for example, NaNO$_3$ bridges. Because AgCl electrodes are designed to work in chloride solutions double salt bridges can be used to avoid incompatibility, i.e., a standard AgCl-KCl agar bridge is extended with a NaNO$_3$ bridge that will face the bath solution containing thallium ions. The same procedure cannot easily be applied to glass microelectrodes, thus they can be simply filled with saturated NaNO$_3$ solution with AgCl electrode in direct contact. The stability of the AgCl/NaNO$_3$ electrode potential and its resistance are less than a AgCl/KCl electrode, especially if big and prolonged currents are applied, but practically, this has not been a problem in our experiments.

3.3.2. Inward Rectifier Currents in Xenopus Oocytes

To our advantage many potassium channels are more permeable to monovalent thallium (Tl$^+$) ions than to K$^+$ (*14–16*), and conduct more current when Tl$^+$ is completely substituted for K$^+$. Figure 2 shows that inward

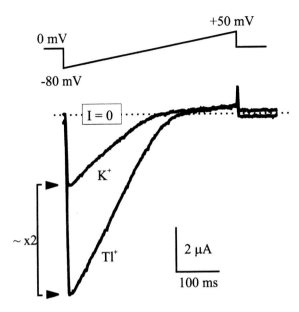

Fig. 2. Cloned inward rectifier potassium channels conduct more current when extracellular K^+ is equimolarly substituted for monovalent thallium, Tl^+. HRK1 (Kir2.3) channels were expressed in *Xenopus* oocytes and ionic currents were recorded using two-microelectrode voltage-clamp in response to ~400 ms voltage ramp from –80 mV to +50 mV in the presence of 100 mM extracellular (a) KNO3 or (b) TlNO3. About a twofold increase of inward current, and a positive shift of reversal potential are observed.

currents through cloned strong inward rectifier potassium channels HIRK1 (Kir2.3) are nearly doubled when 100 mM external K^+ is equimolarly substituted by Tl^+ ions. Interestingly, ionic currents in thallium containing solution usually decline with time, possibly because the formation of TlCl crystals at the inner surface of the membrane which "blocks" the ion-conduction pathway. At high current densities (>20–30 µA per oocyte) and with frequent pulsing, fine white crystals of TlCl are readily observed under a dissecting microscope (not shown). Although prolonged Tl^+ currents may finally cause disruption of the membrane (indicated by appearance of nonselective leak currents), current amplitude may be at least partially restored by keeping oocytes at nonconducting potentials to allow TlCl crystals to dissolve.

3.4. Crystal Growth in Xenopus Oocytes Expressing Potassium Channels

Implementation of the "crystallization method" for visual localization of K^+ channels is shown in Fig. 3A. *Xenopus* oocytes were injected into the

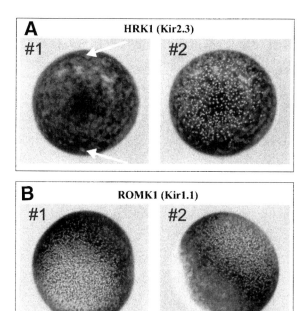

Fig. 3. Crystal growth is determined by the flow of Tl+ ions through K+ channels. **(A)** Images were taken from voltage-clamped oocytes before (#1) and after (#2) ~40 voltage ramps from −80 to +50 mV to cause inward flow of thallium to the cell. The glass microelectrodes are not visible owing to low contrast of the image, but points of electrode insertion are indicated by arrows. **(B)** An oocyte expressing weak inward rectifier ROMK1 channels (Kir1.1) was first injected with ~100 nL of 100 mM KBr (~30 mM final intracellular concentration) ~10-min before exposure to 100 mM TlNO$_3$-min for ~1 min, at which time image #1 was taken. The oocyte was then tilted and photographed again to show the "pseudo-polarized" crystal pattern. Most of the crystals are located in the dark (animal) hemisphere.

animal (dark) hemisphere with 1–5 ng of cRNA encoding Kir2.3 (HIRK1) inward rectifier channels 2 d prior to experimentation. Ionic currents measured at −120 mV in 100 mM KCl extracellular solution usually ranged from 1–20 μA. At least 10 min before exposure to thallium-containing solution (to allow for intracellular diffusion), oocytes were injected with ~100 nL of 30 mM KBr (to bring intracellular concentration to ~ 3 mM). These oocytes could then be incubated in standard extracellular solution supplemented with 3 mM NaBr for up to a few hours prior to experiment. Oocytes were transferred to the recording chamber and voltage-clamped using a standard two-microelectrode voltage-clamp, first in 100 mM K$^+$ solution to check for expression level and leakage currents. Once voltage clamp was established extracellular potassium solution was switched to solution containing 100 mM TlNO$_3$ (NT100, *see* Section 2.). Linear voltage ramps from -80 mV to $+50$ mV (400 msecs) were applied at a frequency of 1–0.75 Hz to produce net inward flow of Tl$^+$ ions, and oocytes were photographed. After a brief period of time, usually less than a minute, a clear patch of multiple white crystals formed on the dark (animal) hemisphere, which could be easily observed under normal light conditions in a dissecting microscope (Fig. 3A). Crystal growth was evidently associated with the presence of potassium channels because no crystals could be observed in (a) uninjected oocytes or in oocytes expressing less than ~0.2 μA of current (at -120 mV) or in (b) expressing oocytes but held at voltages preventing inward currents (from 0 to $+50$ mV).

3.5. Crystals Can Be Generated Without Voltage-Clamping

Electrodiffusion (i.e., diffusion driven not only by concentration gradient but also by applied voltage) of Tl$^+$ ions into the oocytes can be substituted by simple diffusion (no voltage applied) just by appropriate increase of intracellular Br$^-$. Figure 3B shows that patches of white crystals can be easily observed in nonclamped oocytes expressing Kir1.1 (ROMK1) channels, if oocytes are first preinjected with 300 mM bromide (to a final intracellular concentration of about 30 mM) and then simply exposed to 100 mM extracellular Tl$^+$.

We have found that not only inward rectifier potassium channels can be localized by this approach in *Xenopus* oocytes but also voltage-gated K channels (not shown). The limiting factor in many cases is the final concentration of Br$^-$ ions, which should not exceed some reasonable value, which is around 100 mM (intracellularly), or else oocytes rapidly die.

3.6. Functional Channels and TlBr Crystals Are Colocalized

Although crystal growth correlates with the expression of functional potassium channels in *Xenopus* oocytes, it could conceivably be merely a reflection of disturbances in the membrane or in the cytoskeletal network of the oocyte caused by damage during the cRNA injection. In order to prove co-localization of K$^+$ channels and TlBr crystals directly, it is important to correlate experimentally current density with crystal density. We have done this by direct patch clamping of oocytes having crystals using giant patch pipettes. The use of up to 20 μm tip diameter pipettes was necessary because of the macro size of visible crystals. In a few cases we recorded extremely large (up to 20 nA) currents (at -80 mV, 100 mM K$^+$ outside) from membrane patches that contained large visible crystals. By contrast, multiple patches from areas between large visible crystals (i.e., containing only barely identifiable crystals) gave rise to current amplitudes of only about 0.1–0.5 nA, and only leakage currents (<= 50 pA) were observed when areas free of any signs of crystals were patch-clamped.

It is clear that TlBr crystals are arranged in patches, i.e., highly localized to seemingly random parts of the oocyte membrane. Simple experiments using injection of cRNA either into the animal (black) or vegetal (white) poles proved that crystals, and hence channels, are preferentially located at the point of injection *(12)*. We called this trivial phenomenon a "pseudo polarization" of ion channel expression, as opposed to "natural polarization" that might result from the polarized nature of the cell.

3.7. Sensitivity of the "Crystallization Technique"

The sensitivity of the crystallization technique for ion-channel localization is striking. We find that channel-specific crystal growth can be reliably detected from oocytes expressing as little as 100 nS K^+ conductance in 100 mM extracellular K^+. Rough estimation of channel density, assuming 1 pA for single channel current amplitude and 0.5 mm for the average oocyte radius translates to only 1 million channels per whole oocyte or less than 1 (~0.6) channel per square micrometer.

3.8. Confocal Microscopy May Be Used To Observe Out-Of-Focus Crystals and To Enhance Image Contrast

Crystal visualization using a dissecting microscope and standard camera is limited by (1) low image contrast (especially for crystals located on the white, vegetal side), and (2) the low depth of focus, which prevents more detailed analysis of crystal localization and characterization. To overcome these problems, we have used confocal microscopy and exploited the property of TlBr crystals to reflect effectively yellow light (548 nm) generated by an argon laser, as used in standard confocal microscopes (Biorad MR 100). Because of the size of *Xenopus* oocytes, low-power objectives (×4) have to be used to image an entire hemisphere. For the same reason, the iris diaphragm (which determines the vertical or "Z" resolution of the confocal microscope) usually has to be set to higher values (bigger opening) to bring vertical Z resolution to a reasonable value of ~10–50 μm, such that only 10–20 optical sections will be required to cover the whole hemisphere in the vertical direction.

Placing oocytes in a desired and stable position, and artifact-free imaging may take some time. For our recordings we use a simple chamber (Fig. 4). An oocytes is placed in the desired position in a small pit impressed on the surface of soft putty (Fun-Tak®) placed on the bottom of the chamber. The

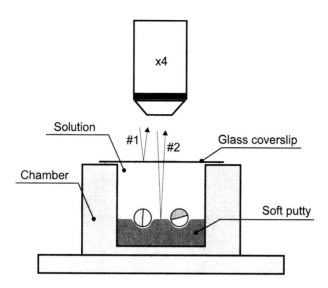

Fig. 4. Simple chamber for confocal imaging of *Xenopus* oocytes. Oocytes are placed in small pits of appropriate size imprinted on a soft water-resistant material (Fun-Tak®). The chamber is filled with solution up to the top and covered with glass cover slip. The cover slip should be far enough (few millimeters) from the top of the oocyte to prevent unwanted reflection (#1). Reflection from the bottom of the chamber (#2) is unavoidable in this arrangement but much less problematic.

solution fills the chamber, which is covered by a piece of glass cover slip at a distance of at least a few mm from the top of the oocyte. This arrangement serves three purposes: (1) because all the space is filled by solution, small movements of the chamber do not cause solution movement, so that oocytes remain stationary; (2) the glass cover slip creates a "flat" surface for perfect imaging; and (3) its distant positioning from the surface of the oocyte does not create unwanted reflection. Imaging close to the surface of the clay is less problematic and artefacts appear only when imaging very close to it.

Figure 5A shows a representative low magnification (×4 objective) projected series of confocal "slices" taken from the vegetal (white) hemisphere of oocytes expressing Kir2.1 (IRK1) channels. Black dots indicate TlBr crystals scattered over the surface of the oocyte. Usually the density of crystals declines in a uniform manner from the point of cRNA injection (pseudo-polarization) but in some cases unusual patterns can be observed (Fig. 5B). Arrowheads in Fig. 5B, in places distant from the point of injection of cRNA and bromide, point to spots of silence. Progressively smaller crystals can be observed by switching to more powerful objectives (Fig. 5C). At higher magnification (×60 objective), it was also possible to observe apparently

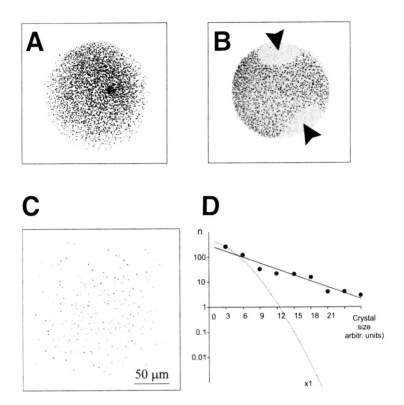

Fig. 5. Reflection confocal imaging of TlBr crystals in Xenopus oocytes. Reflected light from TlBr crystals can be collected at different depths by confocal microscopy to obtain the total projection of the oocyte surface. **(A)** "Piled-up" projection from an oocyte expressing ROMK1 (Kir1.1) channels and treated as described in this chapter to grow TlBr crystals. "Z" resolution (×4.5 objective, iris diaphragm I = 8 in BioRad MR 1000) was set to minimum for the purpose of presentation. **(B)** Unusual distributions of active channels can be observed ("spots of silence") without any visual disturbances in the color pattern of the oocytes (not shown). **(C)** Crystals can be imaged at higher magnification (×60 objective here) and crystal size distribution (arbitrary units) analyzed **(D)**. The size distribution of TlBr crystals can be approximated by an exponential function (note Log scale). Approximations of crystal size based on random distribution (Poisson equation) of ion channels are much steeper functions (×1).

circular and linear paths along which TlBr crystals were located (not shown) but quantitative analysis and interpretation of these patterns is challenging at this time. Crystal size, which should be proportional to the current density, or to the density of K+ channels, is much easier to quantify. We have used a powerful "ImageTool" software (v. 1.27) from UTHSCSA (free access on internet at http://vivaldi.ece.ucsb.edu/courses/ece181b/vision181.html) to estimate the distribution of crystal size. Crystal size does not follow Poisson distribution (which would correspond to random channel distribution, Fig. 5D). Instead, the distribution of crystal size (area) is approximated by an exponential function, the number of crystals of a bigger size is approximately halved with doubling of their size. This discrepancy strongly agues in favor of clustered organization of K^+ channels in *Xenopus* oocytes *(12)*.

4. POSSIBILITIES FOR APPLICATION OF THE CRYSTALLIZATION TECHNIQUE FOR LOCALIZING ION CHANNELS IN CULTURED CELLS

The crystallization technique, employing thallium halide crystal formation, may in principle be extended, by appropriate choice of permeant and counter ions to generate hardly precipitates, to the examination of the distribution of any other ion channels in any cell type. In practice though there are some essential limitations, which make application of this technology challenging if not impossible in cells other than *Xenopus* oocytes. There are some crucial properties of *Xenopus* oocytes, which make them unique in this context: (1) the intracellular milieu of the oocyte represents a practically infinite sink for Tl^+ ions entering from outside, and (2) the intracellular solute composition can be easily varied by simple microinjection of desired solution. In small cells, thallium concentration may increase rapidly, eliminating the initial concentration gradient and preventing localized crystal growth. The total amount of counter ion loaded inside cultured cells may be limiting, so that the total number and size of the crystals could also be very low. The "supersolubility" *(12)* of small crystals will contribute to the problem.

With some modifications the crystallization technique can probably be successfully used for localizing cells expressing specific, pharmacologically or physiologically distinguishable ion channels and receptors *(17)* *(see* Chapter 16). We have found, for example, that Tl_2S crystals can serve as catalytic centers for the common process of reducing Ag^+ to metallic silver, similar to processes used in film development. According to this idea, cells expressing specific Tl^+ permeable channels (K channels, glutamate receptors, etc.) could be loaded with thallium and then exposed to Na_2S (sodium sulfide). Tl_2S crystals would then be formed in cells expressing a specific channel. Cells could then be washed out to remove free sulfur and localized by applying a standard photo-developing solution. Similar technology has been used to localize zinc-enriched synaptic vesicles in brain *(18)*.

5. SOME USEFUL TIPS FOR WORKING WITH CLONED CHANNELS IN *XENOPUS* OOCYTES

Several practical points emerge from these localization studies that should be considered when studying channels expressed in oocytes, because pseudo-polarization of ion channel expression owing to localized cRNA injection appears to be so strong.

1. If the level of expression of an ion channel is low, and macroscopic patch-clamp currents are desired, then cRNA can be injected at one of the poles of the oocyte (i.e., a position that can subsequently be easily recognized), as close to the surface as possible. Then, after 1–2 d of expression, much higher than average density of ionic current should be measurable at designated places.
2. If agonist or blocker of a specific channel is applied to *Xenopus* oocytes expressing channels (receptors) one has to be sure that the channel expressing spot is not facing the bottom of the chamber. If so, then application or withdrawal of the agent may be dramatically slowed down because of slow diffusion from restricted areas.
3. One potential application that follows from the above is that subunit association rates and mechanisms may be studied for multisubunit channels. Different subunits of the channel (or receptor) could be expressed in different parts of the oocyte and then allowed to diffuse along the membrane until meeting each other and forming functional aggregates.

ACKNOWLEDGMENTS

This work was supported by NIH Grant HL 54171 (CGN), AHA SDG Grant 9630291N (ANL), and NIH R21 Grant GM57892–02 (ANL).

REFERENCES

1. Robitaille, R., Bourque, M. J., and Vandaele, S. (1996) Localization of L-type Ca2+ channels at perisynaptic glial cells of the frog neuromuscular junction. *J. Neurosci.* **16,** 148–158.
2. Deerinck, T. J., Levinson, S. R., Bennett, G. V., and Ellisman, M. H. (1997) Clustering of voltage-sensitive sodium channels on axons is independent of direct Schwann cell contact in the dystrophic mouse. *J. Neurosci.* **17,** 5080–5088.
3. Shi, G., Kleinklaus, A. K., Marrion, N. V., and Trimmer, J. S. (1994) Properties of Kv2. 1 K+ channels expressed in transfected mammalian cells. *J. Biol. Chem.* **269,** 23,204–23,211.

4. Flucher, B. E. and Daniels, M. P. (1989) Distribution of Na+ channels and ankyrin in neuromuscular junctions is complementary to that of acetylcholine receptors and the 43 kd protein. *Neuron* **3**, 163–175.

5. Boudier, J. L., Le Treut, T., and Jover, E. (1992) Autoradiographic localization of voltage-dependent sodium channels on the mouse neuromuscular junction using 125I-alpha scorpion toxin. II. Sodium distribution on postsynaptic membranes. *J. Neurosci.* **12**, 454–466.

6. Robitaille, R., Adler, E. M., and Charlton, M. P. (1993) Calcium channels and calcium-gated potassium channels at the frog neuromuscular junction. *J. Physiol. Paris* **87**, 15–24.

7. Pelchen-Matthews, A. and Dolly, J. O. (1989) Distribution in the rat central nervous system of acceptor sub-types for dendrotoxin, a K+ channel probe. *Neuroscience* **29**, 347–61.

8. Froehner, S. C., Luetje, C. W., Scotland, P. B., and Patrick, J. (1990) The postsynaptic 43K protein clusters muscle nicotinic acetylcholine receptors in Xenopus oocytes. *Neuron* **5**, 403–410.

9. Prendergast, F. G. and Mann, K. G. (1978) Chemical and physical properties of aequorin and the green fluorescent protein isolated from Aequorea forskalea. *Biochemistry* **17**, 3448–3453.

10. Gomez-Hernandez, J. M., Stuhmer, W., and Parekh, A. B. (1997) Calcium dependence and distribution of calcium-activated chloride channels in Xenopus oocytes. *J. Physiol. (Lond.)* **502**, 569–574.

11. Pruss, R. M., Akeson, R. L., Racke, M. M., and Wilburn, J. L. (1991) Agonist-activated cobalt uptake identifies divalent cation-permeable kainate receptors on neurons and glial cells. *Neuron.* **7**, 509–518.

12. Lopatin, A. N., Makhina, E. N., and Nichols, C. G. (1998) A novel crystallization method for visualizing the membrane localization of potassium channels. *Biophys. J.* **74**, 2159–2170.

13. Hille, B. (1992) *Ionic Channels of Excitable Membranes*. Sinauer Associates, Sunderland, MA.

14. Hagiwara, S., Miyazaki, S., Krasne, S., and Ciani, S. (1977) Anomalous permeabilities of the egg cell membrane of a starfish in K+- Tl+ mixtures. *J. Gen. Physiol.* **70**, 269–281.

15. Blatz, A. L. and Magleby, K. L. (1984) Ion conductance and selectivity of single calcium-activated potassium channels in cultured rat muscle. *J. Gen. Physiol.* **84**, 1–23.

16. Eisenman, G., Latorre, R., and Miller, C. (1986) Multi-ion conduction and selectivity in the high-conductance Ca++- activated K+ channel from skeletal muscle. *Biophys. J.* **50**, 1025–1034.

17. Engelman, H. S., Allen, T. B., and MacDermott, A. B. (1999) The distribution of neurons expressing calcium-permeable AMPA receptors in the superficial laminae of the spinal cord dorsal horn. *J. Neurosci.* **19**, 2081–2089.

18. Danscher, G. (1996) The autometallographic zinc-sulphide method. A new approach involving in vivo creation of nanometer-sized zinc sulphide crystal lattices in zinc-enriched synaptic and secretory vesicles. *Histochem. J.* **28**, 361–373.

18

Imaging of Localized Neuronal Calcium Influx

Fritjof Helmchen

1. INTRODUCTION

Intracellular Ca^{2+} controls such diverse processes as growth, cell division, contraction, secretion, and cell death. In neurons Ca^{2+} influx triggers neurotransmitter release, causes activation of various enzyme cascades, and regulates gene expression *(1)*. Increases in the intracellular calcium concentration ($[Ca^{2+}]$) also affect membrane excitability and are involved in synaptic plasticity *(2)*. How does Ca^{2+} accomplish this multitude of tasks, often within the same cell? A clue to the answer is the spatial segregation of Ca^{2+} signaling pathways in different cellular compartments *(3)*. This compartmentalization is based on the nonuniform cellular distribution of Ca^{2+}-permeable ion channels, intracellular Ca^{2+}-binding proteins, and Ca^{2+} pumps. Localized Ca^{2+} signaling enormously increases the cells' ability and flexibility to use Ca^{2+} as an intracellular messenger in many parallel ways.

This chapter focuses on optical measurements of localized Ca^{2+} influx in neurons. Ca^{2+} influx occurs through a variety of ion channels, including voltage-gated calcium channels, partially Ca^{2+}-permeable ligand-gated receptor channels, and sensory transduction channels (Table 1). In addition, Ca^{2+} may be released from the endoplasmic reticulum. The subcellular distribution of these various Ca^{2+} sources can be investigated in individual neurons using fluorescent Ca^{2+} indicators *(4)*. The localization of ion channels is indirectly inferred from the localized fluorescence changes caused by the underlying Ca^{2+} currents (Fig. 1). The spatial confinement of Ca^{2+} signals can range from the submicron scale to the coarse segregation of Ca^{2+} entry pathways in different cell compartments *(3,5,6)*. Although Ca^{2+} indicators do not probe channel localization directly (complications to be considered

From: *Ion Channel Localization Methods and Protocols*
Edited by: A. Lopatin and C. G. Nichols © Humana Press Inc., Totowa, NJ

Table 1
Ca²⁺ Entry Routes in Neurons

Class	Type	Blockers
Voltage-gated channels	T	Ni^{2+}
	N	ω-Conotoxin GVIA
	L	1,4-Dihydropyridines
	P/Q	ω-Agatoxin VIA
	R	Ni^{2+}
Ligand-gated channels	GluR (NMDA)[a]	D-APV
	GluR (AMPA)	CNQX
	GluR (kainate)	
	nACh receptor	α-Bungarotoxin
	ATP receptor	
	5-HT₃ receptor	
Release channels	IP₃ receptor	Heparin
	Ryanodine receptor	Ruthenium Red
Transduction channels	cGMP-gated	
	cAMP-gated	Pseudechetoxin
	Mechanoelectrical	Aminoglycoside antibiotics

[a]Glutamate receptor channels (GluRs) are classified in NMDA-, AMPA-, and kainate-type according to their specific agonists.

Abbreviations: NMDA, *N*-methyl-*D*-aspartate; AMPA, α-amino-2-hydroxy-5-methyl-isoxazolepropionate; nACh, nicotinic acetylcholine; 5-HT, 5-hydroxytryptamine (serotonin); cGMP, cyclic GMP; cAMP, cyclic AMP; IP₃, inositol 1,4,5-triphosphate; D-APV, *D*-2-amino-5-phosphonovalerate; CNQX, 6-cyano-7-nitroquinoxaline-2,3-dione.

are the unspecificity of Ca^{2+} indicators for the Ca^{2+} source as well as their mobility), they are extremely useful because they probe the functionally relevant Ca^{2+} current component. The spatiotemporal activation pattern of different Ca^{2+} sources can be studied under relatively physiological conditions and may be linked to specific cellular functions.

2. METHODS

2.1. Fluorescent Calcium Indicators

A broad palette of fluorescent Ca^{2+} indicators is available *(4)*. Most indicators are small organic molecules with a Ca^{2+}-binding site and a fluorophore that changes its fluorescence properties upon Ca^{2+} binding. Most commonly changes in fluorescence emission are measured. Cells are loaded with these dyes either via micropipets or using acetoxymethyl ester

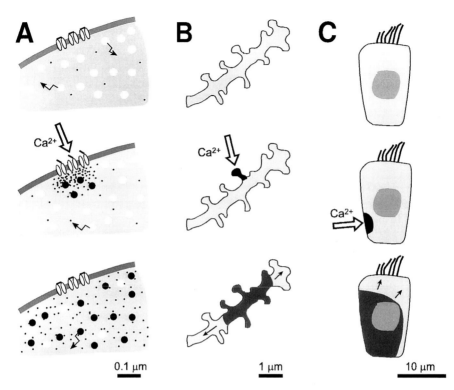

Fig. 1. Ca^{2+} indicators as functional probes of ion channel localization. Schematic illustration of localized fluorescence signals caused by local Ca^{2+} influx and their subsequent diffusional spread on three spatial scales. **(A)** Molecular scale. Calcium ions enter the cytosol through open channels, bind to indicator molecules (solid circles), and cause a change in their fluorescence. Both Ca^{2+} and the indicator diffuse in the cytosol. The domains of high Ca^{2+} concentration collapse within 10–100 µs after channel closure. **(B)** Subcellular scale. Ca^{2+} influx in a small cellular compartment, e.g., a dendritic spine, leads to a localized $[Ca^{2+}]$ increase, which spreads several micrometers within 10–100 ms. **(C)** Cellular scale. Nonuniform Ca^{2+} entry across the plasma membrane induces Ca^{2+} concentration gradients, which dissipate on the 100 ms to seconds time scale.

forms that permeate through membranes but get trapped inside cells after cleavage by endogenous esterases. A second group of indicators are Ca^{2+}-sensitive proteins, including the luminescent photoprotein aequorin *(7)* and fluorescently labeled Ca^{2+}-binding proteins *(4)*. These indicators are genetically encoded and therefore can be targeted to specific cell types or subcellular locations.

2.1.1. High vs Low Affinity

Ca^{2+} indicators differ in their affinity for Ca^{2+} binding. Typically they are divided in high- and low-affinity dyes with dissociation constants of 0.1–1 μM and ≥ 1 μM, respectively. High-affinity indicators are more sensitive to small cytosolic [Ca^{2+}] changes; however, they blunt steep [Ca^{2+}] gradients and may saturate at high [Ca^{2+}] levels near entry sites. Low-affinity dyes are advantageous for visualizing Ca^{2+} entry sites because their fluorescence may change substantially only near the source. In addition, low-affinity dyes generally have a relatively fast Ca^{2+} association rate, which minimizes temporal filtering caused by dye kinetics and enables more accurate measurements of the time course and spread of rapid [Ca^{2+}] signals *(8)*. Commonly used low-affinity dyes are Calcium Green-5N, Oregon Green 488 BAPTA–5N, Mag-Fura-2, and Magnesium Green (all available from Molecular Probes, Oregon).

2.1.2. Mobility

Calcium ions and most Ca^{2+} indicators diffuse throughout the cytosol. The diffusional spread of Ca^{2+} signals not only depends on cell morphology but also on the presence of Ca^{2+} buffers and Ca^{2+} extrusion mechanisms *(6)*. It is important to note that indicators themselves possibly affect the spread of Ca^{2+} signals. For example, a highly diffusible indicator may alter Ca^{2+} compartmentalization severely by acting as an artificial Ca^{2+} shuttle between cellular compartments *(6)*. This problem can be somewhat reduced by application of less mobile dextran-linked indicators *(4)*. Another problem of diffusible dyes is the large background signal associated with bulk cytoplasmic staining, which makes the detection of highly localized fluorescence changes difficult. Several approaches try to overcome this problem by targeting indicators to specific locations in a cell, i.e., by anchoring them next to the channels of interest. For example, aliphatic or lipophilic Ca^{2+} indicators that are favorably incorporated into membranes have been designed by attachment of lipophilic tails to indicator molecules. Except in a few instances *(9,10)*, however, these near-membrane indicators have not been used much so far, probably because of problems with dye loading, unspecific staining, and the relatively low dissociation constants compared to the expected submembranous Ca^{2+} concentrations of >10–100 μM. Alternatively, genetically encoded Ca^{2+}-sensitive proteins, such as aequorin *(7)* and cameleons *(11)*, can be targeted to specific intracellular organelles. Cameleons consist of two mutant variants of green fluorescent protein (GFP) attached to calmodulin *(11)*. Variant forms of cameleon bearing appropriate localization signals have been used to visualize Ca^{2+} dynamics in the nucleus and endoplasmic reticulum of HeLa cells *(11)*; a similar approach should make Ca^{2+} measurements from well-defined subcellular locations in neurons possible.

2.2. Microscopy Techniques

Various imaging techniques have been applied to measure neuronal $[Ca^{2+}]$ in dissociated or cultured cells, in brain slices, whole-brain preparations, and even in intact animals *(12)*. Typically, cells or tissue slices are continuously perfused with extracellular saline in a microscope chamber and microelectrodes or patch pipets are used for dye loading and for simultaneous electrical recordings. Pharmacological substances are either bath-applied or applied locally using additional pipets. Intracellular channel blockers may be included in the electrode solution.

Microscope techniques differ in their lateral and axial spatial resolution, their temporal resolution, and their ability to penetrate into strongly scattering tissue. High spatiotemporal resolution often is desirable for the study of localized Ca^{2+} influx. The spatial and temporal resolution are fundamentally limited by the diffraction limit of the objective and the dye kinetics, respectively. To date, hardly any imaging system achieves maximal resolution in both the spatial and the temporal domain (~1 μm and ~1 ms, respectively) simultaneously (but see, for example, high-speed cameras from PixelVision, Oregon). In most cases, a compromise is necessary, trading resolution in one domain for high resolution in the other (Fig. 2).

2.2.1. Spot Measurements

The average fluorescence from a large area can be measured with a photomultiplier or a photodiode (Fig. 2). This simple method provides submillisecond time resolution. It has been applied, for instance, to study presynaptic Ca^{2+} dynamics in large pools of labeled CNS nerve terminals *(see* below). Because of the massive spatial averaging this method provides a high signal-to-noise ratio. Rapid measurements from more localized regions are possible by restricting the field of illumination (Fig. 2). In the extreme case, the excitation light is focused to a diffraction-limited spot *(13)*.

2.2.2. Imaging Techniques

Two-dimensional images are obtained either by projecting the fluorescence image onto a two-dimensional detector or by scanning of an illuminating spot (Fig. 2). Array detectors include video cameras and charge-coupled device (CCD) cameras. Cooled CCD cameras are particularly well suited for fluorescence imaging because of their high sensitivity, low noise, and large dynamic range. Their image acquisition rate, however,

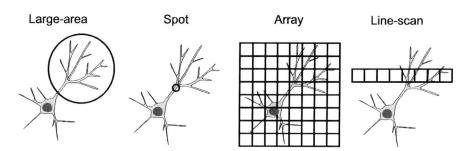

Fig. 2. Different modes of Ca²⁺ imaging. The average fluorescence signal from a large area can be detected with high time resolution. Although this method lacks true spatial resolution, a comparison of Ca²⁺ signaling in large cellular compartments, e.g., dendrites vs soma, is possible by moving the field of view. Fast measurements from small areas (down to the submicron-size) are possible with spot illumination and confocal detection. Two-dimensional images are aquired using either a camera system or a laser-scanning microscope. In the line-scan mode a single line is repetitively scanned, which enables millisceond time-resolution while maintaining spatial resolution in one dimension.

is limited by the relatively slow read-out rate. Many cameras offer "binning" of pixels, which increases the acquisition rate but reduces the spatial resolution. In laser-scanning microscopy a laser beam is focused and scanned over the field of view using galvanometric mirrors or other devices *(14)*. Fluorescence emission is detected with a photomultiplier tube and assigned to the corresponding position. Two major types of laser-scanning microscopes exist. In confocal microscopy a pinhole in front of the detector blocks out-of-focus fluorescence light, which results in a micrometer axial resolution *(12,14)*. Confocal microscopes, however, suffer from relatively low signal-to-noise and problems with photobleaching and photodamage. These problems are reduced in two-photon laser scanning microscopy *(15)*. Two-photon excitation of fluorophores requires simultaneous absorption of two photons that each provide half of the excitation energy. For excitation of common Ca²⁺ indicators wavelengths in the range of 800–900 nm are used. Major advantages of two-photon microscopy are reduced light scattering caused by the longer excitation wavelength and the confinement of the excitation to the focal spot resulting from the nonlinear dependence of two-photon absorption on light intensity. Two-photon microscopy therefore is well suited for measuring Ca²⁺ signals in small structures deep in brain slices or the intact brain *(16,17)*.

2.2.3. Line-Scan Mode

Most camera systems and laser-scanning microscopes cannot reach a millisecond time resolution in full-frame mode. Laser-scanning microscopes in the best cases attain full-frame acquisition at video rate (30 Hz). Higher acquisition rates of up to 1 kHz can be achieved by repetitively scanning only a single line in the so-called "line-scan" mode (Fig. 2). Line-scans are particularly useful to compare rapid Ca^{2+} signals in two (or more) nearby structures, for example in a dendritic spine and its parent dendritic shaft.

2.2.4. Sequential Measurements

Maps of $[Ca^{2+}]$ changes with both high spatial and temporal resolution can be built from a series of sequential measurements in cases in which a reliable cellular response can be stimulated repeatedly. Examples are the Ca^{2+} influx evoked by action potentials or Ca^{2+} currents induced by well-defined voltage steps in whole-cell recordings. Two different approaches are possible. First, spot measurements with high time resolution can be repeated at different locations. For example, spatial profiles of dendritic Ca^{2+} signals have been constructed from sequential measurements at various dendritic positions *(18)*. On a smaller scale $[Ca^{2+}]$ domains near active zones in presynaptic terminals have been mapped using this approach *(13)*. Alternatively, single high-resolution images are acquired in each trial using brief light exposures; an artificial time series of such "snapshots" then is built by varying the delay of the light exposure after the stimulation. Light flashes of 1 ms or less duration can be provided by a pulsed laser or a flash lamp. Pulsed laser imaging, for example, has been used to detect short-lived Ca^{2+} gradients in chromaffin cells and in skeletal muscle *(19)*.

2.3. Optical Measurement of Calcium Influx

Fluorescence signals from Ca^{2+} indicators are expressed as changes from prestimulus level (ΔF) or as relative fluorescence changes $\Delta F/F$ to normalize for spatial inhomogeneities in dye concentration or illumination. How do these fluorescence signals relate to the underlying Ca^{2+} currents and to the spatial distribution of Ca^{2+}-permeable channels? Because intracellular Ca^{2+} is buffered only a small percentage (1% or less) of Ca^{2+} entering the cytosol remains unbound. Ca^{2+} indicators act as buffers themselves and contribute to the cytoplasmic buffering capacity. Depending on the relative concentrations of indicator and endogenous buffers rather different qualities are measured *(20)*: At relatively low concentrations the indicator affects $[Ca^{2+}]$ changes little and essentially reports unaltered $[Ca^{2+}]$ dynamics. At very high concentrations the indicator becomes the dominant buffer and catches virtually all incoming calcium ions. In the latter case $[Ca^{2+}]$ signals are severely distorted but the absolute fluorescence change ΔF is directly proportional to the total Ca^{2+} flux. Excess dye loading therefore can be used to quantify the total Ca^{2+} charge entering a cell compartment after calibration of ΔF in terms of Ca^{2+} charge, e.g., by measuring ΔF evoked by electrically recorded pure Ca^{2+} currents *(21)*. Dye overload for example has been used to determine fractional Ca^{2+} currents through ligand-gated receptor channels in somata *(20–22)* or dendrites *(23)*, and to quantify the presynaptic Ca^{2+} influx during an action potential *(24)*.

The identification and localization of Ca^{2+} sources using Ca^{2+} indicators may be complicated by the following problems. First, multiple Ca^{2+} pathways can be activated nearly simultaneously, resulting in a mixture of Ca^{2+} currents. For example, synaptic activation at excitatory synapses may lead to strong postsynaptic depolarization followed by activation of voltage-gated Ca^{2+} currents. This secondary effect then masks the direct Ca^{2+} influx through glutamate receptors. To study the distribution of a particular source in isolation or to dissect the relative contribution of different pathways, specific blockers of Ca^{2+} sources therefore have to be applied (Table 1). Activation of voltage-gated currents in some cases can be prevented using voltage-clamp of the membrane potential. Second, Ca^{2+} signals spread by diffusion, which often makes it difficult to determine whether $[Ca^{2+}]$ changes at a particular location were caused by local entry or diffusion from a remote site. Analysis of the amplitude of fluorescence signals at various locations alone may not be sufficient to determine the entry site because amplitudes also depend on buffering and surface-to-volume ratio. Often it is useful to compare the risetime of fluorescence signals at nearby locations in order to find the origin of the Ca^{2+} signal. Such an analysis is particularly challenging on the micrometer scale because it requires millisecond time resolution. Line-scans have been particularly useful to determine the location of Ca^{2+} entry on this spatial scale (*see* below). A third point is that the functional activation pattern of Ca^{2+} sources might differ from their anatomical distribution. In other words, Ca^{2+} imaging can only provide positive evidence for the presence of a particular source. The lack of a signal in a cellular compartment does not necessarily mean that the source is not present; it may be there, however, it may not be activated by the experimental stimulation protocol. This aspect of optical imaging clearly distinguishes it from purely anatomical methods and can be considered advantageous because channel activation can be spatially mapped under various conditions. The questions remain, however, which stimulus patterns are physiological and how they can be mimicked during an experiment.

3. LOCALIZED CALCIUM ENTRY IN NEURONS

Neurons are highly polarized cells, typically with one cellular pole that receives and handles input signals and another pole that transfers information to other cells. This cellular polarization is reflected in the compartmentalization of Ca^{2+} signaling *(3)*. Segregation of Ca^{2+} signals is important because Ca^{2+} may serve different functions in different compartments and crosstalk between signaling pathways must be minimized. The following sections give examples of how Ca^{2+} imaging has been used to characterize Ca^{2+} entry pathways in sensory neurons, nerve terminals, and dendrites.

3.1. Sensory Neurons

Ca^{2+} influx in sensory neurons is important for sensory transduction, adaptation, and synaptic transmission (Fig. 3). Fluorescence imaging revealed localized Ca^{2+} signals in sensory neurons of the visual, auditory, vestibular, and olfactory system.

3.1.1. Retinal Cells

Ca^{2+} influx occurs at several stages of signal processing in the retina (Fig. 3A). Photoreceptors respond to light with a transient decrease of a steady cation current through cGMP-gated ion channels in their outer segments. In the dark, Ca^{2+} steadily flows into the outer segments through these channels and is extruded from the cytosol so that $[Ca^{2+}]$ reaches a steady-state level. Upon light exposure $[Ca^{2+}]$ in the outer segments transiently decreases, a phenomenon that has been measured using Ca^{2+} indicators *(25)*. Although cGMP and not Ca^{2+} is the messenger for excitation in photoreceptors, Ca^{2+} modulates the gain of phototransduction and thus is important for light adaptation *(26)*. At the opposite cellular pole, in the synaptic terminals attached to the inner segments, Ca^{2+} entry through L-type Ca^{2+} channels regulates neurotransmitter release onto bipolar and horizontal cells *(27)*. Interestingly, Ca^{2+} extrusion mechanisms in photoreceptors are differentially distributed as well *(28)*. Localized Ca^{2+} influx, furthermore, occurs in bipolar cell terminals where it is mediated by L-type Ca^{2+} currents *(29)*. Ca^{2+} imaging of the intact retina has been difficult because of the interference of the excitation light with retinal light sensitivity. Two-photon microscopy can overcome this problem because photoreceptor activation is minimized at longer excitation wavelengths. A recent study using two-photon excitation reported light-induced dendritic Ca^{2+} responses in ganglion cells and spatially inhomogeneous Ca^{2+} signals in amacrine cell dendrites *(30)*.

3.1.2. Hair Cells

Ca^{2+} influx in hair cells of the vestibular and the auditory system is involved in mechanosensory transduction as well as synaptic transmission *(31,32)*. Mechanical displacements of the hair bundle open mechanosensitive transduction channels in the stereocilia, causing electrical excita-

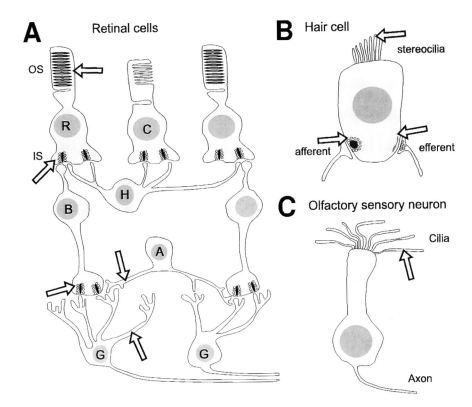

Fig. 3. Localized Ca^{2+} influx in sensory neurons. (**A**) Ca^{2+} enters locally in several retinal cell types. In the rod (R) and cone (C) photoreceptors Ca^{2+} enters the outer segment (OS) through cGMP-gated channels. At the other pole, Ca^{2+} influx into synaptic terminals of the inner segment (IS) promotes graded transmitter release onto retinal bipolar cells (B) and horizontal cells (H). Bipolar cells further transmit the signal to ganglion cells (G) via graded transmitter release controlled by Ca^{2+} influx in their synaptic terminals. Localized dendritic Ca^{2+} influx possibly occurs in amacrine (A) and ganglion cells. (**B**) Several Ca^{2+} entry pathways exist in hair cells of the auditory and vestibular system. Ca^{2+} imaging studies found that Ca^{2+} influx through mechanosensitive transduction channels is located at the tip of the hair bundle stereocilia. At the basolateral membrane, Ca^{2+} influx through clusters of Ca^{2+} channels controls graded release onto afferent fibers. Efferent inhibition involves Ca^{2+} entry through nicotinic ACh receptors and possibly via local release. (**C**) In olfactory sensory neurons, the signal transduction mechanism is located in the cilia at the apex of the cells. It involves the activation of a Ca^{2+}-activated chloride channel after Ca^{2+} entry through cAMP-gated channels. In all these sensory neurons Ca^{2+} is involved in sensory adaptation, in addition to its role in sensory transduction and synaptic transmission.

tion and Ca^{2+} entry (Fig. 3B). The attempts to determine whether transduction channels are located at the base or the tip of stereocilia illustrate the problem of using a diffusible indicator to study localization. Early measurements revealed large fluorescence changes at the base of stereocilia and were interpreted as evidence for a location near the base *(33)*. However, these measurements could not resolve the rapid diffusional spread of Ca^{2+} within stereocilia. Line-scans with almost millisecond time resolution using confocal *(34)* or two-photon microscopy *(35)* later demonstrated that fluorescence initially increases near the tip of stereocilia and subsequently spread towards the base, consistent with a transduction channel location near the tip. Ca^{2+} entry through transduction channels is important in sensory adaptation *(31,32)* and in the amplification of bundle motion *(36)*.

At their basolateral membrane, hair cells form chemical synapses onto afferent dendrites and receive inhibitory efferent synaptic inputs from brainstem neurons (Fig. 3B). Afferent synapses are formed at about 20 specialized "active zones," each of which consists of a dense body with surrounding transmitter-containing vesicles. Ca^{2+} influx through dihydropyridine-sensitive Ca^{2+} channels (Table 1) at these sites causes transmitter release and activation of Ca^{2+}-activated potassium channels, which are involved in resonant tuning of the response to a particular frequency *(31)*. Consistent with the morphology, localized high $[Ca^{2+}]$ domains could be visualized at the basolateral membrane as fluorescence "hot spots" during depolarizing voltage steps in isolated hair cells using confocal microscopy *(37,38)*. At the third major Ca^{2+} signaling site, the efferent cholinergic synapse, Ca^{2+} enters through nACh receptor channels and may be released from submembraneous cisternae *(32)*. Inhibition is caused by the activation of a Ca^{2+}-activated potassium channel. It should be possible to detect "hot spots" of Ca^{2+} entry near efferent synapses.

3.2.3. Olfactory Sensory Neurons

Localized Ca^{2+} signaling is also found in the olfactory receptor neurons in the olfactory epithelium (Fig. 3C). A recent study succeeded in imaging odor-induced Ca^{2+} increases in individual cilia of dissociated salamander olfactory receptor neurons *(39)*. These experiments confirmed that the transduction machinery is located in the cilia. Transduction most likely includes cAMP production after odor-binding to receptors, gating of a cAMP-gated ion channel, and activation of a choride current by Ca^{2+} entering through the cAMP-gated ion channels. Alternatively or in addition, Ca^{2+}-release from IP3-sensitive stores might be involved. Besides being part of the excitation cascade, Ca^{2+} also mediates odorant adaptation by desensitizing cAMP-gated channels *(40)*.

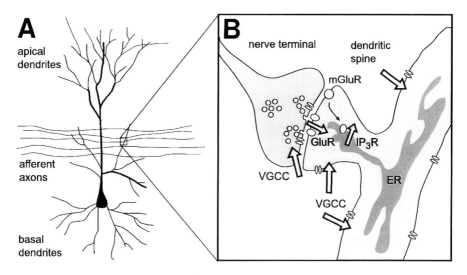

Fig. 4. Pre- and postsynaptic Ca^{2+} entry routes at excitatory synapses in the CNS. (**A**) A nonuniform distribution of different subtypes of voltage-gated Ca^{2+} channels probably exists in dendrites of pyramidal neurons although the total Ca^{2+} channel density may be fairly uniform (*see* text). (**B**) Various Ca^{2+} sources contribute to $[Ca^{2+}]$ elevations on the level of individual synapses. Presynaptic Ca^{2+} influx is mediated by voltage-gated Ca^{2+} channels (VGCC) of the N-, P/Q-, and R-type, and triggers glutamate release. Postsynaptically, several Ca^{2+} entry pathways may be activated, including calcium-permeable glutamate receptors (GluRs), activation of voltage-gated Ca^{2+} channels, and release from the endoplasmic reticulum (ER) through IP_3-receptor channels after activation of metabotropic glutamate receptors (mGluRs).

3.2. Presynaptic Nerve Terminals

3.2.1. Measurements from Individual Nerve Terminals

Several Ca^{2+} pathways are activated during synaptic transmission at central synapses (Fig. 4). On the presynaptic side, action potentials briefly open voltage-gated Ca^{2+} channels and evoke neurotransmitter release *(24)*. Release is thought to depend on high $[Ca^{2+}]$ domains beneath Ca^{2+} channel clusters at release sites *(41,42)*. Freeze-fracture studies and labeling of Ca^{2+} channels with fluorescently tagged blockers provided evidence for such clustering *(43)*. The spatial arrangement of Ca^{2+} channels with respect to exocytotic proteins is crucial for the amount and speed of release because of its steep, nonlinear $[Ca^{2+}]$-dependence. Unfortunately, the relevant spatial scale (ten to hundreds of nanometers) is below the optical resolution limit. Intraterminal $[Ca^{2+}]$ gradients therefore have been resolved in only few preparations. In squid giant presynaptic terminals, Smith et al. *(44)* observed that [Ca^{2+}] increases were largest adjacent to the postsynaptic fiber, consistent with a Ca^{2+} channel localization at active zones. Furthermore, punctuate light emissions were measured in squid terminals with a low-affinity mutant of the luminescent protein aequorin, suggesting discrete Ca^{2+} microdomains *(45)*. [Ca^{2+}] gradients at release sites also have been resolved in hair cells (*see* above) and in adrenal chromaffin cells using pulsed laser imaging *(19)*. More recently, localized [Ca^{2+}] domains were characterized in single nerve terminals of a cultured *Xenopus* neuromuscular junction preparation using a low-affinity indicator and confocal spot detection *(13)*. These measurements corroborated the idea of rapid, high [Ca^{2+}] elevations at release sites; however, experiments in CNS nerve terminals await to be done. As another twist of the multifunctional use of Ca^{2+} the residual [Ca^{2+}] remaining after the collapse of intraterminal Ca^{2+} gradients contributes to short-term synaptic plasticity *(2)*.

3.2.2. Measurements from Pools of Terminals

Large pools of nerve terminals can be labeled by remote uptake of Ca^{2+} indicators in afferent axons *(46)*. In several studies presynaptic Ca^{2+} signals averaged over such pools were measured, e.g., at the CA3-CA1 Schaffer collatorals in hippocampus *(47)*, and at the granule cell Purkinje cell synapse in cerebellum *(48)*. Although lacking subterminal resolution these measurements provide valuable information about presynaptic [Ca^{2+}] dynamics and the pharmacology and modulation of presynaptic Ca^{2+} currents. For example, presynaptic Ca^{2+} influx was found to depend mainly on N- and P/Q-type channels in several CNS preparations *(47,49)*. An additional contribution of R-type channels is likely and has been observed in the "calyx of Held," a giant nerve terminal in the medial nucleus of the trapezoid body (MNTB) in the brainstem *(50)*. In general, presynaptic Ca^{2+} influx at central fast synapses appears to be mediated by N-, P/Q-, and R-type channels, whereas L-type channels predominate in peripheral nerve terminals and in sensory neurons *(51)*.

Average presynaptic fluorescence recordings also have been combined with simultaneous monitoring of release to indirectly probe the distance of different Ca^{2+} channel subtypes from release sites *(51)*. Release was measured using postsynaptic field potential slopes or postsynaptic current amplitudes. The potencies of Ca^{2+} channel subtypes to evoke release were determined from the exponent in the power law relationship between release and average presynaptic [Ca^{2+}]. Consistently, N-type channels were found to be less effective in triggering release than P/Q-type channels at hippocampal synapses *(47)*, at cerebellar parallel fiber synapses *(49)*, and in the calyx of Held *(52)*. Wu et al. *(52)* furthermore found that R-type channels coupled to release with an efficiency similar to N-type channels. Testing different scenarios for the spatial organization of the channels, they concluded that all three subtypes can contribute to release at individual release sites, but that a larger fraction of N- and R-type channels is localized distant from release sites, affecting exocytosis only little. These results were consistent with antibody double labelings of Ca^{2+} channel subtypes and the synaptic vesicle protein synaptotagmin, which demonstrated a higher degree of co-localization with release sites for P/Q-type channels than for N- or R-type channels *(52)*.

3.3. Postsynaptic Calcium Entry

3.3.1. Dendrites and Dendritic Spines

On the postsynaptic side multiple Ca^{2+} routes are present, including Ca^{2+}-permeable receptor channels, voltage-gated channels, and release channels (Fig. 4). Voltage-gated Ca^{2+} channels in dendrites can be activated by backpropagating action potentials, by synaptic potentials, or by regenerative dendritic potentials *(53,54)*. The spatial profile of action potential-evoked Ca^{2+} transients indicates how far action potentials backpropagate in the dendritic tree. Dendritic Ca^{2+} action potentials, for example, have been observed in neocortical layer 5 neurons *(55,56)*. It is difficult to convert dendritic Ca^{2+} transient amplitudes to Ca^{2+} channel densities because they depend on the local membrane potential and surface-to-volume ratio. At least, most of the data are consistent with a fairly uniform total density of Ca^{2+} channels in pyramidal cell dendrites *(57)*. The relative contribution of the different subtypes, however, seems to be inhomogeneous in dendrites. Christie et al. *(58)* compared $[Ca^{2+}]$ transient profiles in hippocampal pyramidal dendrites before and after blocking several types of Ca^{2+} channels. They found a preferential location of high-voltage activated Ca^{2+} channels (L-, N-, and P/Q-type) near the soma and in proximal dendrites, whereas the remaining component (T- and R-type channels) showed a more uniform or distally increased contribution. These results are consistent with direct electrical recordings *(57)* and with immunocytochemical data showing the presence of L-, N-, and P/Q-type channels in pyramidal dendrites *(59–61)*.

Optical detection of dendritic Ca^{2+} influx through receptor channels has been difficult because of the masking effect of voltage-gated Ca^{2+} currents during strong dendritic depolarizations and neuronal firing. In several cases, localized dendritic $[Ca^{2+}]$ transients during subthreshold synaptic potentials were found to be mediated mainly by low-threshold Ca^{2+} channels *(62)*. An NMDA receptor-dependent component of dendritic Ca^{2+} accumulations could be identified in hippocampal neurons by application of D-APV *(63)*.

A different strategy to visualize Ca^{2+} entry through NMDA receptors was to continuously depolarize a postsynaptic neuron to inactivate Ca^{2+} channels and to reverse synaptic currents. Using this approach and focal stimulation, Malinow et al. *(64)* observed hot spots of dendritic Ca^{2+} elevations that were blocked by D-APV. Application of confocal and in particular two-photon microscopy for imaging in brain slices eventually made the investigation of Ca^{2+} entry pathways in individual dendritic spines possible *(16)*. In hippocampal and neocortical neurons a clear NMDA-mediated component of spineous Ca^{2+} influx was resolved *(65–67)*. In some spines a component through nonNMDA receptors may exist as well *(68)*. An important question has been whether voltage-dependent Ca^{2+} channels are located in dendritic spines. Line-scans demonstrated that action potential-evoked Ca^{2+} transients rise as fast in spines as in the parent dendrite *(65,66)*; this is inconsistent with diffusion from the shaft into the spine and suggests that Ca^{2+} channels are present in the spineous membrane, consistent with a report on N-type channels in dendritic spines using fluorescently labeled ω-conotoxin *(60)*. In addition, several recent studies found evidence for synaptically induced Ca^{2+} release in dendritic spines *(69)*. In summary, multiple pathways coexist in spines and it will be necessary to further dissect their relative contribution to Ca^{2+} influx under various conditions. At present it is not clear whether and how the subspinous spatial organization of these sources relates to specific functions, e.g., the induction of long-term plasticity. Unfortunately, rapid Ca^{2+} gradients in spines are almost impossible to resolve with diffusible indicators. Perhaps, specific labeling of various spineous proteins with genetically encoded indicators will allow us to see how Ca^{2+} signals differ at subspinous locations.

3.3.2. MNTB Principal Neurons

On a larger spatial scale, a differential pattern of postsynaptic Ca^{2+} influx through NMDA receptors and voltage-gated Ca^{2+} channels was observed in principal neurons of the MNTB in rat brainstem (Fig. 5). These neurons are covered by large calyx-type nerve terminals (Fig. 5A). A presynaptic action potential evokes glutamate release and the postsynaptic current typically elicits a single action potential in the principal neuron. Postsynaptic Ca^{2+} influx during synaptic transmission mainly occurs through NMDA receptors and voltage-gated Ca^{2+} channels *(22)*. Using a CCD camera system, Bollmann et al. *(22)* found a difference in the spatial pattern of postsynaptic Ca^{2+} influx through these two entry pathways (Fig. 5C,D). It is likely that different sets of proteins are activated by the two Ca^{2+} pathways; the subterminal NMDA receptor-mediated $[Ca^{2+}]$ elevations may be specifically important for synapse stabilization early in development.

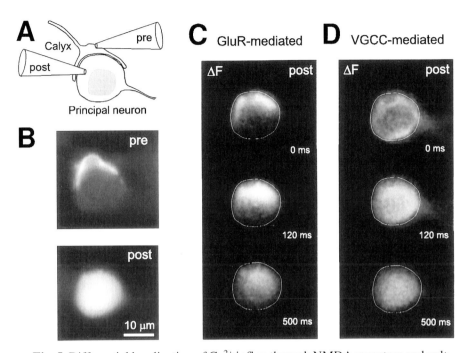

Fig. 5. Differential localization of Ca^{2+} influx through NMDA receptors and voltage-gated Ca^{2+} channels (VGCC) at the giant synapse in the MNTB. (**A**) Schematic of the recording configuration. A simultaneous pre and postsynaptic whole-cell-recording was made from a presynaptic terminal (calyx of Held) and a MNTB principal neuron in a rat brainstem slice. The pre and postsynaptic pipet contained 0.4 mM MagFura-2 and 0.4 mM Oregon Green 488 BAPTA-5N, respectively. The presynaptic membrane potential was recorded in current-clamp mode. Single presynaptic action potentials were evoked by afferent stimulation with a remote bipolar electrode. (**B**) Morphological images of the presynaptic terminal (*top*) and the principal neuron (*bottom*). Pre- and postsynaptic fluorescence were separated by using excitation wavelengths of 380 and 480 nm, respectively. (**C**) In Mg^{2+}-free extracellular solution, a presynaptic action potential evoked a large NMDAR-mediated Ca^{2+} signal that was initially located beneath the presynaptic terminal. Images were aquired at 30 Hz. Difference images (ΔF) are shown at three different times after stimulation. The postsynaptic voltage was clamped to -80 mV and AMPA receptors were blocked. (**D**) Later in the same experiment Na$^+$ and K$^+$ currents were blocked with TTX and TEA. A large Ca^{2+} current evoked by a 40 ms voltage step to -10 mV caused a different pattern of postsynaptic Ca^{2+} influx, comprising the side opposite to the terminal and the postsynaptic axon. Note that in both cases (C) and (D) fluorescence changes almost equilibrated in the cell after 500 ms.

4. CONCLUSIONS

Neurons perform multitasking using the same messenger ion Ca^{2+} by segregating Ca^{2+} signals in different cellular compartments. Optical imaging of fluorescent Ca^{2+} indicators has provided at least qualitative spatial maps of the distribution of various Ca^{2+} sources in many neurons. Notably, this method probes the physiologically relevant activation pattern of Ca^{2+}-permeable ion channels. Application of new indicators as well as improvements in imaging techniques may lead to a refinement of these maps. Fluorescence imaging on the micrometer scale ultimately is limited by the optical resolution; nevertheless, it is useful to determine local values of biophysical parameters, such as diffusion coefficients or Ca^{2+}-buffering capacities. Together with ultrastructural information and a more detailed knowledge about the identity and distribution of Ca^{2+}-binding proteins and Ca^{2+} clearance mechanisms, such values may enable realistic simulations of $[Ca^{2+}]$ dynamics on the molecular scale. Perhaps the greatest challenge, however, will be to further link the observed local Ca^{2+} signals to their downstream biochemical effects in order to understand their functional relevance.

ACKNOWLEDGMENTS

The author thanks Mark Schnitzer for comments on the manuscript and acknowledges support by a postdoctoral fellowship from the Human Frontier Science Program.

REFERENCES

1. Ghosh, A. and Greenberg, M. E. (1995) Calcium signaling in neurons: molecular mechanisms and cellular consequences. *Science* **268,** 239–247.
2. Zucker, R. S. (1999) Calcium- and activity-dependent synaptic plasticity. *Curr. Opin. Neurobiol.* **9,** 305–313.
3. Wang, S. S.-H. and Augustine, G. J. (1999) Calcium signaling in neurons: a case study in cellular compartmentalization, in *Calcium as a Cellular Regulator* (Carafoli, E. and Klee, C., eds.), Oxford University Press, Oxford, UK, pp. 545–566.
4. Tsien, R. Y. (1999) Monitoring cell calcium, in *Calcium as a Cellular Regulator* (Carafoli, E. and Klee, C., eds.), Oxford University Press, Oxford, UK, pp. 28–54.
5. Augustine, G. J. and Neher, E. (1992) Neuronal Ca^{2+} signalling takes the local route. *Curr. Opin. Neurobiol.* **2,** 302–307.
6. Helmchen, F. (1999) Dendrites as biochemical compartments, in *Dendrites* (Stuart, G., Spruston, N., and Hausser, M., eds.), Oxford University Press, Oxford, UK, pp. 161–192.
7. Brini, M., Pinton, P., Pozzan, T., and Rizzuto, R. (1999) Targeted recombinant aequorins: tools for monitoring $[Ca^{2+}]$ in the various compartments of a living cell. *Microsc. Res. Tech.* **46,** 380–389.
8. Sabatini, B. L. and Regehr, W. G. (1998) Optical measurement of presynaptic calcium current. *Biophys. J.* **74,** 1549–1563.

9. Etter, E. F., Kuhn, M. A., and Fay, F. S. (1994) Detection of changes in near membrane Ca^{2+} using a novel membrane associated Ca^{2+} indicator. *J. Biol. Chem.* **269**, 10,141–10,149.

10. Vorndran, C., Minta, A., and Poenie, M. (1995) New fluorescent calcium indicators designed for cytosolic retention or measuring calcium near membranes. *Biophys. J.* **69**, 2112–2124.

11. Miyawaki, A., Llopis, J., Heim, R., McCaffery, J. M., Adams, J. A., Ikura, M., and Tsien, R. Y. (1997) Fluorescent indicators for Ca^{2+} based on green fluorescent proteins and calmodulin. *Nature* **388**, 882–887.

12. Yuste, R., Lanni, F., and Konnerth, A. (eds.) (1999) *Imaging Neurons: A Laboratory Manual.* Cold Spring Harbor Laboratory, Cold Spring Harbor, NY.

13. DiGregorio, D. A. and Vergara, J. L. (1997) Localized detection of action potential-induced presynaptic calcium transients at a Xenopus neuromuscular junction. *J. Physiol. (Lond.)* **505**, 585–592.

14. Pawley, J. B. (ed.) (1995) *Handbook of Biological Confocal Microscopy.* Plenum, New York.

15. Denk, W., Strickler, J. H., and Webb, W. W. (1990) Two-photon laser scanning fluorescence microscopy. *Science* **248**, 73–76.

16. Denk, W., Yuste, R., Svoboda, K., and Tank, D. W. (1996) Imaging calcium dynamics in dendritic spines. *Curr. Opin. Neurobiol.* **6**, 372–378.

17. Denk, W. and Svoboda, K. (1997) Photon upmanship: why multiphoton imaging is more than a gimmick. *Neuron* **18**, 351–357.

18. Schiller, J., Helmchen, F., and Sakmann, B. (1995) Spatial profile of dendritic calcium transients evoked by action potentials in rat neocortical pyramidal neurones. *J. Physiol. (Lond.)* **487**, 583–600.

19. Monck, J. R., Robinson, I. M., Escobar, A. L., Vergara, J. L., and Fernandez, J. M. (1994) Pulsed laser imaging of rapid Ca^{2+} gradients in excitable cells. *Biophys. J.* **67**, 505–514.

20. Neher, E. (1995) The use of fura-2 for estimating Ca buffers and Ca fluxes. *Neuropharmacology* **34**, 1423–1442.

21. Schneggenburger, R., Zhou, Z., Konnerth, A., and Neher, E. (1993) Fractional contribution of calcium to the cation current through glutamate receptor channels. *Neuron* **11**, 133–43.

22. Bollmann, J. H., Helmchen, F., Borst, J. G., and Sakmann, B. (1998) Postsynaptic Ca^{2+} influx mediated by three different pathways during synaptic transmission at a calyx-type synapse. *J. Neurosci.* **18**, 10,409–10,419.

23. Garaschuk, O., Schneggenburger, R., Schirra, C., Tempia, F., and Konnerth, A. (1996) Fractional Ca^{2+} currents through somatic and dendritic glutamate receptor channels of rat hippocampal CA1 pyramidal neurones. *J. Physiol. (Lond.)* **491**, 757–772.

24. Borst, J. G. and Helmchen, F. (1998) Calcium influx during an action potential. *Meth. Enzym.* **293**, 352–371.

25. Ratto, G. M., Payne, R., Owen, R. G., and Tsien, R. Y. (1988) The concentration of cytosolic free calcium in vertebrate rod outer segment measured using Fura-2. *J. Neurosci.* **8**, 3240–3246.

26. Koutalos, Y. and Yau, K.-W. (1996) Regulation of sensitivity in vertebrate rod photoreceptors by calcium. *TINS* **19**, 73–81.

27. Rieke, F. and Schwartz, E. A. (1996) Asynchronous transmitter release: control of exocytosis and endocytosis at the salamander rod synapse. *J. Physiol. (Lond.)* **493**, 1–8.

28. Krizaj, D. and Copenhagen, D. R. (1998) Compartmentalization of calcium extrusion mechanisms in the outer and inner segments of photoreceptors. *Neuron* **21**, 249–256.

29. Protti, D. A. and Llano, I. (1998) Calcium currents and calcium signaling in rod bipolar cells of rat retinal slices. *J. Neurosci.* **18**, 3715–3724.

30. Denk, W. and Detwiler, P. B. (1999) Optical recording of light-evoked calcium signals in the functionally intact retina. *Proc. Natl. Acad. Sci. USA* **96**, 7035–7040.

31. Lenzi, D. and Roberts, W. M. (1994) Calcium signalling in hair cells: multiple roles in a compact cell. *Curr. Opin. Neurobiol.* **4**, 496–502.

32. Jaramillo, F. (1995) Signal transduction in hair cells and its regulation by calcium. *Neuron* **15**, 1227–1230.

33. Ohmori, H. (1988) Mechanical stimulation and fura-2 fluorescence in the hair bundle of dissociated hair cells of the chick. *J. Physiol. (Lond.)* **399**, 115–137.

34. Lumpkin, E. A. and Hudspeth, A. J. (1995) Detection of Ca²⁺ entry through mechanosensitive channels localizes the site of mechanoelectrical transduction in hair cells. *Proc. Natl. Acad. Sci. USA* **92**, 10,297–10,301.

35. Denk, W., Holt, J. R., Shepherd, G. M., and Corey, D. P. (1995) Calcium imaging of single stereocilia in hair cells: localization of transduction channels at both ends of tip links. *Neuron* **15**, 1311–1321.

36. Hudspeth, A. J. (1997) Mechanical amplification of stimuli by hair cells. *Curr. Opin. Neurobiol.* **7**, 480–486.

37. Issa, N. P. and Hudspeth, A. J. (1996) The entry and clearance of Ca²⁺ at individual presynaptic active zones of hair cells from the bullfrog's sacculus. *Proc. Natl. Acad. Sci. USA* **93**, 9527–9532.

38. Tucker, T. and Fettiplace, R. (1995) Confocal imaging of calcium microdomains and calcium extrusion in turtle hair cells. *Neuron* **15**, 1323–1335.

39. Leinders-Zufall, T., Greer, C. A., Shepherd, G. M., and Zufall, F. (1998) Imagning odor-induced calcium transients in single olfactory cilia: specificity of activation and role in transduction. *J. Neurosci.* **18**, 5630–5639.

40. Menini, A. (1999) Calcium signalling and regulation in olfactory neurons. *Curr. Opin. Neurobiol.* **9**, 419–426.

41. Smith, S. J. and Augustine, G. J. (1988) Calcium ions, active zones and synaptic transmitter release. *TINS* **11**, 458–464.

42. Neher, E. (1998) Vesicle pools and Ca²⁺ microdomains: new tools for understanding their roles in neurotransmitter release. *Neuron* **20**, 389–399.

43. Robitaille, R., Adler, E. M., and Charlton, M. P. (1990) Strategic location of calcium channels at transmitter release sites of frog neuromuscular junction. *Neuron* **5**, 773–779.

44. Smith, S. J., Buchanan, J., Osses, L. R., Charlton, M. P., and Augustine, G. J. (1993) The spatial distribution of calcium signals in squid presynaptic terminals. *J. Physiol. (Lond.)* **472**, 573–593.
45. Llinas, R., Sugimori, M., and Silver, R. B. (1992) Microdomains of high calcium concentration in a presynaptic terminal. *Science* **256**, 677–679.
46. Regehr, W. G. and Tank, D. W. (1991) Selective fura-2 loading of presynaptic terminals and nerve cell processes by local perfusion in mammalian brain slice. *J. Neurosci. Meth.* **37**, 111–119.
47. Wu, L. G. and Saggau, P. (1994) Pharmacological identification of two types of presynaptic voltage-dependent calcium channels at CA3-CA1 synapses of the hippocampus. *J. Neurosci.* **14**, 5613–5622.
48. Regehr, W. and Atluri, P. P. (1995) Calcium transients in cerebellar granule cell presynaptic terminals. *Biophys. J.* **68**, 2156–2170.
49. Mintz, I., Sabatini, B. L., and Regehr, W. G. (1995) Calcium control of transmitter release at a cerebellar synapse. *Neuron* **15**, 675–688.
50. Wu, L. G., Borst, J. G., and Sakmann, B. (1998) R-type Ca^{2+} currents evoke transmitter release at a rat central synapse. *Proc. Natl. Acad. Sci. USA* **95**, 4720–4725.
51. Dunlap, K., Luebke, J. I., and Turner, T. J. (1995) Exocytotic Ca^{2+} channels in mammalian central neurons. *TINS* **18**, 89–98.
52. Wu, L. G., Westenbroek, R. E., Borst, J. G. G., Catterall, W. A., and Sakmann, B. (1999) Calcium channel types with distinct presynaptic localization couple differentially to transmitter release in single calyx-type synapses. *J. Neurosci.* **19**, 726–736.
53. Regehr, W. G. and Tank, D. W. (1994) Dendritic calcium dynamics. *Curr. Opin. Neurobiol.* **4**, 373–382.
54. Yuste, R. and Tank, D. W. (1996) Dendritic integration in mammalian neurons, a century after Cajal. *Neuron* **16**, 701–716.
55. Schiller, J., Schiller, Y., Stuart, G., and Sakmann, B. (1997) Calcium action potentials restricted to distal apical dendrites of rat neocortical pyramidal neurons. *J. Physiol. (Lond.)* **505**, 605–616.
56. Helmchen, F., Svoboda, K., Denk, W., and Tank, D. W. (1999) *In vivo* dendritic calcium dynamics in deep-layer cortical pyramidal neurons. *Nature Neurosci.* **2**, 989–996.
57. Magee, J., Hoffman, D., Colbert, C., and Johnston, D. (1998) Electrical and calcium signaling in dendrites of hippocampal pyramidal neurons. *Ann. Rev. Physiol.* **60**, 327–346.
58. Christie, B. R., Eliot, L. S., Ito, K., Miyakawa, H., and Johnston, D. (1995) Different Ca^{2+} channels in soma and dendrites of hippocampal pyramidal neurons mediate spike-induced Ca^{2+} influx. *J. Neurophysiol.* **73**, 2553–2557.
59. Westenbroek, R. E., Ahlijanian, M. K., and Catterall, W. A. (1990) Clustering of L-type Ca^{2+} channels at the base of major dendrites in hippocampal pyramidal neurons. *Nature* **347**, 281–284.
60. Mills, L. R., Niesen, C. E., So, A. P., Carlen, P. L., Spigelman, I., and Jones, O. T. (1994) N-type Ca^{2+} channels are located on somata, dendrites, and a sub-

population of dendritic spines on live hippocampal pyramidal neurons. *J. Neurosci.* **14**, 6815–6824.

61. Westenbroek, R. E., Sakurai, T., Elliott, E. M., Hell, J. W., Starr, T. V. B., Snutch, T. P., and Catterall, W. A. (1995) Immunochemical identification and subcellular distribution of the alpha 1A subunits of brain calcium channels. *J. Neurosci.* **15**, 6403–6418.

62. Eilers, J. and Konnerth, A. (1997) Dendritic signal integration. *Curr. Opin. Neurobiol.* **7**, 385–390.

63. Regehr, W. G. and Tank, D. W. (1990) Postsynaptic NMDA receptor-mediated calcium accumulation in hippocampal CA1 pyramidal cell dendrites. *Nature* **345**, 807–810.

64. Malinow, R., Otmakhov, N., Blum, K. I., and Lisman, J. (1994) Visualizing hippocampal synaptic function by optical detection of Ca²⁺ entry through the N-methyl-D-aspartate channel. *Proc. Natl. Acad. Sci. USA* **91**, 8170–8174.

65. Yuste, R. and Denk, W. (1995) Dendritic spines as basic functional units of neuronal integration. *Nature* **375**, 682–684.

66. Schiller, J., Schiller, Y., and Clapham, D. E. (1998) NMDA receptors amplify calcium influx into dendritic spines during associative pre- and postsynaptic activation. *Nature Neurosci.* **1**, 114–118.

67. Koester, H. J. and Sakmann, B. (1998) Calcium dynamics in single spines during coincident pre- and postsynaptic activity depend on relative timing of back-propagating action potentials and subthreshold excitatory postsynaptic potentials. *Proc. Natl. Acad. Sci. USA* **95**, 9596–9601.

68. Yuste, R., Majewska, A., Cash, S. S., and Denk, W. (1999) Mechanisms of calcium influx into hippocampal spines: heterogeneity among spines, coincidence detection by NMDA receptors, and optical quantal analysis. *J. Neurosci.* **19**, 1976–1987.

69. Svoboda, K. and Mainen, Z. F. (1999) Synaptic [Ca²⁺]: intracellular stores spill their guts. *Neuron* **22**, 427–430.

19

Using Caged Compounds to Map Functional Neurotransmitter Receptors

Diana L. Pettit and George J. Augustine

1. INTRODUCTION

As amply demonstrated by each of the chapters of this volume, location is an integral part of the physiological function of ion channels. Neurotransmitter receptors may represent an extreme example of this important concept, because these receptors must be targeted—within an accuracy of nanometers—in order to detect the release of neurotransmitters from presynaptic terminals. However, it has been challenging to visualize the location of receptors that are within the plasma membrane, as opposed to being within transport vesicles or other intracellular sites. It has been even more challenging to examine the functional properties of selected populations of receptors on the plasma membrane. Here we describe experiments that allow the use of "caged" neurotransmitters for these purposes.

Flash photolysis of caged compounds by UV light is a powerful tool because it offers high spatial and temporal resolution. The UV light beam used to photolyze caged compounds can be focused to less than a μm in diameter, allowing production of caged compound to a very small portion of a cell *(1–6)*. Photolysis also offers very high time resolution; in favorable cases, photolysis occurs within tens of μs, which has made caged compounds the method of choice for determining the kinetics of many biological processes *(7–9)*. Flash photolysis also allows for the focal release of neurotransmitters in a wide spectrum of experimental systems, ranging from dissociated cells to whole animals.

In this chapter, we describe some of the considerations involved in using caged neurotransmitters to map the distribution and function of neurotrans-

From: *Ion Channel Localization Methods and Protocols*
Edited by: A. Lopatin and C. G. Nichols © Humana Press Inc., Totowa, NJ

mitter receptors and also summarize some of our recent experiments that use this approach to define the distribution of neurotransmitter receptors in neurons within hippocampal slices.

2. HARDWARE FOR UNCAGING NEUROTRANSMITTERS

Focal uncaging of neurotransmitters requires a microscope with a suitable recording chamber, a UV light source for uncaging, an imaging system to visualize the neurons, and hardware for focusing and positioning the UV light beam (Fig. 1). Although imaging systems and recording chambers have received substantial attention in the literature, little has been written about the hardware required for local uncaging experiments. For this reason, we will consider these topics in some detail.

Most caged transmitters are photolyzed to their biologically active form by near-UV light (300–400 n*M*). The most commonly used sources of UV light are arc lamps or lasers. Each light source has advantages and the choice of light source is often dictated by the specifics of each application, as well as the amount of funds available. Arc lamps used for uncaging are either continuous-discharge arc lamps or an arc lamp connected to a bank of capacitors (so-called flash lamps; *10*). These lamps are inexpensive; indeed nearly every fluorescence microscope has an arc lamp that requires minimal adaptation (addition of a shutter and perhaps a quartz collector lens) to be suited for photolysis. Arc lamps typically are used when a large uncaging area is desired. With these lamps, an entire specimen can be illuminated or the light can be focused down to spots tens of micrometers in diameter. The main limitation of these lamps is that their light energy is limited. Continuous discharge lamps typically emit a relatively small amount of UV light, with mercury lamps being more powerful that xenon lamps. Flash lamps use the power stored in the capacitor bank to produce a very intense but short-lived flash of UV light. For some applications, it may not be possible to produce enough UV light within a biologically relevant time frame. Despite this problem, arc lamps are economical and reliable UV light sources.

When an uncaging area of a few micrometers or less is required, a laser is the light source of choice. A laser light beam is a highly collimated light source and therefore can be focused down to a very small spot, a few micrometers or less in diameter. Only a few lasers produce a suitable amount of UV light; among these, we and most others have used continuous-discharge argon ion lasers. The laser that we use (Coherent Innova 305) emits

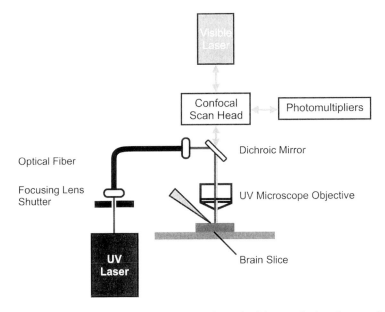

Fig. 1. Diagram of an uncaging setup. Adapted with permission from ref. *5.*

up to 200 mW of UV light at 351–364 nm. As described earlier for the case of continuous-discharge flash lamps, an electronic shutter is needed to control the duration of illumination from such continuous-discharge lasers. Measurements of UV light intensity on our setup indicate that an energy density of 0.01–0.1 $\mu J/\mu m^2$ per flash is sufficient to uncage the neurotransmitter compounds described in this chapter. Other compounds will be photolyzed in proportion to the product of their extinction coefficients and quantum yields. This power level is easily achieved by the use of an argon ion laser; for the laser and coupling system that we have employed, flashes of 1–10 ms are sufficient to achieve these energy levels. The biggest drawbacks of UV lasers are higher purchase costs and increased maintenance hours (relative to a flash lamp). Some of this expense can be offset by the purchase of a refurbished laser, which costs little more than a new flash lamp.

Light can be routed from the UV light source to the specimen by either an optical fiber or a set of mirrors and lenses. The latter is the approach of choice if the UV light must be focused to a diffraction-limited spot. This will produce the smallest possible uncaging area, but limits the possible paths for routing light to the microscope. In addition, mirrors usually require more alignment to keep the light focused. However, mirrors tend to lose less light than other optical elements. For uncaging applications where power is limited, this is a very substantial advantage.

Optical fibers provide great flexibility in routing UV light to a microscope. Typically, a lens is used to focus the output of a laser onto an optical fiber and the output from the fiber is then focused either through the microscope objective or directly onto the specimen. Because of their size, optical fibers usually prevent focusing the light spot to diffraction-limited dimensions (sub-micrometer). The most significant problem associated with the use of optical fibers is that they can attenuate UV signals themselves and coupling of laser output to fibers is rather inefficient. As a result, a significant fraction (50% or more) of the UV light can be lost between the laser and the specimen. Having a laser with an excess of power can remedy this problem.

3. CAGED COMPOUNDS

The choice of caged compound is a critical factor in the success of a flash photolysis experiment. An ideal caged compound should: (1) be stable in the caged form; (2) uncage rapidly and with high efficiency when irradiated by UV light; and (3) neither the free cage nor the caged compound should have any biological actions *(11)*. The design and synthesis of optimal caged compounds remains an ongoing effort, though great strides have been made in recent years.

Restricting the spatial extent of photolysis of caged neurotransmitters is one of the central challenges. In three-dimensional recording chambers, caged neurotransmitter can be found throughout the light beam, meaning that light on its way to and from the targeted portion of the specimen will photolyze caged compound (Fig. 2A). This can greatly reduce the spatial resolution of neurotransmitter application. To improve this situation, we have developed a simple and economical way to eliminate out-of-focus uncaging. Our approach relies on attaching two caging groups to a single molecule. If each cage inactivates the compound, then two photons of light will be required to produce a free molecule of neurotransmitter (Fig. 2B). We call this phenomenon "chemical two-photon uncaging" *(12)* to distinguish it from "optical" two-photon excitation *(13)*, in which two long-wavelength photons are needed to provide sufficient energy to photolyze a single caging group *(14,15)*.

A double-caged compound can be synthesized from any molecule that has two sites where inactivating cages can be attached. Each cage must inactivate the molecule, so that the singly-caged intermediate, produced by partial photolysis of the double-caged compound, will have no biological activity. As a test of the chemical two-photon uncaging concept, we have

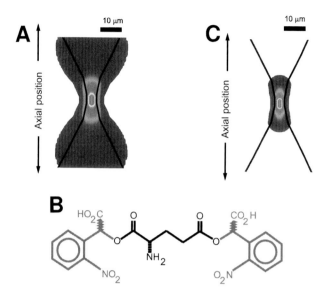

Fig. 2. Theoretical improvement in axial resolution with double-caged glutamate. (**A**) The double cone of a light beam converging to a focus. Values are taken for our experimental setup as described in ref. *5*. The concentration of glutamate produced by uncaging as a function of distance from the focal plane, for single-caged glutamate. (**B**) The structure of double-caged glutamate. The double cone of a light beam converging to a focus. Values are taken for our experimental setup as described in *(5)*. (**C**) The concentration of glutamate produced by uncaging as a function of distance from the focal plane, for double-caged glutamate. Adapted with permission from ref. *12*.

used a double-caged glutamate compound *(12)*. Earlier work established that both the α and γ carboxyl groups of glutamate are inactivated by cages *(16)*, so that suitable double-caged glutamate could be synthesized by adding carboxynitrobenzyl caging groups to each of these two carboxyl groups (Fig. 2B). This compound is now commercially available from the Molecular Probes company. We assume that each caged carboxylate group is photolyzed identically to the analogous mono-carboxynitrobenzyl (single) caged glutamates, which have quantum yields of 0.16–0.21 and half-lives of photolysis that range from 21–80 μs *(16)*.

The main contaminant of commercial preparations of single-caged glutamate is free glutamate. Because glutamate can cause unwanted activation or desensitization of glutamate receptors, this can be a serious problem. By these criteria we have observed spontaneous loss of the caging groups, over time scales of tens of minutes, when using single-caged glutamate. As expected, this is much less of a problem for double-caged glutamate. However, even with double-caged glutamate it is important to minimize loss of the cages during storage and handling.

The requirement for two photons to produce the free, uncaged molecule should improve axial resolution in proportion to the square of the light intensity (Fig. 2C). To predict the efficacy of double-caged compounds, we used the geometry of the light beam on our apparatus (Fig. 1; 5) to calculate the axial distribution of glutamate produced by photolysis of single-caged or double-caged glutamate *(12)*. Our calculations predict that photolysis of single-caged glutamate will produce free glutamate in a large volume while photolysis of double-caged glutamate should produced free glutamate primarily at the focal plane (Fig. 2C). Assuming that electrical current, I, is produced in proportion to glutamate concentration *(17)* the response of a neuron to photolysis of double-caged glutamate ($I_{double}(z)$) is then:

$$I_{double}(z) = \frac{I_0 C r^2_0 p^2}{2} \frac{[1-2^{-2 \, r^2_{cell}/r^2_{spot}(z)}]}{r^2_{spot}(Z)}$$

where C is caged glutamate concentration; p is the probability of photolyzing a single caging group at the center of the focused spot and is proportional to light flash energy, coefficient, and quantum yield; $r_{spot}(z)$ is the radius of the UV light beam at axial position z; ro is the radius of the light spot in the focal plane; r_{cell} is the radius of the neuron; and I_0 is a parameter proportional to the responsiveness of receptors to glutamate. With non-saturating light intensities ($p \ll 1$) and a minimal spot radius $r_0 = 2.8$ μm, this equation predicts that the expected half-maximal depth for the response to photolysis of double-caged glutamate should be 17 μm in our system, a 60% improvement in axial resolution over single-caged glutamate *(12)*. For more intense flashes, the axial resolution of responses should degrade because the nonlinearity of glutamate production is lost as saturation causes the region of maximal glutamate production to become more distributed.Numerical calculations indicate that for p = 0.9, the half-maximal depth for double-caged glutamate will expand to 32 μm *(12)*.

4. 2-PHOTON PHOTOLYSIS OF GLUTAMATE IN BRAIN SLICES

We have tested the utility of chemical two-photon uncaging by applying glutamate onto neurons within brain slices. Our goal was to compare the axial resolution of the double-caged glutamate to that of a conventional,

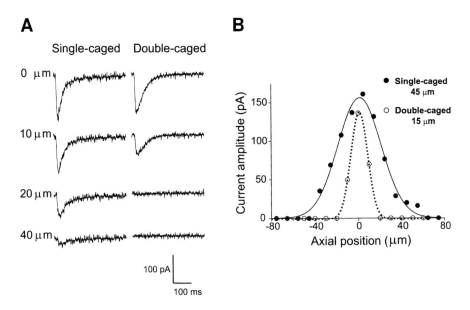

Fig. 3. Double-caged glutamate improves axial resolution. **(A)** Current traces obtained from z-series with single- and double-caged glutamate. **(B)** The peak amplitudes of currents from the z-series in (c), plotted against axial position. The half-width of the gaussian fit for single-caged glutamate is 40 μm and 15 μm for double-caged glutamate. The current amplitudes represent responses taken at +70 to –80 μm from the focal plane, taken at 10 μm steps. All uncaging light flashes were 5 ms in duration. Adapted with permission from ref. *18.*

single-caged glutamate by measurements of glutamate-induced electrical responses in hippocampal CA1 pyramidal neurons *(12)*. Hippocampal slices were prepared from rats 13-18 d old and whole-cell patch clamp recordings were made from the cell bodies of pyramidal neurons. Figure 3A shows recordings of membrane currents evoked by uncaging either single- or double-caged glutamate at various axial positions above or below the neuronal cell body. In both cases, maximal responses occured at the focal plane (z = 0 μm) and dropped off with distance. Strikingly, 20 μm below the focal plane, single-caged glutamate evoked a response, but no response to double caged glutamate was observed. This shows that adding a second cage to glutamate improves axial resolution.

This improvement in axial resolution was quantified by plotting the relationship between the amplitude of glutamate-induced currents and the distance from the focal plane. These relationships could be fit with gaussian functions (Fig. 3B) and the half-width of these functions were used as a

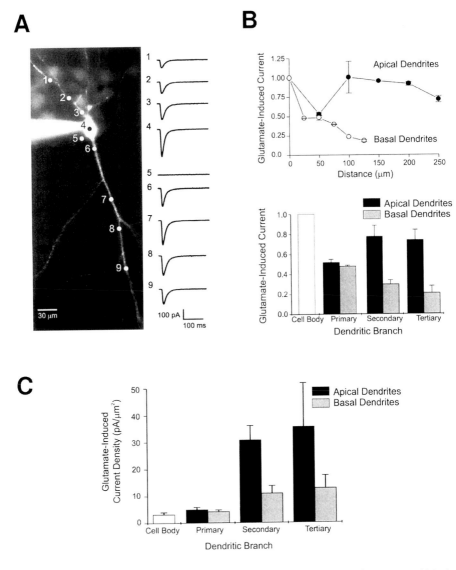

Fig. 4. Non-uniformity of glutamate responses on pyramidal neurons. (**A**) A volume-rendered image of a CA1 pyramidal neuron filled with fluorescent dye via a patch pipet. Circles indicate the position and diameter of the UV light spot used. Traces at right are averages of five responses evoked with 3 ms pulses from the locations indicated by the numbers. Traces 1–3 are responses from basal dendrites, traces 6–9 are responses from apical dendrites. Moving the uncaging spot off the neuron elicited no glutamate response from the neuron (trace 5). (**B**) Relationship between the location of the UV light spot with respect to the some and the ampli-

(continued)

measure of axial resolution. For the case of hippocampal pyramidal neurons, the mean half-width of the gaussian was 43.5 µm ± 5.9 µm for the single-caged compound and 18.7 ± 4.8 µm for the double-caged compound. This is a 57% improvement in axial resolution over single-caged glutamate, in excellent agreement with the theoretical prediction described earlier. Very similar improvements in axial resolution of uncaging were also observed for the case of Purkinje neurons in cerebellar slices *(18)*. In addition, the presence of two caging groups also appears to improve lateral resolution significantly *(19)*. Taken together, these data clearly indicate the utility of chemical two-photon uncaging. Further, such analyses provide a simple empirical test that can be applied to future applications of chemical two-photon uncaging.

One possible complication of the chemical two-photon method is that photolysis of caged glutamate could cause depletion of caged glutamate or accumulation of free glutamate, single-caged glutamate, or carboxynitrobenzyl groups. To test for such phenomena, we have given repeated light flashes while monitoring the stability of the glutamate-induced electrical currents. No changes in the amplitude or time course of responses were observed when the light flashes were repeated at 10-s intervals. This demonstrates that changes in the chemical environment are minimal on a time scale of 10 s and that photoproducts are not accumulating to an appreciable extent. This observation also indicates that free glutamate is cleared out very quickly from brain slices. In fact, we have seen no evidence for buildup of glutamate even when uncaging repeatedly at 500 ms intervals in cerebellar slices. Purkinje cell responses to uncaged glutamate decay over tens of milliseconds *(18)*, suggesting that glutamate is removed over such time scales (*see* also ref. *20*). Other transmitters may not be handled as efficiently as glutamate. For example, light flashes must be separated by tens of seconds to evoke stable responses to photolysis of single-caged GABA in hippocampal slices *(19)*. In the case of caged carbachol, light flashes must be separated by minutes (D. Pettit and J. Yakel, unpublished data), presumably owing to the inability of endogenous cholinesterases to degrade the carbachol. However, with appropriate time intervals it is possible to produce

---

tude of the current induced by glutamate at each location. The peak amplitude of the glutamate-induced currents have been normalized to the amplitude of currents evoked over the cell body of each of the 8 neurons examined. (**C**) The same glutamate responses shown in A, considered as a function of dendritic branch. (**D**) Relationship between the location of the UV light spot and the mean density of the current induced by glutamate at each location, calculated by dividing current amplitude by the area over which glutamate was photoreleased. Adapted with permission from ref. *18*.

stable responses with little variation over hundreds of light flashes. Achieving this condition for a given application requires a careful balance of caged compound concentration and light flash power and frequency.

5. GLUTAMATE RECEPTOR DISTRIBUTION IN PYRAMIDAL CELLS AND INTERNEURONS

We have used local photolysis to determine the spatial distribution of neurotransmitter receptors along hippocampal neurons. In these experiments, neurotransmitter receptors were activated by scanning a spot of UV light (4.6 μm in diameter) along the neuron to generate active neurotransmitter over a restricted region. A fluorescent dye was included in the solution used to fill the recording pipet; when this dye solution diffused from the pipet to the neuronal cytoplasm, it was possible to visualize the processes of these cells during the photolysis experiments (*see* Fig. 1). This approach allowed us to position the light spot as far as 250 μm along apical dendrites and up to 100 μm along basal dendrites of hippocampal pyramidal neurons. By using whole-cell patch-clamp methods to measure electrical currents resulting from uncaging the transmitter at various positions, it is possible to map regional variations in the transmitter responsiveness of individual neurons. To examine currents flowing through transmitter receptors, without contamination by voltage-gated currents, all experiments were done in the presence of (1) tetrodotoxin, to block voltage-gated sodium channels; (2) cesium in the recording pipet to block voltage-gated potassium channels; and (3) cadmium to block calcium channels.

When examining glutamate receptors, the double-caged glutamate compound described above was used to obtain optimal spatial resolution. Responses could be observed when glutamate was generated over any region of CA1 pyramidal neurons (Fig. 4A) *(19)*. In basal dendrites, glutamate response amplitude decreased rapidly as the light spot was moved further from the cell body (Fig. 4A, trace 2). However, the response profile for apical dendrite had a very different pattern. When the uncaging spot was moved to the primary apical dendrite (Fig. 1C, trace 6), the amplitude of glutamate responses decreased in manner similar to that seen in the basal dendrites. But when the uncaging spot was moved even further away, the glutamate responses amplitude increased relative to the response at the primary apical dendrites (e.g., Fig. 4A, trace 7). When plotted as a function of distance or the order of the dendritic branch, it could be observed that the increase in glutamate current amplitude along the apical dendrite was restricted to the secondary and tertiary dendrites (Fig. 4B). This spatial profile did not depend on activation of N-methyl-D-aspartate (NMDA) receptors because it was unaffected by application of APV ($100\ \mu M$), a blocker of NMDA receptors. These data suggest that glutamate receptors, specifically the alpha-amino-3-hydroxy-5-methyl-4-isxazolepropionic acid (AMPA)-type glutamate receptor, distribute heterogeneously over the surface of pyramidal neurons.

Although the UV light spot has a constant diameter, dendritic diameter varies. This results in variations in the area of plasma membrane that is exposed to uncaged glutamate as the spot is scanned along the dendrite. To account for such variations in surface area, we used volume-rendered confocal images of the pyramidal neurons to estimate the diameter of each region of dendrite exposed to the UV light beam. The surface area under each uncaging spot was then calculated by modeling the dendrite as a cylinder with a length identical to the diameter of the UV uncaging light beam *(5,12)*. The density of glutamate-induced electrical current at each site was then determined by dividing the peak amplitude of each current by the area exposed to glutamate.

The density of glutamate-induced currents increased with distance from the cell body (Fig. 4C). Because of the larger surface area of the cell body, current density was higher in the dendrites than in the cell body, and highest in the smallest, most distal dendrites (Fig. 4C) *(19)*. Although current amplitude declined along basal dendrites (Fig. 4A,B), the area of these dendrites declined more steeply so that there was a higher density of glutamate-induced current in their distal regions (Fig. 4C). These data indicate that glutamate receptors are are not uniformly distributed but are targeted to specific regions. In fact, the receptors appear to form a gradient, with the highest point of the gradient in the most distal dendtrites. Perhaps this is a mechanism for amplification of distal dendritic signals.

To test whether this potential amplification mechanism is restricted to pyramidal neurons, we also mapped the distribution of glutamate receptors on interneurons in the CA1 stratum radiatum region. Photolysis of double-caged glutamate produced inward currents similar to those seen in the pyramidal neurons. Decay time constants for these glutamate responses were similar to those calculated for pyramidal cells. The distribution of the interneuronal glutamate responses also was nonuniform, though a spatial pattern differing from that seen in pyramidal cells. Electrical responses could be detected when glutamate was photoreleased over the cell bodies of interneurons, but when the uncaging spot was moved away from the interneuron some, glutamate responses increased in amplitude (Fig. 5A). This increase was observed on all dendrites within a given interneuron; for example, the

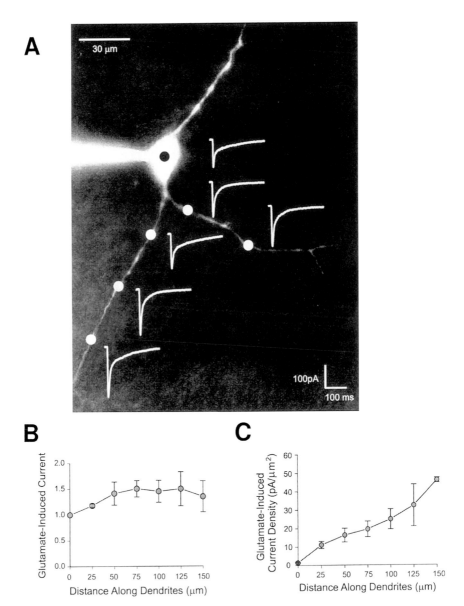

Fig. 5. Nonuniform density of glutamate responses on interneurons. **(A)** A volume-rendered image of a dye-filled interneuron. Circles indicate the position and diameter of the UV light spot used to uncage glutamate and traces indicate averages of five evoked responses at each location. **(B)** Relationship between the location of the UV light spot with respect to the cell body and the amplitude of the current induced by glutamate at each location. The peak amplitudes of the glutamate currents have been normalized to the amplitude of currents evoked over the cell body of each of the 4 neurons examined. **(C)** Relationship between the location of the UV light spot and the density of the current induced by glutamate at each location. Adapted with permission from ref. *18*.

two processes of the interneuron shown in Fig. 5A produced very similar responses.

Although hippocampal interneurons are heterogeneous in their physiological properties *(21–23)*, the pattern of glutamate responsiveness was consistent for all interneurons examined. The absolute amplitudes of glutamate responses of interneuronal dendrites were larger than those of the somata, with dendritic glutamate-induced currents maximally about 150% of those evoked in the cell body (Fig. 5A). Averaged data shown in Fig. 5B is plotted as a function of distance from the cell body (as in Fig. 2A) because the dendrites of these interneurons do not branch extensively. This difference was even more striking when the density of glutamate currents was calculated as described earlier ($n = 4$), with current density increasing as the glutamate was applied to regions farther from the cell body (Fig. 5C). Applying the arguments presented for the glutamate responses of pyramidal cells, we conclude that interneurons also have a pronounced distally-directed gradient of glutamate receptors along the their dendrites.

6. GABA RECEPTOR MAPPING ON PYRAMIDAL CELLS AND LNTERNEURONS

Using a very similar technical approach, we also have been able to map the distribution of functional GABA receptors on hippocampal neurons. Because no double-caged GABA compound has been successfully synthesized, we used single-caged GABA for all mapping experiments. This results in an approx twofold degradation of lateral and axial resolution compared to what would be possible with a double-caged GABA compound *(19)*. Uncaged GABA evoked outward current responses in all regions of pyramidal neurons. The amplitude of GABA responses varied along the length of the dendritic processes in a manner similar to that of the glutamate responses (Fig. 6A). GABA responses decreased in amplitude with increasing distance from the cell body along the basal dendrites (Fig. 6A, traces 3-1). However, as the uncaging spot was moved from the cell body to the primary apical dendrite, the amplitude of GABA responses remained approximately the same as those of the cell body (Fig. 6A, traces 4,6).

To account for differences in the surface area over which GABA was applied, GABA current density was calculated as described earlier for glutamate currents. The highest densities of GABA-induced currents were found in the distal regions of both the apical and basal dendritic trees (Fig. 5C). These data suggest that GABA receptors are distributed in a gradient, with the highest point of the gradient in the most distal dendrites, and that

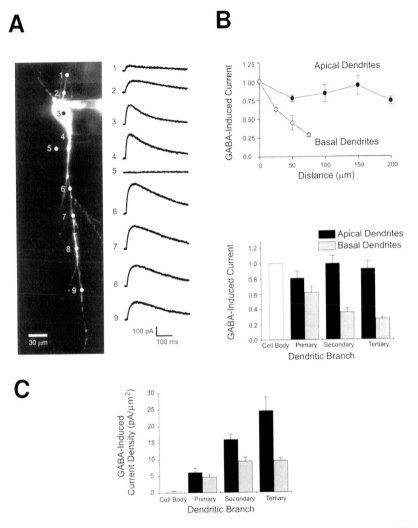

Fig. 6. Nonuniform density of GABA responses on pyramidal neurons. **(A)** A volumerendered image of a CA1 pyramidal neuron filled with fluorescent dye via a patch pipet. Circles indicate the position and diameter of the UV light spot used to uncage GABA. Traces at right are averages of three responses evoked by 5 ms uncaging pulses. Traces 1 and 2 are responses from basal dendrites, whereas traces 4–9 are responses from apical dendrites. **(B)** Relationship between the location of the UV light spot with respect to the cell body and the amplitude of the current induced by GABA at each location. The peak amplitude of the GABAinduced currents have been normalized to the amplitude of currents evoked over the cell body of each of the 6 neurons examined. **(C)** The same data as in **(A)** plotted with respect to dendritic branch. **(D)** Relationship between the location of the UV light spot and the density of the current induced by GABA at each location. Adapted with permission from ref. *18.*

the gradients observed for GABA and glutamate receptors are not owing to a general voltage clamp error. Any unclamped GABA currents would-hyperpolarize the membrane potential, rather than depolarizing it as would be the case for unclamped glutamate currents. Thus, any voltage escape and resultant activation of voltage-dependent conductances, would have opposite effects on the amplitude of currents evoked by the two transmitters. The fact that similar patterns of responses are nonetheless similar on pyramidal cells suggests that the variations in responsiveness arise from genuine increases in receptor density rather than space clamp errors.

The spatial distribution of functional GABA receptors on hippocampal interneurons was markedly different from that of pyramidal cells. Responses to uncaged GABA were a very sensitive function of position and were often undetectable when GABA was photoreleased on dendritic locations only 100 μm away from the cell body (Fig. 7A). As a result, the spatial profile of interneuronal GABA responses declined steeply with distance (Fig. 7B). Calculations of the density of the GABA-induced current reinforce this conclusion; the density of GABAinduced currents showed a spatial distribution that was almost the inverse of that seen for the glutamate responses of these same neurons (Fig. 7C). Given that responses could be observed when glutamate was applied to the distant regions of these cells, the absence of GABA responses in these regions cannot be attributed to electrotonic decrement within the dendrites. Thus, interneurons appear to concentrate their GABA receptors in the perisomatic region.

7. MECHANISMS UNDERLYING REGIONAL VARIATIONS IN TRANSMITTER RESPONSIVENESS

We have used local photolysis of caged neurotransmitters to map the distribution of functional neurotransmitter receptors on pyramidal cells and interneurons in hippocampal slices. These receptors are not uniformly distributed but rather are targeted to specific regions along the dendrites and cell body of these neurons. The spatial profile of the receptors varies depending on the type of neuron and neurotransmitter. We found that CA1 pyramidal neurons have parallel gradients of glutamate and GABA receptors on their dendrites, with the highest density of receptors in the most distal apical and basal dendrites. Interneurons also have an increasing density of glutamate receptors along their dendrites, but these processes have very few functional GABA receptors on their dendrites. Our results are the first to document a distally directed gradient of functional receptors in hip-

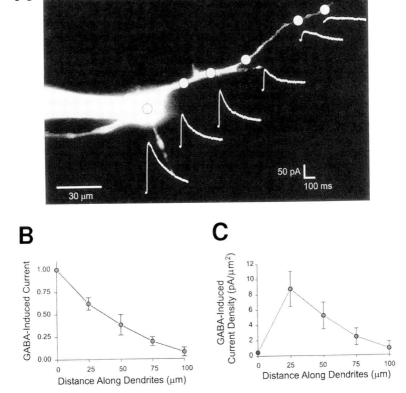

Fig. 7. Nonuniform density of GABA responses on interneurons. **(A)** A volume-rendered image of a dye-filled interneuron. Circles indicate the position and diameter of the UV light spot used to uncage GABA and nearby traces indicate averages of three responses evoked by uncaging at each location. **(B)** Relationship between the dendritic location of the UV light spot and the amplitude of the current induced by GABA at each location. The peak amplitudes of the GABA-induced currents have been normalized to the amplitude of currents evoked over the cell body of the 6 neurons examined. **(C)** Relationship between the location of the UV light spot and the density of the current induced by GABA at each location. Adapted with permission from ref. *18*.

pocampal pyramidal neurons and are consistent with previous anatomical data suggesting that glutamate and GABA receptors/synapses are located along the entire length of the dendrites of these neurons *(23–26)*. Our results complement recent data suggesting a similar arrangement of functional glutamate receptors in cortical pyramidal cells *(27)*.

The spatial variations in GABA and glutamate responses that we observed could arise from a number of different mechanisms. It is possible that our measurements of current amplitude are distorted by poor spatial control of membrane potential during voltage clamping. If this were to occur, distal currents would be preferentially attenuated and slowed because of increased filtering of currents. In addition, loss of voltage control with distance could cause an increase in local depolarization and a decrease in the driving force for ions. Finally, loss of voltage control with distance could result in the activation of voltage-dependent channels on the distal dendrites *(28,29)*. With the possible exception of I_H channels activation during GABA responses *(30)*, all of these effects will yield an underestimate in the magnitude of the observed receptor gradient. Thus, loss of space clamp cannot account for the changes in transmitter responsiveness that we have observed.

It is possible that differences in the unitary conductance and/or affinity of the receptors, rather than the absolute number of these receptors, are responsible for the gradients that we have observed. However, available evidence argues against this possibility. Spruston et al. *(31)* found that the unitary properties of glutamate receptors in the cell body and dendrites of CA1 pyramidal neurons were identical. Although further studies of the unitary properties of dendritic receptors are warranted, it is unlikely that such differences can account for our results.

Although we have attempted to account for variations in surface area, our measurements of dendritic surface area could not take into account dendritic spines because these structures were not well-resolved in our images. If spine density were higher in distal dendrites than in proximal dendrites, the area of distal dendrite membrane exposed to uncaged neurotransmitter would be systematically underestimated and could give rise to the observed gradient of responses. Of course, this mechanism is unlikely to account for the glutamate receptor gradient observed in interneurons because these neurons typically do not have spines. Further, two considerations argue against the possibility that inequities in spine density account for the receptor gradients observed in pyramidal cells. First, the density of spines is apparently uniform along CA1 pyramidal cell dendrites, except for a lower spine density in the most proximal 20–100 μm region of the primary apical dendrite *(32,33)*. Second, any non-uniformities in spine density are quantitatively inadequate to account for most of our results. Estimates suggest 1–3 spines/μm on dendrites of CA1 pyramidal cells *(32,34,35)*; using the upper estimate of 3 spines per micrometer and a surface area of 1.15 μm^2 for a spine *(34)*, the area of spines exposed to uncaged glutamate would be about 16 μm^2. Because the measured surface area of the smallest dendrites was 9 μm^2, the total area for these dendrites could be as great as 25 μm^2 after including the spine membrane. This area is still significantly smaller than the surface area of primary dendrites, which averaged 37 µm². Thus, even in the extreme (and unlikely) case that primary dendrites have no spines, the surface area of a primary dendrite is still larger yet the distal dendrites produce larger responses to uncaged glutamate. By process of elimination, we conclude that the spatial variations in glutamate responsiveness arise from heterogeneity in the distribution of glutamate receptors. We therefore conclude that the density of glutamate receptors must increase with distance along the dendrites of both pyramidal neurons and interneurons and the same must be true for GABA receptors in pyramidal cells but not interneurons.

Whether these receptors are synaptic or extrasynaptic cannot yet be resolved, though it is likely that synaptic receptors dominate, at least on dendrites. Two extreme cases can be considered: the photoreleased transmitter could selectively activate synaptic receptors or could selectively activate extrasynaptic receptors. If only synaptic receptors were activated and the density of synapses is constant along the length of the dendrite *(32)*, then the relevant parameter is the length of dendrite exposed to transmitter rather than the area of dendrite. In this case, because the width of the light spot is the same in all regions, then the relevant parameter to measure is the absolute magnitude of currents generated by uncaged transmitter. We found substantial spatial gradients of responses for glutamate and GABA in the dendrites of pyramidal cells and interneurons. In the case where only extrasynaptic receptors are activated, then the relevant parameter is the area of dendrite exposed to transmitter. We calculated the areas of dendrites and made density estimates which showed steep gradients of transmitter responsiveness. Thus, both types of analysis revealed similar response gradients independent of whether the receptors for these transmitters are synaptic or extrasynaptic.

Assuming the very likely case that some at least of the receptors activated by uncaging are synaptic, our measurements cannot discriminate between a higher number of receptors per synapse and a higher number of synaptic contacts. Currently, there are no measurements of the total number of synaptic contacts along the entire length of a hippocampal pyramidal neuron. As mentioned earlier, spine density appears uniform along the length of pyramidal cell dendrites *(32)*; if spines are proportional to the number of synapses, then synapse density also should be uniform. If synapse density is indeed uniform along pyramidal cell dendrites, then the higher density of functional receptors that we observed is owing to a higher density of receptors per synapse.

Regardless of whether synaptic or extrasynaptic receptors were being activated, our results point to a gradient in the distribution of these receptors. The gradients have not been revealed previously because until now no technique permitted mapping of functional transmitter receptors in central neurons, except in cultured neurons where the distribution of synapses and receptors is altered by cell dissociation. These gradients are likely to be very important for the biology of these neurons.

8. FUNCTIONAL IMPLICATIONS OF DIFFERENTIAL RECEPTOR TARGETING

The enhancement of glutamate responses in the distal dendrites of both pyramidal neurons and interneurons may provide a mechanism that allows neurons to boost excitatory synaptic transmission at distal dendrites. We propose that the gradients of increasing receptor density that we observed may help compensate for the electrotonic filtering properties of dendrites, allowing neurons to accurately code synaptic strength in a location-independent manner. Our results are reminiscent of those obtained by Jack et al. *(36)*, who found that electrical responses recorded from the cell body of spinal motor neurons were constant in amplitude even when synapses were activated at varying electrotonic distances along the dendrites. Variations in receptor density of the sort we have observed could account for such results and could also account for the observation that the amplitude of excitatory field potentials is independent of the location of the synaptic input in hippocampal pyramidal neurons *(37)*.

9. CONCLUSION

Local photolysis of caged neurotransmitters is a practical means of mapping the distribution of neurotransmitter receptors on neurons. This method selectively probes functional receptors on the surface of the cells and can be applied to a wide range of preparations, ranging from dissociated single cells to whole organisms. The limited spatial resolution in photolyzing caged neurotransmitters can be substantially imporved by synthesizing neurotransmitters with two independent light-sensitive cages. Such "chemical two-photon uncaging" makes it possible to apply neurotransmitters over small volumes that approach the size of single synapses. Local photolysis of caged glutamate and GABA reveals pronounced gradients of receptors for these two neurotransmitters on hippocampal pyramidal neurons and interneurons. Further applications of this approach should reveal much more about the targeting of neurotransmitter receptors in the brain.

REFERENCES

1. Mitchison, T. J. (1989) Polewards microtubule flux in the mitotic spindle: evidence from photoactivation of fluorescence. *J. Cell Biol.* **109,** 637–652.
2. O'Neill, S. C., Mill, J. G., and Eisner, D. A. (1990) Local activation of contraction in isolated rat ventricular mlyocytes. *Am. J. Physiol.* **258,** C1165–C1168.
3. Parker, L. and Yao, Y. (1991) Regenerative release of calcium from functionally discrete subcellular stores by inositol trisphosphate. *Proc. R Soc. Lond.* **246,** 269–274.
4. Callaway, E. M. and Katz, L. C. (1993) Photostimulation using caged glutamate reveals functional circuitry in living brain slices. *Proc. Natl. Acad. Sci. USA* **88,** 7661–7665.
5. Wang, S. S.-H. and Augustine, G. J. (1995) Confocal imaging and local photolysis of caged compounds: dual probes of synaptic function. *Neuron* **15,** 755–760.
6. Svoboda, K., Tank, D. W., and Denk W. (1996) Direct measurement of coupling between dendritic spines and shafts. *Science* **272,** 716–719.
7. McCray, J. A. and Trentham, D. R. (1989) Properties and uses of photoreactive caged compounds. *Ann. Rev. Biophys. Biophys. Chem.* **18,** 239–270.
8. Adams, S. R. and Tsien, R. Y. (1993) Controlling cell chemistry with caged compounds. *Ann. Rev. Physiol.* **5S,** 755–784.
9. Hess, G. P., Niu, L., and Wieboldt, R. (1995) Determination of the chemical mechanism of neurotransmitter receptor-mediated reactions by rapid chemical kinetic methods. *Ann. NY Acad. Sci.* **757,** 23–39.
10. Rapp, G. and Guth, K. (1988) A low cost high intensity flash device for photolysis experiments. *Pflugers Arch.* **411,** 200–203.
11. Lester, H. A. and Nerbonne, J. M. (1982) Physiological and pharmacological manipulations with light flashes. *Ann. Rev. Biophys. Bioeng.* **11,** 151–175.
12. Pettit, D. L., Wang, S. S.-H., Gee, K. R., and Augustine, G. J. (1997) Chemical two-photon uncaging: a novel approach to optical mapping of glutamate receptors. *Neuron* **19,** 465-469.
13. Goppert-Mayer, M. (1931) Ueber Elementarakte mit zwei Quantenspruengen. *Ann. Phys.* **9,** 273.
14. Denk, W. (1994) Two-photon scanning photochemical microscopy: mapping ligand-gated ion channel distributions. *Proc. Natl. Acad. Sci. USA* **91,** 6629–6633.
15. Denk, W., Piston, D. W., and Webb, W. W. (1995) In *Handbook of Biological Confocal Microscopy,* 2d ed. (Pawley, J. B., ed.), Plenum, New York, pp. 445–458.
16. Wieboldt, R., Gee, K. R., Niu, L., Ramesh, D., Carpenter, B. K., and Hess, G. P. (1994) Photolabile precursors of glutamate: synthesis, photochemical properties, and activation of glutamate receptors on a microsecond time scale. *Proc. Natl. Acad. Sci. USA* **91,** 8752–8756.
17. Hausser, M. and Roth, A. (1997) Dendritic and somatic glutamate receptor channels in rat cerebellar Purkinje cells. *J. Physiol.* **501,** 77–95.
18. Pettit, D. L. and Augustine, G. J. (2000) Topology of functional neurotransmitter receptors on dendrites of hippocampal neurons. *J. Neurophysiol.* **84,** 28–38.

19. Wang, S. S.-H., Khiroug, L., and Augustine, G. J. (2000) Postsynaptic spread of cerebellar long-term depression revealed with chemical two-photon uncaging. *Proc. Natl. Acad. Sci. USA.* **97,** 8635–8640.

20. Otis, T. S., Kavanaugh, M. P., and Jahr, C. E. (1997) Postsynaptic glutamate transport at the climbing fiber-Purkinje cell synapse. *Science* **277,** 1515–1518.

21. Sik, A., Penttonen, M., Ylinen, A., and Buzsaki, G. (1995) Hippocampal CA1 interneurons: An *in vivo* intracellular labeling study. *J. Neurosci.* **15,** 6651–6665.

22. Acsady, L., Gorcs, T. J., and Freund, T. F. (1996) Different populations of vasoactive intestinal polypeptide-immunoreactive interneurons are specialized to control pyramidal cells or interneurons in the hippocampus. *Neuroscience* **73,** 317–334.

23. Cobb, S. R., Halasy, K., Vida, I., Nyiri, G., Tamas, G., Bubl, E. H., and Somogyi, P. (1997) Synaptic effects of identified interneurons innervating both interneurons and pyramidal cells in the rat hippocampus. *Neuroscience* **79,** 629–648.

24. Craig, A. M., Blackstone, C. D., Huganir, R. L., and Banker, G. (1994). Selective clustering of glutamate and gamma-aminobutyric acid receptors opposite terminals releasing the corresponding neurotransmitters. *Proc. Natl. Acad. Sci. USA* **91,** 12,373–12,377.

25. Mammen, A. L., Huganir, R. L., and O'Brien, R. J. (1997) Redistribution and stabilization of cell surface glutamate receptors during synapse formation. *J. Neurosci.* **17,** 7351–7358.

26. Baude, A., Nusser, Z., Molnar, E., McIlhinney, A. J., and Somogyi, P. (1995) High-resolution immunogold localization of AMPA type glutamate receptor subunits at synaptic and nonsynaptic sites in rat hippocampus. *Neuroscience* **69,** 1031–1055.

27. Dodt, H. U., Frick A., Kampe, K., and Zieglgansberger, W. (1998) NMDA and AMPA receptors on neocrotical neurons are differentially distributed. *Eur. J. Neurosci.* **10,** 3351–3357.

28. Magee, J. C. and Johnston, D. (1995a) Synaptic activation of voltage-gated channels in the dendrites of hippocampal pyramidal neurons. *Science* **268,** 301–304.

29. Magee, J. C. and Johnston, D. (1995b) Characterization of single voltage-gated Na^+ and Ca^{2+} channels in apical dendrites of rat CA1 pyramidal neurons. *J. Physiol.* **481,** 67–90.

30. Magee, J. C. (1998) Dendritic hyperpolarization-activated currents modify the integrative properties of hippocampal CA1 pyramidal neurons. *J. Neurosci.* **18,** 7613–7624.

31. Spruston, N., Jonas, P., and Sakmann, B. (1995) Dendritic glutamate receptor channels in rat hippocampal CA3 and CA1 pyramidal neurons. *J. Physiol.* **482,** 325–352.

32. Trommald, M., Jensen, V., and Anderson, P. (1995) Analysis of dendritic spines in rat CA1 pyramidal cells intracellularly filled with a fluorescent dye. *J. Comp. Neurol.* **353,** 260–274.

33. Bannister, N. J. and Larkman, A. U. (1995) Dendritic morphology of CA1 pyramidal neurones from the rat hippocampus: II. Spine distributions. *J. Comp. Neurol.* **360,** 161–171.

34. Harris, K. M., Jensen, F. E., and Tsao, B. (1992) Three-dimensional structure of dendritic spines and synapses in rat hippocampus (CAT) at postnatal day 15 and adult ages: implications for the maturation of synaptic physiology and long-term potentiation. *J. Neurosci.* **12,** 2685–2705.

35. Ishizuka, N., Cowan, W. M., and Amaral, D. G. (1995) A quantitative analysis of the dendritic organization of pyramidal cells in the rat hippocampus. *J. Comp. Neurol.* **362,** 17–45.

36. Jack, J. J., Redman, S. J., and Wong, K. (1981) The components of synaptic potentials evoked in cat spinal motorneurones by impulses in single group Ia afferents. *J. Physiol.* **321,** 65–96.

37. Andersen, P., Silfvenius, H., Sundberg, S. H., and Sveen, O. (1980) A comparison of distal and proximal dendritic synapses on CA1 pyramids in guinea-pig hippocampal slices *in vitro. J. Physiol.* **307,** 273–299.

Part IV

Atomic Force Microscopy

20

Atomic Force Microscopy of Reconstituted Ion Channels

Hoeon Kim, Hai Lin, and Ratneshwar Lal

1. INTRODUCTION

Ion channels and receptors are specialized biomembrane structures that serve as the interface between opposing compartments (e.g., cytoplasm and extracellular region, cytoplasm and intravesicular region) and toward which most of the regulatory signals are directed. Molecular three-dimensional (3D) structure of channels and receptors are studied primarily by high-resolution imaging techniques, including electron microscopy, electron and X-ray diffractions, and infra-red spectroscopy. These techniques provide insufficient information about the surfaces of channels and receptors, the very sites of molecular interactions with external perturbations, and are usually unsuitable for combining biochemical, electrophysiological, and molecular biological techniques for simultaneous structure-function analyses. An atomic force Microscope (AFM) *(1)* can image the 3D-surface structure of a wide variety of native biological specimens, including reconstituted channels and receptors, in an aqueous medium and with subnanometer resolution (for reviews, *see* refs. *2–4*). An AFM can also manipulate surfaces with molecular precision, i.e., it can nanodissect, translocate, and reorganize molecules on surfaces. AFM imaging in the hydrated condition provides an opportunity for observing biochemical and physiological processes in real time at molecular level and thus can be used for direct molecular structure-function studies. 3D surface topography has been imaged for several ion channels, pumps, and receptors that were: 1) present in isolated native membranes, 2) reconstituted in artificial membrane or, 3) expressed

From: *Ion Channel Localization Methods and Protocols*
Edited by: A. Lopatin and C. G. Nichols © Humana Press Inc., Totowa, NJ

in an appropriate expression system. The present chapter provides a brief summary of imaging molecular structure and function of reconstituted channels and receptors using AFM.

2. PRINCIPLE OF OPERATION

For a detailed treatise on the principle of operation, resolution, and limitations of AFM, *see* ref. *2*.

Briefly, AFM images consist of a series of parallel line contours obtained by scanning the surface of a specimen across a molecularly sharp tip with a small (~a nanoNewton [Nn]) tracking force. The tip is mounted on a microcantilever with a small spring constant. As the tip (or the specimen) is scanned, the net interaction force between the molecules on the probe tip and the sample surface deflects the tip and hence the cantilevered spring. The cantilever deflection is sensed by multi-segmented photodetectors as the relative angular deflection of a laser beam reflected off the back of the mirrored cantilever. The relative deflection is converted to electrical signals by photodetectors. An electronic feedback loop keeps the cantilever deflection and hence the tracking force constant by moving the sample up and down as the tip traces over the contours of the surface (Fig. 1). An image is obtained by plotting the vertical motion (z) of the xyz translator and hence the sample height (z) as a function of specimen lateral position (xy).

Two major factors for the AFM to be applicable to biological imaging are described below.

2.1. Resolution

With AFM, the images are formed by reconstructing the contour of the interaction forces between the probe and the specimen. By selecting a small imaging area and appropriate operating conditions, one can distinguish adjacent structures less than a nanometer apart as the signal-to-noise (S/N) ratio in an AFM image is sufficiently large compared to EM and other techniques. For hard inorganic crystals, atomic resolution is obtained *(5)*. For soft biological specimens such as a living cell, resolution is reduced (for review, *see* ref. *2*). In biological specimens with a high density of protein and limited mobility, such as membranes with channels and receptors, the resolution could be comparable to that for a hard crystal. On many channels and receptors including gap junctions, bacteriorhodopsin, HPI-layer, AChR, Na^+-K^+ ATPase, and porin channels, a subnanometer resolution has been obtained.

2.2. Identity of the Imaged Structures: Correlative Studies

Though AFM could provide, with molecular resolution, surface information of crystalline as well as amorphous materials, it is often difficult to identify the chemical nature of individual components, especially if the surface contains a heterologous population of structures. This is often the case with most of the biological membranes, except in favorable systems like purified membranes and reconstituted channels and receptors (for review, *see* ref. *3*).

For mixed macromolecules, it is essential to obtain comparative information from AFM and alternative techniques, such as EM and X-ray diffraction, biochemical and immunological binding assays, pharmacological labeling, and electrophysiological measurements *(6–9)*. The simple design of AFM allows integration of other techniques, such as fluorescence and laser confocal microscopies (Fig. 1) *(10–12)*, which permit molecular identification using specific markers (Fig. 2).

3. SAMPLE PREPARATION

AFM can operate in aqueous as well as in dry conditions, at ambient temperature and pressure. Physicochemical properties of the sample and sample-support interactions determine or suggest ways under which it can be imaged. on the other hand, imaging conditions influence the choice of substrate, the stability of the specimen with respect to its interaction with the probe, and the preservation of the specimen with respect to its physiological or biochemical functions. For example, it can simply involve getting the sample attached to the support by drying down of samples or adsorption against specially prepared surfaces. A low sample-support interaction would require a low imaging force, otherwise, the tip would sweep the sample away from the support. Originally, graphite (HOPG hydrophobic uncharged), mica (hydrophilic negatively charged) and glass were the supports most routinely used. These supports can also be modified chemically to adjust their hydropathicity, charge density, and their polarity. Today the repertoire has expanded greatly.

The sample support can be modified or coated such that it acts as a ligand for the sample and thus orient the specimen in a defined way. In addition, artificial systems can be used to generate constraints to hold samples. For example, Yang et al. *(13)* incorporated cholera toxins into synthetic phospholipid bilayers followed by covalent crosslinking to image the pentameric structure of the B-subunit.

The most commonly used sample preparation for isolated macromolecules and 2D membrane-bound macromolecules (such as channels and

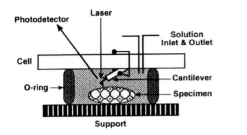

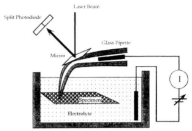

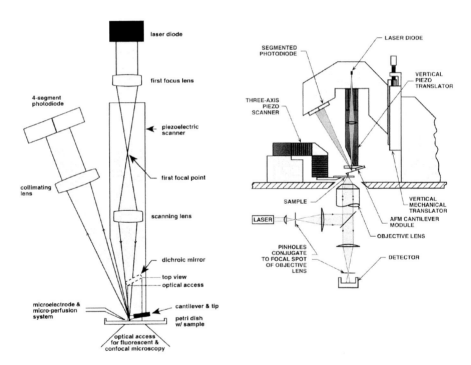

Fig. 1. Top left: Schematics of operation of an AFM. As the tip (integrated to a cantilever) scans the surface of a specimen, the forces from the specimen deflects the tip and hence the cantilever. The deflection is measured by an optical-deflection detection system, using multiple photodetectors. A deflection of the cantilever causes the reflected laser light to fall asymmetrically at photodetectors. A difference signal from them is used in a feedback loop to keep the deflection and (hence the tracking force) constant while the tip scans the specimen. Although imaging hydrated specimens, both the cantilevered tip and the specimen are immersed in a fluid. The surface of the fluid cell is transparent. Bottom left: Schematic of opera-

(continued)

receptors) is a simple adsorption in the presence of appropriate counterions or crosslinking of macromolecules to a chemically modified substratum (such as covalent linking) is *(14,15)*. However, such method may not be suitable to observe structural changes *in situ*. For multilayer systems such as reconstituted vesicles and planer bilayers, they nevertheless can leave the upper portions of the proteins free for conformational changes to occur in response to on-line perturbations.

AFM imaging of 3D reconstituted specimens has been limited. In one such study, a small volume of solution containing reconstituted OmpC microcrystals was mixed with equal volume of the mother liquor *(16)*. Microcrystals were then carefully harvested and transferred on to the substrate, a nitrocellulose paper glued to a 12-mm diameter stainless steel disc. Crystal's flat shape favored its adsorption such that its prominent (100) surface was parallel to the substrate's surface. To remove the debris from the crystal surface, crystals were then washed gently a few times with the fresh mother liquor, the excess fluid was removed using filter papers and the sample was air-dried at room temperature for 1–2 h.

For imaging hydrated crystals, the bottom surface of the crystals were glued to the nitrocellulose filter paper quickly and sufficient amount of mother fluid was added. However, in such condition, crystals were often loosely attached to or became completely detached from the nitrocellulose substrate once the mother liquor was introduced and thus, these crystals were

---

tion of a combined light and AFM. The first focal point is located inside the upper portion of the piezoelectric scanner. After the positions of the lenses are adjusted, the scanning focused spot accurately tracks the cantilever and the zero-deflection signal from the 4-segment photodiode is independent of position within the scan area. One of the key advantages of the new AF*M* is that there is optical access to the sample from above and below. Thus the new AF*M* can be combined with an optical microscope of high numerical aperture. The other key advantage is that because the sample is stationary during scanning and can be large, techniques for on-line perturbations and recordings can easily be incorporate. For details, *see* refs. *12,31*. Top right: Schematic of the combined SICM/AFM. A laser beam reflecting off a mirror glued to the back of a pipet with nanometers-sized hole provides the deflection signal for the topographic image. Intra-pipet and bath electrodes measures electrical currents. For details, *see* ref. *30*. Bottom right: Schematics of a combined atomic force microscope and confocal laser-scanning microscope. The sample is scanned by a boom attached to an xy-piezo tube scanner. Sample topography deflects a microfabricated AFM cantilever. A two-segment photodiode measures the deflection. Below the sample, a confocal microscope system focuses laser light to excite fluorescence in the sample, then collects the emitted light. A scanning probe microscope controller (not shown) displays both the topography and the fluorescence signal. For details, *see* ref. *10*.

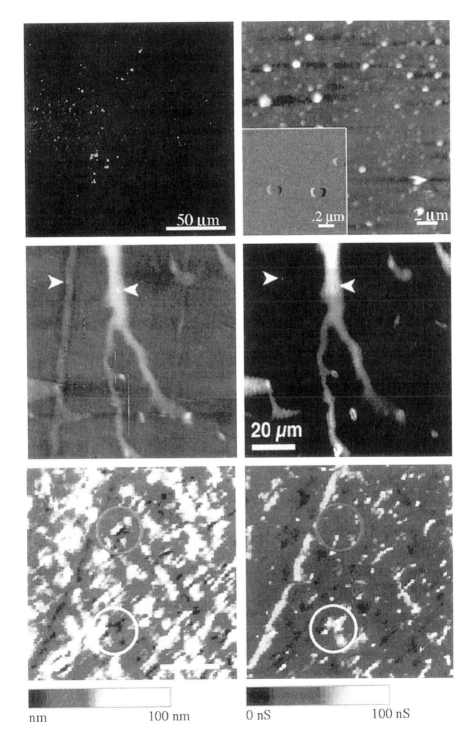

pushed aside by tips during AFM imaging. For those crystals that remained attached to the substrate, no repeatable and high-resolution images were obtained in the presence of mother liquor, possibly because of the high viscosity of the OmpC porin crystal growth medium, which altered the AFM tip movement significantly. Also, alteration of the mother liquor composition was not an option as this led to disordered crystals as revealed by X-ray diffraction analysis. Attempts to adhere 3D crystals to the substrate with organic "glues" (e.g., agarose) damaged the crystal surface and no discernible images were obtained.

4. REPRESENTATIVE EXAMPLES

AFM imaging can provide high-resolution information on noncrystalline aggregates of macromolecules. By using integrated multiimaging systems, the physicochemical identity of these macromolecules can also be ascertained. Another advantages of AFM imaging includes an unambiguous determination of the surface polarity (sidedness) of the sample (for example, a double-bilayered gap junction will always have the cytoplasmic surface

---

Fig. 2. Top panels: Simultaneous immunofluorescence and atomic force microscopy of AβP reconstituted into liposomes. The liposomes were first treated with AβP antibody, and subsequently identified with fluorescein-conjugated secondary antibody. The AβP-carrying liposomes showed strong fluorescence signals (top left). All liposomes with AβP were imaged with AFM simultaneously (top right). For details, *see* ref. *19*. Middle panels: Simultaneous combined AFM and fluorescence-confocal microscopic images. The sample consists of a suspension of fluorescently labeled latex beads that were dried into a gel on a plastic diffraction grating. The lines of the grating are visible in the topographic image (middle left panel) but not in the fluorescence image (middle right panel). The fluorescence image allows a nonfluorescent particle (right arrow) to be distinguished from a fluorescent particle (left arrow), although both appear as raised bumps in the AFM image. For details, *see* ref. *10*. Bottom panels: Simultaneous combined AFM and electrophysiology. Bottom left image shows a contact mode AFM image of a nucleopore synthetic membrane. The bottom right panel shows the associated ionic conductivity image. The line traces below the images show the SICM and AFM signals taken from the solid dark line in the images. The trace from the AFM image shows two pores that appear to be of comparable depth. The associated ionic conductivity show a large difference, implying the pore on the right has a much larger connectivity than the pore on the left. This illustrates how the SICM/AFM allows the functionality as well as the morphology of membrane structures to be studied. For details, *see* ref. *30*.

facing upward) and a more precise measurement of the sample thickness. A few pertinent examples are provided below.

4.1. Purified Channels and Receptors

AFM imaging is not confined to purified native membranes with channels and receptors only. Recent studies show a remarkable advantage of using AFM to image ultrastructure of isolated as well as reconstituted channels and receptors that are present in noncrystalline specimens. A few examples of AFM imaging of isolated as well as reconstituted channels and receptors are discussed below.

4.1.1. Cholera-Toxin B-Oligomers

Yang et al. *(13)* were able to incorporate purified cholera toxin into synthetic phospholipid bilayers by covalent crosslinking. Imaging under an appropriate buffer, they were able to show a pentameric molecular structure of individual cholera toxins. The lateral dimensions of individual subunits as well as the whole complex were comparable to that obtained by other methods. The height of the individual subunits, however, was lower than predicted and could result from the partial embedding of protein in the lipid substrate and/or imaging force-induced compression of the proteins.

Mou et al. *(15)* have imaged isolated cholera-toxin B-oligomers that were anchored to supported bilayers made of DPPC and POPG (Fig. 3). Individual oligomers, their subunit organization, and few missing subunits were clearly resolved at a lateral resolution of ~1 nm. Significantly, the image quality and resolution were comparable in both the fluid phase and the gel phase of the bilayer suggesting that the bilayer fluidity did not introduce any significant perturbation during high resolution imaging. Also, they were able to grow 2D arrays of B-oligomers directly on these model membranes without any special treatment. Thus, isolated channels and receptors can be imaged with AFM without any significant chemical modifications such as crosslinking with the substrate.

4.1.2. Cytotoxin VacA

Czajkowsky et al. *(17)* have imaged cytotoxin VacA, which causes osmotic swelling of endosomes and lysosomes. VacA adsorbed directly to freshly prepared cleaved mica and imaged under buffered solution revealed both dodecamers and tetradecamers. The structural features imaged with AFM were identical to those previously reported. Significantly, these channel-forming oligomers were aggregated in noncrystalline random order. For comparison, when these VacA were adsorbed on supported lipid bilayers, they formed crystalline arrays (*see* below), suggesting a role of protein–lipid interaction in long-range packing of channels and receptors.

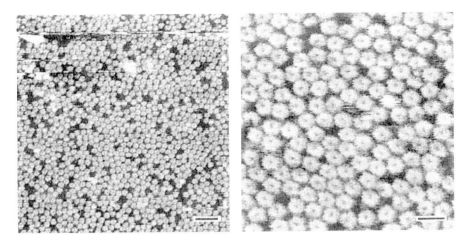

Fig. 3. AFM images of individual cholera toxin B-oligomers that were bound to the gangliosides in a bilayer made of egg-PC by the vesicle fusion method. The full coverage of the bilayer is achieved with 10 mol% GM1. Left panel: medium resolution image of the reconstituted bilayer in the gel phase. Scale bar = 30 nm. Right panel: high-resolution image. The image quality is comparable to that for the gel-phase image (left side), suggesting that the fluidity of the bilayer did not seriously reduce the resolution in AFM images. B-oligomers with both sixfold and fivefold symmetries are visible. Missing subunits are also visible in some B-oligomers. Scale bar = 10 nm. For details, *see* ref. *15*.

VacA cytotoxin was reconstituted with anionic lipid bilayers at acidic pH. The supported bilayer membrane was formed by sequential depositions of two separately prepared monolayers to mica using Langmuir trough *(17)*. The bilayer was then incubated with VacA for 1–2 h at room temperature. The reconstituted membrane was then partially fixed with glutaraldehyde to improve the mechanical stability. AFM imaging show that these reconstituted VacA forms two-dimensional crystals of membrane-associated VacA oligomers. These oligomers are arranged in a hexagonal array with lattice parameters a = b = 22 nm (Y = 60°). The VacA oligomers show sixfold rotational symmetry and has an overall diameter of ~28 nm. Electrophysiological measurements suggest the formation of ion-conducting pore that is pH sensitive.

4.2. Reconstituted Channels and Receptors in 2D Systems

4.2.1. AβP Channels

Amyloid beta protein (AβP) forms plaques in the brain of Alzheimer's disease (AD) patients. However, very little is known about the role of AβPs in such pathology. Rhee et al. *(18)* and Lin et al. *(19)* have examined the activity of $A\beta P_{1-42}$ and $A\beta P_{1-40}$ reconstituted in phospholipid vesicles. Using multimodal AFM, which was a combined light fluorescence-atomic force microscope, they were able to localize AβPs reconstituted in the vesicular membrane. Vesicles reconstituted with AβPs showed strong immunofluorescence labeling with an antibody raised against an extracellular domain of AβP. Vesicles reconstituted without AβPs showed no such labeling.

The combined AFM was used to image the structure of these vesicles. Vesicles were 0.5–1 µm in diameter and were mostly unilammelar. There was no significant difference in the thickness of the vesicles with/without AβPs, suggesting that the extramembranous protrusion of AβPs is very small. Vesicles reconstituted with AβP showed a significant level of $^{45}Ca^{2+}$-uptake, which was inhibited by the monoclonal anti-AβP-antibody and Zn^{2+} but not by the reducing agents Trolox and DTT, indicating that the oxidation of AβP or its surrounding lipid molecules is not directly involved in the AβP-mediated Ca^{2+}-uptake *(19)*. Preliminary AFM images suggest that these AβPs form oligomeric complex with a pore-like features *(20)*.

4.2.2. Staphylococcal α-Hemolysin (αHL)

Staphylococcal α-hemolysin (αHL), a bacterial toxin and a prototype of many toxins, is secreted as a water-soluble monomer which, upon binding to lipid membranes, can self-assemble into oligomeric transmembrane pores. Based on earlier biochemical and structural analyses, these membrane-bound oligomers were believed to be a hexameric conformation. Recent data from biochemical assays and X-ray crystallography, however, show that the αHL oligomers are most likely heptamers. Such anomaly suggests that the techniques used in earlier studies presumably did not have sufficient resolution to properly determine the subunit stoichiometry of this membrane protein. It is most likely that αHL has both heptameric and hexameric conformations. AFM imaging shows that membrane-bound αHLs are hexamers (Fig. 4) *(21)*. It is most likely that αHL forms both hexamers and heptamers in lipid membranes, although the heptamers may form more readily in detergent.

4.2.3. OmpF Porin

Bacterial porins are one of the best studied channel forming membrane proteins. Recently, a number of these porins reconstituted as 2D crystals into DMPC lipid vesicles were imaged, with an AFM, in a fluid environment. DMPC vesicles reconstituted with OmpF porins assume flattened, double bilayer configurations *(22)*. Often, multilammelar vesicles with incremental step membrane thicknesses were apparent in AFM images. Molecular resolution images show the predicted porin trimers as also shown by X-ray crystallography and EM reconstruction. The long-range packing of these trimeric complexes was dependent on the lipid-to-protein ratio.

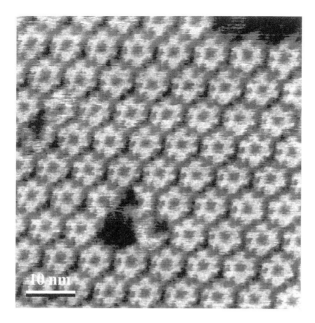

Fig. 4. An unprocessed AF*M* image of reconstituted Staphylococcal α-hemolysin (αHL) channels obtained in solution. Hexameric channels with a central pore-like depression are clearly visible. Some αHL channels with missing subunits are also present. For details, *see* ref. *21*.

OmpF porins showed a mixed hexagonal and rectangular packing, the center to center spacing was consistent with the X-ray diffraction study, and the mixed patterns correlate well with the given protein-to-lipid ratio (0.7).

Significantly, the regularity of protein packing depends on the protein-to-lipid interaction *(3)*. When the protein-to-lipid ratio was changed from 0.5 to 5.0 (by reducing the concentration of lipid at a given protein concentration), the shape and size of the vesicles changed from very large and irregular to small and spherical. In addition, the packing of proteins changed from hexagonal to rectangular (Fig. 5).

Schabert et al. *(23)* were able to resolve fine-details of OmpF porins reconstituted in DMPC vesicles at a protein-to-lipid ratio of 2.0. They were able to resolve rectangular unit cells (a = 13.5 nm and b = 8.2 nm) that comprise two trimers with central pore-like protrusions. Interestingly, two conformations of these channels were observed while imaging at a low force (0.1 n*N*), suggesting that AFM can be used to monitor conformational states of membrane proteins.

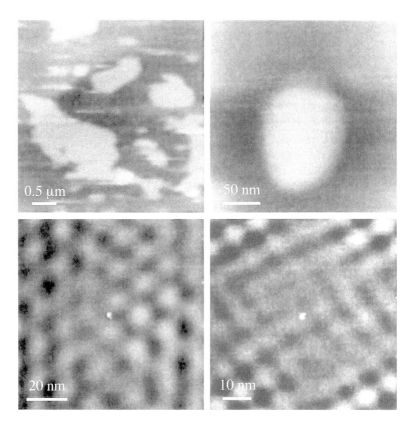

Fig. 5. Images of DMPC vesicle morphology and reconstituted OmpF porins for different protein-to-lipid ratios. The protein concentration was kept constant and the lipid concentration was changed (µg/µg) such that the lipid-to-protein (L/P ratio) varied from 2.0 to 0.2. Top left: Vesicles with L/P ratio of 2.0. The vesicles are large and irregular. Top right: A vesicle with L/P ratio of 0.2. The vesicle is small and oval. Bottom left: Inverse 2-D FFT filtered image of porin channels on the upper surface of a vesicle with a L/P ratio of 2.0. Porins appear to be arranged in a long-range hexagonal order. Bottom right: Inverse 2-D FFT filtered image of porin channels on the upper surface of a vesicle with a L/P ratio of 0.2. Porins appear to be arranged in a long-range rectangular order. For details, *see* ref. *3*.

4.2.4. Bordetella pertussis *Porin*

Lal et al. *(22)* were able to achieve molecular resolution on *Bordetella pertussis* porins that were packed in a quasi-rectangular order. These images also showed a lack of strong long range order, commonly observed for naturally occurring membranes and viewed by EM, indicating that the molecular motion in a native environment and perhaps tip induced perturbations. In

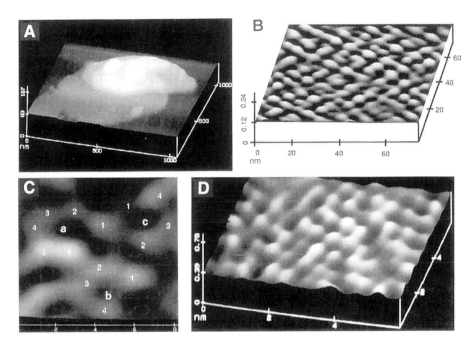

Fig. 6. Reconstituted porin channels imaged with an AFM. (**A**) Reconstituted DMPC lipid vesicles imaged in phosphate-buffered saline (PBS). Note the overlapping multilammelar vesicles. (**B**) Inverse 2D FFT filtered image of *Bordetella pertussis* porin channels reconstituted in DMPC vesicles and imaged under PBS with an AFM. The raw image showed identical pattern but was noisy. Note that the long-range packing is rectangular. Unit cell (~7.9 × 13.8 nm) shows two trimers. The lattice parameters are similar to that reported by EM study. (**C**) Subnanometer resolution unfiltered image (in 3D) showing the fine structures in the individual monomers. Note several bead-like structures and asymmetrically located pores (marked a,b,c). (**D**) Subnanometer resolution images of reconstituted DMPC vesicles without any protein added. Only the filtered image is shown although a similar pattern was visible in the raw data. Individual phospholipid headgroups (~0.5 nm in size; arrowhead) appear to be arranged in a crystalline fashion. For details, *see* ref. *22.*

addition, molecular resolution surface topology of *B. pertussis* porins was obtained for the first time (Fig. 6). The individual trimeric porins were visible. In a few cases, one can see monomeric components that had pore like central depressions and several surrounding bead like protrusions, perhaps the β-sheet folding of polypeptide.

4.2.5. Aquaporins

Aquaporins are ubiquitous membrane channels that allow passage of water and appear to be exclusively water-selective. These channels are involved in osmoregulation and volume control. High-resolution structural analyses and biochemical assays suggest that the membrane-spanning domains of the monomers are highly conserved. Like other transmembrane proteins, the nonmembranous, surface-exposed loops are the least-conserved and provide tissue and species specificity. Scheuring et al. *(24)* have imaged reconstituted aquaporin Z water channels from *Escherichia coli*. They were able to obtain small crystals with or without the N-termini. Using these crystals, they were able to obtain nanometer resolution images of the surfaces and were able to distinguish extracellular vs cytoplasmic faces, as previously recorded for purified gap junctions and hemi gap junctions *(11,24–26)*.

4.3. Reconstituted 3D Crystals of Ion Channels

4.3.1. OmpC Osmoporin 3D Crystals

Imaging molecular structure of 3D crystals of membrane proteins (e.g., channels and receptors) with AFM has been limited. Kim et al. *(16)* have imaged 3D microcrystals of OmpC osmoporin. OmpC osmoporin 3D crystals used in their study was unsuitable for high resolution X-ray diffraction. However, they have large and flat surfaces and thus are ideally suited for AFM imaging. Moreover, the crystals are highly stable and have a large unit cell, so that the crystal parameters are easily recognized.

AFM images of these microcrystals show multilayered crystalline surfaces and the corresponding crystallographic axes. The overall features including the step height and the perpendicular lattices at each surfaces correlate well with the X-ray diffraction data of OmpC crystals: monoclinic $P2_1$ with the unit cell constants a = 117.6 Å, b = 110 Å, c = 298.4 Å, $\beta = 97°$ (Fig. 7). Such a good correspondence between X-ray diffraction and AFM data suggests that the slow and mild air drying of these crystals did not induce significant alterations in the crystal lattices as expected upon crystal dehydration. At the (100) crystal face, individual trimeric protein-detergent complexes were resolved. These results show the potential for studying the molecular structure of microcrystals of integral membrane proteins. This study also suggests that the crystal grew in a fashion of rapid 2D expansion along the bc plane followed by a slow deposition along the a axis, perhaps as a rate-limiting nucleation process.

Thus, imaging 3D crystals in air may be better suited to achieve molecular resolution than in an aqueous medium because, in such preparation, the crystal surface is no longer active in the crystallization process and both the

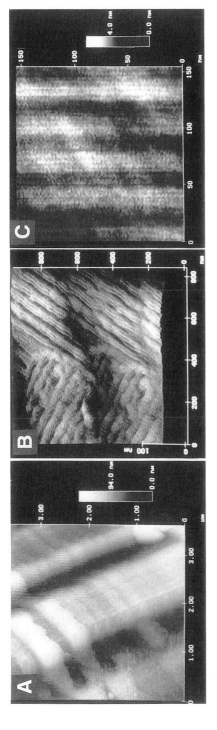

Fig. 7. AFM images of an OmpC 3D crystal. (**A**) A large scan image. The three perpendicular lattices and multiple layers of crystalline membrane surfaces are apparent. (**B**) A low-resolution AFM image of the membrane crystal surface where the two perpendicular lattices at the (100) face of the crystal are visible. Although the crystal surface is very rugged, the lattice system seems to be uninterrupted throughout the scan area. The high-frequency imaging noise (parallel lines at ~45° angle) are also visible. (**C**) A medium resolution (scan size 150 nm × 150 nm) top view AFM image of 2D pattern of substructures. The surface appears folded in the lateral direction (x-axis), whereas the pattern in the longitudinal direction (y-axis) is not immediately visible. The section analysis of the image in y direction shows the pattern spacing of about 20 nm. The section analysis in x-direction shows a clear spacing of 30 nm, which corresponds to cell parameters of the crystallographic c-axis. For details, *see* ref. *16*.

385

intra- and interlayer protein mobility are restricted. Moreover, AFM imaging of air-dried crystals would also be of considerable use in the early stages of a project to grow 3D crystals of membrane proteins suitable for high-resolution X-ray diffraction studies.

4.3.2. Ca-ATPase

Lacapere et al. *(27)* have imaged 3D crystals of Ca-ATPase that were reconstituted from 2D crystalline membranes isolated from sarcoplasmic reticulum vesicles. In their study, the lateral resolution was limited and they were not able to image crystal periodicity on the surface. However, the steps of membrane planes were measured that corresponded to the unit cell spacings. Although imaging under aqueous medium, they observed a significantly greater mobility on the surface, perhaps reflecting the intrinsic flexibility of layers of membrane sheets.

As the spectrum of AFM imaging is expanding, it is becoming clear that molecular resolution can be obtained on noncrystalline specimens in fluid medium. This opens a new avenue for the study of molecular structure of biological macromolecules such as ion channels and receptors that can be isolated and anchored properly on a suitable substrate and or reconstituted in an appropriate bilayer.

5. FUNCTIONAL ASSAY IN RECONSTITUTED SYSTEMS

Significant advantages of AFM over conventional high resolution microscopy is that AFM allows imaging under an aqueous environment and AFM can be combined with other techniques for simultaneous or successive structure-function studies. Such potentials of AFM have just began to be used for biological studies.

Butt et al. *(28)* have simultaneously imaged the structure of purple membrane, measured ion transport through the membrane, and examined the electrical properties of the membrane. Dietz et al. *(29)* have measured electric charge transfer through synthetic ultrafiltration membranes. And, Proksch et al. *(30)* have simultaneously imaged the surface structure of nuleopore filters and measured electrical current passing across the filter through pores of different diameters. For these studies, they developed a combined scanning ion-conductance microscope, which can record electrical activity while imaging the 3D structure of various membranes.

AFM has also been used to image dynamic physical properties in response to specific agonists/antagonists. For example, the change in viscoelasticity of AβP-reconstituted vesicles were recently measured *(18)*. The stiffness of the AβP-containing vesicles was significantly higher in the presence of calcium and the stiffness change was prevented in the presence of zinc, Tris, and anti-AβP antibody but not in the presence of Trolox and DTT. Thus the stiffness change is consistent with the vesicular uptake of Ca^{2+}. These findings provide additional biophysical evidence that $AβP_{1-42}$ forms calcium-permeable channels.

6. CONCLUSION

The simple design and invariance to the operating environment allows AFM to be integrated with other techniques for simultaneous structure-function correlational studies. The integration of the AFM and fluorescence microscope is one such exciting development *(31)*. Other combinations, specifically a combined near-field differential scanning optical microscope with AFM *(32)* and the AFM-based NMR imaging *(33)* provide promising avenues for 3D structural analysis of individual channels and receptors without the need of crystallization and related complications. New cryo-atomic force microscope, developed by Shao and his collaborators *(9)* will provide a significant impetus for high resolution and even atomic resolution imaging of channels and receptors, both isolated and those present in cell membranes.

The studies of ion channels and receptors in their native hydrated states has potential for direct structure-function studies, including short-, and long-term molecular interactions with various ligands (e.g., antibodies, toxins, drugs).

ACKNOWLEDGMENTS

We thank Dr. Zhifeng Shao for providing images of cholera-toxins and α-hemolysin. Supported by a grant from the National Institute of Health (GM-NIA 05620) (RL).

REFERENCES

1. Binnig, G., Quate, C. F., and Gerber, C. (1986) Atomic force microscope. *Phys. Rev. Lett.* **56,** 930–933.
2. Lal, R. and John, S. A. (1994) Biological application of atomic force microscopy. *Am. J. Physiol.* **266,** C1–C21.
3. Lal, R. (1998) Imaging molecular structure of channels and receptors with an atomic force microscope. *Scan. Microsc.* **10,** 81–96.
4. Yang, J. and Shao, Z. F. (1995) Recent advances in biological atomic force microscopy. *Micron* **26,** 35–49.

5. Ohnesorge, F. and Binnig, G. (1993) True atomic resolution by atomic force microscopy through repulsive and attractive forces. *Science* **260,** 1451–1456.

6. Lal, R. and Yu, L. (1993) Molecular structure of cloned nicotinic AChR receptors expressed in xenopus oocyte as revealed by atomic force microscopy. *Proc. Natl. Acad. Sci. USA* **90,** 7280–7284.

7. Kordylewski, L., Saner, D., and Lal, R. (1994) Atomic force microscopy of freeze-fracture replicas of rat atrial tissue. *J. Microscopy* **173,** 173–181.

8. Parbhu, A. N., Bryson, W. G., and Lal, R. (1999) Disulfide bonds in the outer layer of keratin fibers confer higher mechanical rigidity: correlative nanoindentation and elasticity measurement with an AFM. *Biochemistry* **38,** 11,755–11,761.

9. Han, W., Mou, J., Yang, J., and Shao, Z. F. (1995) Cryo atomic force microscopy: a new approach for biological imaging at high resolution. *Biochemistry* **34,** 8216–8220.

10. Hillner, P. E., Walters, D. A., Lal, R., Hansma, H. G., and Hansma, P. K. (1995) Combined atomic force and confocal laser scanning microscope. *J. Micro. Soc. Am.* **1,** 123–126.

11. Lal, R., John, S. A., Laird, D. W., and Arnsdorf, M. F. (1995) Heart gap junction preparations reveal hemiplaques by atomic force microscopy. *Am. J. Physiol.* **268,** C968–C977.

12. Lal, R. and Proksch, R. A. (1997) Multimodal imaging with atomic force microscopy: combined atomic force, light fluorescence, and laser confocal microscopy and electrophysiological recordings of biological membranes. *Int. J. Imaging Syst. Technol.* **8,** 293–300.

13. Yang, J., Tamm, L., Tillack, T., and Shao, Z. F. (1993) New approach for atomic force microscopy of membrane proteins: imaging of cholera toxin. *J. Mol. Biol.* **229,** 286–290.

14. Karrasch, S., Dolder, M., Schabert, F., Ramsden, J., and Engel, E. (1993) Covalent binding of biological samples to solid supports for scanning probe microscopy in buffer solution. *Biophys. J.* **65,** 2437–2446.

15. Mou, J., Yang, J., and Shao, Z. F. (1995) Atomic force microscopy of cholera toxin B-oligomers bound to bilayers of biologically relevant lipids. *J. Mol. Biol.* **248,** 507–512.

16. Kim, H., Garavito, M. J., and Lal, R. (2000) Atomic force microscopy of three-dimensional crystal of membrane protein, OmpC porin. *Colloids Surfaces B: Biointerfaces* **19,** 247–355.

17. Czajkowsky, D. M., Iwamoto, H., Cover, T. L., and Shao, ZF. (1999) The vacuolating toxin from *Helicobacter pylori* forms hexameric pores in lipid bilayers at low pH. *Proc. Natl. Acad. Sci. USA* **96,** 2001–2006.

18. Rhee, S. K., Quist, A. P., and Lal, R. (1998) Amyloid beta protein(1–42) forms calcium permeable, Zn^{2+}-sensitive channel. *J. Biol. Chem.* **273,** 13,379–13,382.

19. Lin, H., Zhu, Y. J., and Lal, R. (1999) Amyloid beta protein (1–40) forms calcium permeable, zinc-sensitive pores in reconstituted lipid vesicles. *Biochemistry* **38,** 11,189–11,196.

20. Lin, H., Alig, T, Zasazdinski, J., and Lal, R. (2000) Amyloid beta protein (1–42) (AβP) forms tetrameric pores in lipid bilayers: an atomic force microscopy study. *Biophys. J.* **78,** 177A.

21. Czajkowsky, D. M., Sheng, S., and Shao, Z. F. (1998) Staphylococcal α-hemolysin can form hexamers in phospholipid bilayers. *J. Mol. Biol.* **276,** 325–330.

22. Lal, R, Kim, H., Garavito, R. M., and Arnsdorf, M. F. (1993) Molecular resolution imaging of outer membrane channels reconstituted in an artificial bilayer. *Am. J. Physiol.* **265,** C851–C856.

23. Schabert, F. A., Henn, C., and Engel, A. (1995) Native *E. coli* OmpF porin surfaces probed by atomic force microscopy. *Science* **268,** 92–94.

24. Scheuring, S., Ringler, P., Borgnia, M., Stahlberg, H., Muller, D. J., Agre, P., and Engel, A. (1999) High resolution AFM topographs of the *Escherichia coli* water channel aquaporin Z. *EMBO J.* **18,** 4981–4987.

25. Hoh, J., Lal, R., John, S. A., Revel, J.-P., and Arnsdorf, M. F. (1991) Atomic force microscopy and dissection of gap junctions. *Science* **253,** 1405–1408.

26. John, S. A., Saner, D. A., Pitts, J., Finbow, M., and Lal, R. (1997) Atomic force microscopy of arthropod gap junctions. *J. Struct. Biol.* **120,** 22–31.

27. Lacapere, J. J., Stokes, D. L., and Chatenay, D. (1992) Atomic force microscopy of 3-dimensional membrane-protein crystals — Ca-ATPase of sarcoplasmic reticulum. *Biophys. J.* **63,** 303–308.

28. Butt, H.-J., Seifert, K., Fendeler, K., and Bamberg, E. (1993) Characterizing solid supported membranes with the atomic force microscope. *Biophys. J.* **64,** A14.

29. Dietz, P., Hansma, P. K., Herrmann, K.-H., Inacker, O., and Lehmann, H.-D. (1991) Atomic force microscopy of synthetic ultrafiltration membranes in air and under water. *Ultramicroscopy* **35,** 155–159.

30. Proksch, R. A., Lal, R., Hansma, P. K., Morse, D., and Stucky, G. (1996) Imaging the internal and external pore structures of membrane in fluid: tapping mode scanning ion conductance microscopy. *Biophys. J.* **71,** 2155–2157.

31. Hansma, P. K., Drake, B., Grigg, D., Prater, C. B., Yasher, F., Gurley, G., et al. (1994) A new, optical-lever based atomic force microscope. *J. Appl. Phys.* **76,** 796–799.

32. Toledo-crow, R., Yang, P., Chen, Y., and Vaez-Iravani, M. (1992) Near-field differential scanning optical microscope with atomic force regulation. *Appl. Phys. Lett.* **60,** 2957–2959.

33. Ruger, D., Yannoni, C. S., and Sidles, J. A. (1992) Mechanical detection of magnetic resonance. *Nature* **360,** 563–566.

21

Imaging the Spatial Organization of Calcium Channels in Nerve Terminals Using Atomic Force Microscopy

Hajime Takano, Marc Porter, and Philip G. Haydon

1. INTRODUCTION

For many years there has been much interest in identifying the spatial relationship between the organization of calcium channels and the sites for the release of chemical neurotransmitter (for a recent review, *see* ref. *1*). During this time, the debate has been fostered by biophysical studies concerning the relation between calcium and transmitter release. Many studies, for example, have asked whether multiple calcium ions are required for the release of neurotransmitter. With the frequent observation of an apparent cooperative relation between calcium influx and stimulated release, and the demonstration of very short latencies between calcium influx and the onset of the evoked synaptic potential/current, there has been much debate about the organization of calcium channels with respect to the secretory apparatus. Questions that frequently surface are how many channels surround a vesicle, is calcium influx through multiple calcium channels necessary for the release of neurotransmitter, and how closely do calcium channels cluster at a release site? Although these questions frequently surface, there have been few successful attempts to define the spatial organization of calcium channels in nerve terminals. This paucity of information is not owing to a lack of effort, but rather because of technical challenges that are associated with working within the limited space of a nerve terminal.

The goal of this chapter is to discuss one approach that has yielded some answers to these questions. We discuss the use of atomic force micrscopy

From: *Ion Channel Localization Methods and Protocols*
Edited by: A. Lopatin and C. G. Nichols © Humana Press Inc., Totowa, NJ

(AFM) to investigate the organization of the calcium channels in nerve terminals, and additionally, provide a discussion of other scanning-probe microscopy methods that hold promise for the future.

As has so frequently been the case, the squid giant synapse yielded the first clear insights into questions regarding the relation between sites of calcium influx and synaptic transmission *(2,3)*. In this preparation the presynaptic terminals are highly accessible for experimentation. The large presynaptic axon branches into a series of fingers that innervate postsynaptic dendrites. Because of the experimental accessibility of the system, fluorescent ion indicators can be readily microinjected into the presynaptic axon, and following diffusion, the dye fills the presynaptic terminals where relative changes in calcium can be monitored following the stimulation of presynaptic axons. Stimulation of the presynaptic axon evoked elevations of calcium in the presynaptic axon terminal in a heterogeneous manner consistent with the maximum influx sites being located in the presynaptic axon membrane *(2)*. Studies using a low-affinity form of the luminescent calcium indicator, n-aequorin-J, revealed highly localized puncta of luminescent emission at presynaptic sites adjacent to the postsynaptic membrane *(3)*. Despite the importance and elegance of these functional studies, they fail to provide high-resolution details about the organization of channels in the nerve terminal. Additionally, because the optical assays are limited in resolution by the Abbe diffraction limit, it was not possible to achieve structural resolution at a finer level than about 250 nm. Because a synaptic vesicle is of the order of 40–50 nm in diameter, and calcium channels are about 8–16 nm in diameter *(4)*, methods are required that have at least one order of magnitude greater resolution than the diffraction limit in order to reveal necessary organizational principles.

To achieve subdiffraction resolution, techniques are required that using different principles than objective-based optics. Freeze-fracture data suggest that calcium channels cluster in parallel rows adjacent to the sites of vesicle exocytosis *(5)*. These freeze fracture images demonstrated rows of intramembranous particles that have been interpreted as rows of calcium channels. Although this might be the case, interpretation of the data is complex because these particles could not be labeled to confirm identity.

In order to identify the organization of calcium channels, it is necessary to be able to tag, or label the channel, and to be able to interrogate the system with methods that are not limited by a resolution of 250 nm. To tag the channel, we used a modification of the general approach that was first demonstrated to disclose the location of presynaptic calcium channels at frog neuromuscular junction *(6)*. Fluorescently labeled ω-conotoxin (ω-CgTx), an N-type calcium channel binding peptide that was originally isolated from the venom of the marine snail *Conus geographus (7–11)*, labels the calcium channels of the presynaptic terminal at the neuromuscular junction. When double-label experiments were performed, it was demonstrated that the calcium-channel labeling matched the positioning of postsynaptic acetylcholine receptors *(6)*, indicating that calcium channels cluster in the nerve terminal in a manner consistent with a localization in the release face of the membrane. These results provided the starting point to begin to address the nature of the calcium channel organization because the tag had the possibility of identifying the location of the channel.

Instead of using a fluorescently conjugated ω-CgTx to label calcium channels, we used biotinylated ω-CgTx, which selectively labels the calcium channel, and then labeled the toxin by reacting the preparation with avidin-coated gold particles *(12)*. To study the location of the gold particles, and thus of the calcium channels, we then applied the technique of AFM which can, with appropriate samples, image with atomic scale resolution. In the following paragraphs, we discuss the fundamental basis of AFM and its application to the study of calcium-channel location, as well as highlight some of the strengths and weaknesses of this approach.

2. ATOMIC FORCE MICROSCOPY

The atomic force microscope is a direct descendent of the scanning tunneling microscope (STM) that was invented in 1981 *(13)* (for review, *see* ref. *14*). In effect, the atomic force microscope is a profilometer as shown in Fig. 1. A pyramidal tip that is attached to the end of a flexible cantilever (Fig. 1A,B) locally interacts with the sample that is moved under the tip in a raster scan fashion by piezo-control. As the tip encounters changes in underlying topography, the cantilever bends, and an optical beam, that is reflected off the backside of the cantilever (Fig. 1A), detects this motion. The movement of the optical lever is detected by a position-sensitive split photodiode. The instrument can be operated in two modes, either in a feedback mode where small optically detected movements of the cantilever are used to control compensating z-piezo movements (constant force), or where the system is used open loop and the deflections of the cantilever are converted into forces. For imaging calcium-channel locations, we used the constant force mode, because it is preferable to exert the minimum force at the tip-sample microcontact.

AFM can provide very high-resolution structural information. For example, Fig. 2 shows an image of gold atoms with nanometer resolution.

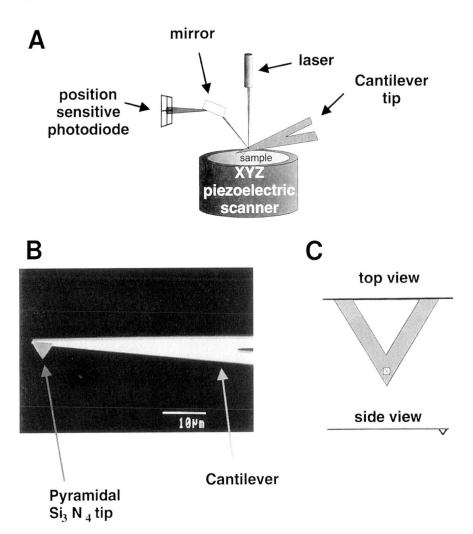

Fig. 1. (**A**) The principal components for an optical lever type AFM. The laser beam is reflected off the back of the cantilever onto a position sensitive photodiode. (**B**) Scanning electron micrograph of a pyramidal tip at the end of a microfabricated silicone nitride cantilever. (**C**) Schematics of a silicon nitride cantilever.

The possibility that this technique could provide such resolution on biological samples attracted the interests of many researchers. However, early studies with either fixed or living cells demonstrated that although exciting images could be achieved *(15–20)*, it was difficult to approach the resolu-

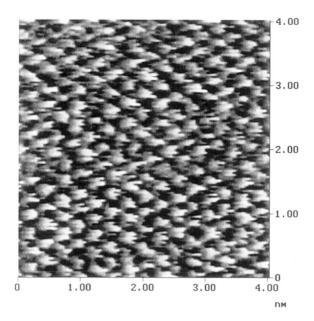

Fig. 2. AFM (lateral force) image (4 nm × 4 nm) of gold on mica. Gold was vapor deposited onto freshly cleaved mica and was annealed at 300°C for 5 h; this process yields a surface composed of large (100–200 nm) atomically smooth gold crystallites.

tion of samples such as that shown in Fig. 2. This disconnect in resolution is likely owing to two reasons. First, cells are highly compliant materials in comparison to monolayers of atoms molecules or crystals. Second, the high resolution seen in Fig. 2 probably requires the repetitive nature of the crystalline array of molecules

Before leaving this brief discussion of AFM, it is worth noting that this technique also provides some very exciting possibilities for studying biomolecules. One of the great powers of AFM that was not initially exploited by biologists was the ability to precisely measure forces *(14)*. In addition to imaging, as discussed earlier, one can also operate the AFM in a mode in which the pyramidal tip is moved in the z dimension over any given x, y position. With appropriate biomolecules attached to the pyramidal tip and the substrate, forces of molecular interaction can be measured. This was first shown to have utility in studies where the force to rupture a single biotin and avidin bond was measured *(21)*. Subsequently, the method has been used very successfully to measure changes in compliance of mast cell granules *(22)*, and to identify properties of the muscle protein titan *(23)*.

3. THE CHICK CILIARY GANGLION CALYX NERVE TERMINAL AND CALCIUM CHANNEL LABELING

In order to apply AFM to the study of calcium channels, it is essential that we have direct access to the release face of the nerve terminal so that pyramidal tip of the microscope can directly access the channels. This is a challenging problem because the release face is normally directly opposite to the postsynaptic cell. However, Elis Stanley has demonstrated that it is possible to dissociate the nerve terminal from the postsynaptic cell *(24–31)*. In chick embryos at d 15, the presynaptic innervation of the ciliary ganglion is in the form of a large calyx that ensheaths a large portion of the postsynaptic cell. After enzymatic treatment, it is possible to dissociate presynaptic calycees from the postsynaptic cell. The challenge, however, is to distinguish functional terminals from detritus in the resulting mixture. Of critical importance for this approach was the ability to use a vital stain of living nerve terminals. 4-Di-2-Asp selectively labels presynaptic terminals and maintains labeling if the dissociated terminal is still functional. This method has been critically evaluated in studies where acetylcholine release and single calcium-channel opening was simultaneously monitored *(24)*.

In studying the location of calcium channels, we first identified isolated nerve terminals and recorded their position on the microscope coverslip by using labeled grids that had been affixed to the underside of the coverslip *(12)*. Subsequently, the sample was processed by addition of biotinylated ω-CgTx, and after washing and incubation with avidin gold, the preparation was fixed in 4% paraformaldehyde. After washing in phosphate-buffered saline (PBS), the sample was transferred to the stage of an atomic force microscope. In our original work, we used a Digital Instruments Nanoscope III for these studies. However, newer generation instruments that are integrated with inverted microscopes would be preferable for this type of study because they would permit the user to locate the previously identified nerve terminal with relative ease.

Throughout the processing of biological samples for use in AFM, it is critical that they retain hydration. We found that when samples are dehydrated, the plasma membrane collapses onto the internal contents of the cell, leading to complex topography. This makes the interpretation of images difficult when one is searching for gold particles against a background of the cell surface topography. However, when samples retain hydration, the surface topography is much less tortuous, making the identification of gold particles possible.

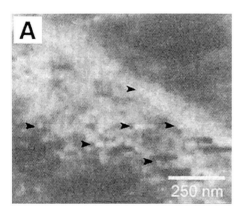
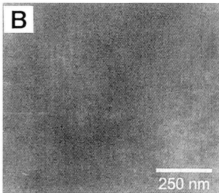

Fig. 3. Binding of gold particles to calcium channels. (**A,B**) 1 μm² area of b-ω-CgTx/gold (A) and ω-CTx preblocked (B) calyx scans. Examples of particles are indicated by arrowheads. All images were scanned in PBS. Adapted with permission from ref. *12*.

4. IMAGING GOLD PARTICLES ON THE CELL SURFACE

Having performed the labeling of samples with biotin-ω-CgTx followed by avidin gold, examination with AFM reveals cluster of particles. Although much of the sample contains few particles, we identified regions where clusters of up to about 150 particles per μm² were identified *(12)*. We presume that these clusters of particles correspond to the locations of release sites and thus N-type calcium channels. We were particularly excited by the quantitative agreement between these labeling studies and physiological records of calcium-channel activity, which also suggested that channels cluster and that clusters can contain similar channel densities *(27)*.

In channel-tagging studies, controls were particularly important in order to determine whether apparent particles result from the presence of gold or from the biological sample itself (Fig. 3). Thus we scanned unlabeled samples, and samples that had been incubated with ω-CgTx prior to applying biotin-ω-CgTx. Finally, we also scanned samples that had been labeled with biotin-ω-CgTx, but prior to addition of avidin gold. After collecting an image, the gold particle was then reacted with the sample and was demonstrated to label regions of the nerve terminal that did not previously contain particles. These types of controls are extremely important so that one can be certain that the labeling is specific and not owing, for example, to existing topographic features of the nerve terminal *per se.*

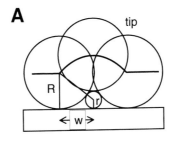

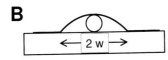

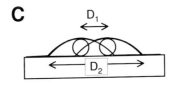

Fig. 4. Real and apparent shapes in AFM images. (**A**) Owing to the finite tip radius (R), the apparent shapes are wider in width compared to the original particle that has a radius of r. (**B**) Apparent shapes of spherical particles; for example, the tip radius R = 20 nm and the particle radius r = 1 nm give the apparent particle width (2w) of ~18 nm. Note that height should reflect the real particle height of 2r. (**C**) When two particles exist at a separation distance of D_1 and tip radius is not small enough to distinguish the individual particles, the apparent shapes have a width (D2) with two peaks. Importantly the separation distance of those two peaks D_1 is the same as the separation distance of the particles.

5. IMAGES OBTAINED WITH AFM RESULT FROM A CONVOLUTION OF THE TIP AND SUBSTRATE

In order to interpret the pattern of gold labeling on the surface of a nerve terminal, it is important to be able to understand the mechanism that generates image contrast. With AFM, although one can detect inter-atomic spacing (Fig. 2), this does not mean that all samples will provide the same information. In fact, because the image that is generated is owing to a convolution of the pyramidal tip and the sample, it is very difficult to measure the diameters of structures. Figure 4 demonstrates some of the concerns related to this issue. If one is imaging a sphere with the AFM tip, interactions between the tip and sample occur prior to the tip becoming centered over the sphere. This leads to inaccurate measurements of the diameter of the sphere *(32)*. The height measure is, however, very accurate. Because of this problem with measuring widths, it is difficult to confirm that a particle detected on the surface of a nerve terminal has the correct dimensions of the applied gold particles and reaffirms the importance of the labeling controls discussed earlier. Although the diameter of a particle cannot be measured well, it is possible to measure the center-to-center spacing of particles to indicate the relative organization of the channel (Fig. 4C).

6. THE SPACING OF CALCIUM CHANNELS IN THE NERVE TERMINAL

Given that it is possible to measure distances between individual particles, we asked whether we could gain insights into the organization of the calcium channels in nerve terminals with this approach. The center of each particle in each image was identified and we determined the distance to the nearest neighboring particle. Figure 5 demonstrates the results of this analysis and shows that the predominate mode is located at 40 nm, with harmonics at 20 nm increments. Because we were restricted to using 30 nm gold particles in this study (it is difficult to readily identify smaller particles on the surface of a cell), we feel that it is likely that calcium channels are actually separated by about 20 nm *(12)*, a value that corresponds well with the approximate diameter of calcium channels *(4)*.

The application of AFM to the study of ion-channel organization has clearly demonstrated that the channels are clustered and are likely to be at extremely high density in the nerve terminal. Thus, even though the opening of one channel can stimulate neurotransmitter release, channels are present at a sufficient density to permit calcium entry through more than one channel (if they are simultaneously gated) to contribute to the stimulation of exocytosis.

7. FUTURE PROSPECTS FOR THE USE OF NANOTECHNOLOGY IN STUDIES OF CALCIUM CHANNEL ORGANIZATION

Some of the frustrating aspects of the use of AFM for studying calcium channel organization are that it is difficult to achieve high-resolution measurements of particle widths and it is not possible to determine the co-localization of the secretory apparatus and the calcium channels. To overcome

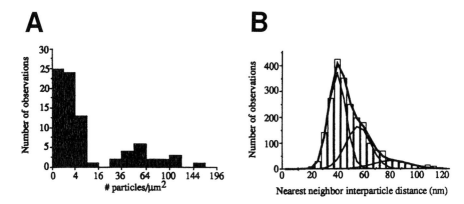

Fig. 5. Analysis of gold-particle distribution. **(A)** Frequency histograms of particle density per 1 μm² field. Note there are two modes to this distribution, a very low and high density of particles. The high-density mode probably corresponds to calcium channels at synaptic sites. **(B)** Frequency histograms of particle nearest-neighbor analyses from all preparations (2273 particles). Note that although a mode is identified at 40 nm particle spacing, additional modes at 60 and 80 nm suggest that channels are in fact spaced at 20 nm intervals. Because the gold particles used in the study were 30 nm in diameter, it was not possible to resolve this closer spacing. Adapted with permission from ref. *12*.

these limitations, there are two emerging developments that may facilitate this type of study. First, the use of carbon nanotubes attached to the tip of the cantilever in order to enhance the lateral resolution of AFM *(33,34)*. Second, the development of a subdiffraction resolution optical method opens the possibility for double-labeling studies in the near future. In near-field scanning optical microscopy (NSOM) samples are excited using illumination that passes along an optical fiber that has an extremely small exit aperture *(35–41)*. The resolution of optical information achieved with this method is regulated by the diameter of this exit aperture (about 50 nm). In the physical sciences this method has proven effective for studying single molecules. Potentially, NSOM could be applied to biological samples also. However, the transfer of the technique into this area has been slow, in large part because of difficulties associated with working with hydrated, soft, thick samples (i.e., cells). Over the past several years, significant progress has been made with this method in biology *(42–53)* and we have recently demonstrated that we can reliably image with sub-diffraction resolution from hydrated cells (Haydon et al., unpublished data). Because we have also demonstrated that we can illuminate calcium indicator contained within living cells *(55)*, we anticipate that it will not be long until this high-resolution optical approach can be used to monitor local calcium accumulation immediately beneath ion channels. Thus, with this method and further developments in nanotechnology, we expect that it will become possible to double-label vesicles and monitor single-vesicle exocytosis while recording the local calcium accumulation that stimulates membrane fusion.

ACKNOWLEDGMENTS

The authors work is supported by grants from the Roy J. Carver Charitable Trust, Muscatine, Iowa, the National Institutes of Health, the U.S. Department of Energy, and the National Science Foundation.

REFERENCES

1. Stanley, E. F. (1997) The calcium channel and the organization of the presynaptic transmitter release face. *Trends. Neurosci.* **20,** 404–409.
2. Smith, S. J., Buchanan, J., Osses, L. R., Charlton, M. P., and Augustine, G. J. (1993) The spatial distribution of calcium signals in squid presynaptic terminals. *J. Physiol. Lond.* **472,** 573–593.
3. Llinas, R., Sugimori, M., and Silver, R. B. (1992) Microdomains of high calcium concentration in a presynaptic terminal. *Science* **256,** 677–679.
4. Witcher, D. R., De Waard, M., Sakamoto, J., Franzini-Armstrong, C., Pragnell, M., Kahl, S. D., et al. (1993) Subunit identification and reconstitution of the N-type Ca2+ channel complex purified from brain. *Science* **261,** 486–489.
5. Pumplin, D. W., Reese, T. S., and Llinas, R. (1981) Are the presynaptic membrane particles the calcium channels? *Proc. Natl. Acad. Sci. USA* **78,** 7210–7213.
6. Robitaille, R., Adler, E. M., and Charlton, M. P. (1990) Strategic location of calcium channels at transmitter release sites of frog neuromuscular synapses. *Neuron* **5,** 773–779.
7. McIntosh, J. M., Olivera, B. M., and Cruz, L. J. (1999) Conus peptides as probes for ion channels. *Methods Enzymol.* **294,** 605–624.
8. Olivera, B. M., et al. (1990) Diversity of Conus neuropeptides. *Science* **249,** 257–263.
9. Gray, B. W. R., Olivera, B. M., and Cruz, L. J. (1988) Peptide toxins from venomous Conus snails. *Annu. Rev. Biochem.* **57,** 665–700.
10. Olivera, B. M., Cruz, I. J., deSnatos, V., LeChemiuant, G. W., Griffin, D., Zeikus, R., et al. (1987) Neuronal calcium channel antagonists. Discrimination between calcium channel subtypes using omega-conotoxin from Conus magus venom. *Biochemistry* **26,** 2086–2090.
11. Olivera, B. M., Cruz, I. J., de Santos, V., Le Cheminant, G. W., Griffin, D. Zeikus, F., et al. (1985) Peptide neurotoxins from fish-hunting cone snails. *Science* **230,** 1338–1343.
12. Haydon, P. G., Henderson, E., and Stanley, E. F. (1994) Localization of individual calcium channels at the release face of a presynaptic nerve terminal. *Neuron* **13,** 1275–1280.

13. Binnig, G., Rohrer, H., Gerber, C., and Weibel, E. (1981) *Phys. Rev. Lett.* **49,** 57.

14. Takano, H., Kenseth, J. R., Wong, S., O'Brien, J. C., and Porter, M. D. (1999) Chemical and biochemical analysis using scanning force microscopy. *Chem. Rev.* **99,** 2845–2890.

15. Haydon, Lartius, R., Parpura, V., and Marchese Ragona, S. P. (1996) Membrane deformation of living glial cells using atomic force microscopy. *J. Microsc.* **182,** 114–120.

16. Parpura, V., Haydon, P. G., and Henderson, E. (1993) Three-dimensional imaging of living neurons and glia with the atomic force microscope. *J. Cell Sci.* **104,** 427–432.

17. Parpura, V., Doyle, R. T., Basarsky, T. A., Henderson, E., and Haydon, P. G. (1995) Dynamic imaging of purified individual synaptic vesicles. *Neuroimage* **2,** 3–7.

18. Hoh, J. H. and Schoenenberger, C. A. (1994) Surface morphology and mechanical properties of MDCK monolayers by atomic force microscopy. *J. Cell Sci.* **107,** 1105–1114.

19. Hansma, H. G. and Hoh, J. H. (1994) Biomolecular imaging with the atomic force microscope. *Annu. Rev. Biophys. Biomol. Struct.* **23,** 115–139.

20. Henderson, E., Haydon, P. G., and Sakaguchi, D. S. (1992) Actin filament dynamics in living glial cells imaged by atomic force microscopy. *Science* **257,** 1944–1946.

21. Florin, E. L., Moy, V. T., and Gaub, H. E. (1994) Adhesion forces between individual ligand-receptor pairs. *Science* **264,** 415–417.

22. Parpura, V. and Fernandez, J. M. (1996) Atomic force microscopy study of the secretory granule lumen. *Biophys. J.* **71,** 2356–2366.

23. Rief, M., Gautel, M., Oesterhelt, F., Fernandez, J. M., and Gaub, H. E. (1997) Reversible unfolding of individual titin immunoglobulin domains by AFM [see comments]. *Science* **276,** 1109–1112.

24. Stanley, E. F. (1993) Single calcium channels and acetylcholine release at a presynaptic nerve terminal. *Neuron* **11,** 1007–1011.

25. Stanley, E. F. (1993) Presynaptic calcium channels and the transmitter release mechanism. *Ann. NY Acad. Sci.* **681,** 368–372.

26. Stanley, E. F. (1992) The calyx-type synapse of the chick ciliary ganglion as a model of fast cholinergic transmission. *Can. J. Physiol. Pharmacol.* **70(Suppl.),** S73–S77.

27. Stanley, E. F. (1991) Single calcium channels on a cholinergic presynaptic nerve terminal. *Neuron* **7,** 585–591.

28. Stanley, E. F. and Goping, G. (1991) Characterization of a calcium current in a vertebrate cholinergic presynaptic nerve terminal. *J. Neurosci.* **11,** 985–993.

29. Stanley, E. F. and Cox, C. (1991) Calcium channels in the presynaptic nerve terminal of the chick ciliary ganglion giant synapse. *Ann. NY Acad. Sci.* **635,** 70–79.

30. Stanley, E. F. and Atrakchi, A. H. (1990) Calcium currents recorded from a vertebrate presynaptic nerve terminal are resistant to the dihydropyridine nifedipine. *Proc. Natl. Acad. Sci. USA* **87,** 9683–9687.

31. Stanley, E. F. (1987) Light microscopic visualisation of the presynaptic nerve terminal calyx in dissociated chick ciliary ganglion neurons. *Brain Res.* **421,** 367–369.

32. Vesenka, J., Manne, S., Giberson, R., Marsh, T., and Henderson, E. (1993) Colloidal gold particles as an incompressible atomic force microscope imaging standard for assessing the compressibility of biomolecules. *Biophys. J.* **65,** 992–997.

33. Wong, S. S., Harper, J. D., Lansbury, P. T., and Lieber, C. M. (1998) Carbon nanotube tips: high resolution probes forimaging biological systems. *J. Am. Chem. Soc.* **120,** 603,604.

34. Dai, H., Hafner, J. H., Rinzler, A. G., Colbert, D. T., and Smalley, R. E. (1996) Nanotubes as nanoprobes in scanning probe microscopy. *Nature* **384,** 147–150.

35. Hwang, J., Tamm, L. K., Bohm, I., Ramalingham, T. S., Betzig, E., Edidin, M. (1995) Nanoscale complexity of phospholipid monolayers investigated by near-field scanning optical microscopy. *Science* **270,** 610–614.

36. Ambrose, W. P., Goodwin, P. M., Martin, J. C., and Keller, R. A. (1994) Alterations of single molecule fluorescence lifetimes in near-field optical micorscopy. *Science* **265,** 364–367.

37. Betzig, E. and Chichester, R. J. (1993) Single molecules observed by near-field scanning optical microscopy. *Science* **262,** 1422–1425.

38. Betzig, E. and Chichester, R. J. (1992) Near-field optics: microscopy, spectroscopy, and surface modification beyond the diffraction limit. *Science* **257,** 189–195.

39. Kopelman, R. and Tan, W. (1993) Near-field optics: imaging single molecules. *Science* 1382–1384.

40. Trautman, J. K., Macklin, J. J., Brus, L. E., and Betzi, E. (1997). Near-field spectroscopy of single molecules at room temperature. *Nature* **369,** 40–42.

41. Trautman, J. K., et al. (1971) Image contrast in near-field optics. *J. Appl. Physics* 4663

42. Marchese-Ragona, S. P. and Haydon, P. G. (1997) Near-field scanning optical microscopy and near-field confocal optical spectroscopy: emerging techniques in biology. *Ann. NY Acad. Sci.* **820,** 196–206.

43. Bui, J. D., et al. (1999) Probing intracellular dynamics in living cells with near-field optics. *J. Neurosci. Methods* **89,** 9–15.

44. Nagy, P., Zelles, T., Lou, H. J., Gallion, V. L., Phillips, M. I., Tan, W. (1999) Activation-dependent clustering of the erbB2 receptor tyrosine kinase detected by scanning near-field optical microscopy. *J. Cell Sci.* **112,** 1733–1741.

45. Lewis, A., Radko, A., Ben Ami, N., Palanker, D., and Lieberman, K. (1999) Near-field scanning optical microscopy in cell biology. *Trends. Cell Biol.* **9,** 70–73.

46. Shiku, H. and Dunn, R. C. (1999) Near-field scanning optical microscopy. *Anal. Chem.* **71,** 23A–29A.

47. Subramaniam, V., Kirsch, A. K., and Jovin, T. M. (1998) Cell biological applications of scanning near-field optical microscopy (SNOM). *Cell Mol. Biol. (Noisy-le-grand)* **44,** 689–700.

48. Meixner, A. J. and Kneppe, H. (1998) Scanning near-field optical microscopy in cell biology and microbiology. *Cell Mol. Biol.* **44,** 673–688.

49. Hwang, J., Gheber, L. A., Margolis, L., and Edidin, M. (1998) Domains in cell plasma membranes investigated by near-field scanning optical microscopy. *Biophys. J.* **74,** 2184–2190.

50. Ben-Ami, N., et al. (1998) Near-field optical imaging of unstained bacteria: comparison with normal atomic force and far-field optical microscopy in air and aqueous media. *Ultramicroscopy* **71,** 321–325.

51. Bui, J. D., et al. (1999) Probing intracellular dynamics in living cells with near-field optics. *J. Neurosci. Methods* **89,** 9–15.

52. Subramaniam, V., Kirsch, A. K., and Jovin, T. M. (1998) Cell biological applications of scanning near-field optical microscopy (SNOM). *Cell Mol. Biol.* **44,** 689–700.

53. Ben-Ami, N., et al. (1998) Near-field optical imaging of unstained bacteria: comparison with normal atomic force and far-field optical microscopy in air and aqueous media. *Ultramicroscopy* **71,** 321–325.

54. Haydon, P. G., Marchese Ragona, S., Basarsky, T. A., Szulczewski, M., and McCloskey, M. (1996) Near-field confocal optical spectroscopy (NCOS): subdiffraction optical resolution for biological systems. *J. Microsc.* **182,** 208–216.

22

Nanoarchitecture of Plasma Membrane Visualized with Atomic Force Microscopy

Hans Oberleithner, Hermann Schillers, Stefan W. Schneider, and Robert M. Henderson

1. ATOMIC FORCE MICROSCOPY

The atomic force microscope (AFM) was developed in 1986 *(1)*. Like the scanning-tunnelling microscope (STM) that preceded it, the AFM is a scanning-probe microscope. These instruments differ from "conventional" optical and electron microscopes because they work by moving a probe back and forth across a surface and recording features as the probe encounters them. Scanning-probe microscopes thus produce images that are not compromised by the limitations of the wavelengths of the various types of electromagnetic radiation. This means that very high resolution can be obtained. In some cases, studying physically hard samples down to atomic resolution, but with softer samples, the maximum resolution is at present in the order of 1 and 0.1 nm in the lateral and vertical directions, respectively. The probe of the STM is made from a conductive material and the instrument works by measuring a current — the "tunnelling current" between the probe and the sample. Thus, the STM is suitable for use only to study electrically conductive materials. The AFM, on the other hand, can be used on nonconducting specimens. As a result of the high resolution and the fact that it can be used on samples under fluid, the AFM (which was originally designed with applications in physical sciences in mind) soon attracted interest among biological scientists *(2)* as a tool for imaging cellular and subcellular structures under physiological or near-physiological conditions and to study dynamic features of molecular behavior at high resolution in "real time" under these

From: *Ion Channel Localization Methods and Protocols*
Edited by: A. Lopatin and C. G. Nichols © Humana Press Inc., Totowa, NJ

conditions. Biological work using the AFM has shown considerable growth throughout the 1990s *(3)*. As a result, partly owing to technical innovations, the realization that useful images could be obtained under fluid, together with the ready availability of microscopes from a number of manufacturers, the field has moved on and expanded far beyond that envisaged when the instrument was developed.

The AFM probe is typically made from a pyramidal crystal of silicon nitride (Si_3N_4) deposited onto a gold-coated, flexible cantilever. A sample is prepared on a flat substrate and moved so that it makes contact with the probe. The sample is then moved back and forth in a raster pattern and the probe is deflected vertically as features in the sample move under it. The movement is controlled by a series of piezoelectric drivers and the control is such that the probe can be positioned in either horizontal "x" or "y" dimensions or in the vertical "z" dimension very accurately (in the subnanometer scale). In some microscopes, especially those designed for use with biological specimens, the probe is mounted on the bottom of the piezo assembly, and is itself moved across the sample, which remains static. This means that the sample can be simultaneously observed using an inverted optical microscope and the AFM. With both configurations of the AFM, a low-powered laser is focused onto the cantilever and is reflected onto a series of photomultiplier detector elements. As a result, when the probe scans across a surface and meets some sort of obstacle, the cantilever is deflected, changing the reflected angle of the laser beam, and therefore affecting the signal detected by the photomultipliers. The photomultiplier's signals are fed into a computer, which then constructs a three-dimensional image from the information received. The principle of the AFM is therefore quite simple, and its implementation is dependent on the availability of suitable sensitive photomultipliers and piezo control mechanisms.

In constructing an image with the AFM, the probe normally has to make contact with the specimen. This means that as it moves across it can distort the sample (and thus produce misleading images) because it normally applies both vertical and lateral force. This is particularly important when using AFM on biological specimens (which are relatively soft compared with many specimens studied in the physical sciences), and it is therefore important that the force applied to the sample by the probe can be minimized. This is partly achieved by the cantilevers upon which the probes are mounted having very low spring constants. This means that as the probe moves across a sample, it can be deflected vertically by features it might encounter without the danger of the cantilever being so stiff that it sweeps away all obstacles in its path. In addition, the force can be reduced by fine adjustment of the microscope at the start of an experiment. This is achieved by means of a "force curve." To construct the force curve, the probe is held stationary (in the horizontal directions) on the substrate with the tip oscillating vertically. As the probe and substrate make contact (during the downward moving "approaching" phase of the probe), the cantilever bearing the probe is deflected, and this deflection is registered by the photomultipliers. As the probe and substrate are drawn apart (during the "withdrawal" phase) the cantilever is again deflected, returning to its original position, but often being further deflected as a consequence of the probe "sticking" to the substrate—a result of the adhesion forces (which may be chemical, electrostatic, or even magnetic) between probe and substrate. These adhesion forces are a consequence of the way in which the AFM works. By examination and by adjustment of the force curve, they can be minimized in such a way that excessive vertical forces are not applied to the sample. In addition, adhesive forces between probe and substrate are reduced considerably if imaging is conducted under fluid — a medium that is often to be preferred in biological imaging. Besides adjustment of the microscope to optimize image generation, the force curve also provides a useful measure of the degree of attraction between probe and substrate and may thus be used to distinguish different areas of the same sample if they have different physical characteristics. The AFM may be used to obtain data using various different "modes" of recording. The "conventional" use of the AFM described earlier is known as "contact mode." The probe applies constant force while it scans and the tip and piezoelectric drivers are connected via a feedback loop circuit to move the probe and substrate towards and away from each other to maintain the constant force. This leads to a representation of the height of topographical features in the image obtained ("height mode" recording). Because the feedback loop is driven by changes in cantilever deflection, it is also possible to monitor these deflection signals and use them to construct an image. This type of data collection is called "deflection mode" recording and it typically produces images in which edges of features are emphasized (which can be useful under some conditions) but gives no quantitative data on height. Contact mode recording, with either or both height and deflection images, is very effective under many circumstances, but even when vertical forces are minimized using the force curve, the application of lateral force as the probe is drawn across the surface of the sample is unavoidable and this can also distort the image produced. If the force applied is excessively high, the sample can even be damaged or perhaps pushed around the substrate by the probe, which behaves like a small snowplow. If the applied force is too low, then the probe can bounce off the sample as it moves over topographical features. These limitations can be overcome by setting the tip oscillating vertically at a high frequency while scanning normally in the x-y direction, a mode of recording known as "tapping mode." The reflected signal from the cantilever detected by the photomultipliers then describes a sine wave, the amplitude of which is altered as the probe moves over any physical feature on the surface. The tapping mode technique results in much lower lateral (and also vertical) forces being applied to the sample compared with those seen in contact mode recording and produces concomitantly clearer images with less scope for distortion of samples. Tapping mode was originally only possible on dry samples imaged in air or a vacuum, but even under these conditions the adhesive forces between a dry sample and the probe can be such that distorted images can result. To circumvent this problem, the technology has been developed that makes it possible to make tapping mode recordings under fluid *(4,5)*.

Although there are a number of different ways in which images can be obtained in AFM, they are all dependent on the types of probes used. A consideration therefore arises in choosing the type of tips on probes used in imaging experiments. Although for most purposes a tip with a conventional pyramidal profile produces good images and force information, various types of other probes with tips of different aspect ratios can be produced. Under certain circumstances, it is important to use probes that have a sharper profile, effectively tapering at a sufficiently acute angle at the tip so that they are able to penetrate small crevices in the sample. If unable to do so, fine details of the structure may be lost in the image. Various techniques have been adopted to optimize tip profiles. Probes are commercially available that have been sharpened or that have sharply tapering columns of Si_3N_4 deposited at their ends to improve resolution, but the sharper the tip, the more difficult it is to make, and this is reflected in the price. A recent development of potential importance has been the production of Si_3N_4 probes that have had carbon "nanotubes" attached to their tips *(6)*. These nanotubes are long (up to 1 μm) and thin (1–5 nm in diameter at the tip), optimizing image production by their ability to gain access to small recesses in surfaces without exerting large forces.

The possibility of scanning native biological samples under physiological conditions *(7)* opened a new field for biological and medical research and a wide range of biological samples has been studied successfully under native conditions *(8–10)*. Nevertheless, scanning of biological preparations is still challenging owing to the large height fluctuations of the sample and the high scanning forces (about 1.0 nN) applied by the AFM tip onto the sample surface. As a result, the resolution that may be achieved of soft materials, such as living cells, is rather limited.

To gain information about the arrangement of proteins in the native plasma membrane, we established some methods for scanning the plasma membrane surface with high resolution. In the first approach, we excised small plasma membrane patches (of the type used in the patch-clamp technique) and then transferred them on freshly cleaved mica coated with poly-L-lysine *(11)*. By scanning these plasma membrane patches firmly attached to mica, we avoided the problems of cell elasticity, height fluctuations, and cell motility.

2. IMAGING EXTRACELLULAR PLASMA MEMBRANE OF CULTURED KIDNEY CELLS

In this approach we attached the intracellular side of the plasma membrane to mica *(11)*. Experiments were performed on Madin Darby Canine kidney (MDCK) cells (American Type Culture Collection, No. CLL 34 ATTC, Bethesda, MD). Cells were grown on coverslips and then transferred to the stage of an inverted microscope for patch-clamp experiments. Modified Ringer solution: 140 mM NaCl, 5 mM KCl, 1 mM MgCl$_2$, 1 mM CaCl$_2$, 5 mM glucose, 10 mM HEPES, pH 7.4) was used for both patch-clamp and AFM experiments. Patch pipets were filled with KCl solution containing 140 mM KCl, 1 mM MgCl$_2$, 1 mM CaCl$_2$, 10 mM HEPES, pH 7.4.

Patch clamp experiments were performed as described by Hamill et al. *(12)*. We applied this technique for gaining a "gigaseal." Pipets, pulled from glass capillaries (ringcaps® 50 µL, Hirschmann Laborgeräte, Eberstadt, Germany; pipet puller: BB-CH, Mecanex, Genf, Switzerland), had resistances of 3–5 MΩ when filled with 140 mmol/L KCl solution. Their external tip diameter was 2–3 µm. For monitoring seal resistance, we used an arrangement consisting of a patch-clamp amplifier (EPC 7, List-Electronic, Darmstadt, Germany), an 8-pole Bessel filter (902 LPF, Frequency Devices Inc. Haverhill, MA), a pulse generator (Grass S 44 Stimulator, Grass Instruments) and an oscilloscope (HM 208, Hameg GmbH, Frankfurt, Germany). After obtaining a seal (in the range of 1–5 GΩ), the plasma membrane patch was excised in the inside-out configuration and transferred on mica. Because freshly cleaved mica offers a clean and atomically flat surface, it is a suitable substrate for AFM experiments. Sheets of freshly cleaved mica (G 250-1, Plano, Marburg, Germany) attached to double-sided tape were coated with poly-L-lysine (0.1 g/L, Serva, Heidelberg, Germany) to increase adhesion of plasma-membrane patches.

The transfer of the inside-out patches was described recently in detail *(11)*. In short, after obtaining a gigaseal, the excised plasma membrane patch located in the pipet's tip was moved out of the bath solution and lowered gently onto the coated surface of the mica, thus transferring the patch. The successful transfer was evaluated electrically by submerging the (now empty) pipet tip into the bath solution and measuring the pipet's electrical resistance. After the transfer the patches were allowed to dry but they were re-hydrated for AFM experiments.

A BioScope (Digital Instruments, Santa Barbara, CA) was used for the AFM. The BioScope was mounted onto an inverted optical microscope (Axiovert 100, Zeiss, Oberkochen, Germany), which allowed optical control of the scanning process. Scanning was performed in either contact or tapping mode. In the latter, the tip was tuned to a frequency of about 30 kHz. Both scanning modes were performed in air and in fluid. All experiments were performed using V-shaped Si_3N_4-cantilevers with integrated pyramidal tips and spring constants of 0.06 N/m (Digital Instruments). Scanning forces were in the range of several nN in contact mode, and less than 1 n*N* in tapping mode. By applying high scan forces (up to 100 n*N*) on purpose, we were able to penetrate the plasma membrane completely. These artificial defects were used to measure the exact height of the membrane patch.

For an approximate calculation of the possible molecular weight of the observed membrane proteins, we used the simplified model of a sphere embedded in the lipid bilayer assuming integral proteins penetrating the entire bilayer. This model has been described in detail elsewhere *(11)*. In short, the diameter of this sphere ($\varnothing$) was calculated by adding the height of the protein protruding from the bilayer (h) and the measured thickness of the bilayer itself: $\varnothing = h + 4.7$ nm.

Owing to the geometry of the scanning tip, the lateral dimensions of any scanned object are usually overestimated *(13)*. We assumed that the scanning tip and the membrane-embedded protein are both noncompressible spheres. Thus, the overestimation of the protein's lateral dimension and the expected width can be calculated *(11)*. Using the equation for the volume of a sphere ($V = \frac{4}{3}r^3\pi$) with the protein radius r, we can calculate the volume of a single protein V_{prot}. The molecular weight M_0 can then be calculated *(14)*:

$$M_0 = (N_0 / V_1 + d \cdot V_2) \cdot V_{prot}$$

In this equation N_0 is the Avogadro constant ($6.022 \cdot 10^{23}$ mol^{-1}), V_1 is the partial specific volume of the protein (0.74 cm^3/g), V_2 is the specific volume of water (1 cm^3/g), and d is a factor describing the extent of hydration for air-dried proteins (0.4 mol H_2O/mol protein).

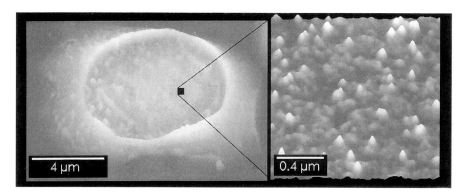

Fig. 1. Apical plasma membrane patch (extracellular side) of a MDCK cell spread on mica and imaged using AFM in air. An overview of the patch is given in the image on the left. High magnification of the plasma membrane (on the right) shows multiple proteins protruding from the lipid bilayer.

About one-third of the successfully transferred patches was found usable for further experiments. Scratches on the mica surface, caused by the patch pipet, and salt crystals in the region of contact between pipet and mica gave helpful hints when searching for the transferred patch by AFM.

A typical patch is shown in Fig. 1. The surface areas of these patches varied from 40–200 μm^3. By increasing the scanning force (up to 100 nN) in a small area near the center of the patch, an artificial defect could be produced in the membrane. Using cross-section analysis, the height of the membrane patch could be exactly determined at such spots. The thickness of the membrane averages 4.7 ± 0.06 nm ($n = 100$) matching the predicted value for a lipid bilayer. This indicates that the membrane is spread out flat on mica in this central area of the patch.

In such flat areas, a lateral and vertical resolution of 5 and 0.1 nm, respectively, can be achieved, which is an improvement compared to the resolution achievable on whole cells. At this resolution the patch surface which represents the extracellular side of the cell membrane shows multiple protrusions (= proteins). They appear with a density of about 90/μm^2, with heights (above bilayer) between 1 and 9 nm and with apparent lateral dimensions between 20 and 60 nm. Frequency distribution (500 protrusions analyzed) shows a peak for the protrusion height at about 3 nm. Patches and protrusions on the surface could be scanned for hours without any detectable damage at scanning forces in the range of 1–10 nN.

After re-hydration, the patch morphology did not change dramatically. The arrangement of the membrane proteins showed no visible changes. The heights of the bilayer and the protrusions increased slightly. The measured value for the bilayer thickness was 5.5 ± 0.08 nm ($n = 75$). A comparison of the protrusions in air and fluid showed that their heights had increased by about 0.3–0.5 nm (which represents about 5% of the total protein height). The main reason for this slight increase in height when scanned in fluid could be the reduction of the applied scanning force to less than 1 nN.

To estimate the molecular weight of these proteins we used the model of a sphere described earlier. The calculated values ranged from 50–710 kDa. The peak value of about 3 nm matches an estimated molecular weight of about 125 kDa.

Although this method allowed a reasonable resolution of the native plasma-membrane surface structure, there are still problems to be solved. As biological membranes undergo changes during drying *(15)*, we have to expect artificial changes in the membrane patch. For example, the distribution and arrangement of the different components could be altered during the drying process or the interaction between proteins and lipids could be changed and function disturbed. Although we did not detect any changes after the re-hydration of the patches, modifications of the proteins and the lipid bilayer cannot be excluded, and may occur at the molecular scale. However, drying of the patches before re-hydration was necessary for the sufficient attachment of the plasma membrane to mica.

3. IMAGING INTRACELLULAR PLASMA MEMBRANE OF CULTURED KIDNEY CELLS

In another approach, we attached the extracellular side of the plasma membrane to freshly cleaved mica. As a "membrane glue" we used iberiotoxin (IBTX), a potent blocker of calcium-activated potassium channels *(16)*. This toxin molecule carries positive net-charges and thus binds to both the negatively charged mica surface and the negatively charged extracellular domain of calcium-activated potassium channels present in the plasma membrane of MDCK cells *(17)*.

After attachment to IBTX coated mica the cell was "ripped off," leaving the inner side of the plasma membrane exposed to the bath solution. Integral or membrane-associated proteins facing the cell interior became therefore accessible for imaging with AFM. Using this "inside-out" membrane preparation, it was also possible to study native proteins undergoing structural changes when exposed to ATP. This trinucleotide is known to bind to a variety of membrane proteins and to change the structural conformation of ROMK channels *(18)*, a member of a potassium-channel family identified in kidney *(19)*. Using this approach, we identified clusters of proteins in their native environment and elicited ATP-induced changes in cluster conformation.

The crucial steps for membrane isolation have been described previously *(20)*. In short, small pieces of mica were glued on round glass coverslips with a two-component adhesive. Prior to the experiment the most upper sheet of mica was cleaved off, thereby providing an atomically flat (and absolutely clean) mica surface. Then, the freshly exposed mica surface was coated with 20 nM IBTX (Alomone Labs, Jerusalem, Israel) dissolved in cytosolic solution. The coating procedure was as follows: 20 µL of IBTX containing solution was pipetted on mica. A few minutes later the droplet was removed and the mica surface carefully washed with distilled water. The positively charged IBTX firmly bound to the negatively charged mica surface. Coating with IBTX was necessary for two reasons: first, to neutralize the negative net charges of the mica surface and second, to "glue" the plasma membrane of MDCK cells to mica via the strong interaction of the toxin with the K^+-channel. In a next step, MDCK cells grown on glass coverslips were washed with modified Ringer solution and pressed ("sandwiched") upside-down onto the IBTX-coated mica surface. Two minutes later, the glass coverslip was ripped off the mica surface. The plasma membrane usually remained attached to the IBTX-coated mica with its cytosolic side facing upwards. The membrane preparation was kept in cytosolic solution until experimentation.

First, noncoated and IBTX-coated mica surface (without attached plasma membranes) were scanned in cytosolic solution in order to show adhesion of IBTX to mica. Noncoated mica is atomically flat and a mean roughness (i.e., the mean height of all surface structures analyzed in a single AFM image) of 40 ± 0.4 pm was measured. This value reflects the natural roughness of the mica surface and "background noise." In contrast, IBTX coated mica showed multiple small protrusions assumed to be clustered IBTX molecules. Mean roughness was 99 ± 2 pm. This indicated that IBTX bound to mica. From the known molecular mass of iberiotoxin (4213 D) the volume of an individual toxin molecule could be calculated according to the equations used previously *(14)*. The calculated molecular volume of one single IBTX molecule is 5.3 nm³. Considering the measured heights and radii of visible IBTX-clusters, we estimated the number of IBTX molecules per area and thus assessed the density of IBTX-coating. We calculated a minimum of 15,000 IBTX molecules per µm². This number indicated that IBTX coating was sufficient to offer enough binding sites for the potassium channels of the plasma membrane of the MDCK cells.

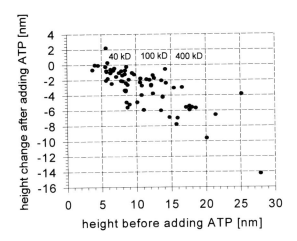

Fig. 2. Dissociation of plasma-membrane protein clusters in response to 1 m*M* ATP studied with AFM in membrane patches of MDCK cells in physiological buffer. The change in absolute height (in nm) induced by ATP is plotted as a function of absolute height (in nm) measured before ATP application.

Successfully stripped membranes were scanned and height analysis was done using the mica surface as the reference level. The extracellular side was attached to IBTX-coated mica while the cytosolic side was accessible to the AFM tip. The membrane was bathed in cytosolic solution. Proteins protruded from the inner side of the plasma membrane into the cytosolic fluid. They had mean heights of 9.6 nm ± 0.02 (n = 880). As expected for protein clusters, they were highly heterogeneous in height.

Protein clusters were sensitive to ATP. Although in the absence of ATP protein clusters exhibited rather smooth surfaces, multiple peaks appeared within minutes of ATP exposure. A first distinct decrease in height was exerted already with an ATP concentration of 300 μmol/L. This effect was most pronounced after rising ATP concentration to 1 mmol/L. The decrease in height clearly depended upon the absolute height of the protein cluster before ATP exposure. As documented in Fig. 2, there was a strong correlation between height change and absolute height: the larger (and thus higher) the protein cluster, the more pronounced the ATP-induced decrease in height. Time-course experiments revealed that the first onset of the height change occurred after 30 s of ATP addition. The process was finished after about 4 min.

The experiments show that plasma-membrane proteins (and/or membrane-associated) proteins form clusters in their natural environment. These clusters may represent specific families with a different and varying number of family members. It is rather unlikely that the clusters were artefacts caused by the membrane preparation. Membranes were kept in electrolyte solution mimicking the composition of the cytosol in order to reduce drying artefacts. Observed protein clusters most likely represent functional units (i.e., families of proteins) within the plasma membrane whose members interact with each other. However, it is at present not possible to distinguish between integral plasma-membrane proteins, membrane-associated proteins, and cytoskeletal structures associated with the membrane. Thus, the protein cluster, as detected by AFM, could be composed of several as yet unidentified molecular structures. The fact that physiological concentrations of hydrolyzable ATP led to pronounced rearrangements in cluster conformation reveals that energy is required to "organize" a protein cluster. Obviously, ATP is necessary to maintain a specific "nanoarchitecture" of a cluster to allow its adequate function. It was, at first sight, rather surprising that proteins were able to rearrange in a membrane firmly attached to mica by iberiotoxin. However, the "ATP-induced rearrangement hypothesis of membrane proteins" receives support by the view that most likely the iberiotoxin-sensitive potassium channels represent only a small portion of one individual protein cluster and thus lateral movements of the individual proteins within a cluster could occur in the nanometer range.

4. IMAGING INTRACELLULAR PLASMA MEMBRANE OF *XENOPUS LAEVIS* OOCYTE

In a third approach, we imaged the cytoplasmic side of oocyte plasma membranes. We developed a method to spread patches of oocyte plasma membrane "inside-out" on glass, rendering them suitable for AFM scanning *(21)*.

The experiments were performed on *Xenopus laevis* oocytes (stage V), which were obtained as described *(22)* and stored in Barth medium (87 mM NaCl, 1 mM KCl, 1.5 mM CaCl$_2$, 0.8 mM MgSO$_4$, 2.4 mM NaHCO$_3$, 5 mM HEPES, pH 7.4, containing 100 IU/mL penicillin and 100 μg/mL streptomycin). The oocytes were mechanically defolliculated 1 h after collagenase treatment (1 mg/mL, type D collagenase, Boehringer, Mannheim) and then incubated for 2 h in Barth medium. Removal of the vitelline membrane was performed by hypertonic shrinkage in potassium aspartate buffer (10 min; 200 mM K-aspartate, 20 mM KCl, 1 mM MgCl$_2$, 10 mM EGTA, 10 mM HEPES, pH 7.4) followed by mechanical stripping similar as previously reported *(23)*. The oocyte plasma membrane was stained with FM1-43 (0.1 μM in Barth medium; Molecular Probes, Eugene, OR) for 1 min and then rinsed with Barth medium twice.

The glass coverslips used had grids (CELLocate®; Eppendorf, Hamburg), which helped to locate an individual plasma membrane patch. The coverslips were cleaned by treatment for 1 h with concentrated $H_2SO_4/30\%$ H_2O_2 (9:1), rinsed three times with double-distilled H_2O and twice with acetone. 40 μL of an aqueous solution of poly-L-lysine (0.01% [w/v], Sigma, Deisenhofen, Germany) was applied to the clean side of each glass coverslip and removed 10 min later. Coated coverslips were then baked for 1 h at 60°C.

After removal of the vitelline membrane and staining with FM1-43, the oocyte was transiently attached to the coated glass for a minute and then removed. The plasma-membrane patch remaining on the glass surface was rinsed with H_2O, air-dried, and located by fluorescence microscopy.

AFM experiments were performed in contact mode using a Nanoscope III Multimode-AFM (Digital Instruments, Santa Barbara, CA) with an E-type scanner (maximal scan area:15 × 15 μm). Glass coverslips were attached to stainless steel discs with double-sided adhesive tape and mounted in the commercially available fluid cell (Digital Instruments) without using the o-ring. V-shaped oxide sharpened cantilevers with spring constants of 0.06 N/m were used for scanning in air. Images (512 × 512 pixels) were captured with scan areas between 1 and 25 μm^2 at a scan rate of 12 Hz (12 scan lines/s). Images were processed using the Nanoscope III software (Digital Instruments). Particle counting and 3D presentation were performed with SPIP software (Scanning probe image processor, Image Metrology, Lyngby, Denmark).

Examination of coverslips by fluorescence microscopy revealed large patches of inside-out oriented plasma membrane, areas without membrane and small regions with relatively high structures. For AFM experiments areas showing the outline of a membrane were chosen so that height of plasma membrane and proteins could be determined. Figure 3 shows the top view of a 7.5 μm^2 scan area, containing plasma-membrane fragments attached to poly-L-lysine-coated glass. White spots covering the membrane are proteins protruding into the intracellular space. The broken line in the upper part of Fig. 3 corresponds to the profile line in the lower part. Basically three different height levels could be determined: the first level is a height value of about 1.5 nm caused by poly-L-lysine coating. The second level corresponds to the 5 nm-height of the plasma membrane. The third level indicates the height of the proteins (5–15 nm) protruding from the inner surface of the plasma membrane. The same oocyte plasma membrane patch is shown in Fig. 4 as a 3D color-coded view of the three different levels. Poly-L-lysine coated glass is shown in blue, the lipid bilayer membrane is shown in turquoise, and the membrane proteins are shown in brown.

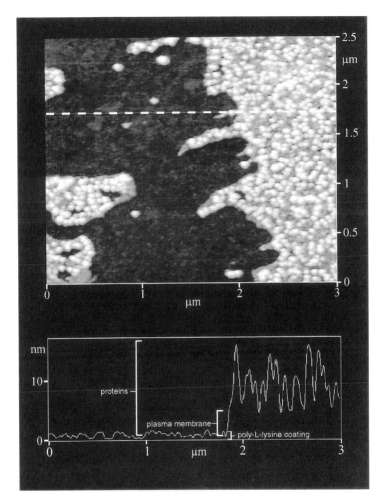

Fig. 3. Plasma membrane of *Xenopus laevis* oocyte spread on glass and studied by AFM in air. View of a membrane patch (cytosolic side) attached to poly-L-lysine coated glass. White spots covering the membrane are proteins, protruding into the intracellular space. The broken line in the upper part corresponds to the profile line in the lower part. In the lower part of the figure the first height level is about 1.5 nm caused by poly-L-lysine coating. The second level corresponds to the 5 nm-height of the lipid bilayer. The third level (bracket) indicates the height of the proteins (up to 15 nm) protruding from the inner surface of the plasma membrane.

Figure 5 shows a complex scenario indicating high plasticity of plasma membranes. The image shows lipid membrane (arrow 4) attached to the glass support (arrow 1) but lacking proteins. It further shows membrane proteins

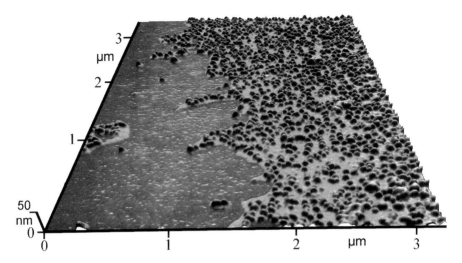

Fig. 4. Plasma membrane of *Xenopus laevis* oocyte spread on glass and studied by AFM in air. 3D color-coded view of Fig. 3. Poly-L-lysine coated glass is shown in blue, the lipid bilayer membrane is shown in turquoise, and the membrane proteins are shown in brown.

(arrow 3) firmly attached to poly-L-lysine coating (arrow 2) but lacking lipid bilayer. Such a scenario is obviously caused by incomplete poly-L-lysine coating. Membrane proteins do need coating for attachment to glass whereas lipid membrane components do not. In Fig. 5, on the left, multiple planes of bilayers in a lamellar arrangement are visible. The first plateau is a membrane of 5 nm in height (arrow 4), while the second plateau (arrow 5) represents two lipid bilayers (10 nm in height) on top of the first (total height measured from the glass support = 15 nm). A fourth phospholipid bilayer (5 nm in height; total height in ref. to glass surface = 20 nm) is visible in the image on the far left (arrow 6).

Figure 6 shows the color-coded three-dimensional image of the membrane pattern explained in Fig. 5. Black corresponds to the glass surface and blue to poly-L-lysine coating. Brown spikes are plasma-membrane proteins, turquoise indicates the first lipid bilayer, orange the next two lipid bilayers, and finally yellow corresponds to the fourth lipid bilayer on the top.

Figure 7 shows a histogram of plasma-membrane protein distribution in relation to measured protein heights and calculated molecular weights. Measurements were exclusively taken from the intracellular aspect of the plasma membrane. Molecular volumes were estimated from protein heights measured by AFM. Molecular weights were then calculated from the respective

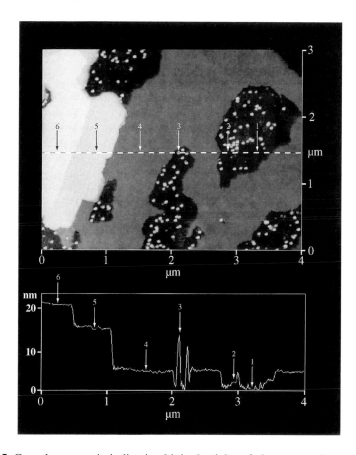

Fig. 5. Complex scenario indicating high plasticity of plasma membrane of *Xenopus laevis* oocyte spread on glass and studied by AFM in air. Lipid membrane is visible (arrow 4), attached to the glass support (arrow 1) but lacking proteins. Furthermore, the image shows membrane proteins (arrow 3) firmly attached to the poly-L-lysine coating (arrow 2) but lacking lipid bilayer. In the left part of this figure multiple planes of bilayers in a lamellar arrangement are visible. The first plateau is a membrane of 5 nm in height (arrow 4), while the second plateau (arrow 5) represents two lipid bilayers (10 nm in height) on top of the first (the total height measured from the glass support = 15 nm). A fourth phospholipid bilayer (5 nm in height; total height in ref. to glass surface = 20 nm) is visible in the image on far left (arrow 6).

volume. We found a wide range of different molecular weights. Surprisingly, we did not find cytoskeletal structures attached to the intracellular surface of the plasma membrane. We assume that binding between cytoskeletal structures and membrane proteins was disrupted during the process of membrane excision, leaving behind the membrane proteins embed-

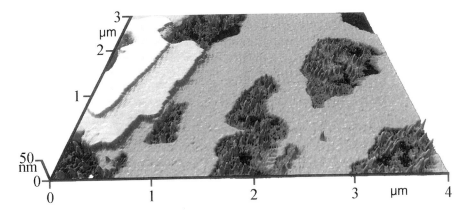

Fig. 6. Complex scenario indicating high plasticity of plasma membrane of *Xenopus laevis* oocyte spread on glass and studied by AFM in air. Color-coded three-dimensional image of the membrane pattern is explained in Fig. 5. Black corresponds to glass surface and blue to poly-L-lysine coating. Brown spikes are plasma-membrane proteins, turquoise indicates the first lipid bilayer, orange the next two lipid bilayers, and finally yellow corresponds to the fourth lipid bilayer on top.

ded in the lipid bilayer firmly attached to the coated glass surface. However, we cannot exclude the possibility that membrane proteins were pulled off the lipid bilayer mediated by firmly bound cytoskeletal structures leaving behind membrane lacking cytoskeletal bound proteins.

Most frequently we found plasma-membrane protein structures with about 10 nm for protein height (cytoplasmic domains: 5 nm in height). The proteins differed from each other in height and shape. Some were hardly detectable, others were up to 20 nm in height. Because plasma membrane height is 5 nm, we could not detect proteins smaller than 5 nm, i.e., membrane-embedded proteins. The apparent shape of the proteins was conical. This was most likely owing to the fact that lateral dimensions of the base of individual proteins were overestimated as a result of AFM-tip geometry *(11)*. Usually membrane fragmentation occurred in our experiments, which in turn was likely to be owing to an imbalance of the forces between poly-L-lysine coating, proteins, and lipid components. There are some "rules" that in general can be drawn from the images. First, membrane proteins need poly-L-lysine coating for firm attachment on glass. Second, the lipid bilayer is stable only when the protein density of the membrane is high. The pure lipid component of plasma membrane is not normally robust enough to survive scanning. Third, poly-L-lysine coating facilitates protein attachment but, at the same time, decreases the affinity for lipid membrane to stick to glass. This

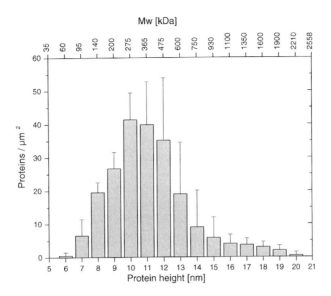

Fig. 7. Histogram of the plasma-membrane protein distribution (intracellular side) in relation to measured protein heights and calculated molecular weights. Mean values and SEM (*n* = 10) are given.

phenomenon could explain the inhomogeneous distribution of lipid membrane and membrane proteins. Another reason why membrane proteins seem necessary for stabilizing the lipid bilayer could be the hydrophobic interaction between phospholipids and the transmembrane domains of the proteins. Finally, high-protein density shields the lipid bilayer from the strong lateral scanning forces applied by the AFM-tip. We assume that the affinity of the phospholipids for uncoated glass is higher then the lipids" affinity for poly-L-lysine. This apparently results in a flow of the lipid bilayer away from proteins (attached to poly-L-lysine) towards naked glass. The hydrophobic interactions between phospholipids and proteins are usually strong enough to hold the lipids back. However, when membrane proteins occur at low density in the lipid membrane, hydrophobic interactions are rare, and thus lipids flow off.

Modelling plasma-membrane proteins as spherical structures protruding from the lipid bilayer allowed an estimation of their possible molecular weights *(11)*. Proteins ranged from 35–2000 kDa with a peak value of 280 kDa. The most frequently found protein structure (40 proteins per μm²) had a total height of 10 nm (including the intramembrane domain). This indicates an apparent lateral dimension of the cytoplasmic domain of about 40 nm (NB: lateral dimensions are usually overestimates owing to the geometry of

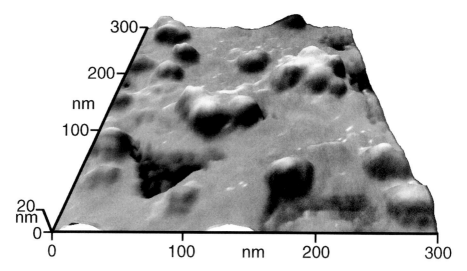

Fig. 8. Plasma membrane patch of *Xenopus laevis* oocyte imaged by AFM in air (size: 0.09 µm²). Monomeric and multimeric membrane proteins are visible (brown) in native plasma membrane (turquoise). Blue spots indicate defects in the lipid bilayer.

the AFM tip, and thus are not used for volume calculations) and an estimated molecular weight of 280 kDa.

5. CONCLUSIONS

Atomic force microscopy is a potentially valuable tool for imaging plasma membrane at the nanometre scale. Membrane proteins can be detected in their physiological environment (i.e., a lipid bilayer) at the single molecule level. The current resolution in terms of molecular mass is about 60 kDa. Using antibodies, it should in the near future be feasible to identify individual proteins. This should open the possibility of understanding the formation of protein clusters in the membrane. Currently, we can only describe proteins in the membrane in terms of molecular mass and gross substructure (Fig. 8). So far we cannot identify them and thus cannot elucidate the meaning of clusters. The major goal is therefore the identification of individual molecules using AFM.

ACKNOWLEDGMENTS

The study was supported by the "Interdisziplinäre Zentrum für Klinische Forschung," IZKF (A8&C11).

REFERENCES

1. Binnig, G. and Quate, C. F. (1986) Atomic force microscope. *Phys. Rev. Lett.* **56(9),** 930–934.
2. Hansma, P. K., Elings, V. B., Marti, O., and Bracker, C. E. (1988) Scanning tunneling microscopy and atomic force microscopy: application to biology and technology. *Science* **242,** 209–216.
3. Hansma, H. G. and Pietrasanta, L. (1998) Atomic force microscopy and other scanning probe microscopies. *Curr. Opin. Chem. Biol.* **2,** 579–584.
4. Hansma, P. K., Drake, B., Grigg, D., Prater, C. B., et al. (1994) A new, optical-lever based atomic force microscope. *J. Appl. Phys.* **76,** 796–799.
5. Putman, C. A. J., Van der Werf, K. O., De Grooth, B. G., Van Hulst, N. F., et al. (1994) Tapping mode atomic force microscopy in liquid. *App. Phys. Lett.* **64,** 2454–2456.
6. Dai H, Hafner, J. H., Rinzler, A. G., Colbert, D. T., et al. (1996) Nanotubes as nanoprobes in scanning probe microscopy. *Nature* **384,** 147–150.
7. Drake, B., Prater, C. B., Weisenhorn, A. L., Gould, S. A. C., et al. (1989) Imaging crystals, polymers, and processes in water with the atomic force microscope. *Science* **243,** 1586–1589.
8. Hoh, J. H. and Hansma, P. K. (1992) Atomic force microscopy for high-resolution imaging in cell biology. *Trends. Cell. Biol.* **2,** 208–213.
9. Shao, Z. and Yang, J. (1995) Progress in high resolution atomic force microscopy in biology. *Q. Rev. Biophys.* **28,** 195–251.
10. Henderson, R. M. and Oberleithner, H. (2000) Pushing, pulling, dragging and vibrating renal epithelia using atomic force microscopy. *Am. J. Physiol. BOED,* **278,** T689–T701.
11. Larmer, J., Schneider, S. W., Danker, T., Schwab, A., et al. (1997) Imaging excised apical plasma membrane patches of MDCK cells in physiological conditions with atomic force microscopy. *Pflügers Arch.* **434,** 254–260.
12. Hamill, O. P., Marty, A., Neher, E., Sakmann, B., et al. (1981) Improved techniques for high-resolution current recording from cell-free membrane patches. *Pflügers Arch.* **391,** 85.
13. Allen, M. J., Hud, N. V., Balooch, M., Tench, R. J., et al. (1992) Tip-radius-induced artifacts in AFM images of protamine-complexed DNA fibers. *Ultramicroscopy* **42–44,** 1095–1100.
14. Schneider, S. W., Lärmer, J., Henderson, R. M., and Oberleithner, H. (1998) Molecular weights of individual proteins correlate with molecular volumes measured by atomic force microscopy. *Pflügers Arch.* **435,** 362–367.
15. Crowe, J. H., Hoekstra, F. A., and Crowe, L. M. (1992) Anhydrobiosis. *Ann. Rev. Physiol.* **54,** 579–599.
16. Candia, S., Garcia, M. L., and Latorre, R. (1992) Mode of action of iberiotoxin, a potent blocker of the large conductance Ca^{2+}-activated K+ channel. *Biophys. J.* **63,** 583–590.
17. Schwab, A., Westphale, H.-J., Wojnowski, L., Wünsch, S., et al. (1993) Spontaneously oscillating K+ channel activity in transformed Madin-Darby canine kidney cells. *J. Clin. Invest.* **92,** 218–223.

18. Henderson, R. M., Schneider, S., Li, Q., Hornby, D., et al. (1996) Imaging ROMK1 inwardly rectifying ATP-sensitive K+ channel protein using atomic force microscopy. *Proc. Natl. Acad. Sci. USA* **93,** 8756–8760.

19. Ho, K., Nichols, C. G., Lederer, W. J., Lytton, J., et al. (1993) Cloning and expression of an inwardly rectifying ATP-regulated potassium channel. *Nature* **362,** 31–38.

20. Ehrenhoefer, U., Rakowska, A., Schneider, S. W., Schwab, A., and Oberleithner, H. (1998) Atomic force microscopy detects ATP-sensitive protein clusters in the plasma membrane of transformed MDCK cells. *Cell Biol. Intern* **21(11),** 737–746.

21. Schillers, H., Danker, T., Schnittler, H. J., and Oberleithner, H. (2000) Plasma membrane plasticity of *Xenopus laevis* oocyte imaged with atomic force microscopy. *Cell Physiol. Biochem.,* **10,** 99–107.

22. Madeja, M., Musshoff, U., Kuhlmann, D., and Speckmann, E. J. (1991) Membrane currents elicited by the epileptogenic drug pentylenetetrazole in the native oocyte of *Xenopus laevis. Brain. Res.* **553,** 27–32.

23. Choe, H. and Sackin, H. (1997) Improved preparation of Xenopus oocytes for patch-clamp recording. *Pflügers Arch.* **433,** 648–652.

23

Dynamic AFM of Patch Clamped Membranes

Kenneth Snyder, Ping C. Zhang, Frederick Sachs

1. INTRODUCTION

The investigative power of a single technique can be significantly enhanced by the simultaneous addition of a second, independent technique. This is especially true for the combination of atomic force microscopy (AFM) and patch-clamp recording for the study of biological systems because each technique has the ability to observe dynamic molecular events under physiological conditions. Merging these approaches will have direct application in examining structures in which mechanical and electrical parameters are paramount; for example, the study of mechanosensitive ion channels (MSCs), flexoelectricity (mechanical/electrical coupling), and outer-hair-cell electromotility. In addition, subtle advantages of this arrangement can be beneficial in studying related problems of membrane mechanics and voltage- and ligand-sensitive ion-channel physiology. Correlating mechanical and electrical interactions on a molecular level has only been attempted in a few instances. This chapter introduces our attempt to create a setup of standard components that allows concurrent use of both methods without limiting the practical use of either technique individually. We discuss experimental results exploiting this setup and consider the possibilities for further applications. We will begin with a review of some history of use of AFM and patch-clamp (summarized in Table 1).

2. BACKGROUND

2.1. Patch-Clamp and MSCs

Patch-clamp recording has been described as the "best biophysical technique for the study of ion channels for over 40 years" (1). In its current

From: *Ion Channel Localization Methods and Protocols*
Edited by: A. Lopatin and C. G. Nichols © Humana Press Inc., Totowa, NJ

Table 1
Summary of Patch-Clamp Scanning Force Microscope Applications

Patch-Clamp

Applications	Identification and classification of all types of ion channels based on biophysical properties
	Whole cell measurements allow clarification of the relative importance and physiological role of a specific type of ion channel in a given cell type.
	Capacitance measurements yield current density and assessment of endocytotic and exocytotic activity
	Instantaneous manipulation of membrane voltage or current.
Limitations	The number of channels in a patch or whole cell is not known.
	Response time of pressure pulses is limited.
	Local variation of membrane tension during pressure steps is unknown.
	Natural membrane structure is altered during patch formation.
	Lack of consistent sealing protocols might cause variability in biophysical parameters.
	Mechanical properties estimated using micropipet aspiration are confounded by the mechanics of patch adhesion.

AFM

Applications	High-resolution topographic images of biological samples (membranes and proteins). Images of ion channels yield important substructure (subunits, pore diameter, binding sites).
	Dynamic observation (directly image conformational changes).
	Ability to apply small forces and make elasticity measurements.
	Ability to chemically modify the tip and make images or force spectroscopy.
	Use as a nanotool to cut, push, or pull in a controlled way.
Limitations	Low lateral resolution when imaging unsupported biological samples.
	Difficulty locating object of interest within bilayers or on cell surface.
	Undefined contact area between tip and sample (pressure) when doing elasticity measurements. Can be overcome by using linker molecules of known stiffness to pull on supported membranes.
	Limited understanding of tip sample interactions.

context, the term "patch-clamp" refers to using micropipets to record electrophysiological properties in either voltage-clamp or current-clamp mode with a tight seal between the pipette and the membrane. In voltage-clamp

Table 1 (cont.)
Summary of Patch-Clamp Scanning Force Microscope Applications

AFM/Patch-Clamp	
Applications	Use of micropipet as support for imaging of biological membranes.
	Comparison of independent measures of channel density and surface area (electrical and topographic estimates).
	Correlation of dynamic topological detail of ion channels with ionic currents (i.e., correlate conductance with number of subunits, pore size, conformational changes, and binding events).
	Use of patch-clamp to identify channels of interest for AFM imaging.
	Clarification of patch morphology by imaging substructure on inner or outer membranes of patch.
	Tool of choice for the study of mechanoelectric transduction (i.e., application of force directly to MSC while monitoring channel conductance).
	Tool of choice for studying electromechanical transduction (i.e., flexoelectricity, OHC electromotility)
	Estimates of membrane mechanics using well-defined probe sample adhesion points (especially if using linkers to specific proteins in the membrane).

mode, the experimenter sets the voltage across the membrane while recording the ionic current necessary to maintain that voltage. Alternatively, transmembrane current can be manipulated while monitoring the membrane potential (current-clamp mode). This latter mode mimics the physiological response of a cell. The size of the membrane "patch" can range from an isolated patch (single-channel recording) to an entire cell membrane (whole-cell recording). The whole-cell configuration provides the average response of all channels in a cell, whereas single-channel recordings can report the individual behavior of a few channels. Clearly, the relative importance and physiological role of a given ion channel in a specific cell type can subsequently be assessed by identifying its contribution to whole-cell currents. Although the actual number of ion channels in a given recording (whole-cell or single-channel) is not known, estimates can be made using stochastic analysis *(2)*. Patch-clamp recording offers flexibility in experimental design with the ability to concurrently perfuse cells (extracellularly or intracellularly) with pharmacological probes or solutions of varying composition as well as applying pressure (tension) pulses via the micropipet holder. Using these methods, it has been possible to measure the biophysical properties of ion channels (conductance, voltage/concentration/tension-dependence, ion selectivity, kinetics, and pharmacological profile). Dynamic parameters are obtained by measuring properties over time (i.e., latency of channel opening/closure, adaptation, inactivation, and desensitization). Free software exists to invert the Markov series of data points to the best fitting state model with the appropriate molecular rate constants (www.qub.buffalo.edu). Additionally, by normalizing with respect to cell membrane capacitance (which is indicative of plasma membrane surface area), we can calculate current density as well as exocytotic and endocytotic activity (3,4). Furthermore, by using molecular biological techniques, we can estimate the importance of specific residues or regions of the protein. Hence, patch-clamp recording has been directly responsible for clarifying gating mechanisms and characterization of all types of ion channels (voltage-, ligand-, mechano-gated).

The investigation of time-dependent ion channel properties relies, in general, on the ability to deliver an instantaneous stimulation pulse in order to resolve fast events. Many of the fine details of the dynamics of voltage gated channels have been clarified because that the patch-clamp is capable of applying voltage pulses with submicrosecond rise times. Similar progress has been achieved with ligand-gated channels using high-speed solution exchange systems (5–7). However, the application of fast-pressure steps during patch-clamp recording is more problematic because the rise time for pressure pulses is limited to ~1 ms (8) and cytoskeletal viscosity will resist rapid changes in dimensions.

Some of the motivation for doing combined AFM and patch-clamp comes from our interest in MSCs. These ubiquitous channels are found in all cell types from prokaryotes to humans (reviewed in refs. 9–12). They function as transducers, converting cortical membrane tension into an ionic signal (12,13). Although the tension needed to open a MSC might be transmitted by the bilayer alone (14), other components such as the cortical cytoskeleton or extracellular matrix may also be functionally linked to the channels. There are a variety of MSCs with different gating properties (some are stretch-activated while others are stretch-inactivated) and selectivity (nonselective, cation selective, K^+-selective, and Cl^- selective) (12). Although MSCs have been activated by osmotic swelling of the cell, the most direct method is to apply pressure to the suction port of the pipet holder (15–17). The analysis of MSCs in natural membranes is confounded by the fact that tension in the various heterogeneous elements of the cortex is not directly measurable. Currently, mean tension is calculated by estimating membrane curvature from high-resolution images of a membrane patch (18). Although, this method provides an approximation of the mean tension in the membrane, it fails to clarify the local tension sensed by the channel.

Each patch-clamp recording begins with the use of suction to produce a high resistance seal between a biological membrane and the micropipet. It is worth noting that *(1)* little information is available about the mechanism of seal formation and *(2)* sealing protocols alter membrane substructure (i.e., cytoskeletal attachments) which in turn may modify channel properties. Comparison of whole-cell, outside-out, inside-out, cell-attached, and whole-cell patch-clamp configurations have shown inconsistencies (especially for MSCs) *(19–22)*.

Pressure pulses used to assess membrane mechanics (micropipet aspiration) alter the amount of membrane in the pipet *(18,23)*. These measurements generally serve as qualitative measures of the material properties because membranes are not homogeneous. In tight seals, the boundary condition of adhesion of membrane to the pipet wall adds to apparent stiffness of the membrane *(24)*.

2.2. Atomic Force Microscopy

In 1989, Drake et al. *(25)* used the AFM to resolve surface features of nonbiological samples under a variety of conditions, including buffer solutions. This demonstrated that the AFM might be used to image biological samples under physiological conditions. Since then a great deal of effort has gone into optimizing the AFM for use in the biological sciences, focusing mainly on increasing image resolution while decreasing sample damage *(26,27)*. High-resolution images have been obtained from a variety of biological samples including: artificial lipid bilayers *(28)*, isolated secretory vesicles *(29)* and intact cell membranes *(30–35)*. Images have also been obtained from DNA *(36,37)*, isolated proteins *(33,38)* and ion channels (reviewed in refs. *39,40*) including gap junctions *(41–44)*, acetylcholine receptors *(39)* and nuclear pores *(45–49)*.

AFM is basically a tool for measuring surface profiles. A sharp tip at the end of a microfabricated cantilever is drawn over the sample while the height of the tip is recorded with Angstrom precision. By scanning the tip over the sample in a raster, a three-dimensional image can be generated. There are two recording modes: constant force, in which the deflection of the cantilever is held constant; and constant height, in which interaction forces modulate the height of the cantilever. Another imaging modality is tapping mode *(27,50)* in which the tip is oscillated and may only touch the sample briefly at the bottom of each swing. In this mode, lateral traction forces are avoided at the expense of reduced the lateral resolution.

It is important to note that AFM images contain mixed topographic and elasticity information about the sample. This information must be independently separated by either comparing AFM images with those obtained by another imaging techniques (i.e., SEM), by fixing the sample or by doing force/distance experiments at each imaging point in order to measure local elasticity. Fine positioning of the cantilever relative to the sample is usually accomplished with a piezoelectric device, and cantilever deflection is most commonly detected using a reflected laser beam and photodetector (optical lever).

Because cantilever deflections are produced by local interaction forces between the tip and sample (i.e., van der Waals forces, hydrophobic interactions, hydration forces), experimental conditions play a major role in image resolution. A problem of interpreting AFM images is the limited understanding of what factors affect the interaction between the tip and the sample *(51)*. Even in tapping mode, the mechanism(s) of image generation and their interpretation are only partially understood owing to the complexity of the adhesive and viscous interaction between the oscillating AFM tip and the specimen *(52)*.

The lateral resolution in AFM images depends on the intrinsic rigidity of the sample, the size and shape of the AFM tip, and the depth of compression and lateral drag on the sample during imaging. Because, most biological samples are soft, softer than the cantilevers *(53)*, images of unsupported samples usually have poor lateral resolution. Also, higher resolution images require a smaller contact areas (sharper tips), creating higher pressures that deform the sample under study. Various methods have been employed for increasing sample rigidity including adsorption of the sample on mica, making 2D crystals and covalent immobilization. Using these techniques, image resolution has been improved to 1–2 nm laterally and 1–2 Å vertically *(54–57)*. Shao and co-workers have imaged bacterial toxins such as cholera and pertussis toxin B oligomers revealing a pentameric structure with a 1 nm central opening *(58)*. Czajkowsky and Shao (1998) *(59)* have packed α-hemolysin onto a supported lipid bilayer and produced images at 1 nm lateral resolution that revealed a hexameric structure. This level of topographic detail can be used to clarify the number of subunits in a specific ion channel, the size of channel pore, and location of binding sites. By optimizing electrolytes and recording conditions, they imaged the surfaces of bacteriorhodopsin molecules with 0.5 nm lateral resolution. Loops that connect the α helices as well as certain lipid head groups were resolved. As with all microscopies, contrast agents are useful for obtaining high resolution data. Chemically modifying cantilevers and labeling cells with identifiable objects is an area of intense study *(60)*.

The most exciting applications of AFM in biology take advantage of its ability to work dynamically under water *(27,35,40,61,62)*. It is possible to observe time-dependent changes in the inner surface of the hexagonally packed intermediate (HPI) layer from the cell envelope of *Deinococcus radioduras (63)* and conformational changes of the bacterial porin OmpF induced by pH changes and electric fields *(55,56)*.

In addition to imaging surfaces, the AFM can measure and manipulate local mechanical properties. The AFM tip has been used as a nanotool to cut chromosomes *(64)*, disrupt protein complexes in a controlled fashion *(65)*, and induce reversible conformational changes of single loops of purple membranes *(66)*. It has been used to mechanically stimulate cells *(62,67,68)* as well as make time-resolved one-dimensional elasticity measurements of single molecules *(53,69–71)*. For these latter studies, molecules are attached to the cantilevers and substrates by adsorption or specific chemical reactions. Making compliance measurements using force spectroscopy of single molecules removes the need to estimate the contact area between the AFM tip and the sample.

2.3. AFM/Patch-Clamp

AFM and patch-clamp have been used either sequentially or simultaneously. The sequential approach has the advantage that the probability of success with separate measurements is higher and discrete off-the-shelf components are available. No commercial system is available that readily allows for simultaneous AFM/patch-clamp measurements. The major disadvantage of the sequential analysis is the loss of time-correlated information. Although there are few experiments utilizing simultaneous recording, we feel that this approach will prove to be the most powerful.

The first combined AFM/patch-clamp was developed by Haberle et al. in 1991. Although no electrical recordings were made, they used a micropipet to support living cells for AFM imaging and achieved the first images of biological membranes with a lateral resolution less than 100 nm. By modifying their AFM cantilever detection system from a scanning tunneling microscope (STM) to an optical lever, the same group *(31)* was able to achieve images with a lateral resolution better than 20 nm. The authors predicted the use of the new setup for observation of immune reactions, the formation of cell pores, and endo- and exocytosis.

In 1994, Oberleithner et al. *(45)* applied sequential AFM and patch-clamp recording to quantify the number of nuclear pore complexes (NPCs) in Madin-Darby canine kidney (MDCK) nuclei. They used the AFM images to estimate surface area and NPC density and showed the surface area estimates were similar to results obtained using DIC microscopy. (It would have been informative if they had also used membrane capacitance as an estimator of area.) They concluded that the increase in nuclear conductance associated with application of aldosterone was owing to an increase in NPC density while the biophysical properties of individual NPCs remained unchanged. To resolve a discrepancy between estimates of channel diameter from conductance measurements (~11 nm) and AFM images, which showed pore sizes of 40–50 nm, it was postulated that either a major portion of the central channel was electrically blocked, or that these channels were undergoing dynamic conformational changes.

Bustamante et al. *(72)* was the next group to use patch-clamp and AFM imaging capabilities in series to study NPCs. They hoped to clarify details of TATA-binding protein (TBP) association with the NPC. A transient reduction of NPC single-channel conductance with TBP was hypothesized to be associated with the translocation of TBP. AFM images of the NPC pore did not display a prominent plug, which agreed with this interpretation. Patch-clamp recordings identified an increased open probability and slight increase in conductance with administration of TBP. In analogous AFM studies, the timing of binding events of the TBP molecule to the outer rim of the pore on the cytoplasmic agreed with the timing from patch-clamp observations of TBP binding. Thus, it was concluded that TBP molecules bound to the cytosolic side of NPCs, conferring an increased mean conductance and stability to the channel. A correlation between binding events, changes in pore size, and conductance changes was not possible, either because the TBP binding events interfered with topographic images or the conductance changes corresponded to diameter changes which were beyond the resolving capability of the microscope. Although these experiments illustrate the advantage of combining AFM and patch-clamp, the conclusions would have been more significant if the events were monitored simultaneously.

In 1995, Horber et al. *(73)* extended their previous work *(31)* by imaging extracellular and cytoplasmic sides of excised membrane patches with the AFM. A common feature seen on all membrane patches were fibers, believed to be cytoskeletal structures, extending from the glass pipette toward the center of the patch. By imaging broken patches they attempted to address how membranes form high resistance "gigaseals" with the glass of the pipette. The images showed fibers still fixed to the rim together with an aggregation of globular structures of up to 100 nm in size. In addition to these observations, they presented preliminary work on the mechanical properties of inside-out patches. When a negative pressure (25 mbar) was applied to the inside of the pipet, AFM images showed that only the central part of a patch moved up the pipette. They estimated membrane stiffness using micropipette aspiration and compared their results with AFM elasticity measurements on a whole cell *(74)*, and found aspiration estimates to be about 30 times stiffer. They concluded that because AFM can apply forces very locally, the deformation depth is correlated in a different way to the applied force than with aspiration. Patches have a disrupted cytoskeleton *(75–77)*. Thus, with micropipette aspiration more of the membrane-glass attachment is involved and this may lead to higher stiffness values. It should be noted that coating the pipette with bovine serum albumin (BSA) prior to aspiration experiments could reduce this problem. Horber et al. conclude by discussing initial experiments with MSCs of oocyte membranes in which the probability of opening could be influenced by pressure applied through the pipet or force applied with the cantilever (although no data is shown for the force application by the AFM). The nonuniform curvature produced by suction on outside-out patches was not be expected from images of cell-attached or inside-out patches *(18,78)*. Horber et al. *(79)* predicted that it should be possible to use this approach to activate single MSCs (while simultaneously verifying this with membrane current measurements) and further suggested that this technique will ultimately allow an estimate of the force needed to gate a single MSC. This work highlights the potential benefits of the simultaneous approach.

Mosbacher et al. *(80)* and Horber et al. *(24)* repeated the aforementioned experiments showing that suction pressure caused reversible indentations in the center of outside out patches. They also suggested using AFM rather than optical microscopy to image patch shapes for estimating mean tension. (The dimensions of outside-out patches are not observable in the optical microscope because of diffraction by the pipette tip). Both groups briefly described experiments in which voltage pulses (± 100 mV for 1 or 2 s) applied to a membrane vesicle held by a patch pipette produced movement of the membrane visible by the AFM. These movements were detected only in the center of the membrane indicating that only the most elastic part of the vesicle could react to the voltage steps. They suggested that measurement of such voltage-dependent movements might be useful for studying voltage gated ion channels.

In 1997, Larmer et al. *(81)* used the patch-clamp to isolate a section of membrane for AFM imaging. However, no channel activity was recorded. They simply hoped to gain information about the arrangement and distribution of proteins within the plasma membrane. To minimize problems of cell and membrane elasticity affecting the images, the patch was transferred from the pipet to freshly cleaved mica coated with poly-L-lysine. The sample was allowed to dry for a period of time and then rehydrated before imaging. The surface areas of these patches varied from 40 to 200 μm^2. These surprisingly large areas were justified by referencing the large "Ω"-shaped DIC images of cell-attached patches *(18)*. The authors observed bumps they interpreted as protein clusters as well as single proteins, but none of the proteins could be identified. They suggested further experiments using specific markers (i.e., antibodies) to aid protein identification. Inferring native structures from such abused membranes *(82)* is subject to significant errors, but the group was unsuccessful in obtaining adequate adhesion to the mica without drying.

Danker et al. *(83)*, expanded upon Larmer et al.'s *(81)* approach to NPCs by using patch-clamp recording to select membrane patches of special interest for further investigation with the AFM. They extended the technique by attempting to find out if the native structure of the nuclear membrane was preserved in membrane patches. From electrophysiological data *(45,72)*, NPCs are expected to have a large conductance and a single patch should contain 10–100 NPCs. Thus, one would not expect patches of the nuclear membrane to form "gigaseals." Nonetheless, they are frequently observed. This suggests that either NPCs are not present or else they are shut. The limiting factor in this study was the extensive time needed to find a transferred membrane patch with the AFM. The AFM images suggested that a "complete" NE was included in the patch and that this configuration correlates with the appearance of typical electrical signals from the nuclear envelope *(84)*. Although NPC structure was not preserved in a way that allowed measuring NPC density, the finding of NPCs in the patch supports the hypothesis that they could be the source of the patch-clamp currents *(72)*. The authors observed different membrane configurations in different samples. If these were not owing to drying the membrane as part of the transfer protocol but indeed occurred at the tip of the patch pipet, it could help to explain conflicting results from electrophysiological recordings. Again, this illustrates the utility of dual AFM/patch recording.

In 1998, Mosbacher et al. *(85)* attempted a careful analysis of the voltage-dependent movement observed previously *(73,80)*. Intact cells were used in these experiments, taking advantage of the additional support provided by the cytoskeleton. Voltage-dependent movement was identified in both control cells (HEK293), as well as cells transfected with *Shaker* K$^+$ channels. Results indicated a linear dependence of the movement on the carrier voltage amplitude, ~0.4 nm/mV, over the range of ± 50 mV (as far as was examined), and an inverse relationship between membrane conductance and movement (arguing against electro-osmotic fluxes as the source of movement). Because the movement was unexpected, the investigators did many control experiments looking for artifactual origins of the movement. No voltage dependent movement was detected when: (a) the voltage was turned off; (b) the AFM tip was moved away from contact with the membrane; (c) the cantilever touched the glass tip of an open patch pipette; (d) the cantilever was placed in front of an open pipette; or (e) the cantilever was placed in direct contact with the silver wire electrode. Similar voltage dependence was observed using cantilevers with different spring constants suggesting a source compliance lower than the cantilevers. For control cells, there was no significant correlation between the holding potential and the amplitude of the movement. However, when the cells were transfected with a noninactivating mutant of the *Shaker* K^+ channel, there was an inverse relationship between the holding potential and the size of the modulated movement. Interestingly, after 30-s depolarizations, the voltage-induced movement of transfected cells only reappeared when we held the cell for several minutes at -80 mV. Mosbacher et al. suggested the converse flexoelectric effect *(86–88)* as the motive source. Flexoelectricity is the coupling of surface charge density (or polarization) with bending (Fig. 1) *(89,90)*. It is perhaps significant that Todorov et al. have observed a flexoelectric sensitivity in bilayers similar to what was observed here, ~2 nm/mV. The flexoelectric sensitivity of transfected cells may have increased and showed a dependence on the holding potential because of the large saturating dipole moment of the *Shaker* channels. The slow inactivating response to continued depolarization could have been a result of the substantial ionic current flow causing K^+ efflux and shrinkage of the cell, pulling the cell surface away from the cantilever. It was estimated that observed K^+ currents could shrink the cell diameter by ~200 nm in 20 s. Mosbacher et al. predicted that the influence of such currents might be removed using K^+ channel blockers, nonconducting mutants, or by varying the command pulse duration to minimize flux in favor of gating movements. Additionally, because AFM cantilever deflections can be caused by topography changes as well as from stiffness changes, these results could just as easily have been owing to changes in membrane stiffness caused by alterations of the transmembrane field. Flexoelectric movements are a new source of contrast for imaging membranes.

Recently, Iwamoto et al. *(91)* used AFM and patch-clamp in parallel to estimate the subunit stoichiometry in the VacA toxin, believed to form a Cl^- channel. Patch-clamp data suggested that the channel is most likely a hexamer. AFM data shows a central hexagonal ring surrounded by six peripheral domains. Although neither experiment is conclusive on its own, but taken together they strongly suggest a hexameric structure.

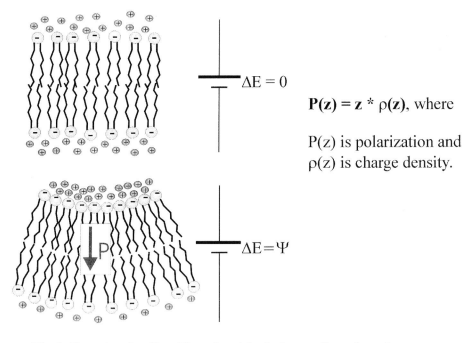

$$P(z) = z * \rho(z), \text{ where}$$

P(z) is polarization and
$\rho(z)$ is charge density.

Fig. 1. Flexoelectric effect. Flexoelectricity is the coupling of membrane curvature with the electric field.

Most recently, Bett and Sachs *(92)* used the flat surface of an AFM cantilever to squeeze cells while simultaneously recording whole-cell currents. A step displacement elicited a current that activated rapidly and then inactivated. Although the position of the stimulus probe was accurately known, the compliance of the cell wasn't measured making it difficult to determine whether the inactivating current was owing to adaptation of membrane tension (i.e., by cytoskeletal reorientation) or perhaps decreased stimulus force owing to a plastic change in cell height. Using cytoskeletal reagents and a complete AFM setup to monitor application force over time will clarify this issue. This chapter illustrates that it is possible to mechanically stimulate a cell using an AFM and simultaneously record whole-cell currents.

A summary of potential AFM/patch applications is listed in Table 1.

3. EXPERIMENTAL SETUP

We have developed a patch-clamp AFM that requires minimal modifications to commercially available products, allows independent use of either technique, and is readily customized. Two approaches have been used for simultaneous AFM/Patch recordings. The first, used by Haberle et al. *(30)*, Horber et al. *(31,73)*, and Mosbacher et al. *(80,85)*, consisted of a fixed probe and a scanned sample. The micropipette was mounted on a piezo positioner, and after a patch was formed, the pipette (the sample) was moved in a raster. This arrangement requires extra shielding of the patch pipette from the high voltages applied to the piezo, a rigid coupling between the piezo and pipette holder, and it limits the use of the AFM to samples that can be held by a micropipette (also limiting the area of membrane than can be imaged). The other arrangement was developed by Langer et al. *(93)*. In this approach, the piezo moved the cantilever while the pipette remained fixed on a micromanipulator. This setup was built into an upright microscope and required design of a special sample chamber. An inverted microscope is better suited for AFM/patch-clamp because of clearance above the sample for placement of pipettes and a perfusion system. Both of these setups used custom designed AFM hardware, electronics, and software.

We chose to purchase an inexpensive commercial AFM (Nomad™, Quesant Instrument Corp., Agoura Hills, CA 91301; www.quesant.com) that came with extensive software and source codes, schematics and outputs of key low-level signals. The Nomad is portable so the tip is scanned relative to the sample. Our major alteration to the scope mechanics was a redesign of the aqueous immersion scanhead. We created clearance for the patch pipette and replaced the corrosion-prone metal components with a glass-coated acrylic immersion cone *(94)*. With this arrangement, the cantilever is held in place using a small amount of adhesive (Kwick-Cast™, World Precision Instruments, Sarasota, FL 34240, www.wpiinc.com). This biocompatible silicone elastomer cures in 5 min, allowing sufficient time for adjustment of the tip position and can be peeled off the scanhead surface using a small amount of ethanol (note that the front of our scanhead is protected by glass so the ethanol is never directly in contact with the acrylic). We also replaced one of the coarse positioning micrometers with a microstepping lead screw (New Focus, Inc., Santa Clara, CA 94041; www.newfocus.com) to allow higher resolution Z positioning.

Quesant's customization package allows the user to manipulate the instrument via external inputs, record the outputs and modify the source codes, most of which are in Visual Basic. The Nomad has a coaxial optical path so that the AFM's descanning optics can also serve as a condenser with an NA = 0.1 (Fig. 2) and can utilize the normal light source of an inverted microscope. We have added a set of relay lenses to the illumination path to improve phase-contrast imaging, although in practice there is sufficient contrast without these lenses (Fig. 2). High-resolution transmitted-light imag-

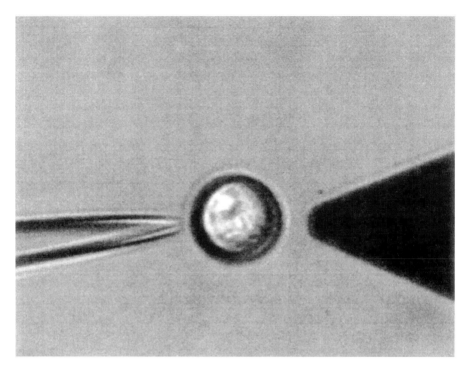

Fig. 2. Image through AFM lens system. Illustration of image quality using 20×
objective and AFM lens system as microscope condensor. Picture shows AFM cantilever (right), micropipet (left), and HEK293 cell. Micropipet tip is ~2 microns in
diameter.

ing is not important because the cantilever always covers the region of interest. Placing a green filter between the objective and the eyepiece allows
visualization of the AFM laser spot on the cantilever without being too
bright. Once the laser is focussed on the tip, we switch to a blue filter that
blocks all the laser reflections to improve video recording. A narrow band
filter can be placed in front to the photodetector to minimize interference
from room lights and the microscope illumination, although we have not
found this to be necessary in practice.

The key to any AFM setup is mechanical stability. It is important to support the entire apparatus on a vibration isolation table to reduce low-frequency vibrations (1–100 Hz). If you are not working on the basement/
ground floor, you may also consider suspending a rigid table from the ceiling with bungee cords that will provide inexpensive vertical and horizontal
isolation. Acoustical vibrations are the other primary source of parasitic
noise, and it is useful to purchase or build a sound-proof enclosure. The

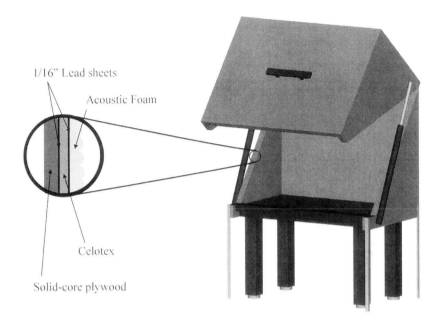

Fig. 3. Acoustic box design. The box surrounds the vibration isolation table. There is a small gap between the air table and the acoustic foam, allowing the table to float freely. The base of the box can be sealed below the air table for complete acoustic isolation. The gas cylinders must be oriented in this manner to allow easy opening and closure of the box. A 4" piano hinge runs along the upper back edge of the box. Two small holes were cut in the box for the fiber-optic cables and wires. Lead sheeting was flapped over the holes and sealed with liquid foam.

enclosure simplifies operation during normal working hours as well as removing air currents that cause low-frequency drift. Commercial acoustic shrouds are expensive so we built our own (Fig. 3).

We made a five-sided plywood box that surrounds our air table, but stands on its own feet. The top and front open up away from the user. We used gas cylinder trunk lifts (NAPA Auto Parts, www.napaonline.com) to support the top and make opening and closing the top gentle despite the weight, ~500 lbs. The box consists of 5 layers (outside to inside): 1" solid-core plywood, 1/16" lead sheeting (McMaster-Carr, Cleveland, OH 44101-4930, www.mcmaster.com) Celotex acoustical ceiling tiles, 1/16" lead, and acoustic foam (McMaster-Carr, Cleveland, OH 44101-4930, www.mcmaster.com). Grounding the lead provides a Faraday cage. To further minimize mechanical noise, it is important to stabilize all mechanical components coupled to the AFM. The wing plates that hold the patch-pipette manipulator must be rigidly mounted to the body of the microscope. Because the micropipette will be connected to the sample, the holder must be short and stiff *(95)*. We use ½" long micropipettes. If a standard pipette holder is used, we suggest thick rubber gaskets to stabilize the micropipettes for drift and movement with pressure/suction pulses. We prefer the capillary-coupled KCl pipette holder (ALA Scientific Instruments, Westbury, NY, www.alascience.com *[96]*). The goal of placing the manipulator relative to the AFM is to have the cantilever and pipette opposite one another, reducing the risk of breaking pipette tips and allowing maximum mobility of either apparatus throughout the field of view.

The AFM, micropipette, and sample must be capable of independent movement and we have used two different methods. In the first method (Fig. 4, setup 1), we built a ½" thick aluminum bridge that spans the body of the microscope. The micrometer feet of the AFM fit into holes in the bridge to secure it in place. These holes (a cone, a plane, and a groove) are kinematically arranged to prevent rotation of the base with rotation of the lead screws while avoiding resting strain (Fig. 4). The bridge is actually a sliding stage coupled to the microscope via vacuum grease so that the AFM axis can be translated relative to the optical microscope stage. The sample (cover slip) is translated or rotated on a commercial gliding stage (Nikon, Melville, NY 11747-3064, www.nikon.com).

The second arrangement (Fig. 4, setup 2) replaces the gliding bridge with a separate x-y manipulator that translates the base of the AFM. Both arrangements allow simple positioning with minimal machine work. It is important that the micropipette manipulator has low drift and allows remote control enabling work with a closed shroud. We use an MP-285 micromanipulator (Sutter Instrument Co., Novato, CA 94949; www.sutter.com) that provides the additional benefit of programmable paths that permit placing the micropipette under the cantilever without breaking the tip.

A good method for measuring system stability is to collect AFM tip height data from a single point for 2–3 min while operating the patch-clamp. We do checks when the AFM probe is in contact with the bottom of the sample chamber (a cover slip) and freely suspended. The standard deviation from a Gaussian curve fit to the histogram of z heights gives the rms noise (in our setup, the mechanical noise is below 3 Å). Additionally, while the AFM is scanning the surface of a cell or patch, the patch-clamp noise should be monitored. By using a common ground for the patch-clamp and AFM, the patch-clamp noise is ~600 fA in a 3kHz bandwidth. This noise is higher than a standard patch recording because the shallow angle of approach places more of the pipette under water increasing its capacitance.

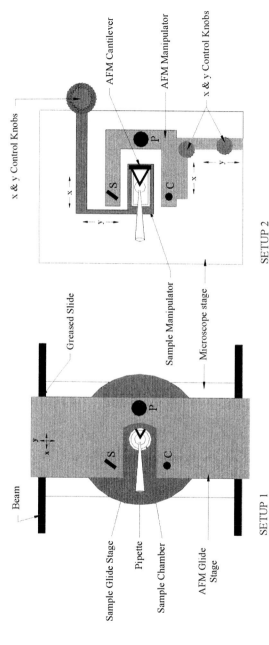

Fig. 4. AFM glide stage and mechanical stage. In SETUP 1, the AFM glide stage translates along a pair of aluminum beams connected to the base of the microscope. In SETUP 2, the sample and AFM stages are translated independently with mechanical controls. After positioning the sample, the manipulator is moved out of contact with the sample chamber, eliminating the effect of drift of the translation stage. Magnets are used to hold the AFM stage and sample chamber in contact with the microscope stage. S, P, and C represent the slot, plane, and cone holes of the kinematic mount for the AFM.

To optically visualize the sample with the acoustic enclosure shut, we use an inexpensive (~$50) PCI frame grabber (Hauppauge Co., Hauppauge, NY 11788; www.hauppauge.com) connected to a CCD camera on the video port. Hauppauge software allows us to view the image on the computer monitor. We prefer LCD monitors to eliminate electrical noise from the flyback transformer. With this arrangement, we can simultaneously record AFM and light microscopy images (transmitted and/or epifluorescence) directly to the hard disk or to sVHS videotape. The pipette can also be visually repositioned with the acoustic enclosure shut. In order to achieve similar control of the AFM, we designed a Visual Basic Form that allows mouse movements to position the AFM tip in x-y (available on our web site, www.sachslab.buffalo.edu). The form records the x-y position so that the experimenter can keep track of the locations where force-distance or other one-dimensional measurements were made.

With the shroud closed, the temperature inside the box tends to increase owing to the halogen and mercury light sources. This is a problem for stable AFM operation so we moved both lamp housings outside the box and use fiberoptics, either 1-mm quartz or 3-mm liquid-filled light guides (Oriel, Stratford, Ct, www.oreil.com), to supply light to the microscope. Figure 5 shows the inverted microscope adapted with a fiber-optic input for transmitted light. This is a true-to-scale representation of SETUP1, illustrating the amount of room between the collecting lens on the inverted microscope and the top of the AFM. Setup 2 offers even more room because we eliminated the thick AFM glide stage. Figure 5 also shows other system modifications.

It is possible to use the unmodified Quesant software and manually control the patch-clamp. Alternatively, Quesant's customization package adds 3 additional DACs and ADCs that can control the AFM and patch-clamp. We use a third method, accessing the AFM's electronics with a data acquisition board (PCI MIO 16 E, National Instruments, Inc., Austin, TX, 78759-3504; www.ni.com) using LabVIEW™ (National Instruments, Inc.), a graphical programming environment for data acquisition. Our VI's (Virtual Instument software) are available on our web page, www.sachslab.buffalo.edu. The VIs control every aspect of our setup, including the patch-clamp, AFM, pressure clamp, and perfusion system. The interface allows the user to select voltage protocols to send to the patch pipette while simultaneously monitoring the AFM photodetector outputs or, alternatively, sending waveforms to drive the AFM probe in x, y, or z while monitoring pipette current. A modulating z input can also be used for force application, elasticity measurements, or tapping-mode imaging. AFM image data is recorded using Quesant's software and can be exported in many different formats.

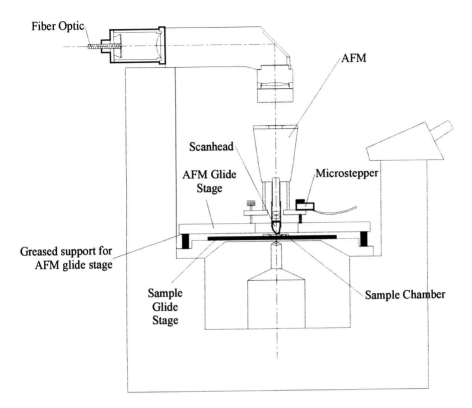

Fig. 5. Placement of the AFM in the optical axis of the inverted microscope. Modifications to the system are highlighted in bold (scanhead, microstepper, and mounting for the fiber optic).

It is important to visually observe cells while scanning, especially when the cells are not flat, because the compliance of the cell is higher than the cantilever and the cell can be observed to move visually when there is little output from the photodetector. We use the softest cantilevers available, the 0.01 *N*/m from ThermoMicroscopes (the old Park Instruments; Sunnyvale, CA 94089; info@thermomicro.com) to allow us to minimally perturb the sample.

To further minimize the force, we designed and built new cantilevers (Fig. 6) *(97)*. These cantilevers consist of a short hinge region that increases the sensitivity of optical detection methods because motion at the tip is magnified by 2 L/l, where L is the path length from the tip to the photodetector, and l is the length of the hinge region. In commercial cantilevers with low spring constants (~0.01 *N*/m), l can be ~ 500 µm. For our cantilevers, l is 20

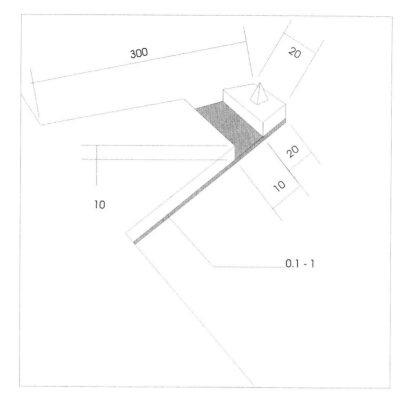

Fig. 6. New cantilever design. All dimensions are in microns.

μm. This allows us to increase our spring constant to reduce its thermal noise without decreasing the sensitivity of the detection system

$$dz = \sqrt{k_B T / k}$$

where dz is the cantilever displacement, k is cantilever stiffness, k_B is Boltzman's constant, and T is temperature. Alternatively, the bandwidth can be increased at the same static compliance.

4. VOLTAGE STIMULUS EXPERIMENTS

The new patch-clamp scanning force microscope was first used to study the voltage dependent membrane movement reported by Mosbacher et al. *(80,85)*. As pointed out previously, transduction of mechanical inputs into ionic signals is quite common for MSCs, but the converse, turning voltage into movement, is rarely observed outside auditory outer hair cells *(98)*. It is known that changes in the transmembrane electric field may cause changes in the conformation of the lipid bilayer *(87)*. A wide range of experiments infer conformational changes of voltage-sensitive ion channels during electrical stimulation, and Mosbacher et al. (1998) may have measured this movement superimposed on the voltage-dependent background membrane movement using HEK293 cells transfected with the *Shaker* K$^+$ channels. To perform measurements on single channels, the background voltage-dependent movement of the membrane must be understood.

4.1. Methods

4.1.1. Electrophysiology and AFM

We used standard patch-clamp recording conditions. HEK 293 cells were grown on acid-washed #1 glass coverslips 2 d before recording. The cells were placed in a recording chamber and superfused with normal extracellular solution containing 167 mM NaCl, 5.6 mM KCl, 11 mM HEPES, 0.6 mM CaCl$_2$, 0.6 mM MgCl$_2$, pH 7.4 (NaOH). Recording and ground pipettes were filled with a solution containing 150 mM KCl, 10 mM EGTA, 5 mM HEPES, pH 7.4 (KOH). The pipettes had tip resistances of 3–5 MΩ. Electrophysiological recordings were carried out using an AXOPATCH-1B (Axon Instruments Inc., Foster City, CA 94404, www.axon.com). LabVIEW VIs were used to generate voltage pulses for the patch pipette and to record whole cell currents and AFM tip movements. To follow the fast cell-movement response, we used the AFM in constant height mode rather than constant force that requires feedback. The photodetector signal was obtained directly from the AFM's electronic interface unit and passed through a tunable low pass filter with the bandwidth set between 0.1 kHz and 1 kHz and digitized at 25 kHz.

4.1.2. Experimental Procedure

The AFM was calibrated and positioned near the surface of a cell of interest. To calibrate the distance vs photodetector (PD) output, we placed the tip in contact with the cover slip and measured the piezo movement (previously calibrated) to compensate for a known error signal. Probe sensitivity was examined before and after each experiment and only if the values were similar were the data retained. The probe tip was then placed near the surface of the cell. After measuring the pipette resistance, the pipette was advanced to the cell making a gigaseal that was broken to create the whole-cell mode. The AFM tip was then advanced toward the cell surface using the microstepper until within the range of the piezo (~4 µm). The piezo was then slowly advanced until reaching a prescribed contact force (in most cases <1 nN). Alternatively, we sometimes used the Quesant engage form with feedback parameters set low (~50). The approach was extremely gentle so as not to disturb the seal. Only cells with seal resistances of >2GΩ were used for quantitative experiments to minimize series resistance artefacts. Different voltage protocols were then sent to the voltage clamp while monitoring the AFM photodetector voltage.

4.1.3. Results

Depolarization and hyperpolarization produced, respectively, outward and inward movements of the membrane. Figure 7 shows the movement of the cantilever requires touching the membrane. The movement varied linearly with the change in membrane potential (Fig. 8), but was insensitive to the holding potential. The differential sensitivity was ~ 1Å/mV calculated from experiments where the mean contact force was ~0.7 nN (Fig. 8D). This sensitivity is similar to the 4 Å/mV reported by Mosbacher et al. *(85)*, and 2 Å/mV reported by Todorov et al. *(87,88)*. The sensitivity increased with the mean contact force and eventually saturated (Fig. 9). It is also important to note that membrane movement and ionic current were uncorrelated, suggesting the motor mechanism is not electro-osmotic.

In some cases, the movement response showed two time constants. These time constants were independent of potential and the fastest one exceeded that of the free cantilever in solution. (Note that the frequency response of a cantilever depends on the compliance of the sample. On hard substrates the cantilever is supported at both ends and the resonant frequency is approximately that of the second harmonic of the free cantilever. In free solution, the lowest frequency response is the first harmonic. The frequency response of the cantilever in contact with a deformable sample lies between these two figures.) The slow response of the cells may represent viscoelastic relaxation of the cytoskeleton. We sometimes observed adaptation during a voltage step (Fig. 9A) that continued after removal of the pulse indicative of plastic defomation (i.e., cytoskeletal modulation or lipid flip-flop).

4.1.4. Discussion

This work shows that the AFM can resolve sub-Angstrom movements with sub-millisecond time resolution from intact cells under voltage clamp. As suggested in Mosbacher et al. *(85)*, the voltage dependent membrane movement can be explained by flexoelectricity. The equations for flexoelectricity predict a movement on the order of ~1 Å/mV. We are currently in the process of studying the origin of the two time constants and the adaptation using cytoskeletal reagents.

The flexoelectric effect provides a unique method for determining the contact force while scanning cells. At low forces, the fit of the data in Fig.

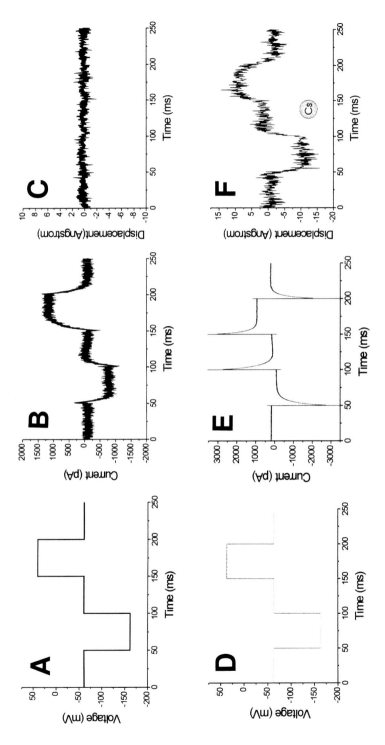

Fig. 7. Voltage-induced membrane movement. (**A,D**) Stimulus voltage; (**C,F**) Membrane movement. In cell #1, there was no movement when the probe was positioned just over the cell. In cell #2, 10 Å of movement was detected when the cell was indented with 0.7 nN of mean force. In (**F**), the crystal diameter of a cesium atom (5.2 Å) is shown to emphasize the scale of the membrane movement.

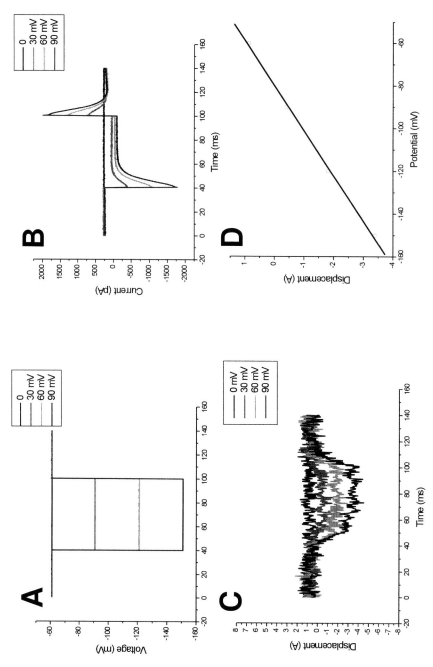

Fig. 8. Effect of voltage on membrane movement. Steady-state displacement *vs* command voltage. (**A**), (**B**), and (**C**) show the membrane potential, ionic current, and membrane movement from the same cell (average of 20 sweeps). (**D**) Illustrates that the movement is linear with voltage.

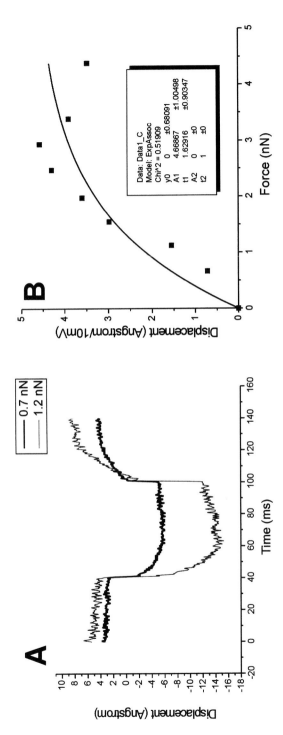

Fig. 9. Effect of contact force on voltage sensitivity. Panel (**A**) shows two representative membrane displacements (average of 50 sweeps) with fast and slow components. The curve in the right panel is the sensitivity as a function of mean force, which in turn is a monotonic function of the insertion depth.

449

9B, is F(nN) = 2.6*Z'(Å/mV), where F is the mean force and Z' is the voltage sensitivity. A modulating voltage provides an exquisitely sensitive measure of the applied force. A phase lock amplifier tuned to the carrier signal will reduce the random noise dramatically because it is only sensitive to a narrow frequency band and only to a defined phase within that band. In our setup, with the phase lock tuned to 500Hz and a bandwidth of 15Hz, the noise level is equivalent to 10fN! The flexoelectric effect offers the possibility of producing AFM images via a new contrast modality, with extremely low contact force and still maintaining the high lateral resolution of contact mode imaging.

A long-range goal is to link covalently the AFM tip to a movable part of the extracellular domain of a cloned voltage-sensitive channel while applying voltage protocols in order to measure voltage-dependent movements of the channel. If we can record both movement and channel current from a molecule, we may be able to separate states that are aggregated in either modality alone; i.e., all closed states do not have the same conformation.

Preliminary work shows that there are few free sulfhydryl groups on the cell surface so that cysteine mutants can in principle be detected. We have measured the adhesion strength between a cantilever tip labeled with a maleimide linker and a cover slip with free sulfhydryl groups. We have also measured the adhesion between chemically modified tips and active groups on the cell surface.

4.1.5. Preparation of Cantilevers with Sulfhydryl Groups

Silicon nitride cantilevers (ThermoMicroscopes, Sunnyvale, CA 94089; www.park.com) were cleaned in a cationic surfactant substitute for dichromic acid (10% RBS-35, Pierce Chemical, Rockford, IL, www.piercenet.com) for 15 min, concentrated HNO_3 for 15–30 min, and rinsed with deionized water and ethanol. 3-mercapto-propyl-trimethoxy-silane (United Chemical Technologies, Bristol, PA 19007, www.unitedchem.com) films were formed by immersing the chips in 94% acidic methanol (0.15 M acetic acid), 3.7% H_2O and 2.3% saline for 30 min at room temperature under nitrogen, followed by three rinses with absolute ethanol and drying with nitrogen. The cantilevers were then stored under nitrogen until use. Sulfhydryl groups we attached to cover slips using similar procedures.

4.1.6. Preparation of Cantilevers with Active Maleimide Linkers

Cantilevers were cleaned as above. The cleaned tips were immersed into a solution of 1% (3-aminopropyl) triethoxysilane (APTES, Aldrich, Milwaukee, WI 53233, www.sigma-aldrich.com) in ethanol for about 30 min at room temperature under nitrogen, followed by three rinses with absolute ethanol times and drying under nitrogen. The cantilevers were then put into a 5 m*M* solution of the hetero-bifunctional crosslinker (NHS-PEG-MAL, Shearwater Polymers Inc., Huntsville, AL 35801, www.swpolymers.com) in a 1:4 DMSO/ethanol mixture for 2 h under nitrogen. The tips were again rinsed with ethanol three times and dried with nitrogen. The tips were then stored under nitrogen until use.

4.1.7. Chemical Modification of HEK293 Cells

We added free maleimide groups to the extracellular surface of intact HEK293 cells for testing local compliance using SH-derivatized cantilevers. We incubated the cells in a 5 m*M* solution of the hetero-bifunctional crosslinker (NHS-PEG-MAL, Shearwater Polymers, Huntsville, AL 35801, www.swpolymers.com) in PBS, pH 7.4, for 1–2 h. The cells were then rinsed three times with PBS.

4.1.8. AFM Procedure

The AFM tip was advanced into the sample to a contact force ~1 n*N*. The tip remained in contact with the sample for a defined period of time, 30–120 s. As the tip was withdrawn from the surface, we tracked the photodetector Z voltage looking for deflections associated with forming and breaking bonds. Tips with NHS-PEG3400-MAL linkers were tested on coverslips with free sulfhydryl groups. The force curve (Fig. 10A) shows a large negative peak as the cantilever is pulled away from the surface, and several smaller negative peaks appear after further withdrawing the tips. The step-like force change relaxing the cantilever about 0.5–1 n*N*, which is likely to correspond to the breaking of a single covalent bond. It is important to point out that the step-like force change only appears when the tip sits on the surface for more than 30 s. If the tip is withdrawn immediately after making contact, there is no specific adhesion and the force curve looks like Fig. 10B. This curve is similar to that observed with plain coverslips. These results suggest that the association rate for making covalent bonds between the functionalized tip and coverslip is significant, in practice requiring tens of seconds to minutes. Obviously ligand-binding densities will also play a role in association kinetics.

To pull on membrane proteins, we added MAL groups to the cell surface. We treated HEK293 cells with NHS-PEG-MAL in PBS solution at pH 7.4. The reaction-linked amino groups on the cell surface to the NHS group of NHS-PEG-MAL, producing an active maleimide group. Figure 11 shows the cantilever response when the tip, with free sulfhydryl groups, was retracted after contacting the surface of the modified cells for >30 s. Because the cells are much softer than the coverslip, the negative peak is broad. More

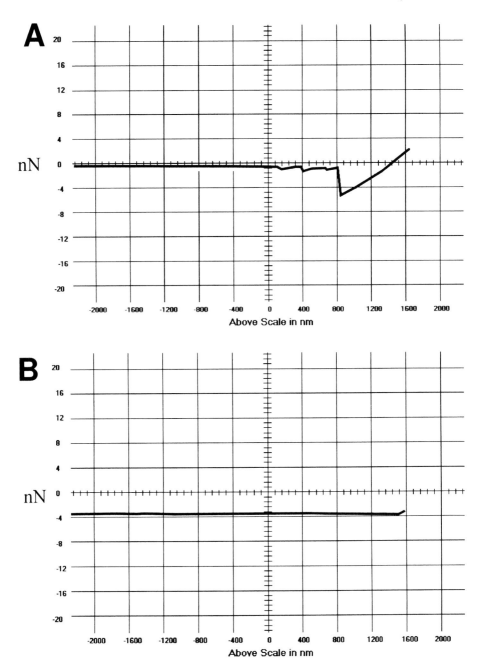

Fig. 10. Force spectroscopy on functionalized cover slips. (**A**) shows the retraction force curve of a maleimide linker attached to the cantilever tip and SH groups on a cover slip after a 60 s reaction time. (**B**) is the force curve after < 30 s contact. The minimal adhesion is similar to unfunctionalized cover slips.

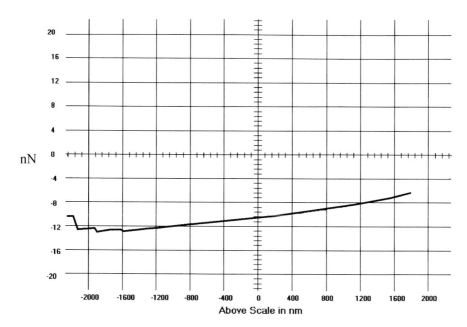

Fig. 11. Force spectroscopy on functionalized HEK cells. Retraction force curve of SH activated cantilevers bonded to HEK cells labeled with maleimide linkers.

importantly, the force curve contains several step-like changes similar to the covalent binding of the cantilever to the sulfhydryl groups on the coverslip. As a control experiment, we also examined the force curve when the cantilever was immediately withdrawn after touching the cell surface, giving little time for a reaction. This response was showed no step-like changes in the force curve. It should be possible to form a covalent bond between a specific sulfhydryl group, i.e., cysteine, and a maleimide linker. Once this attachment is made, we can track dimensional changes of a specific molecule.

5. CONCLUSIONS

The combination of AFM and patch-clamp can, in principal, allow us to record two dependent variables from the same single molecule. Simultaneous recording by both instruments allows the necessary time correlations for understanding the causal relationship of the kinetics as well as providing fundamental physical parameters. We look forward to using force and voltage as independent sources of free energy to study channel and membrane biophysics.

ACKNOWLEDGMENTS

We would like to thank Dr. Asbed Keleshian and Dr. Steven Besch for their thoughtful comments on the manuscript.

REFERENCES

1. Hille, B. (1992) *Ionic Channels of Excitable Membranes.* Sinauer Associates Inc., Sunderland, MA.
2. Horn, R. (1991) Diffusion of nystatin in plasma membrane is inhibited by a glass- membrane seal [published erratum appears in *Biophys. J.* **60(4)**, 985]. *Biophys. J.* **60**, 329–333.
3. Fernandez, J. M., Neher, E., and Gomperts, B. D. (1984) Capacitance measurements reveal stepwise fusion events in degranulating mast cells. *Nature* **312(5993)**, 453–455.
4. Joshi, C. and Fernandez, J. M. (1989) Capacitance measurements: an analysis of the phase detector technique used to study exocytosis and endocytosis. *Biophys. J.* **56**, 1153–1162.
5. Dilger, J. P., Brett, R. S., Poppers, D. M., and Liu, Y. (1991) The temperature dependence of some kinetic and conductance properties of acetylcholine receptor channels. *Biochim. Biophys. Acta* **1063**, 253–258.
6. Sachs, F. (1999) Practical limits on the maximal speed of solution exchange for patch- clamp experiments. *Biophys J.* **77**, 682–690.
7. Besch, S. D. and Sachs, F. (2000) *A Compact, High Speed, Air Pressure Servo.* In press.
8. Mcbride, D. W. and Hamill, O. P. (1995) A fast pressure-clamp technique for studying mechanogated channels, in *Single-Channel Recording* (Sakmann, B. and Neher, E., eds.), Plenum, New York, pp. 329–340.
9. Martinac, B. (1993) Mechanosensitive ion channels: biophysics and physiology. *Thermodynamics of Cell Surface Receptors* (Jackson, M., ed.), CRC Press, Boca Raton, FL, pp. 327–351.
10. Sachs, F. (1992) Stretch sensitive ion channels: an update, in *Sensory Transduction* (Corey, D. P. and Roper, S. D., eds.), Rockefeller University Press, Society General Physiology, NY, pp. 241–260.
11. Sackin, H. (1995) Stretch activated ion channels. *Kidney Int.* **48**, 1134–1147.
12. Sachs, F. and Morris, C. (1998) Mechanosensitive ion channels in non specialized cells, in *Reviews of Physiology and Biochemistry and Pharmacology* (Blaustein, M. P., et al., eds.), Springer, Berlin, pp. 1–78.
13. Sokabe, M. and Sachs, F. (1992) Towards a molecular mechanism of activation in mechanosensitive ion channels, in *Advances in Comparative and Environmental Physiology,* vol. 10 (Ito, F., ed.), Springer-Verlag, Berlin, pp. 55–77.
14. Sukharev, S., Sigurdson, W., Kung, C., and Sachs, F. (1999) Energetic and spatial parameters for gating of the bacterial large conductance mechanosensitive channel, MscL. *J. Gen. Physiol.* **113**, 525–539.

15. Hamill, O. P., Marty, A., Neher, E., Sakmann, B., and Sigworth, F. J. (1981) Improved patch-clamp techniques for high-resolution current recording from cells and cell-free membrane patches. *Pflugers Arch. Eur. J. Physiol.* **391,** 85–100.

16. Guharay, F. and Sachs, F. (1984) Stretch-activated single ion channel currents in tissue-cultured embryonic chick skeletal muscle. *J. Physiol. (Lond.)* **352,** 685–701.

17. Yang, X. C. and Sachs, F. (1989) Block of stretch-activated ion channels in *Xenopus* oocytes by gadolinium and calcium ions. *Science* **243,** 1068–1071.

18. Sokabe, M., Sachs, F., and Jing, Z. (1991) Quantitative video microscopy of patch clamped membranes: stress, strain, capacitance and stretch channel activation. *Biophys. J.* **59,** 722–728.

19. Small, D. L. and Morris, C. E. (1994) Delayed activation of single mechanosensitive channels in Lymnaea neurons. *Am. J. Physiol.* **267,** C598-C606.

20. Hamill, O. P. and McBride, D. W., Jr. (1992) Rapid adaptation of single mechanosensitive channels in *Xenopus* oocytes. *Proc. Natl. Acad. Sci. USA* **89,** 7462–7466.

21. Suchyna, T. M., Johnson, J. H., Clemo, H. F., Huang, Z. H., Gage, D. A., Baumgarten, C. M., and Sachs, F. (2000) Identification of a peptide toxin from *Grammostola spatulata* spider venom that blocks stretch activated channels. *J. Gen. Physiol.* **115,** 583–598.

22. Fahlke, C. and Rudel, R. (1992) Giga-seal formation alters properties of sodium channels of human myoballs. *Pflugers Arch.* **420,** 248–254.

23. Hochmuth, R. M. (2000) Micropipette aspiration of living cells. [Review] [34 refs]. *J. Biomechanics* **33,** 15–22.

24. Horber, J. K., Mosbacher, J., Haberle, W., Ruppersberg, J. P., and Sakmann, B. (1995) A look at membrane patches with a scanning force microscope. *Biophys. J.* **68,** 1687–1693.

25. Drake, B. Prater, C. B. Weisenhorn, A. L., Gould, S. A., Albrecht, T. R., Quate, C. F., et al. (1989) Imaging crystals, polymers, and processes in water with the atomic force microscope. *Science* **243,** 1586–1589.

26. Radmacher, M., Hillner, P. E., and Hansma, P. K. (1994) Scanning nearfield optical microscope using microfabricated probes. *Rev. Sci. Instrum.* **65,** 2737–2738.

27. Hansma, H. and Hoh, J. (1994) Biomolecular imaging with the atomic force microscope. *Ann. Rev. Biophys. Biomol. Struct.* **23,** 115–139.

28. Lal, R., Kim, H., Garavito, R. M., and Arnsdorf, M. F. (1993) Imaging of reconstituted biological channels at molecular resolution by atomic force microscopy. *Am. J. Physiol.* **265,** C851–C856.

29. Jena, B. P., Schneider, S. W., Geibel, J. P., Webster, P., Oberleithner, H., and Sritharan, K. C. (1997) Gi regulation of secretory vesicle swelling examined by atomic force microscopy. *Proc. Natl. Acad. Sci. USA* **94,** 13,317–13,322.

30. Haberle, W., Horber, J. K., and Binnig, G. (1991) Force microscopy on living cells. *J. Vac. Sci. Technol. B* **9,** 1210–1213.

31. Horber, J. K., Haberle, W., Ohnesorge, F., Binnig, G., Liebich, H. G., Czerny, C. P., et al. (1992) Investigation of living cells in the nanometer regime with the scanning force microscope. *Scan. Microsc.* **6,** 919–929.
32. Henderson, E. (1994) Imaging of living cells by atomic force microscopy. *Prog. Surface Sci.* **46,** 39–60.
33. Henderson, R. M., Schneider, S., Li, Q., Hornby, D., White, S. J., and Oberleithner, H. (1996) Imaging ROMK1 inwardly rectifying ATP-sensitive K+ channel protein using atomic force microscopy. *Proc. Natl. Acad. Sci. USA* **93,** 8756–8760.
34. Radmacher, M. (1997) Measuring the elastic properties of biological samples with the AFM. *IEEE Eng. Med. Biol.* **16,** 47–57.
35. Schneider, S. W., Yano, Y., Sumpio, B. E., Jena, B. P., Geibel, J. P., Gekle, M., and Oberleithner, H. (1997) Rapid aldosterone-induced cell volume increase of endothelial cells measured by the atomic force microscope. *Cell Biol. Int.* **21,** 759–768.
36. Fritzsche, W., Takac, L., and Henderson, E. (1997) Application of atomic force microscopy to visualization of DNA, chromatin, and chromosomes. [Review] [65 refs]. *Crit. Rev. Eukaryotic Gene Exp.* **7,** 231–240.
37. Hansma, H. G., Kim, K. J., Laney, D. E., Garcia, R. A., Argaman, M., Allen, M. J., Parsonsand, S. M. (1997) Properties of biomolecules measured from atomic force microscope images: a review. [Review] [59 refs]. *J. Struct. Biol.* **119,** 99–108.
38. Yang, Y., Sweeney, W. V., Schneider, K., Chait, B. T., and Tam, J. P. (1994) Two-step selective formation of three disulfide bridges in the synthesis of the C-terminal epidermal growth factor-like domain in human blood coagulation factor IX. *Protein Sci.* **3,** 1267–1275.
39. Lal, R. and Yu, L. (1993) Atomic force microscopy of cloned nicotinic acetylcholine receptor expressed in Xenopus oocytes. *Proc. Natl. Acad. Sci. USA* **90,** 7280–7284.
40. Lal, R. and John, S. A. (1994) Biological applications of atomic force microscopy. [Review]. *Am. J. Physiol.* **266,** C1–21.
41. John, S. A., Saner, D., Pitts, J. D., Holzenburg, A., Finbow, M. E., and Lal, R. (1997) Atomic force microscopy of arthropod gap junctions. *J. Struct. Biol.* **120,** 22–31.
42. Lal, R. (1996) Imaging molecular structure of channels and receptors with an atomic force microscope. *Scan. Microsc.* **10(Suppl.),** 81–95.
43. Lal, R., John, S. A., Laird, D. W., and Arnsdorf, M. F. (1995) Heart gap junction preparations reveal hemiplaques by atomic force microscopy. *Am. J. Physiol.* **268,** C968–C977.
44. Hoh, J. H., Sosinsky, G. E., Revel, J. P., and Hansma, P. K. (1993) Structure of the extracellular surface of the gap junction by atomic force microscopy. *Biophys. J.* **65,** 149–163.
45. Oberleithner, H., Brinckmann, E., Schwab, A., and Krohne, G. (1994) Imaging nuclear pores of aldosterone-sensitive kidney cells by atomic force microscopy. *Proc. Natl. Acad. Sci. USA* **91,** 9784–9788.
46. Folprecht, G., Schneider, S., and Oberleithner, H. (1996) Aldosterone activates the nuclear pore transporter in cultured kidney cells imaged with atomic force microscopy. *Pflugers Arch. Eur. J. Physiol.* **432,** 831–838.

47. Schneider, S., Folprecht, G., Krohne, G., and Oberleithner, H. (1995) Immunolocalization of lamins and nuclear pore complex proteins by atomic force microscopy. *Pflugers Arch. Eur. J. Physiol.* **430,** 795–801.
48. Perez-Terzic, C., Pyle, J., Jaconi, M., Stehno-Bittel, L., and Clapham, D. E. (1996) Conformational states of the nuclear pore complex induced by depletion of nuclear Ca^{2+} stores. *Science* **273,** 1875–1877.
49. Wang, H. and Clapham, D. E. (1999) Conformational changes of the in situ nuclear pore complex. *Biophys. J.* **77,** 241–247.
50. Radmacher, M., Fritz, M., and Hansma, P. K. (1995) Imaging soft samples with the atomic force microscope: gelatin in water and propanol. *Biophys. J.* **69,** 264–270.
51. Wagner, P. (1998) Immobilization strategies for biological scanning probe microscopy. [Review] [58 refs]. *FEBS Lett.* **430,** 112–115.
52. Korchev, Y. E., Bashford, C. L., Milovanovic, M., Vodyanoy, I., and Laband, M. J. (1997) Scanning ion conductance microscopy of living cells. *Biophys. J.* **73,** 653–658.
53. Merkel, R., Nassoy, P., Leung, A., Ritchie, K., and Evans, E. (1999) Energy landscapes of receptor-ligand bonds explored with dynamic force spectroscopy. *Nature* **397,** 50–53.
54. Engel, A., Lyubchenko, Y., and Muller, D. (1999) Atomic force microscopy: a powerful tool to observe biomolecules at work. [Review] [39 refs]. *Trends Cell Biol.* **9,** 77–80.
55. Schabert, F. A., Henn, C., and Engel, A. (1995) Native Escherichia coli OmpF porin surfaces probed by atomic force microscopy. *Science* **268,** 92–94.
56. Muller, D. J. and Engel, A. (1999) Voltage and pH-induced channel closure of porin OmpF visualized by atomic force microscopy. *J. Mol. Biol.* **285,** 1347–1351.
57. Muller, D. J., Sass, H. J., Muller, S. A., Buldt, G., and Engel, A. (1999) Surface structures of native bacteriorhodopsin depend on the molecular packing arrangement in the membrane. *J. Mol. Biol.* **285,** 1903–1909.
58. Yang, J., Mou, J., and Shao, Z. (1994) Structure and stability of pertussis toxin studied by in situ atomic force microscopy. *FEBS Lett.* **338,** 89–92.
59. Czajkowsky, D. M. and Shao, Z. (1998) Submolecular resolution of single macromolecules with atomic force microscopy. [Review] [40 refs]. *FEBS Lett.* **430,** 51–54.
60. Fisher, T. E., Marszalek, P. E., Oberhauser, A. F., Carrion, V., and Fernandez, J. M. (1999) The micro-mechanics of single molecules studied with atomic force microscopy. [Review] [35 refs]. *J. Physiol.* **520 Pt 1,** 5–14.
61. Shao, Z., Yang, J., and Somlyo, A. P. (1995) Biological atomic force microscopy: from microns to nanometers and beyond. [Review] [134 refs]. *Annu. Rev. Cell. Dev. Biol.* **11,** 241–265.
62. Fritz, M., Radmacher, M., and Gaub, H. E. (1994) Granula motion and membrane spreading during activation of human platelets imaged by atomic force microscopy. *Biophys. J.* **66,** 1328–1334.
63. Muller, D. J., Baumeister, W., and Engel, A. (1996) Conformational change of the hexagonally packed intermediate layer of Deinococcus radiodurans monitored by atomic force microscopy. *J. Bacteriol.* **178,** 3025–3030.

64. Thalhammer, S., Stark, R. W., Muller, S., Wienberg, J., and Heckl, W. M. (1997) The atomic force microscope as a new microdissecting tool for the generation of genetic probes. *J. Struct. Biol.* **119,** 232–237.
65. Fotiadis, D., Muller, D. J., Tsiotis, G., Hasler, L., Tittmann, P., Mini, T., et al. (1998) Surface analysis of the photosystem I complex by electron and atomic force microscopy. *J. Mol. Biol.* **283,** 83–94.
66. Muller, D. J., Buldt, G., and Engel, A. (1995) Force-induced conformational change of bacteriorhodopsin. *J. Mol. Biol.* **249,** 239–243.
67. Schoenenberger, C. A. and Hoh, J. H. (1994) Slow cellular dynamics in MDCK and R5 cells monitored by time-lapse atomic force microscopy. *Biophys. J.* **67,** 929–936.
68. Radmacher, M., Fritz, M., Kacher, C. M., Cleveland, J. P., and Hansma, P. K. (1996) Measuring the viscoelastic properties of human platelets with the atomic force microscope. *Biophys. J.* **70,** 556–567.
69. Rief, M., Gautel, M., Oesterhelt, F., Fernandez, J. M., and Gaub, H. E. (1997) Reversible unfolding of individual titin immunoglobulin domains by AFM [see comments]. *Science* **276,** 1109–1112.
70. Florin, E. L., Rief, M., Lehmann, H., Ludwig, M., Dornmair, C., Moy, V. T., and Gaub, H. E. (1995) Sensing specific molecular interasctions with the Atomic Force Microscope. *Biosens. Bioelectron.* **10,** 895–901.
71. Moy, V. T., Florin, E. L., and Gaub, H. E. (1994) Adhesive forces between ligand and receptor measured by Afm. *Colloids Surfaces A-Physicochem. Eng. Aspects* **93,** 343–348.
72. Bustamante, J. O., Liepins, A., Prendergast, R. A., Hanover, J. A., and Oberleithner, H. (1995) Patch clamp and atomic force microscopy demonstrate TATA-binding protein (TBP) interactions with the nuclear pore complex. *J. Membr. Biol.* **146,** 263–272.
73. Horber, J. K., Mosbacher, J., and Haberle, W. (1995) Force microscopy on membrane patches, in *Single-Channel Recording* (Sakmann, B. and Neher, E., eds.), Plenum, New York, pp. 375–393.
74. Hoh, J. H. and Schoenenberger, C. A. (1994) Surface morphology and mechanical properties of MDCK monolayers by atomic force microscopy. *J. Cell Sci.* **107 ,** 1105–1114.
75. Sokabe, M. and Sachs, F. (1990) The structure and dynamics of patch-clamped membranes: a study by differential interference microscopy. *J. Cell Biol.* **111,** 599–606.
76. McEwen, B. F., Song, M. J., Ruknudin, A., Barnard, D. P., Frank, J., and Sachs, F. (1990) Tomographic three dimensional reconstruction of patch clamped membranes imaged with the high voltage electron microscope. *XII Intl. Cong. El. Microsc.* 522–523 (Abstract).
77. Ruknudin, A., Song, M. J., and Sachs, F. (1991) The ultrastructure of patch-clamped membranes: a study using high voltage electron microscopy. *J. Cell Biol.* **112,** 125–134.
78. Akinlaja, J. and Sachs, F. (1998) The breakdown of cell membranes by electrical and mechanical stress. *Biophys. J.* **75,** 247–254.
79. Horber, J. K. H., Mosbacher, J., Haberle, W., Ruppersberg, J. P., and Sakmann, B. (1995) A look at membrane patches with a scanning force microscope. *Biophys. J.* **68,** 1687–1693.

80. Mosbacher, J., Haberle, W., and Horber, J. K. (1996) Studying membranes with scanning force microscopy and patch-clamp. *J. Vac. Sci. Technol.* B **14**, 1449–1452.

81. Larmer, J., Schneider, S. W., Danker, T., Schwab, A., and Oberleithner, H. (1997) Imaging excised apical plasma membrane patches of MDCK cells in physiological conditions with atomic force microscopy. *Pflugers Arch. Eur. J. Physiol.* **434**, 254–260.

82. Crowe, J. H. and Crowe, L. M. (1982) Induction of anhydrobiosis: membrane changes during drying. *Cryobiology* **19**, 317–328.

83. Danker, T., Mazzanti, M., Tonini, R., Rakowska, A., and Oberleithner, H. (1997) Using atomic force microscopy to investigate patch-clamped nuclear membrane. *Cell Biol. Int.* **21**, 747–757.

84. Bustamante, J. O. (1994) Nuclear electrophysiology. *J. Membr. Biol.* **138**, 105–112.

85. Mosbacher, J., Langer, M., Horber, H., and Sachs, F. (1998) Voltage-dependent membrane displacements measure by atomic force microscopy. *J. Gen. Physiol.* **111**, 65–74.

86. Petrov, A. G. (1999) *Lyotropic State of Matter: Molecular Physics and Living Matter Physics.* Gordon & Breach Publishing Group, Amsterdam.

87. Todorov, A. T., Petrov, A. G., and Fendler, J. H. (1994) 1st observation of the converse flexoelectric effect in bilayer-lipid membranes. *J. Phys. Chem.* **98**, 3076–3079.

88. Todorov, A. T., Petrov, A. G., and Fendler, J. H. (1994) Flexoelectricity of charged and polar bilayer-lipid membranes studied by stroboscopic interferometry. *Langmuir* **10**, 2344–2350.

89. Petrov, A. G., Ramsey, R. L., and Usherwood, P. N. (1989) Curvature-electric effects in artificial and natural membranes studied using patch-clamp techniques. *Eur. Biophys. J.* **17**, 13–17.

90. Petrov, A. G., Miller, B. A., Hristova, K., and Usherwood, P. N. (1993) Flexoelectric effects in model and native membranes containing ion channels. *Eur. Biophys. J.* **22**, 289–300.

91. Iwamoto, H., Czajkowsky, D. M., Cover, T. L., Szabo, G., and Shao, Z. (1999) VacA from Helicobacter pylori: a hexameric chloride channel. *FEBS Lett.* **450**, 101–104.

92. Bett, G. C. L. and Sachs, F. (2000) Activation and inactivation of mechanosensitive currents in the chick heart. *J. Membr. Biol.* **173**, 237–254.

93. Langer, M. G., Offner, W., Wittmann, H., Flosser, H., Schaar, H., Haberle, W., et al. (1997) A scanning force microscope for simultaneous force and patch-clamp measurements on living cell tissues. *Rev. Sci. Instr.* **68**, 2583–2590.

94. Snyder, K., Besch, S. D., Zhang, P. C., and Sachs, F. (2000) Hardware and software modifications of the Quesant AFM for use in biology. In press.

95. Sachs, F. (1995) A low drift micropipette holder. *Eur. J. Physiol.* **429**, 434–435.

96. Snyder, K. V., Kreigstein, A. and Sachs, F. (1999) A convenient electrode holder for glass pipettes to stabilize electrode potentials. *Eur. J. Physiol.* **438**, 405–411.

97. Beyder, A., Snyder, K. V., and Sachs, F. (2000) New AFM cantilever for low force applications in liquids. In press.

98. Ashmore, J. F. (1987) A fast motile response in guinea-pig outer hair cells: the cellular basis of the cochlear amplifier. *J. Physiol. (Lond.)* **388**, 323–347.

24

Localizing Ion Channels with Scanning Probe Microscopes: A Perspective

Daniel M. Czajkowsky and Zhifeng Shao

1. INTRODUCTION

It is now widely appreciated in cell biology that there are two significant modes, beyond synthesis and degradation, by which the cell can regulate its enzymes: covalent modification and subcellular localization. The former mode may be studied with isolated components, and so may be investigated, to great detail, under a variety of well-controlled conditions. However, the localization of proteins must be studied within the context of the more complicated environment of a cell, and as such, is much more technically challenging. Clear examples of the importance of the subcellular location of proteins on the proper functioning of a cell is well-known in the membrane channel field, with the clusters of channels in the opposing membranes of a synapse or the aggregates of channels within the nodes of Ranvier. However, as studies of rafts (domains within the plasma-membrane-enriched in selected lipids and proteins [1]) have demonstrated, active control of the spatial distribution of membrane proteins, lipids, and cytosolic components at the level of the plasma membrane is likely to be a general mechanism underlying many cellular processes.

Scanning-probe microscopes (SPMs) provide a new repertoire of tools to investigate the surface structure and distribution of biological macromolecules (2,3). These instruments generate images of a given sample by a fundamentally different mechanism than traditional microscopes: rather than relying on a combination of lenses (and thus subject to the limitations prescribed by wave optics), images are produced by detecting the local tip-

From: Ion Channel Localization Methods and Protocols
Edited by: A. Lopatin and C. G. Nichols © Humana Press Inc., Totowa, NJ

sample interactions as a very sharp tip raster scans in close proximity to the specimen. The most commonly used microscope of this family is the atomic force microscope (AFM) *(4)*, where the tip is usually the apex of a glass-like Si_3N_4 pyramid affixed to one face of a very soft cantilever. Operated in the contact mode, the submicroscopic changes in the topography of the sample cause the scanning cantilever, which is in direct contact with the sample, to deflect accordingly, and by monitoring these deflections, the surface contour of the specimen can be determined. Because the most common scheme to detect these deflections (by reflecting a laser off of the opposite face of the cantilever) can be performed as well in liquid as in air, there are few restrictions to the possible imaging environments for this type of instrument.

The AFM would thus appear well-poised to provide information about the distribution of channels and other components in cellular membranes under a host of biologically relevant conditions. There are, however, two limitations that have precluded the widespread application of the AFM to this end: the difficulty to identify a particular set of molecules from within a heterogeneous field based on topography alone and the inherent softness or flexibility of living cells. The former might be circumvented, as will be discussed later, using specific labels that can be easily recognized by the AFM, but the latter appears to be a more serious limitation: the sample must be sufficiently rigid and laterally immobile to be able to deflect the tip significantly. However, as is well known, the plasma membrane of an intact cell is easily deformed and its membrane proteins are highly mobile. As a consequence, most of those AFM studies that have successfully imaged membrane proteins within a cell surface have studied cells under conditions where they are more rigid and less responsive to the lateral forces of the tip; namely, the cells have been imaged in air or at cryogenic temperatures. These studies, still, have provided information at exquisite resolution that has been either suggested or verified using less direct but more physiological assays. Yet it is because of this difficulty that this chapter will not only describe some of the more interesting and useful results that have been achieved with AFM at its current stage of technological development, but will also, in the end, describe other imaging modes and other SPMs that will likely prove useful in those studies specifically designed to localize ion channels within the cellular membrane.

2. DISCRIMINATION BASED ON TOPOGRAPHY

2.1. Room Temperature AFM

In most cases, there is really only one, at times difficult, step to prepare samples for AFM: adsorption of the specimen to a very flat substrate. After this is achieved, the sample is then simply placed either on a piezo-stage (beneath a stationary cantilever) or under a scanning cantilever (above an immobile stage), depending on the brand of microscope.

The most commonly used substrate for AFM is the atomically flat and slightly negatively charged surface of mica. Charged biological samples often adsorb either directly to mica or to a mica substrate first coated with polylysine or spermidine (a simple incubation with a ~1 mM solution of either cationic molecule followed by a thorough wash with water and drying in air). Owing to this dependence on electrostatic interactions, it may be necessary to scan quickly a few samples under different salt concentrations to determine if a particular ionic composition will be critical for imaging. For those samples that do not adhere well to mica, there are a few recent studies that have fabricated new, reasonably flat substrates (polyvinyl phenyl ketone) and furan polymers with surface roughness features of 0.3 and 0.15 nm rms, respectively *[5]*) and others that have used the more hydrophobic HOPG graphite surface *(6,7)*. In addition, there is also an earlier report describing procedures to link covalently several biological samples to a functionalized substrate *(8)*.

Figure 1 is an example of the higher level of resolution that may be achieved in solution with AFM, here of the hexameric chloride channel from *Helicobacter pylori*, VacA, reconstituted into a pure lipid bilayer *(9)*. Although its mechanism of incorporation into membranes has yet to be fully described, it is likely that VacA, a water-soluble oligomer at neutral pH, binds to membranes as a monomer at low pH, and then rapidly self-assembles into transmembrane hexamers. To prepare these samples, the lipid bilayer was first deposited onto mica using a Langmuir trough and the protein was then added directly to the bilayer. Figure 1A shows the resulting randomly distributed ensemble of VacA rings within the supported bilayer that is routinely produced by this method. Higher resolution images were difficult to achieve with these samples, likely owing to the high lateral mobility of the membrane protein in the bilayer. Interestingly, neutralizing the pH was sufficient to induce two-dimensional (2D) crystallization of these hexamers, and the patches of crystal could be imaged to a much higher resolution (Fig. 1B). The best resolution that has been achieved with these samples is ~8 Å (D.M.C. and Z.S., unpublished results), which is among the highest obtained of 2D crystals of membrane proteins by AFM to date *(10,11)*.

This level of resolution was possible not only because of the close-packed nature of the sample (a common property among the high-resolution images published so far *[3]*) but also because of the high level of rigidity of the mica substrate immediately below the bilayer. When a similar protein-rich mem-

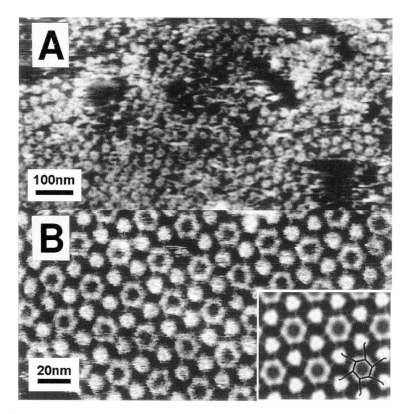

Fig. 1. High-resolution AFM images of the hexameric chloride channel from *H. pylori*, VacA, in pure lipid membranes *(9)*. (**A**) The addition of water-soluble VacA proteins to supported membranes at low pH produced a sample characterized by a random distribution of VacA rings associated with the bilayer. (**B**) Subsequently neutralizing the pH to ~7.0 induced the formation of 2D crystals of these VacA hexamers, which were imaged to greater detail. The inset is a processed image, including a line diagram illustrating a single hexamer within the crystal.

brane is not immediately supported by a rigid substrate (as is the case when imaging proteins within the membrane of an intact cell), it has been difficult to resolve unambiguously individual membrane proteins.

Figure 2 is a state-of-the-art image of the surface of a live cell in solution in a study designed to investigate the mechanical properties of the cell as it moves *(12)*. These cells were simply plated on a Petri dish and imaged in growth medium. The image, however, was obtained in the deflection mode, where, although the tip still follows the sample topography, the contrast presented depicts the magnitude of height changes, and thus emphasizes edges

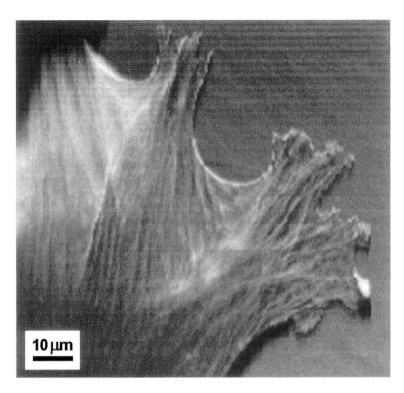

Fig. 2. State-of-the-art AFM image of a living 3T3 fibroblast *(12)*. This image was generated with the deflection mode, which highlights edges within the sample. Although the stress fibers at the leading edge of the cell can be clearly discerned in this image, individual membrane proteins are difficult to identify, likely owing to the softness of the cytoplasm. Image courtesy of Dr. M. Radmacher.

within the sample. As can be seen in this image, the stress fibers beneath the intact membrane are clearly observed at the leading edge of the cell but there is no contrast easily interpretable as membrane proteins, undoubtedly in large part because of the softness of the cytoplasm.

In general, membrane proteins may be observed with an AFM in cells that have been first fixed and then air-dried. As originally demonstrated by Jovin and co-workers *(13)*, a recent study showed that the surface distribution of membrane proteins (here, the HLA class I and II molecules) could be investigated by AFM in conjunction with electron microscopy (EM) *(14)*. These proteins were distinguished over similarly shaped structures in the topographs with the use of 15- or 30-nm gold-labeled antibodies. By comparing the average distance between these labels with that predicted strictly from a completely random distribution, the authors concluded that HLA class II molecules were clustered at the surface of the T- and B-lymphoma cells.

The advantage of using electron-dense gold labels in EM is clear; the use of similar labels in AFM, although helpful to compare directly with EM, does not take full advantage of surface contour information provided by the AFM. Although such large labels can be detected by AFM, there is still, in the end, a problem with distinguishing between these labels and surface structures of a similar size, even with the proper controls. A perhaps more useful set of labels for AFM would be those with an easily identifiable shape, say a ring or a star, which could likewise be attached to antibodies directed against specific surface proteins. Such labeling has yet to be developed but should be possible using, for example, appropriately designed polymers or monocrystals *(15)*.

It should be mentioned that there was one report *(16)* investigating exocytosis at the apical cell surface of isolated pancreatic acinar cells, where in addition to observing several pits (which were, interestingly, approximately the diameter of dislodged microvilli *[17]*), the topographs were characterized by a random distribution of globular protrusions of various sizes across the membrane. Although the authors were primarily investigating the changes in diameter of the pits during exocytosis and did not further characterize these heterogeneous protrusions, it may be that a study of such a surface with antibodies or labels against specific ion channels may reveal a nonrandom distribution, perhaps associated with the edges of the pits. The apical surface of these cells is distinguished by an extensive cytoskeletal network immediately below the cell membrane, which may provide the mechanical support to image membrane proteins under solution.

Further along this line of thought, an earlier study *(18)* claimed that the plasma membrane of living cells should actually appear stiffer when using AFM in the tapping mode *(19–21)* (also called intermittent or AC mode in the literature). In this mode, the cantilever oscillates vertically while scanning, so that the tip contacts the sample for only a brief time during each cycle. This intermittent tip-sample interaction reduces the lateral force imposed by the tip on the specimen during scanning, and hence this mode is better suited for samples that are too laterally mobile for contact-mode imaging. This brief tip-sample contact also reduces the oscillation amplitude, and by monitoring the amount by which the sample must be raised or lowered to maintain a predetermined reduction in this amplitude, the topography of the sample is determined. According to this earlier report *(18)*, after bringing the tip into contact with the sample, a sudden further displacement of the sample at first deflected the cantilever by a similar amount as the sample was raised, as would occur if the sample was incompressible. Over a timescale of milliseconds though, the deflection of the cantilever decreased and then reached a plateau. As a result, the authors argued that for a tip-sample contact time of less than 1 ms (as in the case of the tapping mode) the cell membrane would appear to be a hard surface, and that it is only for longer contact times that the softness of the cytoplasm becomes significant. These results suggest that there may be a set of imaging parameters in the tapping mode that might best allow an opportunity to resolve individual protein components within the membrane of a living cell. However, the effectiveness of this approach remains to be demonstrated.

2.2. CryoAFM

This requirement for a mechanically robust biological sample was the impetus to develop an AFM that could image biological specimens at cryogenic temperatures, where it was believed such samples would become more rigid. Although there were several prototypes, only one has been successfully applied to biological samples *(22–24)*. This successful design involves suspending a specially designed AFM above a large pool of liquid nitrogen within a Dewar. By adjusting the distance between the microscope and the pool, the temperature may be changed from room temperature down to ~79K. A remarkable aspect of this design is that, because contaminants accumulate over time at the coldest location (the pool of liquid nitrogen in this cryoAFM), the sample in the microscope actually becomes cleaner with time.

A typical sample is prepared at room temperature within a sealed box perfused with nitrogen gas. After depositing a small volume of the sample onto mica, the specimen is rinsed, usually with a low ionic-strength buffer to prevent excessive deposition of salt. The solution is then dried with a stream of nitrogen gas, and subsequently lowered into the suspended AFM within the Dewar. This simple sample preparation procedure has proved quite versatile; all biological samples, from multisubunit proteins to chromatin and whole cells, that have been prepared in this way, have been imaged by cryoAFM. In fact, samples which did not bind to mica with sufficient strength for room temperature AFM have been adsorbed tightly enough following the aforementioned procedure for cryoAFM *(24)*.

Figure 3 shows cryoAFM images, taken in the contact mode, of a rabbit red blood cell membrane, first lightly fixed with glutaraldehyde (0.05% for a few seconds) to prevent cell lysis during the rinse with the low ionic-strength solution *(23)*. The characteristic dimple within the large structure in Fig. 3A clearly identifies the cell within the field. Imaging the cell surface

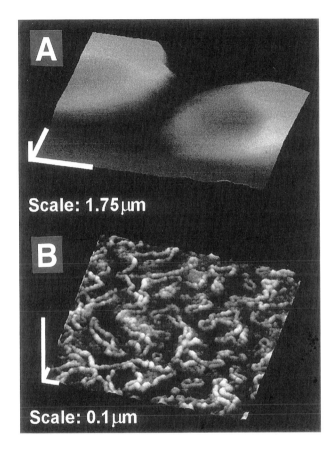

Fig. 3. CryoAFM images of rabbit erythrocytes *(23)*. (**A**) A large-scale image shows two cells within the field, each with the characteristic dimple. (**B**) A smaller scan-size image of the cell surface reveals linear clusters of 5–7 nm protrusions across the membrane. How these are related to the underlying cytoskeleton has yet to be determined.

at a higher resolution (Fig. 3B) revealed a series of linear clusters composed of ~5–7 nm globular protrusions scattered across the surface. A recent theoretical analysis suggested that the cytoskeletal network beneath an erythrocytic membrane should produce a barrier to membrane proteins *(25)*. Interestingly, the accumulation of membrane proteins at these barriers (portrayed in this recent report) resembles the punctate pattern observed in this cryoAFM image. How these surface structures in the cryoAFM images relate to the underlying cytoskeleton has not yet been thoroughly investigated. This initial study, though, clearly shows that even at this early stage of development, cryoAFM possesses the resolving power to localize membrane proteins within the native cellular membrane to a resolution of better than 10 nm.

Furthermore, future technical developments will undoubtedly improve the capability of cryoAFM for investigating cells. For example, it should be possible to include a quick freeze/deep etching chamber within the cryoAFM, which may not only allow the native cellular surface to be probed without the use of chemical fixation, but should also, with controlled fracture and etching, permit investigations into the underlying cytoskeletal arrangements. In addition, the resolution that can be achieved with cryoAFM has been steadily improving and will likely continue to do so. At the moment, 3–5 nm resolution can be routinely obtained with individual proteins or complex molecular assemblies. With the use of nanotube tips *(26,27)* or by implementing different AFM modes, it is anticipated that the imaging power of cryoAFM can be improved to better than 10 Å.

3. DISCRIMINATION BASED ON TIP-SAMPLE INTERACTIONS

The earlier discussion centered almost entirely on the use of AFM to provide high-resolution topographic information of biological samples. However, changes in the sample contour need not be the only mechanism by which contrast is generated with an AFM. This section describes some of the other imaging modes that may be useful when applied to imaging intact cell surfaces in solution.

Ion channels are likely unique among membrane proteins in possessing extra-membranous, highly charged vestibules, which are believed to enhance the accumulation of permeating ions *(28,29)*. Spatially resolving the charge distribution over the cell surface may thus allow the identification of ion channels. Early on, it was recognized that the Si_3N_4 tip used in a typical AFM is actually slightly negatively charged at neutral pH *(30)*. Two recent studies have exploited this property to generate a map of the relative charge distribution of biological samples in solution *(31,32)*.

The set of images depicted in Fig. 4, taken in the tapping mode, reveal high-resolution images of DNA bound to positively charged bilayer, which is directly adsorbed onto the mica substrate *(31)*. The contrast in Fig. 4A is topographic, whereas that in Fig. 4B is predominantly electrostatic. Notice that in Fig. 4B, the mica substrate and the polyanionic DNA are both bright relative to the cationic bilayer. Although not fully understood, the electrostatic information is provided by monitoring the time delay between the cantilever oscillation and that of the driving source, often referred to as the

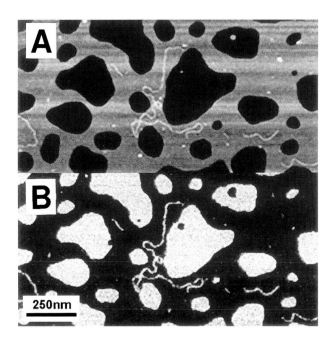

Fig. 4. Tapping-mode AFM images of DNA bound to a positively charged lipid membrane that is adsorbed to the negatively charged mica substrate *(31)*. **(A)** Topographic image generated by analyzing the change in the oscillation amplitude of the cantilever during scanning. **(B)** Phase-mode image, obtained simultaneously, reveals the surface charge distribution of the sample to a similar resolution as the topographic image.

phase mode (which should not be confused with phase imaging in an optical microscope). This phase-imaging capability is now a standard feature on many commercially available AFMs. Even though there are many unknown variables, such as exact tip size and charge, which makes quantitation of the observed charge density challenging, it should be possible to determine relative differences in local charge densities within the same sample or to observe changes in the magnitude of electrostatic interaction at one region over time. Because the strength of this interaction is dependent on ion concentration (through the strength of screening), an exciting possibility of this imaging mode is to identify the changes in the local ion concentration over a cluster of channels while they are opening and closing.

This electrostatic interaction between the tip and sample can also be determined by monitoring the deflections of the cantilever at a single x,y-location while the sample is raised and lowered, in the so-called force mode. The long range nature of the electrostatic forces perturb the tip at distances

greater than direct, van der Waals contact. By analyzing the extent of cantilever deflection at different concentrations of salt while scanning the sample,
in a procedure referred to as D-minus-D imaging, it is possible to characterize the relative charge distribution of biological samples in solution *(32)*.
Although this method does not yet have the resolution comparable to that of
the phase images, it has the advantage of being able to better quantitate the
relative charge density.

This reliance on the force curve to map out different regions of the sample
is also at the heart of a technique called force mapping *(33,34)*. Derived
from the initial investigations by Gaub and others *(35–39)*, this method
involves adsorbing a particular ligand (or antibody) directly to the tip and
scanning the functionalized tip over a sample containing the appropriate
receptor (or antigen). For those regions of the sample where the receptors
are suitably oriented with the labeled tip, there is an increased interaction,
and by monitoring the extent of this interaction across the sample, the distribution of the receptor or antigen is determined. It may also be possible to
use antibodies or other labels (for example, specific toxins) that would react
with only a particular state (say the open state) of a channel so that a map of
the channels only in this state may be generated.

This force mapping was recently demonstrated using a tip labeled with
antibodies against lysozyme to probe a sample of the protein adsorbed onto
mica *(34)*, as shown in Fig. 5, obtained in the tapping mode. In Fig. 5A, a
typical topographic image is presented showing little contrast owing to the
extremely dense multilayered (and hence likely soft) sample. In striking
contrast, images of the same sample with the antibody-labeled tip were characterized by a particulate pattern of various sized bright spots (Fig. 5B). The
increased interaction between the appropriately oriented antigen-antibody
pair reduced the amplitude of cantilever oscillations as would a thicker
region (in the usual tapping mode), and so, like the thicker region, produced
a brighter region in the image. The addition of free antibody to the solution
resulted in a reduced contrast, consistent with the contrast being predominantly determined by the specific antibody-antigen tip-sample interaction
(Fig. 5C). This mechanism of determining the distribution of specific protein molecules is in its infancy, but the ability to localize ion channels should
be already possible.

It should be mentioned though that labeling of the tip in a well-defined
manner is still technically challenging, and moreover, it may, in the end, be
difficult to unambiguously distinguish between specific and nonspecific
interactions (which might both be changed when the labeled tip binds to free
antigen). Use of better chemically defined tips (such as nanotubes *[26,27]*)

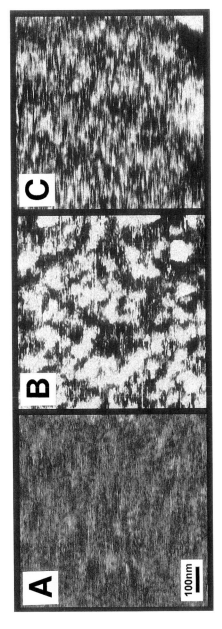

Fig. 5. Force mapping with tapping mode AFM (*34*). (**A**) Topographic image of the multilayered sample of lysozyme adsorbed to mica. There is little contrast in this image, likely owing to the softness of the specimen. (**B**) Imaging a similar sample with a tip that is labeled with antibodies against lysozyme reveals a punctate pattern of bright dots. The stronger interaction between the appropriately oriented antibodies on the tip and antigens in the sample decrease the oscillation amplitude of the cantilever, and thus appear as brighter regions of the sample. (**C**) Consistent with this interpretation, adding free antibodies to the solution resulted in images with reduced contrast. Image courtesy of Dr. P. Hinterdorfer.

and careful controls, such as a range of antibodies to the specific protein, should prove useful in this regard.

4. OTHER SCANNING PROBE MICROSCOPES

Both the successes and shortcomings of the AFM in biology have fueled the development of other, less perturbing SPM modalities. One with great potential in the study of cells is the near-field scanning optical microscope (NSOM) *(40)*. Here, a very small tapered optical fiber is scanned over a fluorescently labeled specimen. Light emitted from the end of the fiber illuminates only the local region of the sample immediately below the end of the fiber, thereby surpassing the diffraction limit of traditional optical microscopy. By scanning such a light source at a constant height above the sample, the distribution of appropriately labeled surface molecules can be determined to a resolution of ~50–100 nm or even better *(41)*. Methods to label specific proteins as well as to detect fluorescence from single molecules are highly advanced and can be combined to provide unparalleled identification of proteins within the cellular membrane. The most challenging aspect about the use of this technique for solution studies is finding a reliable method by which the distance between the optical probe and the sample surface can be controlled. Without such a method, the image would reflect, in an unknown manner, both the spatial distribution of fluorophores as well as the local sample height variations (because those fluorophores closer to the tip would receive greater illumination). At the moment, the tip-sample distance is determined in most investigations by monitoring the resonant amplitude of the fiber driven laterally, which decreases markedly when the tip experiences an increased shear force near the surface of the sample. Although the distance may be controlled with this method to subnanometer resolution in air, the sensitivity is much worse in solution owing to the much greater viscosity. Consequently, when imaging in solution with this shear-force height detection scheme, both the tip and the sample are usually irreversibly damaged shortly after engagement.

Yet, the images in Fig. 6 demonstrate the power of such a microscope even when imaging in air *(42)*. Figure 6A shows the topographic image of the cell surface determined by monitoring the changes in the shear force on the cantilever. The image in Fig. 6B shows the distribution of a fluorescently labeled lipid (Biodipy-PC), whereas that in Fig. 6C reveals the distribution of fluorescent antibodies against the class I MHC molecules. By analyzing such images, the authors were able to not only determine the average cluster size of each of the labeled species but to also determine the degree of corre-

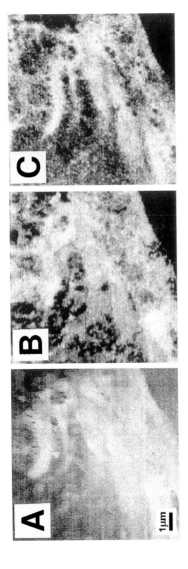

Fig. 6. High resolution NSOM images of human skin fibroblasts, taken in air *(42)*. **(A)** The topography of the sample is obtained by monitoring the shear force on the laterally vibrating optical fiber. **(B)** The distribution of the fluorescently labeled lipid, Biodipy-PC, within the cell membrane. **(C)** The distribution of the fluorescent antibody against class I MHC molecules in the same region of the sample as in (B). In both (B) and (C), the regions of brighter contrast reflect areas of greater fluorescence intensity. Not only can each of these components of the cellular membrane be localized by this approach, but their relative spatial correlation can also be easily determined. Image courtesy of Dr. M. Edidin.

474

lation of the two types of domains. Similar studies with two different membrane proteins have also been performed to a resolution of better than 100 nm *(43)*. These results foster the hope that, when it becomes possible to image in solution, the distribution of many different components of the cell membrane may be simultaneously visualized in real time to a resolution of better than 50 nm.

Another SPM that has not achieved popularity but may be well-designed for imaging live cells is the scanning ion conductance microscope (SICM) *(44,45)*. In this instrument, the tip is made of a small pipet that can be pulled by commercially available instruments to various sizes with high reproducibility. The current through this pipet is monitored while scanning over the sample. Because the conductance drops sharply near a surface (owing to the more restricted pathway for ion movement), this mechanism of monitoring height variations is quite powerful. The image in Fig. 7 shows murine melanocytes imaged by such an instrument with a pixel resolution of 100 nm *(45)*. It is likely that by stimulating the opening of selected ion channels within the cell surface, the distribution of these channels could be clearly identified with similar resolution.

These solution-filled pipets are transparent to light from near IR to near UV. If the outer surface of such a pipet is coated by a light opaque material, such as aluminum, it should be possible to use these coated pipets as a light conduit to guide the light to the tip for use as a near field optical probe (Fig. 8) *(46)*. Thus, such an instrument would be an NSOM with a height regulator provided by the change in current through the pipet, which should allow routine operation in aqueous solution. The optical and topographical resolution of such a design would ultimately depend on the ability to manufacture small apertures. The standard pipet puller should be able to produce probes as small as 50 nm, although nanofabrication of the pipets may improve this even further.

In addition to straightforward optical imaging, such a system can also be used to perform fluorescence resonance energy transfer (FRET) imaging *(47)*. For this purpose, the opaque coating on the pipet would not be necessary; the tip can be labeled with the acceptor and the sample can be labeled with the donor, with the light source provided by epi-illumination. It should be possible, with such an instrument, to observe conformational changes in a donor-labeled channel, in addition to determining its spatial distribution across a cell surface.

Another extension of this idea is to use multibarrel pipets as the probe. In this case, one of the barrels can be used as the height control, while the others can be adopted to collect other signals. For example, one barrel can be filled with a carbon fiber, which, as has been demonstrated *(48)*, can be

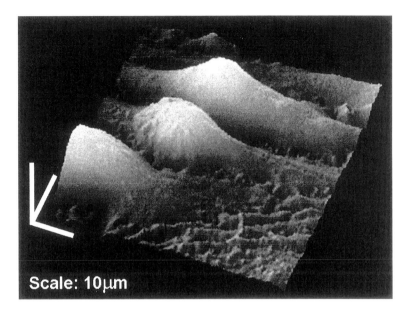

Scale: 10μm

Fig. 7. SCIM image of living murine melanocytes *(45)*. By monitoring the current through a small pipet scanned in close proximity to the sample, images of cell surfaces can be determined to a pixel resolution of 100 nm. The distribution of open ion channels within the plasma membrane should also be possible with this approach. Image courtesy of Dr. Y. Korchev.

used to detect small concentrations of catecholamines. Alternatively, the end of a different barrel may be covered with a membrane containing a channel (such as the glycine receptor) that is gated by a secreted molecule, so that changes in the current within this barrel would simultaneously identify the particular locations of secretion. The spatial resolution with such a device may not achieve values better than 200 nm, but these additional signals may provide a direct, more complete and variegated description of cellular events than is hitherto possible.

5. PERSPECTIVES

At the moment, the most commonly used SPM in biology, AFM, although capable of incredibly detailed images of rigidly supported samples in solution, does not appear capable of resolving, in the contact mode, individual proteins within the plasma membrane of living cells (except perhaps in a few cell systems). This difficulty, undoubtedly, is predominantly owing to the softness of the cytoplasm. Although the technology continues to develop

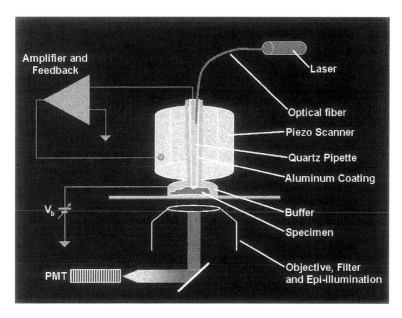

Fig. 8. Schematic diagram of a combined NSOM-SCIM *(46)*. The glass pipet used in SCIM can be converted into a conduit for light by coating it with a light opaque material such as aluminum. The small aperture at the end of the coated pipet can then be used as an NSOM probe, where the sample height is monitored by the ionic conductance through the pipet. High resolution near-field optical imaging should thus be possible in solution. For FRET-NSOM, the metal coating is not required.

(including the recent construction of small cantilevers that are expected to allow similar resolution at a much shorter acquisition time *[49]*), it is not clear if these improvements will, in the end, allow imaging with the lighter forces necessary for cellular specimens. The early suggestion of a stiffer cellular membrane when using the tapping mode should be studied further, as there may indeed be particular technical parameters (for example, oscillation amplitude and frequency as well as rate of scanning) that may make the imaging of these samples possible.

However, as discussed here, there are four more promising approaches to obtain such information using an SPM. First, force mapping with the AFM appears to be best poised to localize ion channels within the membrane of intact cells to high resolution. The methods to label the tip and to prepare the cells are both established, and so it is likely only a matter of time before results begin to accumulate with this approach. Secondly, the recently developed SICM (though not yet commercially available) can generate images of live cells by a mechanism that is dependent upon a property which ion channels can change: the local extracellular concentration of ions. Hence, this approach seems perfectly suited to detect the opening of ion channels, as well as their distribution within the cell membrane. Thirdly, contact-mode AFM imaging of cells in air or at cryogenic temperatures using appropriate labels has already been demonstrated to be a reliable technique for determining the spatial distribution of membrane proteins. Future developments, particularly with the cryoAFM, will likely not only reveal ever more detailed information about the distribution of proteins at the cell surface, but also how this organization is related to the underlying cytoskeleton as well as to the other structures deeper within the cell.

Yet the most effective of the SPMs in investigations of cell surfaces, combining better than 100 nm resolution with the simultaneous identification of many different cellular components, is likely going to be the NSOM. The images obtained in air already surpass the resolution possible with conventional optical microscopy. The conversion of the pipet used in SICM to one capable of locally emitting light may produce an instrument that is, at last, sufficiently powerful to illuminate the entire cellular membrane of living cells with single-molecule resolution.

ACKNOWLEDGMENTS

We wish to thank Drs. Manfred Radmacher, Peter Hinterdorfer, Michael Edidin, and Yuri Korchev for supplying images presented in this chapter. This work was supported by grants from the American Heart Association, the National Institutes of Health, and the National Science Foundation.

REFERENCES

1. Brown, D. A. and London, E. (1998) Functions of lipid rafts in biological membranes. *Annu. Rev. Cell Devel. Biol.* **14,** 111–136.
2. Hansma, H. G. and Pietrasanta, L. (1998) Atomic force microscopy and other scanning probe microscopies. *Curr. Opin. Chem. Biol.* **2,** 579–584.
3. Shao, Z., Mou, J., Czajkowsky, D. M., Yang, J., and Yuan, J.-Y. (1996) Biological atomic force microscopy: what is achieved and what is needed. *Adv. Phys.* **45,** 1–86.
4. Binnig, G., Quate, C. F., and Gerber, Ch. (1986) Atomic force microscope. *Phys. Rev. Lett.* **56,** 930–933.
5. Linder, A., Weiland, U., and Apell, H.-J. (1999) Novel polymer substrates for SFM investigations of living cells, biological membranes, and proteins. *J. Struct. Biol.* **126,** 16–26.

6. Scheuring, S., Müller, D. J., Ringler, P., Heymann, J. B., and Engel, A. (1999) Imaging streptavidin 2D crystals on biotinylated lipid monolayers at high resolution with the atomic force microscope. *J. Microsc.* **193**, 28–35.

7. Kowalewski, T. and Holtzman, D. M. (1999) *In situ* atomic force microscopy of Alzheimer's β-amyloid peptide on different substrates: new insights into the mechanism of β-sheet formation. *Proc. Natl. Acad. Sci. USA* **96**, 3688–3693.

8. Karrasch, S., Dolder, M., Schabert, F., Ramsden, J., and Engel, A. (1993) Covalent binding of biological samples to solid supports for scanning probe microscopy in buffer solution. *Biophys. J.* **65**, 2437–2446.

9. Czajkowsky, D. M., Iwamoto, H., Cover, T. L., and Shao, Z. (1999) The vacuolating toxin from *Helicobacter pylori* forms hexameric pores in lipid bilayers at low pH. *Proc. Natl. Acad. Sci. USA* **96**, 2001–2006.

10. Engel, A., Lyubchenko, Y., and Müller, D. (1999) Atomic force microscopy: a powerful tool to observe biomolecules at work. *Trends Cell Biol.* **9**, 77–80.

11. Czajkowsky, D. M. and Shao, Z. (1998) Submolecular resolution of single macromolecules with atomic force microscopy. *FEBS Lett.* **430**, 51–54.

12. Rotsch, C., Jacobson, K., and Radmacher, M. (1999) Dimensional and mechanical dynamics of active and stable edges in motile fibroblasts investigated by using atomic force microscopy. *Proc. Natl. Acad. Sci. USA* **96**, 921–926.

13. Damjanovich, S., Vereb, G., Schaper, A., Jenei, A., Matho, J., Pascual Starink, J. P., et al. (1995) Structural hierarchy in the clustering of HLA class I molecules in the plasma membrane of human lymphoblastoid cells. *Proc. Natl. Acad. Sci. USA* **92**, 1122–1126.

14. Jenei, A., Varga, S., Bene, L., Matyus, L., Bodnar, A., Bacso, Z., et al. (1997) HLA class I and II antigens are partially co-clustered in the plasma membrane of human lymphoblastoid cells. *Proc. Natl. Acad. Sci. USA* **94**, 7269–7274.

15. Bruchez, M., Moronne, M., Gin, P., Weiss, S., and Alivisatos, A. P. (1998) Semiconductor nanocrystals as fluorescent biological labels. *Science* **281**, 2013–2016.

16. Schenider, S. W., Sritharan, K. C., Geibel, J. P., Oberleithner, H., and Jena, B. P. (1997) Surface dynamics in living acinar cells imaged by atomic force microscopy: Identification of plasma membrane structures involved in exocytosis. *Proc. Natl. Acad. Sci. USA* **94**, 316–321.

17. Darnell, J., Lodish, H., and Baltimore, D. (1990) *Molecular Cell Biology*. Scientific American Books, Inc., NY.

18. Putman, C. A., van der Wert, K. O., de Grooth, B. G., van Hulst, N. F., and Greve, J. (1994) Viscoelasticity of living cells allows high resolution imaging by tapping mode atomic force microscopy. *Biophys. J.* **67**, 1749–1753.

19. Zhong, Q., Inniss, D., Kjoller, K., and Elings, V. B. (1993) Fractured polymer/silica fiber surface studied by tapping mode atomic force microscopy. *Surf. Sci. Lett.* **290**, L688–L692.

20. Hansma, P. K., Cleveland, J. P., Radmacher, M., Walters, D. A., Hillner, P. E., Bezanilla, M., et al. (1994) Tapping mode atomic force microscopy in liquids. *Appl. Phys. Lett.* **64**, 1738–1740.

21. Lantz, M. A., O'Shea, S. J., and Welland, M. E. (1994) Force microscopy imaging in liquids using ac techniques. *Appl. Phys. Lett.* **65**, 409–411.

22. Han, W., Mou, J., Sheng, J., Yang, J., and Shao, Z. (1995) Cryo atomic force microscopy: a new approach for biological imaging at high resolution. *Biochemistry* **34,** 8215–8220.
23. Zhang, Y. Y., Sheng, S., and Shao, Z. (1996) Imaging biological structures with the cryo atomic force microscope. *Biophys. J.* **71,** 2168–2176.
24. Zhang, Y. Y., Shao, Z., Somlyo, A. P., and Somlyo, A. V. (1997) Cryo-atomic force microscopy of smooth muscle myosin. *Biophys. J.* **72,** 1308–1318.
25. Boal, D. H. and Boey, S. K. (1995) Barrier-free path of directed protein motion in the erythrocyte plasma membrane. *Biophys. J.* **69,** 372–379.
26. Hafner, J. H., Cheung, C. L., and Lieber, C. M. (1999) Growth of nanotubes for probe microscopy tips. *Nature* **398,** 761,762.
27. Hafner, J. H., Cheung, C. L., and Lieber, C. M. (1999) Direct growth of single-walled carbon nanotube scanning probe microscopy tips. *J. Am. Chem. Soc.* **121,** 9750,9751.
28. Cai, M. and Jordan, P. C. (1990) How does vestibule surface charge affect ion conductivity and toxin binding in a sodium channel? *Biophys. J.* **57,** 883–891.
29. Adcock, C., Smith, G. R., and Sanson, M. S. P. (1998) Electrostatics and the ion selectivity of ligand-gated channels. *Biophys. J.* **75,** 1211–1222.
30. Hoh, J. H., Revel, J.-P., and Hansma, P. K. (1992) Tip-sample interaction in atomic force microscopy: I. Modulating adhesion between silicon nitride and glass. *Nanotechnology* **2,** 119–122.
31. Czajkowsky, D. M., Allen, M. J., Elings, V., and Shao, Z. (1998) Direct visualization of surface charge in aqueous solution. *Ultramicrosccopy* **74,** 1–5.
32. Heinz, W. F. and Hoh, J. H. (1999) Relative surface charge density mapping with the atomic force microscope. *Biophys. J.* **76,** 528–538.
33. Hinterdorfer, P., Baumbartner, W., Gruber, H. J., Schilcher, K., and Schindler, H. (1996) Detection and localization of individual antibody-antigen recognition events by atomic force microscopy. *Proc. Natl. Acad. Sci. USA* **93,** 3477–3481.
34. Raab, A., Han, W., Badt, D., Smith-Gill, S. J., Lindsay, S. M., Schindler, H., and Hinterdorfer, P. (1999) Antibody recognition imaging by force microscopy. *Nature Biotech.* **17,** 902–905.
35. Florin, E.-L., Moy, V. T., and Gaub, H. E. (1994) Adhesion forces between individual ligand-receptor pairs. *Science* **264,** 415–417.
36. Moy, V. T., Florin, E.-L., and Gaub, H. E. (1994) Intermolecular forces and energies between ligands and receptors. *Science* **266,** 257–259.
37. Lee, G. U., Chrisey, L. A., and Colton, R. J. (1994) Direct measurement of the forces between complementary strands of DNA. *Science* **266,** 771–773.
38. Dammer, U., Popescu, O., Wagner, P., Anselmetti, D., Güntherodt, H.-J., and Misevic, G. N. (1995) Binding strength between cell adhesion proteoglycans measured by atomic force microscopy. *Science* **267,** 1173–1175.
39. Boland, T. and Ratner, B. D. (1995) Direct measurement of hydrogen bonding in DNA nucleotide bases by atomic force microscopy. *Proc. Natl. Acad. Sci. USA* **92,** 5297–5301.

40. Betzig, E. and Chichester, R. J. (1993) Single molecules observed by near field scanning optical microscopy. *Science* **262,** 1422–1425.
41. Zenhausern, F., Martin, Y., and Wickramasinghe, H. K. (1995) Scanning interferometric apertureless microscopy: optical imaging at 10 Ängstrom resolution. *Science* **269,** 1083–1085.
42. Hwang, J., Gheber, L. A., Margolis, L., and Edidin, M. (1998) Domains in cell plasma membranes investigated by near-field scanning optical microscopy. *Biophys. J.* **74,** 2184–2190.
43. Enderle, Th., Ha, T., Ogletree, D. F., Chemla, D. S., Magowan, C., and Weiss, S. (1997) Membrane specific mapping and colocalization of malarial and host skeletal proteins in the *Plasmodium falciparum* infected erythrocyte by dual-color near-field scanning optical microscopy. *Proc. Natl. Acad. Sci. USA* **94,** 520–525.
44. Proksch, R., Lal, R., Hansma, P. K., Morse, D., and Stucky, G. (1996) Imaging the internal and external structure of membranes in fluid: TappingMode scanning ion conductance microscopy. *Biophys. J.* **71,** 2155–2157.
45. Korchev, Y. E., Bashford, C. L., Milovanovic, M., Vodyanoy, I., and Lab, M. J. (1997) Scanning ion conductance microscopy of living cells. *Biophys. J.* **73,** 653–658.
46. University of Virginia Patent Foundation: www.uvapatentfoundation.org.
47. Vickery, S. A. and Dunn, R. C. (1999) Scanning near-field fluorescence resonance energy transfer microscopy. *Biophys. J.* **76,** 1812–1818.
48. Albillos, A., Dernick, G., Horstmann, H., Almers, W., Detoledo, G. A., and Lindau, M. (1997) The exocytotic event in chromaffin cells revealed by patch amperometry. *Nature* **389,** 509–512.
49. Viani, M. B., Schaffer, T. E., Paloczi, G. T., Pietrasanta, L. I., Smith, B. L., Thompson, J. B., et al. (1999) Fast imaging and fast force spectroscopy of single biopolymers with a new atomic force microscope designed for small cantilevers. *Rev. Sci. Instr.* **70,** 4300–4303.

Index